CALCIUM-REGULATING HORMONES
and
CARDIOVASCULAR FUNCTION

Edited by

M.F. Crass, III
Texas Tech University
Lubbock, Texas

Louis V. Avioli
Washington University School of Medicine
St. Louis, Missouri

CRC Press
Boca Raton   Ann Arbor   London   Tokyo

Library of Congress Cataloging-in-Publication Data

Calcium-Regulating Hormones and Cardiovascular Function / edited by M. F. Crass, III, Louis V. Avioli.
      p.   cm.
    Includes bibliographical references and index.
    ISBN 0-8493-8661-6
    1. Calcium-regulating hormones—Physiological effect.   2. Calcium-regulating hormones—
Pathophysiology.   3. Hypertension—Endocrine aspects.   4. Cardiovascular system—Diseases—Endocrine
aspects.   I. Crass, III, M. F. (Maurice F.)   II. Avioli, Louis V.
    [DNLM: 1. Parathyroid Hormone—metabolism.   2. Calcium—metabolism.   3. Cardiovascular System—
physiology.   4. Hypertension—drug therapy.   5. Vitamin D—metabolism. WK 300 C144 1994]
    QP572.C33C35   1995
    612.1—dc20   94-18413
                                                                                                  CIP

Preface

Seventy years of research by numerous investigators have led to the conclusion that calcium-regulating hormones and peptides exert important effects on the cardiovascular system. Many of these effects are direct or independent of changes in plasma calcium values. In addition, and from a pathophysiologic perspective, alterations in circulating levels of parathyroid hormone, 1,25-dihydroxyvitamin D_3, and other peptide and steroid calcium-regulating substances have been implicated in abnormal cardiovascular function. Although several journal reviews have been written on these and related subjects, many investigators felt that a volume that dealt exclusively with the cardiovascular actions of the calcium-regulating hormones and peptides was needed. It is hoped that *Calcium-Regulating Hormones and Cardiovascular Function* will meet this need. Each of the contributors to the book has a background of many years of research in one or more of the subject areas. Thus, the volume provides the reader with critical and in-depth views of the cardiovascular actions and associated mechanisms of action and signalling pathways of each of the calcium-regulating hormones and peptides.

The first chapter enables the reader to review the current status of all of the calcium-regulating hormones and peptides in terms of structure, synthesis, secretion, metabolism, mechanisms of target cell activation, and, in concise fashion, the functions in classic and nonclassic target cells. A strong molecular biology orientation has been given to the subject matter. The authors of this review have also provided an extraordinarily comprehensive bibliography that will be valuable to investigators and students working in the area.

The remainder of the chapters address the cardiovascular actions of the calcium-regulating hormones and peptides in health and disease.

Chapter 2 draws together extensive literature on the vasoactive and cardioactive properties of parathyroid hormone in terms of cardiodynamics and blood pressure regulation at the systemic level and blood flow at the regional level. Local actions of the hormone, as elucidated *in vitro* using vascular and cardiac muscle preparations, are reviewed along with discussion of related mechanisms of signal transduction. This discussion leads logically to Chapter 3, which describes detailed studies and convincing evidence for the modulating actions of parathyroid hormone on calcium channels in both vascular smooth muscle cells and cardiac myocytes.

Chapter 5 discusses the rationale for a second vasoactive substance in the parathyroid glands and the discovery of a parathyroid hypertensive factor. The authors provide a comparison of the biochemical and physiological characteristics of parathyroid hormone and parathyroid hypertensive factor.

Knowledge of the actions of parathyroid hormone-related protein in both normal and pathophysiological settings is developing at a rapid rate. Characterization of the local production of the protein, receptor interactions, and actions in a variety of normal tissues is occurring at a rapid rate. The potentially important roles for the parathyroid hormone-related protein in regulating vascular smooth muscle activity and cardiac muscle function are examined critically in an extensive review by key investigators in Chapter 6.

Chapters 7 and 8 pertain to the functions of $1,25(OH)_2D_3$ in blood vessels and heart, respectively. Actions of the steroid hormone on vascular smooth muscle contraction via both direct and indirect mechanisms and interrelationships with calcium metabolism and hypertension are addressed. The effects of $1,25(OH)_2D_3$ on regulation of cardiac contractile function, including effects on morphology and gene expression, are clearly and expertly discussed. In addition, an epidemiological view of the risk of cardiovascular disease in the context of the effects of seasonal, latitude, and altitude variations as well as ultraviolet radiation exposure is discussed in Chapter 9.

The strong vasodilator effects, cardiac actions, and potential regulatory roles of calcitonin gene-related peptide are critically reviewed in Chapter 10. The authors discuss prospective roles for the neuropeptide in both normal and pathophysiologic areas of cardiovascular function.

Chapter 11 examines the roles that the calcium-regulating hormones play in cellular calcium homeostasis in cardiovascular tissues in contrast with their roles in maintenance of a constant plasma calcium concentration. The authors emphasize the effects of the hormones and peptides on intracellular calcium ion concentrations and the use of calcium in cellular events as differentiated from effects on acquisition, storage, and release of calcium by the cell. In addition, the potential importance of sex steroids as calcium-regulating hormones at the cellular level is discussed.

Insulin has calcium-regulating effects in vascular smooth muscle, resulting in altered intracellular calcium concentrations and vascular tone. In Chapter 12, the authors relate these and other effects, such as the mitogenic properties of insulin in association with insulin-like growth factors, to the atherosclerosis and hypertension often characteristic of hyperinsulinemia/insulin resistant states of type II diabetes and obesity.

In the final chapter, a clinical scientist examines current knowledge of the roles of calcium-regulating hormones and peptides in hypertension, emphasizing how their actions may alter regulation of blood pressure and how variations in circulating levels of the hormones contribute to alterations in cellular cations and, accordingly, to the development of different forms of hypertension.

Since all biomedical scientists, both basic and clinical, recognize the ubiquitous involvement of calcium in biological systems, be they contractile, secretory, or other, the editors hope, indeed predict, that *Calcium-Regulating Hormones and Cardiovascular Function* will be a useful reference not only for cardiovascular scientists, but for investigators in other fields as well.

M. F. Crass, III, Ph.D.
Louis V. Avioli, M.D.

The Editors

Maurice F. Crass, III, Ph.D., is Professor of Physiology in the School of Medicine at Texas Tech University Health Sciences Center at Lubbock, Texas. He received his B.S. and M.S. degrees from the Department of Zoology, University of Maryland, College Park, in 1957 and 1959, respectively. He obtained his Ph.D. degree from the Department of Physiology at the Vanderbilt University School of Medicine, Nashville, Tennessee, in 1965. Dr. Crass was an Instructor of Physiology and a postdoctoral fellow of the Tennessee Heart Association at Vanderbilt in 1966. After doing postdoctoral work at the University of Florida College of Medicine, Gainesville, he was appointed Assistant Professor of Physiology and of Medicine at the University of Florida in 1969. He became an Assistant Professor and then Associate Professor of Biochemistry and of Medicine at the University of Nebraska College of Medicine, Omaha, in 1970 and 1973, respectively. He became an Associate Professor of Physiology in 1973 and Professor of Physiology in 1981 at Texas Tech University School of Medicine, and Adjunct Professor, Department of Food and Nutrition, Texas Tech University College of Human Sciences. Dr. Crass is a member of the American Physiological Society, the Society for Experimental Biology and Medicine, the International Society for Heart Research, the Western Pharmacology Society, and the American Heart Association Councils on Circulation and Basic Science.

Dr. Crass has been principal investigator on research grants from the National Institutes of Health, American Heart Association, American Diabetes Association, and private industry. He has published over 100 papers and has been senior editor on three books. His current research interests are in cardiovascular physiology of aging, gender differences in cardiovascular function, and the actions of calcium-regulating hormones on heart and vascular function.

Louis V. Avioli, M.D., is the Shoenberg Professor of Medicine and Director of the Division of Bone and Mineral Diseases at Washington University School of Medicine located at The Jewish Hospital of St. Louis. He is also an attending physician at Barnes Hospital, St. Louis Children's Hospital, and The Jewish Hospital. In addition, he serves as a consultant at the Shriners Hospital for Crippled Children–St. Louis Unit and St. John's Mercy Medical Center. Dr. Avioli graduated *magna cum laude* from Princeton University and received his medical degree in 1957 from Yale University. He is the founder and past president of the American Society for Bone and Mineral Research and has been elected to the American Association for the Advancement of Science. Dr. Avioli is the recipient of the Andre Lichtwitz International Prize (1979); the American College of Nutrition Award (1987); the American Society of Bone and Mineral Research's William F. Neuman Award (1988); the U. S. Endocrine Society's Robert H. Williams Distinguished Leadership Award (1990); and in 1992 both the John M. Kinney Annual International Award for Nutrition and Metabolism and the American Academy of Orthopedic Surgeons' Kappa Delta Award. In January 1994, Dr. Avioli was named as one of the "Fifty Leaders in the St. Louis Health Industry".

Dr. Avioli has written or co-authored over 270 articles and research papers and has contributed to more than 100 texts and edited volumes. He has served as a contributing editor and member of the editorial boards of such scientific journals as the *Journal of the American Medical Association*, the *Journal of Clinical Endocrinology*, the *American Journal of Medicine*, *Archives of Internal Medicine*, the *Journal of the American Society of Bone and Mineral Research*, the *Journal of Laboratory and Clinical Medicine*, *Metabolic Bone Disease and Related Research*, the *Journal of Endocrinological Investigations*, and the *Italian Journal of Mineral and Electrolyte Metabolism*. He continues to be editor-in-chief of *Calcified Tissue International*, a position held since 1979. Dr. Avioli has been recognized internationally by the presentation of numerous awards and honorary degrees.

Contributors

Louis V. Avioli, M.D.
Schoenberg Professor of Medicine
Division of Bone and Mineral Diseases
Washington University School of Medicine
St. Louis, Missouri

Mario Barbagallo, M.D., Ph.D.
Associate Professor
Universita di Palermo
Faculte di Geriatria e Gerontologia
Palermo, Italy

Christina G. Benishin, Ph.D.
Associate Professor
Department of Physiology
University of Alberta
Edmonton, Alberta
Canada

Nadji Boulebda, Ph.D.
Ouled-Driss
Souk Ahras
Algeria

Richard Bukoski, Ph.D.
Associate Professor
Department of Internal Medicine
Hypertension and Vascular Research
University of Texas Medical Branch
Galveston, Texas

Roberto Civitelli, M.D.
Assistant Professor of Medicine
Division of Bone and Mineral Diseases
Washington University School of Medicine
St. Louis, Missouri

M. F. Crass, III, Ph.D.
Professor of Physiology
Department of Physiology
School of Medicine
Texas Tech University Health Sciences Center
Lubbock, Texas

Donald J. DiPette, M.D.
Professor of Medicine
Department of Internal Medicine, and
    Vice Chairman for Educational Affairs
Division of General Internal Medicine
Section of Hypertension
University of Texas Medical Branch
Galveston, Texas

Alexis Gairard, Ph.D.
Professor
Pharmacologie Cellulaire et Moléculaire
CNRS
Faculté de Pharmacie
Université Louis Pasteur
Strasbourg, France

Edward Karpinski, Ph.D.
Associate Professor, Faculty of Medicine
Department of Physiology
University of Alberta
Edmonton, Alberta
Canada

Richard Z. Lewanczuk, M.D., Ph.D.
Assistant Professor
Departments of Physiology and Medicine
University of Alberta
Edmonton, Alberta
Canada

G. Allen Nickols, Ph.D.
Science Fellow
Molecular Pharmacology Department
Monsanto Corporate Research
St. Louis, Missouri

Timothy D. O'Connell
Department of Pharmacology
University of Michigan
Ann Arbor, Michigan

Peter K. T. Pang, Ph.D., D.Sc.
Professor
Department of Physiology
University of Alberta
Edmonton, Alberta
Canada

Fanny Pernot, Ph.D.
Maître de Conférences
Pharmacologie Cellulaire et Moléculaire
CNRS
Faculté de Pharmacie
Université Louis Pasteur
Strasbourg, France

Patsy A. Perry, Ph.D.
Associate Professor
College of Nursing
Arizona State University
Tempe, Arizona

Jeffrey L. Ram, Ph.D.
Professor of Physiology
Departments of Internal Medicine
    and Physiology
Wayne State University School of Medicine
Detroit, Michigan

Lawrence M. Resnick, M.D.
Professor of Medicine and
    Director of Hypertension
Division of Endocrinology and Hypertension
Wayne State University School of Medicine
University Health Center
Detroit, Michigan

Robert Scragg, MBBS, Ph.D.
Senior Lecturer in Epidemiology
Department of Community Health
University of Auckland
Auckland, New Zealand

Jie Shan, Ph.D.
Postdoctoral Fellow and Research Associate
Department of Physiology
University of Alberta
Edmonton, Alberta
Canada

Robert U. Simpson, Ph.D.
Associate Professor of Pharmacology
Department of Pharmacology
University of Michigan
Ann Arbor, Michigan

James R. Sowers, M.D.
Professor of Medicine and Physiology
Departments of Internal Medicine and Physiology
Wayne State University School of Medicine
Detroit, Michigan

Paul R. Standley, Ph.D.
Assistant Professor of Medicine and Physiology
Departments of Internal Medicine and Physiology
Wayne State University School of Medicine
Detroit, Michigan

Mark A. Thiede, Ph.D.
Senior Research Scientist
Department of Cardiovascular
    and Metabolic Diseases
Pfizer Central Research
Groton, Connecticut

Bruno Van Overloop, Ph.D.
Maître de Conférences
Pharmacologie Cellulaire et Moléculaire
CNRS
Faculté de Pharmacie
Université Louis Pasteur
Strasbourg, France

Sunil J. Wimalawansa, M.D., Ph.D.
Associate Professor of Medicine
Department of Internal Medicine
Division of General Internal Medicine
University of Texas Medical Branch
Galveston, Texas

Table of Contents

1

The Biochemistry and Function of Calciotropic Hormones

Roberto Civitelli and Louis V. Avioli

CONTENTS

0-8493-8661-6/95/$0.00+$.50
© 1995 by CRC Press Inc.

I. STRUCTURE, SYNTHESIS, SECRETION, AND METABOLISM

A. Parathyroid Hormone

Parathyroid hormone (PTH), which is secreted by each of four parathyroid glands, has as its primary role the maintenance of the normal level of circulating calcium and inorganic phosphate. The final hormonal product derives from the sequential enzymatic cleavage of a precursor gene product consisting of 115 amino acids which is first synthesized as preproPTH and then successfully cleaved to proPTH (90 amino acids) and the final active hormone PTH, which consists of 84 amino acids (Figure 1).[1] The 34 amino acids of the amino terminus of the active hormone is essential for normal biological activity of the PTH. Stepwise shortening of the carboxyl terminus from position 34 toward the amino terminus results in a progressive decline in potency until position 25 is reached. This 1-34 region of the PTH molecule is subdivided into a short activation domain (amino acids 1-6) and a longer receptor binding domain (amino acids 7-34). Amino acids 25-31 in the PTH molecule represent the minimal structural requirements for detectable receptor occupancy. Mutational analysis of PTH at the amino (N)-terminus confirmed earlier data suggesting that the receptor-binding domain is located between amino acids 24 and 31, but that an important contribution is also provided by an amphipatic α-helix in the carboxyl (C)-terminus region of the molecule.[2]

The heterogeneity of circulating PTH arises by proteolysis of the 84-amino acid polypeptide into two or more fragments. The intact PTH molecule is in fact rapidly degraded with a plasma half-life of <4 min,[3] and in normal humans only 5 to 30% of the circulating immunoreactive PTH (iPTH) is represented by the intact 1-84 PTH molecule. C-terminus biologically inactive fragments remain in the circulation five to ten times longer than the intact hormone, and they account for the remaining 70 to 95% of the detectable iPTH profile.[4,5] C-terminus fragments are primarily generated by cleavage of the intact hormone in the liver and the parathyroid gland itself,[6-10] with a small contribution from the kidney.[11,12] N-terminus fragments circulate at very low concentrations in normal individuals, but increase in hyperparathyroid states.[4,5] Recent observations suggest that while the kidney clears N-terminus PTH fragments at the same rate as C-terminus peptides by filtration, the liver clears N-terminus fragments faster than the intact hormone, and it does not metabolize C-terminus fragments at all.[13] Thus, the different hepatic clearance may account for the differences in the circulating levels of N- and C-terminus PTH fragments.

Developments in hormonal isolation, purification, and accurate quantitation by specific radioimmunoassay (RIA) procedures, based on the ability of the hormones to competitively inhibit the binding of ^{131}I-labeled hormone to specific antibody, have contributed not only to a verification of the existing hypothesis that circulating ionized calcium is the primary physiologic determinant of PTH secretion, but also to a more fundamental understanding of the role of PTH in a variety of skeletal disorders. However, when one considers that circulating fragments may be detected by one antiserum but not by a second and that the PTH fragments may be cleared from the circulation at rates that differ from those for the intact, recently secreted hormone, then entirely different impressions could be gathered concerning not only absolute concentrations of hormone, but also rates of hormonal disappearance. Thus, interpretation of data that define the regulation of hormonal secretion and subsequent metabolism in various clinical disorders depends on the characterization of the particular antiserum used in the RIA.[14]

Parathyroid hormone is secreted continuously at normal plasma calcium levels in a pulsatile fashion,[15,16] with peak plasma levels occurring in the early morning hours (i.e., 1800 and 0200 h) and troughs at 1000 and 2000 h.[17,18] Circadian patterns of "intact" iPTH differ between the sexes, with an earlier rise and greater increase at night observed in men.[18] In individuals with hyperfunctioning parathyroid glands (i.e., primary hyperparathyroidism), the amplitude

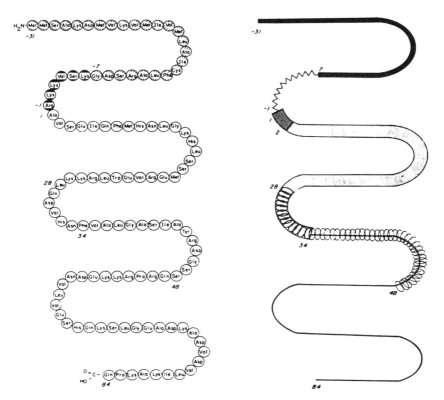

FIGURE 1 Molecular structure of PTH. The bovine sequence is illustrated. The physiologic function of each sequence is indicated at right. The *wide solid line* indicates leader sequence (position –31 through –7). The *saw-toothed* region is the proparathyroid sequence (positions –6 through –1). Fully active portion comprises amino acids 1-34. Positions 1 and 2 (*hatched*) are essential for activation of the cAMP system and most biologic effects. Regions 3-34 (*stippled*) contain the structural determinant for receptor binding and activation of the phospholipase C system. Regions 28-34 and 34-48 (*coil*) are produced by enzymatic cleavage. The biologically inactive C-terminus region (positions 48-84) is indicated by a *narrow solid line*. (From Habener, J. F., Rosenblatt, M., and Potts, J. T., Jr., *Physiol. Rev.,* 64, 985, 1984. Originally appeared in Rosenblatt, M. *Pathobiology Annual,* II, 53, 1981. With permission.)

of the PTH "pulses" is increased. The latter, in addition to an impaired feedback regulation in PTH secretion,[19] often results in progressive hypercalcemia.

Parathyroid hormone regulates calcium homeostasis and phosphate metabolism by a complex interaction of its effects on bone remodeling, the renal excretion of calcium and phosphate, and, indirectly, via vitamin D-activated intestinal calcium absorptive mechanisms. The renal effects of PTH are detected within minutes of its administration, and the skeletal effects (i.e., increments in blood calcium) within hours, although within 5 min following PTH injection increased cellular activity is detectable in bone. The intestinal response, achieved indirectly by way of a stimulated bioactivation of vitamin D, requires days or even weeks to become apparent.[20] The biological events that coordinate the varied and complex cellular responses to PTH are detailed subsequently in this chapter.

In the absence of vitamin D, PTH regulation of either the intestinal absorption of calcium or the mobilization of skeletal calcium by PTH is blunted.[21,22] In contrast, the renal tubular effects of PTH[23] are relatively independent of vitamin D. The so-called permissive role of vitamin D for PTH-induced bone resorption possibly involves a change in the availability of calcium to bone cells, because calcium administration in the absence of vitamin D mimics its effect.[24] In this regard, magnesium ion also appears to be permissive for maximal PTH activity, because the blunted or limited skeletal and renal response to PTH and hypocalcemia, often associated with clinical hypomagnesemia, can be reversed by magnesium administration.[25,26]

Although a multitude of factors have been implicated to regulate the synthesis, intracellular processing, and secretion of PTH,[15,27-39] PTH release is tightly regulated solely if not primarily by extracellular ionized calcium concentration. In humans, changes in blood-ionized calcium concentrations as small as 0.4 mM result in rapid and significant alterations in PTH secretion. The proportional regulation of PTH secretion, which represents an excellent example of a biological "feedback control" mechanism, occurs via an inverse sigmoidal relationship between PTH and ionized calcium concentrations over a defined narrow range of circulating *total* calcium concentration (i.e., 7.5 to 11.0 mg/dl).[40,41] Accumulated evidence indicates that the coordinated response of parathyroid cells to relatively small changes in extracellular ionized calcium is controlled by a membrane calcium-sensing receptor.[42,43] This calcium sensor has been recently cloned in bovine parathyroids, and its structure is similar to that of a G protein-coupled hormone receptor (see below), with a large extracellular domain and seven transmembrane spanning regions.[44] Mutations of the calcium-sensing receptor cause abnormalities of the calcium set point for PTH secretion leading to hypercalcemia, e.g., some inborn errors of calcium metabolism, such as familial hypocalciuric hypercalcemia and neonatal severe hyperparathyroidism.[45] The vitamin D metabolite $1,25(OH)_2D_3$ inhibits PTH secretion by inhibiting its synthesis at the level of gene transcription,[46,47] and a vitamin D response element has been identified in the 5'-flanking region of the PTH gene,[48] thus providing a molecular basis to the negative feedback control of $1,25(OH)_2D_3$ on PTH secretion.

B. Parathyroid Hormone-Related Protein

Parathyroid hormone-related protein (PTHrP), which is immunologically different but biologically similar to PTH, has been isolated from a variety of malignant tumors[49-53] and identified as primarily responsible for "humoral" hypercalcemia of malignancy.[54] the PTHrP contains 141 amino acids and, although its amino acid sequence is substantially different from PTH, eight of the first 13 amino acids of PTHrP are identical to PTH (Figure 2).[55,56] This homology probably accounts for the ability of PTHrP to interact with PTH receptors[1,55] in classic PTH target tissues such as bone and kidney and to mimic the skeletal response to PTH.[57-59] In fact, the molecular cloning of identical cDNAs encoding a human PTH/PTHrP receptor from bone and kidney provides excellent evidence for a single PTH/PTHrP receptor in both target tissues.[60] The PTHrP gene is a complex transcriptional unit that via alternative splicing produces messenger RNAs (mRNAs) that encode three related PTHrP proteins which may activate separate and distinct receptors (Figure 3).[56,61] Utilizing region-specific immunoassays in addition to immunoradioactive assays, circulating forms of PTHrP consist primarily of large N-terminus (1-74) and C-terminus (109-138) peptides in equimolar concentrations.[54] The exact structure of the secretory form of the peptide is unknown. C-terminus fragments of PTHrP that inhibit osteoclastic bone resorption[62] also accumulate in renal failure.[54,63] Although the physiological significance of PTHrP is still conjectural at best, because circulating PTHrP levels in healthy individuals (when detected) are much lower than PTH,[51,64,65] the tissue distribution of PTHrP is extensive. Parathyroid hormone-related protein or its transcripts or both are expressed in the (CNS)[66] and in cardiovascular,[67,68] uterine,[1] pancreas,[70] and pituitary[1] tissues, and an O-glycosylated form of PTHrP is made by keratinocytes.[1,61] Parathyroid hormone-related protein concentrations in milk are 10,000 times normal circulating levels and 1000-fold higher than the average plasma concentration in hypercalcemic cancer patients.[71]

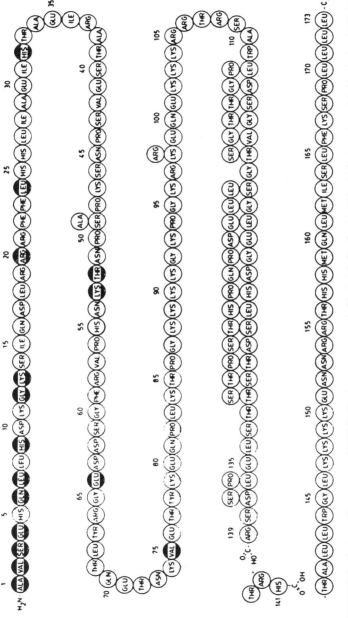

FIGURE 2　Amino acid sequence of PTHrP. The human sequence is illustrated. Blackened circles indicate amino acids identical to PTH. The alternative C-terminus sequences of the human PTHrP isoforms of 139, 141, and 173 amino acids are shown. (Reprinted by permission of the publisher from Goltzman, D., Hendy, G. N., and Banville, D., *Trends Endocrinol. Metab.*, 1, 39, copyright 1989 by Elsevier Science, Inc.)

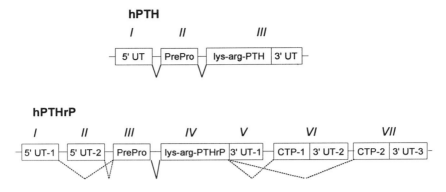

FIGURE 3 Structure of human parathyroid hormone (hPTH) and parathyroid hormone-related peptide (hPTHrP) genes. Exons joined by solid lines are utilized constitutively, those joined by dashed lines are combinatorial. The PTH gene, located in chromosome 11, is constituted by three exons (roman numerals) which encode, respectively, a 5' untranslated region (5'UT), a preproPTH fragment cleaved before secretion, and the PTH sequence, preceded by the Lys-Arg prohormone cleavage site. A 3' untranslated region (3'UT) also exists. The more complex PTHrP gene is located on chromosome 12 and is composed of seven exons. The first 139 amino acids of PTHrP are encoded by exon IV. Alternative splicing of the mRNA produces transcripts that contain carboxyl terminus peptides (CTP) of either 2 or 34 amino acids (exons VI and VII, respectively), thus accounting for three different species of PTHrP. Different 3' untranslated regions (3'UT) follow downstream of the hormone sequence. (Reprinted by permission of the publisher from Goltzman, D., Hendy, G. N., and Banville, D., *Trends Endocrinol. Metab.*, 1, 39, copyright 1989 by Elsevier Science, Inc.)

C.   Calcitonin

Calcitonin, a hormone isolated from the human thyroid gland, is a single-chain, 32-amino acid polypeptide with a molecular weight of 3600 (Figure 4). Twelve species of calcitonin have been isolated to date and common features include a 1-7 amino terminus disulfide bridge, a C-terminus proline amide residue, and a glycine at residue 28. In all 12 calcitonin species, five of the nine N-terminus residues are also identical.[72] The calcitonin gene encodes two distinct hormones: a 141-amino acid precursor for calcitonin and a 128-amino acid precursor for a calcitonin gene-related peptide, which are produced by alternative splicing of mRNA.[73] Messenger RNA processing is relatively tissue specific in that calcitonin is the main product of the thyroid and calcitonin gene-related peptide, the primary product of neurons (Figure 5). Biologically active "fragments" of calcitonin have not yet been identified, and metabolic alterations in the structure of the peptide result in complete biological inactivation. The increase in *in vivo* biological potency of salmon calcitonin relative to other forms, including human, may result from its relative resistance to metabolic degradation or the fact that skeletal and renal receptors for calcitonin have a high apparent affinity for salmon calcitonin.[74]

Calcitonin is produced by the mitochondria-rich parafollicular or C-cells of the thyroid and is secreted in response to elevations in circulating ionized calcium levels. Parafollicular C-cells have been demonstrated to migrate embryologically from the ultimobranchial body, an endodermally derived structure. Additional factors known to influence the rate of calcitonin excretion include glucagon and other gastrointestinal hormones.[75-79] Other tissue sources of calcitonin include the pituitary, a variety of neuroendocrine cells, and carcinomatous lesions such as medullary thyroid carcinoma and small cell lung cancer.[80,81]

The physiological significance of calcitonin on calcium homeostasis of humans is not as well established as that of PTH.[82-84] Calcitonin is inactivated primarily in the kidney and to some extent in muscle or bone or both.[74,85] Available RIA techniques are sensitive enough to detect the elevated calcitonin levels of patients with medullary carcinoma[73,86] and decreased production rates in osteoporotic females.[87] Divergent findings of various investigators regard-

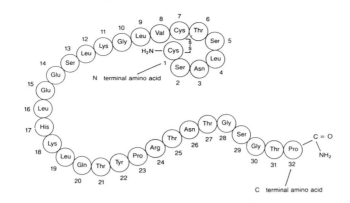

FIGURE 4 Molecular structure of calcitonin. (From *Miacalcic Calcitonin-Sandoz: A Profile of Sandoz's Salmon Calcitonin,* Meditext Ltd., London, 1989, 13. With permission.)

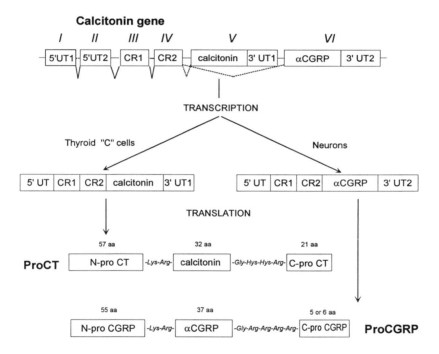

FIGURE 5 Structure and processing of the calcitonin gene. The calcitonin gene is composed of 6 exons which encode both calcitonin (exon V) and calcitonin gene-related peptide α (α-CGRP, exon VI). Two 5′ untranslated regions (5′UT) and two sequences common to both peptides (CR1 and CR2) are encoded by the first four exons. Tissue-specific alternative splicing of the mRNA produces two different transcripts encoding either procalcitonin (proCT) or proCGRP. Both N- and C-terminus propeptides are cleaved before secretion. The C-terminus calcitonin propeptide (C-proCT) is also called katacalcin.

ing age- and sex-related changes in either secreted or circulating calcitonin in adults[88-93] may be explained either by the heterogeneity of immunoassayable circulating calcitonin (iCT), the varying affinity of different antibodies for binding sites on the human calcitonin molecule,[94] and the observations that nonmonomeric as well as monomeric forms of iCT are biologically active.[72,91] Whereas in normal human adults the hypocalcemic effect of injected calcitonin is small, the hypocalcemic activity of exogenously administered calcitonin in young growing animals and in children with increased bone turnover is often dramatic.[95] Although the physiologic role of calcitonin in children or adolescents is also unclear, a significant rise in blood iCT occurs between ages 6 and 12 coupled with a fall in iPTH.[96] Thus, calcitonin may condition skeletal remodeling in the growing child by modulating the rate of bone resorption, and thereby the supply of calcium from bone to extracellular fluids. In this regard, it should be noted that glucocorticoid suppression of longitudinal growth in children has been associated with decreased circulating calcitonin levels.[97] As a result of its ability to suppress bone resorption, pharmacological doses of calcitonin have been used successfully to decrease bone turnover in Paget's disease of bone[98] and the rate of bone loss in postmenopausal osteoporotic syndromes.[99]

D. Calcitonin Gene-Related Peptide

Two calcitonin gene-related peptides (α- and β-CGRP), in addition to the islet amyloid protein (amylin) and calcitonin, comprise the so-called calcitonin family of regulatory peptides.[100] β-Calcitonin gene-related peptide is the product of a separate gene, but is almost identical to α-CGRP, differing by only three amino acids.[101,102] α- and β-CGRP have been identified in plasma and cerebrospinal fluid (CSF);[103,104] both peptides have similar biologic properties.[101,105] α-Calcitonin gene-related peptide, a 37-amino acid peptide derived from alternate splicing of the calcitonin/CGRP gene primary transcript,[106] has been identified in brain, thyroid, heart, smooth muscle of blood vessels, and nerve fibers.[100,107,108] The presence of CGRP in the spinal cord, in addition to plasma and CSF, is consistent with its assumed ability to function as a "neurotrophic hormone".[103,104] Superphysiologic doses of CGRP are also hyperglycemic.[48] Because CGRP-containing neurons have been identified in the heart,[107] and because CGRP has been localized in periadventitial nerves of the vascular system, the peptide is also considered an essential regulator of cardiovascular function and vascular tone.[109-113] As such, the hypotensive response to CGRP is dose dependent[114] and mediated primarily by adenosine 3':5'-cyclic phosphate (cAMP)-dependent mechanisms[112] and hyperpolarization of vascular smooth muscle membranes.[113] Although calcitonin and CGRP have minimal sequence homology, the molecules are similar in size and each contain a disulfide bridge at the N-terminus and an amidated C-terminus end. These structural similarities may account for the ability for both calcitonin and CGRP to bind to each other's receptor[115-117] and to produce similar *in vitro*[118] or *in vivo*[117,119] biological responses utilizing multiple signal-transducing mechanisms in target cells.[118,120]

E. 1,25(OH)$_2$D$_3$

It is now well established that the metabolic activation of vitamin D is essential to its biologic expression in both animals and humans. In fact, the term "vitamin D" is inappropriate, because the endogenous production of vitamin D$_3$ by the skin, its distribution by the bloodstream to kidney, liver, intestine, and bone, its biomolecular action through stimulated protein synthesis, and the negative feedback regulative control of its metabolism all resemble hormonal rather than dietary vitamin activity.

Vitamin D$_3$ is a secosteroid in which the B-ring of the cyclopentanoperhydrophenanthrene structure is cleaved (Figure 6). The vitamin is normally produced in the epidermal layer of skin as a result of the photoconversion of 7-dehydroxycholesterol (7-DHC) to "previtamin D$_3$", utilizing radiation of wavelengths in the ultraviolet B (UVB) (280 to 320 nm) portion of the electromagnetic spectrum.[121] Once formed, the previtamin D$_3$ undergoes either photoconversion to lumisterol, tachysterol, and 7-DHC or a heat-induced ionization to vitamin D$_3$. At body temperature, 50% conversion of previtamin D$_3$ to vitamin D$_3$ occurs within 28 h, with 80% conversion completed within 4 d.[121] The conversion of previtamin D$_3$ to vitamin D$_3$ is blunted by aging and skin pigmentation.[121] The endogenous production rate of vitamin D$_3$ in humans

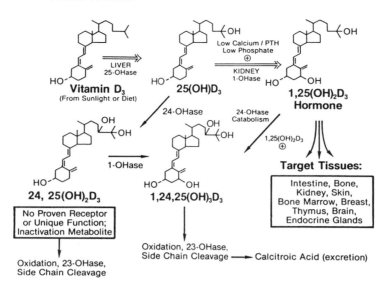

FIGURE 6 Metabolic pathways of the vitamin D endocrine system. (From MacDonald, P. N., Dowd, D. R., and Haussler, R., *Sem. Nephrol.*, 14(2), 101, 1994. With permission.)

is unknown, but it must be at least equivalent to the minimum vitamin D dietary dose of 200 to 400 IU that is essential daily to cure vitamin D-deficiency rickets, as it has been observed that UV skin irradiation alone is curative in this regard.[122]

Following the photochemical conversion of 7-DHC to vitamin D_3, the preformed vitamin D_3 is absorbed into the subepidermal microcirculation and transported in plasma to the liver and target organs bound noncovalently to a specific globulin, DBP (vitamin D binding protein).[123,124] Dietary vitamin D_3 or vitamin D_2, which behaves metabolically like vitamin D_3, are absorbed primarily from the duodenum and jejunum into lymphatic channels, with both bile salts and intraluminal lipids permissive in this regard. Although lipoproteins are not quantitatively important for the transport of vitamin D_3 in plasma, most of the vitamin absorbed from the intestine of animals and humans is transported in lymph by chylomicrons.[125] The site of transfer of vitamin D_3 from chylomicrons to its specific plasma transport protein has not been established, although it appears likely that the liver is fundamental for this transformation. The absorbed vitamin D (i.e., vitamins D_2 and D_3) then admixes with endogenously synthesized vitamin D_3 and is either sequestered into storage depots such as adipose tissue and muscle by specific tissue-binding proteins or is metabolically transferred by the liver where it is subjected to the first of two successive hydroxylations.[125] It seems likely that these tissue-binding proteins also play a role in the regulation of the metabolism of vitamin D and its metabolites.[126-129] In humans, circulating vitamin D levels normally range between 8 and 45 ng/ml.[130] Whereas at normal plasma concentrations vitamin D disappears with a biologic half-life of 19 to 25 h, its metabolic disposal is conditioned by the state of vitamin D nutrition and plasma concentrations, with high and low circulating levels resulting in a decrease and increase, respectively, in the plasma disappearance rate. A hepatic cytochrome P-450-containing 25-hydroxylase enzyme complex converts endogenously synthesized and dietary vitamin D to 25-hydroxylated derivatives (subsequently designated 25-OHD$_3$).[131,132] The enterohepatic circulation of vitamin D is negligible and insignificant amounts of oral vitamin D are excreted in bile as 25-OHD$_3$. The liver converts most of the vitamin D to highly polar (primary glucuronides) substances that are biologically inactive. Also, 25-OHD$_3$ circulates bound to a globular protein that is indistinguishable from that which binds the parent vitamin D with a biologic half-life of approximately 12 d.[127]

Circulating levels of 25-OHD in normal subjects living in the U.S.[128] range between 15 and 30 ng/ml. Reported lower mean circulating 25-OHD levels of 15 to 16 ng/ml in adults from the U.K.[133,134] and seasonal as well as age-related variations in serum levels of healthy individuals[134,135] presumably reflect both the higher dietary intake of vitamin D and the greater sunshine exposure in the U.S. because of its more southerly latitudes. A direct correlation exists between circulating maternal and fetal 25-OHD$_3$ concentrations.[136] Not only does 25-OHD$_3$ represent the major circulating form of vitamin D, but this metabolite accumulates in skeletal tissue,[137] and, in pharmacological doses, stimulates calcium absorption and bone resorption without further structural modification.[138,139] 25-OHD$_3$ also increases the proximal renal tubular reabsorption of calcium, sodium, and phosphate. This effect of 25-OHD$_3$ on phosphate excretion is antagonistic to the phosphaturic effect of PTH.[140,141]

Whereas the metabolic fate of 25-OHD$_3$ in intestine, bone, and extraskeletal storage depot sites (i.e., adipose tissue and muscle) is ill defined, it is further hydroxylated in the proximal and convoluted tubule of the kidney nephron to either 1,25-dihydroxycholecalciferol [1,25(OH)$_2$D$_3$] or 24,25-dihydroxycholecalciferol [24,25(OH)$_2$D$_3$] by either 1α- or 24-cytochrome P-450 hydroxylating enzymes, respectively.[124] Vitamin D deficiency or excess PTH stimulate 1α-hydroxylation. In the vitamin D replete state, 24-hydroxylation predominates. Whereas circulating 25-OHD$_3$ reflects body stores and the availability of vitamin D, 1,25(OH)$_2$D$_3$ is primarily responsible for the biological activity of vitamin D. The renal 1α-hydroxylation of 25-OHD$_3$ is also regulated by a variety of other factors that include intracellular concentrations of potassium, calcium, inorganic phosphate, prostaglandins, and cAMP, as well as gonadal hormones, calcitonin, and pH.[123,124,133,142-146] Thus, unlike the hepatic hydroxylation of vitamin D which is not subjected to particularly tight regulation, the renal conversion of 25-OHD$_3$ to 1,25(OH)$_2$D$_3$ is regulated by a sensitive servocontrol mechanism modulated primarily by circulating calcium, PTH, and the inorganic phosphate content of renal cortical cells.[123,147,148] This biofeedback control mechanism functions as follows: any tendency toward hypocalcemia acts as a stimulus for PTH secretion; the latter, either directly or by depleting renal cortical inorganic phosphate concentration (or both), stimulates the hydroxylation of 25-OHD$_3$ to 1,25(OH)$_2$D$_3$; the increment in circulating 1,25(OH)$_2$D$_3$ in turn completes the negative feedback of hormonal control by stimulating the intestinal absorption and bone resorption of calcium.[123,130] As a consequence, the circulating ionized calcium levels are raised to normal and PTH secretion returns to the basal state. On the other hand, any tendency for serum calcium to increase slows the rate of PTH release, the latter resulting in decreased 1,25(OH)$_2$D$_3$ and elevated 24,25(OH)$_2$D$_3$ production, with a subsequent decrease in both the resorption of bone and intestinal calcium absorption essential to normalize blood calcium levels. 1,25(OH)$_2$D$_3$ also reduces the renal production of 1,25(OH)$_2$D$_3$ and stimulates the production of 24,25(OH)$_2$D$_3$.[149,150] In contrast, 24,25(OH)$_2$D$_3$ appears to exert no effect on the conversion of 25-OHD$_3$ to 1,25(OH)$_2$D$_3$. Once synthesized by the kidney, 1,25(OH)$_2$D$_3$ can be deactivated by a variety of enzymatic oxidations and hydroxylations, particularly at carbons 23, 24, and 26, to form a variety of metabolites. These include 1,24,25(OH)$_3$D$_3$, 1,23,25(OH)$_3$D$_3$, 24 keto-1,23,25(OH)$_3$D3, 1,23,25(OH)$_3$D$_3$, 1,25(OH)$_2$D$_3$-23-26 lactone, and the water-soluble 1α(OH)24,25,26-tetranor-23 (COOH) vitamin D$_3$ (calcitonoic acid).[151] Although varying degrees of biological activity have been demonstrated for many of the 1,25(OH)$_2$D$_3$ metabolites, 1,25(OH)$_2$D$_3$ is much more potent than any of its metabolites when subjected to comparative *in vitro* or *in vivo* biological testing.[83,152-156] 1,25(OH)$_2$D$_3$ circulates with a biologic half-life of 24 h at concentrations of 25 to 33 pg/ml in adults.[157-159] Normal children have higher plasma levels of 49 to 66 pg/ml.[157]

1,25(OH)$_2$D$_3$ is the only vitamin D metabolite that functions in a physiological fashion to regulate the intestinal transport of calcium via a series of genomic and nongenomic biological events, detailed subsequently in this chapter. Thus, we should consider vitamin D$_3$ primarily as an inert reservoir substance, $25\text{-}OHD_3$ as the major circulating biologically active metabolite, and $1,25(OH)_2D_3$ as the metabolite with maximal biologic activity, which, together with PTH (and probably calcitonin), normally regulates the intestinal absorption of calcium and the growth and remodeling of bone.[123-125]

In addition to the effects of $1,25(OH)_2D_3$ on the classic target tissues of intestine, kidney, and bone, a large variety of nontraditional target tissues have been identified as sites for the $1,25(OH)_2D_3$ "receptor", with an ever-increasing panorama of $1,25(OH)_2D_3$ "effects" recorded.[160] A unifying hypothesis proposed to explain the special and diverse effects of $1,25(OH)_2D_3$ on myocardial contractibility, vascular tone, hepatic regeneration, PTH secretion, and the proliferation of hematopoietic cells, keratinocytes, fibroblasts, and thymocytes considers $1,25(OH)_2D_3$ essential for the regulation of intracellular calcium in a rapid and nongenomic fashion, in addition to its ability to modulate genomic events via traditional steroid interactive pathways.[161]

II. MECHANISMS OF TARGET CELL ACTIVATION

A. Receptors

1. PTH/PTHrP

Despite the limited structural homology between PTH and PTHrP, the similarity of their physiologic actions and direct *in vitro* studies suggested that the two hormones should bind the same receptor in bone and kidney target cells.[162] The recent cloning of the gene encoding a receptor that binds both PTH and PTHrP in osteoblasts and kidney cells[60,163] has confirmed this assumption at a molecular level. The identification of the receptor has also allowed the resolution of a number of issues related to the biochemistry of PTH signal transduction and cell activation that could be addressed only indirectly by receptor binding studies. The PTH/PTHrP receptor, along with the calcitonin[164,165] and the secretin receptors,[166] represent a new family of G-protein-linked peptide hormone receptors whose tertiary structure resembles that of the β-adrenergic receptors. They are monomeric proteins, with seven transmembrane-spanning domains, an extracellular N-terminus, and a long C-terminus tail.[60,163] Despite this similarity, <10% sequence homology is shared with other G-protein-linked receptors. This family of receptors has now expanded to include recently cloned receptors for vasoactive intestinal peptide,[167] glucagon-like peptide 1,[168] and growth hormone-releasing hormone.[169]

Pharmacologic analyses of various PTH and PTHrP ligands to the PTH/PTHrP receptor have suggested possible species and tissue differences in receptor affinities. For example, some shortened analogues exhibit higher affinity to bovine renal membranes than to rat osteosarcoma cells,[162,170] whereas intact PTH was found to bind with more affinity to osteosarcoma cells than to canine renal membranes, perhaps via middle and C-terminus regions.[171] Furthermore, different affinities to PTHrP peptides were observed for renal membranes of different species,[162,172,173] implying the existence of organ-specific receptors that can explain differences in ligand binding or activation of signal transduction mechanisms or both. The recent cloning of identical human cDNAs that encode for both renal and bone PTH/PTHrP receptors has unambiguously established that identical receptors are expressed by the major PTH target cells.[60]

Stable transfection of either the cloned PTH/PTHrP or calcitonin receptors into cells that normally do not express either receptor have demonstrated that both are coupled to multiple signaling systems, in particular the adenylyl cyclase and phospholipase C pathways.[174,175] This finding has practically refuted the hypothesis of two types of PTH receptors that was originally proposed on the basis of the demonstration of alternative signal transduction mechanisms activated by the hormone in target cells.[176] As explained in more detail later, coupling to different second messenger systems probably occurs through different G-proteins, a characteristic feature of this family of peptide hormone receptors.[175,177,178] On the other hand, the possible presence of a different receptor for the middle or C-terminus regions of PTH is still unresolved. This hypothesis emerged from binding studies showing that C-terminus fragments of PTH could displace a significant fraction of the full-length PTH-(1-84),[179] whereas N-terminus fragments were unable to completely prevent binding of the intact hormone.[171] Although most of the actions of PTH can be reproduced by N-terminus peptides, the demonstration that in particular conditions and cell models C-terminus fragments can induce physiologic effects such as stimulation of alkaline phosphatase[180] suggests that a binding site specific for the middle portion or the C-terminus end of the molecule may exist, in addition to the cloned PTH/PTHrP receptor.

Similarly, the hypothesis of a different receptor for non-PTH-like domains of PTHrP has been proposed on the bases of observations demonstrating biphasic effects of PTHrP-(1-141) on mixed osteoblast-osteoclast populations and clearly inhibitory actions on isolated osteoclasts.[62,181] Structure-function analysis has located the osteoclast inhibitory site in the 107 to 111 region, close to the C-terminus of PTHrP, a peptide sequence that has been called osteostatin.[182] These findings raise intriguing possibilities for the physiologic role of PTHrP, and open an interesting avenue for the design of molecules able to interfere with the bone resorptive process.

Bone and kidney are the major, classic target tissues for PTH, and receptors are abundant in these organs. However, physiologic responses or binding sites to PTH or PTHrP (or both) have also been reported in other tissues such as vascular smooth muscle [183] (see also subsequent chapters), gastrointestinal cells,[184] mononuclear cells,[185,186] thymic lymphocytes,[187] chondrocytes,[188] dermal fibroblasts,[189] and keratinocytes.[64,190] Parathyroid hormone-like activity also has been found in the brains of several species[191] and in the stimulation of cAMP described in glial cells,[192] as well as adrenocorticotropes.[193] While the relevance of PTH/PTHrP actions on the cardiovascular system is clarified in the following chapters, the physiologic significance of PTH and PTHrP effects on such a variety of nonclassic target cells remains to be elucidated. In bone, PTH receptors are expressed by mature osteoblasts,[194,195] although most binding sites are present in less differentiated cells located in the intertrabecular space of the bone marrow, usually referred to as preosteoblasts.[196] The existence of heterogeneous target sites for PTH, also confirmed in osteogenic cell cultures,[197,198] may imply that different actions of the hormone are mediated by different cell subtypes, perhaps through different hormone sensitivities or signal transduction pathways or both.[196,198]

2. Calcitonin

It is probably not entirely coincidental that both the PTH/PTHrP and the calcitonin receptors have been cloned at the same time, using similar strategies.[163,164] As in the case of the PTH/PTHrP receptor, the cloned calcitonin receptor is functionally coupled to cAMP stimulation, but the deduced amino acid sequence is not similar to any of the known receptors that span the plasma membrane seven times, and couple to G-proteins.[164] Although the PTH/PTHrP receptor is about 100 amino acids longer than the calcitonin receptor, the two sequences share 32% identity and 56% homology.[164] These structural similarities, along with the analogous postreceptor mechanisms of cell activation, identify a unique family of peptide hormone receptors. The subsequent cloning of a human calcitonin receptor has offered an opportunity to understand the evolutionary pathway of this family of receptors.[165] The human calcitonin receptor differs in binding affinity and amino acid sequence from the receptor cloned from a porcine cell line, although they are obviously closely related.[164] By comparing the sequences of the known peptide receptors, Gorn et al.[165] established that the receptors for calcitonin, PTH/PTHrP, and secretin represent an evolutionary branch that originates from an ancestor common to the larger β-adrenergic receptor family (Figure 4). In fact both families exhibit the same evolutionary distance from the cAMP receptor, which mediates chemotaxis and aggregation of *Dictyostelium discoideum,*[199] and is thought to represent the progenitor of these two families of peptide hormone receptors.[165] The most notable homologies among the calcitonin, PTH/PTHrP, and secretin receptors are located in the transmembrane spanning domains, which in turn differ from other G-protein-linked receptors.[200] Other common features include a potential N-terminus glycosylation site and a few key residues at sites thought to be essential for ligand binding.[165] It is possible that these features may account for some characteristic biologic properties common to these receptors such as activation of multiple G-proteins[175,177,178] and cell cycle regulation of ligand-induced responses.[201,202]

Although opposites for most biologic effects, PTH and calcitonin share similar target tissues, i.e., bone and kidney.[203,204] Calcitonin predominantly inhibits bone resorption, acting directly on the osteoclast,[205] and in kidney it enhances calcium excretion in tubule cells.[206] While calcitonin may bind to some osteoblastic cell lines,[207,208] evidence of a direct effect on osteoblasts is still very controversial.[209] As in the case of PTH, calcitonin receptors are distributed to many tissues other than bone and kidney. Calcitonin binding has been reported in male gonadal and germinal cells,[210-212] placenta,[213] lungs,[214] some tumoral cells,[215,216] and lymphoid cells.[217,218] Interestingly, and similar to PTH, the brain and the pituitary may also be target tissues for calcitonin.[219,220] Evidence also exists that calcitonin may interfere with gastrointestinal secretions, but that this action may not be mediated by direct binding to gastrointestinal cells.[221] The physiologic significance of calcitonin receptors in many of these tissues still requires definition, but it is possible that some of its effects in extraskeletal and extrarenal tissues may be mediated by cross-reactivity with receptors of hormones related to calcitonin, such as α- and β-CGRP and amylin. Ligand-binding studies suggest that these peptides possess high affinity specific receptors, but at high concentrations they may in fact cross-react with receptors for the other structurally similar peptides.[115,222]

3.   Vitamin D

Cloning of the receptor that binds $1,25(OH)_2D_3$ (vitamin D receptor) has preceded the description of the receptors for the peptide hormones discussed earlier.[223-225] The vitamin D receptor is a member of the steroid hormone receptor superfamily,[226] its closest relative being the thyroid hormone receptor.[224,227] Accordingly, the receptor is primarily a nuclear protein, where it functions as a transactivating factor.[228] Although this protein is universally termed "vitamin D receptor", in reality it binds $1,25(OH)_2D_3$, the metabolite with hormonal activity, with much higher affinity than any other vitamin D metabolites.[224] As a member of the steroid receptor family, the vitamin D receptor is a DNA-binding protein, with a typical highly conserved DNA-binding domain located near the N-terminus of the molecule and a hormone-binding domain at the carboxyl end.[226,228] Transcriptional regulation occurs via the highly variable N-terminus domain, which may also be involved in regulating DNA binding. The DNA-binding domain possesses the two characteristic "zinc-finger" loops, which mediate the interaction with specific sites of the DNA.[228] Although the precise mechanisms of protein-DNA interaction are not totally known, it is believed that upon binding to $1,25(OH)_2D_3$, the vitamin D receptor undergoes conformational changes that increase its affinity for DNA.[227] The occupied vitamin D receptor interacts with vitamin D-responsive DNA elements of responsive genes, thus acting as a *trans*-activator.[228]

Although its main actions are directed toward the regulation of extracellular calcium homeostasis, probably no other hormonal receptor is so widely distributed in tissues as the vitamin D receptor. This broad distribution reflects the myriad of actions that have been attributed to $1,25(OH)_2D_3$ in nonclassic target tissues (see Reference 124 for a detailed review of tissue distribution and actions of vitamin D). Using traditional biochemical methods and steroid autoradiography, binding sites have been found in almost every tissue in which they have been sought, with very few exceptions. Tissues in which binding sites or actions of vitamin D metabolites or both have been described include the hematopoietic, lymphatic, and reproductive systems, as well as most endocrine glands, the skin, the liver, the lungs, and, of course, skeletal and smooth muscle.[124] Tissue-related differences in receptor affinity and selectivity have been reported, but these may reflect species differences or variable sensitivity and specificity of the assay used. Initial screening of tissues for the expression of the cloned vitamin D receptor seems to confirm the hypothesis that a single receptor mediates the protean actions of vitamin D metabolites in the different target cells.[124]

While most postreceptor effects of $1,25(OH)_2D_3$ are mediated by the nuclear vitamin D receptor and require gene transcription regulation, immediate cellular responses, notably those on intracellular Ca^{2+} homeostasis, are probably independent of genomic regulation, and appear to be mediated by interactions of $1,25(OH)_2D_3$ with the plasma membrane.[229] Evidence of the nongenomic actions of vitamin D metabolites has culminated in a search for the molecular mechanisms that initiate and perpetuate this unconventional signal transducing mode for a steroid hormone. An earlier hypothesis, which implicated changes in a membrane fluidity, was based on the fact that secosterols can be incorporated into the lipid bilayer of the cell membrane, thus altering its physical properties.[230-232] Supporting this so-called "liponomic" hypothesis are the demonstrations that $1,25(OH)_2D_3$ is able to reverse some abnormalities in fluidity and lipid composition of brush-border membranes from enterocytes of vitamin D-deprived rats,[233] and that vitamin D metabolites can stimulate transfer of phosphatidylcholine from unilamellar liposomes to acceptor brush-border membrane vesicles.[234] On the other hand, a number of observations seem to indicate the existence of a membrane resident receptor or binding site for vitamin D metabolites. Evidence for this hypothesis includes the specificity of $1,25(OH)_2D_3$ effects on cytosolic Ca^{2+} homeostasis when compared to other metabolites,[235,236] the inhibition by the inactive $1\beta,25(OH)_2D_3$ epimer of $1\alpha,25(OH)_2D_3$ on phospholipid metabolism,[237] the potential involvement of a G protein in mediating the effect on $[Ca^{2+}]_i$,[237] and the efficacy of $1,25(OH)_2D_3$ on $[Ca^{2+}]_i$ of cells without detectable vitamin D receptors.[236] The latter finding, however, is still controversial, because in some cell systems the presence of a functional surface binding site is required for rapid actions of vitamin D metabolites.[238,239] The rapid activation of inositol phospholipid turnover reported by several investigators after cell exposure to $1,25(OH)_2D_2$[236,237,240-244] lends further support to the idea of a surface receptor, as activation of phosphoinositol metabolism in most cases occurs through the enzymatic breakdown of membrane-associated phospholipids.[245] Despite the many efforts expended to explore this issue, no direct evidence for a surface receptor for $1,25(OH)_2D_3$ exists. Therefore, whether this putative receptor is the same as the cloned nuclear receptor or as a different protein with vitamin D binding capacity remains to be determined.

B. Signal Transduction

Hormone binding to its receptor initiates an event cascade that leads to activation of effector enzymes and generation of second messengers. These soluble molecules or ions activate kinases, and through them the hormonal signal is ultimately transduced into gene expression. Despite their different biologic actions, the peptide hormones PTH, PTHrP, and calcitonin activate similar signal transducing systems, namely the cAMP and the Ca^{2+} message systems. As noted above, the steroid hormone $1,25(OH)_2D_3$ is capable of inducing rapid, nongenomic changes in cytosolic Ca^{2+} homeostasis. Thus, it appears that all the major calciotropic hormones with bone resorptive activity share at least one common intracellular signaling system. This consideration may bear important consequences for the transduction of the resorptive signal to the osteoclasts.

1. PTH and PTHrP

Because PTH and PTHrP activate the same receptor, the mechanisms of signal transduction are very similar, if not identical. Since the characterization of the chemical structure of PTH, production of cAMP was considered the major early event induced by the hormone in target cells, following receptor binding.[246,247] Activation of adenylyl cyclase has thus been considered the classic second messenger for PTH, and this action has been used to define the biological activity of PTH and PTHrP.[248] This concept, which was accepted as dogma for years, was based on the fact that the essential biologic actions of PTH, i.e., induction of hypercalcemia and stimulation of bone resorption, could be mimicked by increasing cellular cAMP levels.[249,250]

Bone resorption could also be stimulated by artificially increasing $[Ca^{2+}]_i$.[251,252] In addition, PTH fragments that are inactive on adenylyl cyclase could mimic some of the biologic action of PTH,[253,254] and PTH regulation of phosphate transport in kidney epithelia was in part independent of cAMP production.[255,256] These observations implicated alternative second messenger pathways for some PTH actions in target cells. Later results of experiments performed by several groups confirmed this hypothesis, demonstrating that PTH rapidly and transiently increases $[Ca^{2+}]_i$ in a variety of cell models, including kidney proximal tubule and osteoblastic cells.[176,257-261] Controversy continues regarding the mechanisms by which PTH increases $[Ca^{2+}]_i$. While some investigators stress the importance of an influx of extracellular Ca^{2+} as the cation source for this effect of PTH,[176,259] in most experimental systems the hormone appears to mobilize Ca^{2+} from intracellular storage pools.[258,260-262] Rapid production of inositol 1,4,5-triphosphate (InsP$_3$) has been repeatedly observed after cell exposure to PTH,[262-266] and suggests the activation of a phospholipase C pathway. Activation of adenylyl cyclase and phospholipase C ultimately results in the activation of the two respective protein kinases, A and C. These final steps of the signal transduction cascade activated by PTH also have been described as occurring in several cell models.[267-272]

The homology between PTHrP and PTH at the N-terminus predicted similar signal transduction mechanisms for the two hormones. Subsequent studies have in fact confirmed this premise, establishing that, like PTH, PTHrP stimulates both the adenylyl cyclase and the phospholipase C systems, thus producing cAMP[273-275] and rapid increases of $[Ca^{2+}]_i$.[59] In most, if not all, circumstances the two hormones have proven to be equipotent for the activation of second messenger pathways. Similar structure-function correlates also have been demonstrated by using shortened N-terminus fragments of both hormones.

Thus, PTH and PTHrP can activate two effector enzymes, adenylyl cyclase and phospholipase C. Although it has been well established that both pathways are activated by the same receptor, it is appropriate to assume that the hormonal signal must divide after hormone receptor binding. This branching of the hormonal signal may occur via receptor coupling to multiple G-proteins, a phenomenon also observed for other members of the PTH/PTHrP family of peptide hormone receptors. Guanosine triphosphate (GTP)-binding proteins, or G-proteins, are heterotrimers, composed of α-, β-, and γ-subunits, and becomes activated following hormone receptor binding. Activation involves binding of the α-subunit to GTP and separation from the β γ complex. The GTP-bound α-subunit then activates a specific effector enzyme, depending on the class of G proteins involved in signal transduction.[276] The adenylyl cyclase system is controlled by stimulatory (G_s) and inhibitory (G_i) proteins, whereas phospholipase C is linked to G_q.[276] While the G-proteins involved in PTH or PTHrP action have not been defined at the molecular level, experimental evidence suggests that both G_s and G_i are present in osteoblasts, because both cholera and pertussis toxins significantly interfere with PTH actions on the cAMP system and on bone resorption.[269,277-279] A G-protein also mediates the activation of phospholipase C by PTH and PTHrP, because GTP analogues mimic this hormonal effect, which is also pertussis toxin sensitive.[266,280]

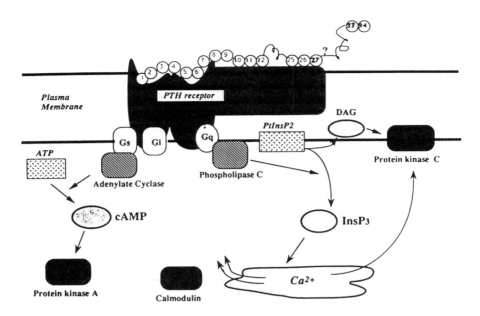

FIGURE 7   Model of PTH signal transduction. The first 2 amino acids of the N-terminus are coupled to adenylyl cyclase through stimulatory (G_s) and inhibitory (G_i) guanosine triphosphate-binding proteins. Activation of adenylyl cyclase leads to cAMP production and stimulation of protein kinase A, which dissociates into its regulatory and catalytic subunits. Phospholipase C is activated by a domain beyond the first 3 amino acids, presumably through a different G-protein, tentatively indicated as G_q. Phospholipase C catalyzes the hydrolysis of phosphatidylinositol 3,4-bisphosphate (PtInsP$_2$) into diacylglycerol (DAG) and InsP$_3$. DAG, in turn, activates PKC, whereas InsP$_3$ mobilizes Ca^{2+} from intracellular storage pools. Increased [Ca^{2+}]$_i$ activates calmodulin and synergizes with protein kinase C. (From Fujimori, A., Cheng, S.-L., Avioli, L. V., and Civitelli, R., *Endocrinology*, 130(1), 29, 1992, © The Endocrine Society. With permission.)

Structure-function studies of PTH and PTHrP signal transduction using truncated peptides have demonstrated that the first two amino acids are essential for the activation of adenylyl cyclase,[253,281,282] while the ability to induce InsP$_3$ and [Ca^{2+}]$_i$ increases, and the activation of protein kinase C (PKC) can be linked to a different domain of the molecule. Additional studies have apparently located the activation of this second messenger pathway to a domain of PTH that includes amino acids 25-34.[272] As discussed below, evidence suggests that the same domain may be responsible for the mitogenic action of the hormone in chondrocytes[188] and possibly in lymphocytes,[187] whereas cAMP production is invariably associated with the inhibition of mitogenesis.[283-285] The analysis of structure and function relationships has led to the definition of a model of PTH signal transduction which implies a single receptor and multiple second messengers generated by coupling to different G-proteins, as illustrated in Figure 7. According to this model, hormone binding can occur even in the absence of the first six amino acids, but full biologic action requires the integrity of the N-terminus.[269] Amino acids 1 and 2 mediate adenylyl cyclase activation, but in the absence of these two residues, the signal can still flow through the phospholipase C/PKC system. The observations that different sites of PTH and PTHrP molecules may mediate different biologic actions has led to the definition of "PTH/PTHrP polyhormones"[286] which has potentially useful implications for the design of hormonal analogues with specific biological activities.

Technological advances have recently permitted an extension of signal transduction studies to single cells in live monolayer cultures, which represents a more physiologic condition when compared to stimulation of cells in suspensions. Using osteogenic sarcoma cells, members of our group have defined the heterogeneous nature of the hormonal response. While [Ca^{2+}]$_i$

transients were observed only in a subgroup of cells, rapid production of cAMP was more homogeneous from cell to cell.[198,287] More recent results suggest that the $[Ca^{2+}]_i$ response to PTH may be more frequent in cells in S phase as compared to cells in G1 phase of the cell cycle.[202] These observations offer new insights into the mechanisms by which the hormone affects cell proliferation and activity. They suggest that hormonal input signals may be modulated from within the cell, thus configuring a sort of "intracrine" regulation via the intracellular pacemaker activity of the cell cycle engine.

2. Calcitonin

As anticipated above, the similarities between the PTH/PTHrP and the calcitonin receptors presumably account for similar mechanisms of signal transduction in target cells. Accordingly, calcitonin activates both the adenylyl cyclase and the Ca^{2+} message systems. While activation of the former pathway has been recognized in bone and kidney,[204,205,288] the existence of a second signaling system was postulated on the basis of a lack of detectable cAMP response in certain systems (i.e., the brain), despite significant hormone binding sites[289,290] or in the face of clear biologic responses.[291] Subsequently, acute increments in $[Ca^{2+}]_i$ have been reported in renal tubules[292] and more recently in single live osteoclasts[293-295] following exposure to calcitonin. Rapid generation of InsP$_3$ and activation of PKC also have been demonstrated in calcitonin-responsive cells[201,265] or in cells transfected with the cloned porcine calcitonin receptor.[175] Thus, cellular mechanisms essential for transducing the response to calcitonin are very similar to those observed for PTH.

The two signaling pathways are activated by calcitonin through two distinct G-proteins. Production of cAMP is mediated by a cholera toxin-sensitive G_s protein,[293] while the effect on $[Ca^{2+}]_i$ and PKC is sensitive to pertussis toxin, implying the involvement of a protein of the G_i class.[201] Interestingly, activation of either signaling system is cell cycle dependent, and may lead to opposite biologic responses.[201] Thus, production of cAMP occurs in G2 phase via G_s, whereas PKC is activated through G_i in S phase.[201] As noted above, cell cycle-dependent activation of the Ca^{2+} message system has been observed for PTH.[202]

The effect of calcitonin on $[Ca^{2+}]_i$ has been analyzed in detail in isolated osteoclasts. The increase in $[Ca^{2+}]_i$ is biphasic, with an initial peak attended by the release of Ca^{2+} from intracellular stores. This event is followed by a sustained phase, probably secondary to the entry of extracellular Ca^{2+}.[175,294] The initial rapid phase is probably mediated, at least in part, by the production of InsP$_3$, as demonstrated in calcitonin-responsive osteoblastic cells.[265] However, this finding has not been confirmed in the osteoclast, which is considered to be the classic calcitonin target cell. In some cell systems the initial rapid phase is not seen, and the effect is limited to a slow, sustained rise of $[Ca^{2+}]_i$.[265,295] As noted subsequently in this chapter, the ability to alter $[Ca^{2+}]_i$ of osteoclasts is relevant to the physiologic action of the hormone, because osteoclast function is directly regulated by the intracellular concentration of this ion.[296]

3. Vitamin D

Binding of the occupied vitamin D receptor to vitamin D responsive elements has been investigated using the osteocalcin gene promoter as a model. Theoretically, the osteocalcin gene represents the best candidate for these studies, because $1,25(OH)_2D_3$ stimulates osteocalcin production both *in vivo* and *in vitro*. The *cis*-acting vitamin D responsive element, which is localized in the promoter region of the osteocalcin gene, is composed of two complex palindromic sequences separated by three base pairs,[297-299] a structure similar to other steroid hormone responsive elements.[299] This DNA sequence is very specific for the occupied vitamin D receptor, and it does not bind other steroid hormone receptors.[299] Although $1,25(OH)_2D_3$ binding is necessary for the receptor to function as a *trans*-acting factor, a nuclear factor appears to be required for gene activation, as *in vitro* expressed vitamin D receptor does not bind to the response elements, even in the presence of $1,25(OH)_2D_3$, unless cell extract is added.[300] Although the observations accumulated with the osteocalcin gene promoter may indeed represent a general mechanism by which vitamin D metabolites regulate gene expression, this premise still requires experimental proof for other genes.

More controversial are the signal transduction mechanisms that lead to changes in intracellular Ca^{2+} homeostasis induced by $1,25(OH)_2D_3$. Earlier studies demonstrated rapid changes in cell membrane Ca^{2+} transport induced by $1,25(OH)_2D_3$ in intestinal[301,302] and other cell systems,[303] thus implying a rapid and direct action on $[Ca^{2+}]_i$. Direct measurement of $[Ca^{2+}]_i$ using fluorescence techniques confirmed that $1,25(OH)_2D_3$ acutely increases $[Ca^{2+}]_i$ in many target cells, including osteoblasts,[236,261,304] hepatocytes,[305] parathyroid cells,[306] and enterocytes.[244] As it occurs for all the other peptide calciotropic hormones, the action of $1,25(OH)_2D_3$ on $[Ca^{2+}]_i$ is very rapid. Although the rise in $[Ca^{2+}]_i$ is sometimes transient with return to baseline,[236] in most cases after the initial $[Ca^{2+}]_i$ spike a new, higher steady state is reached.[244,261,304] This biphasic effect most likely represents the summation of an early Ca^{2+} release from intracellular storage pools and a sustained influx of extracellular Ca^{2+} through Ca^{2+} channels. This mechanism, similar to that described above for calcitonin, is supported by demonstrations that Ca^{2+} channel blockers only partially inhibit the acute $[Ca^{2+}]_i$ spike,[198] whereas in nominally Ca^{2+}-free media only the sustained phase of the $[Ca^{2+}]_i$ rise is abolished.[244] In addition, $1,25(OH)_2D_3$ rapidly and transiently induces the production of $InsP_3$, having a time course closely similar to the changes in $[Ca^{2+}]_i$.[236,238,244] Production of $InsP_3$[236,238,244] and diacylglycerol[236] implies activation of phospholipase C as the initial event in the cellular response to $1,25(OH)_2D_3$. As a consequence, activation of PKC — the expected end point of the signal cascade initiated by phospholipase C activity — has been described in colonocytes.[244] Paralleling these studies, the direct demonstration of the opening of an L-type Ca^{2+} channel by $1,25(OH)_2D_3$ has been obtained by electrophysiological studies.[235] The latter experiments also confirmed the higher potency of $1,25(OH)_2D_3$, as compared to less hydroxylated compounds. The lack of activity of $24,25(OH)_2D_3$[235,236] may suggest that while 1α-hydroxylation is required for the activation of the Ca^{2+} message system, 24-hydroxylation may be inhibitory.

Alternative hypotheses to explain the rapid action of $1,25(OH)_2D_3$ on $[Ca^{2+}]_i$ have also been proposed. $1,25(OH)_2D_3$ stimulates the production of lysophosphatidylinositol in hepatic cells.[237,241] Because lysophosphatidylinositol also mobilizes Ca^{2+} from intracellular stores, the rapid effect of $1,25(OH)_2D_3$ on hepatocyte $[Ca^{2+}]_i$[305] could be mediated by the activation of phospholipase A rather than phospholipase C in this cell system.[237,241] A rapid, presumably nongenomic, and selective stimulation of cyclic guanosine monophosphate (cGMP) by $1,25(OH)_2D_3$ has been observed in human skin fibroblasts[239] and renal cortical membranes.[307] Although the effects were obtained only in cells bearing vitamin D receptors, these convincing results are difficult to interpret with respect to our current understanding of the biologic action of $1,25(OH)_2D_3$. Likewise, although recently $1,25(OH)_2D_3$-induced Ca^{2+} transport in intestinal epithelial cells has been shown to be inhibited by protein kinase A (PKA) antagonists,[308] the attenuation of hormone-induced cAMP responses by $1,25(OH)_2D_3$ observed in osteoblastic cells is probably mediated via the genomic action of $1,25(OH)_2D_3$.[309]

III. CELLULAR ACTIONS

A. Functions in Classic Target Cells

1. Bone

PTH. One of the major paradoxes of bone biology is the fact that PTH, $1,25(OH)_2D_3$, and other factors that stimulate osteoclastic-mediated bone resorption have their respective receptors or binding sites on osteoblasts rather than on osteoclasts. This premise implies that the biologic effect of PTH and other factors that function in a similar manner is indirect and transduced from the osteoblast to the osteoclast.[310] The accumulated evidence suggests that this may occur via the secretion of a soluble factor by the osteoblasts. The hypothesis of a osteoblast-osteoclast "coupling factor" was initially supported by the pioneering work of Chambers and McSheehy,[311] who demonstrated that while osteoblasts were necessary for osteoclasts to excavate resorption pits on devitalized bone slices under stimulation with PTH, direct contact between the two cell types was not required. Medium conditioned by osteoblasts in the presence of PTH was sufficient to stimulate pit formation by isolated osteoclasts.[312] Similar results were reported for $1,25(OH)_2D_3$,[313] prostaglandin E_2 (PGE_2),[314] interleukin-1 (IL-1), and tumor necrosis factor (TNF).[315] However, with the exception of preliminary reports[316,317] the nature of the "coupling factor" that mediates the resorptive activity of PTH, as well as that of other factors, remains elusive. The lagging progress in this area may reflect both the difficulty in identifying the appropriate cell systems and species differences. Thus, other hypotheses remain open, including a direct osteoblast-osteoclast contact through cell adhesion molecules and metabolic and electric coupling through gap junctions.[318] Not only does PTH stimulate gap junction expression and function in osteoblasts,[319] but the possibility has not been excluded that cross-talk between bone-forming and bone-resorbing cells may occur at a stage earlier than terminally differentiated cells.

In addition to its classical effect on bone resorption, PTH also has been shown to function as an "anabolic hormone" in certain conditions *in vivo*. Anabolic effects have been observed after intermittent administration of PTH fragments to rats and humans, resulting in increased cancellous bone formation.[320-324] Despite these *in vivo* observations, experiments designed to identify the effects of PTH on osteoblast function which could translate into increased bone formation have given inconsistent results. For example, depending on the cell system employed, alkaline phosphatase, a marker of osteoblast differentiation, is increased,[325] unaffected,[326] or decreased[327] by PTH. Likewise, while PTH is a potent inhibitor of mitogenesis in osteogenic sarcoma cells,[283,284] it may stimulate cell proliferation in human bone cell cultures.[328] Although some of these discrepancies may be explained by the activation of different second messenger systems by different domains of the PTH molecule, the results of most *in vitro* studies are consistent with the inhibition of both collagen synthesis[329-331] and osteoprogenitor cell differentiation into functional osteoblasts[332] by PTH. While it is difficult to envision a unifying hypothesis that would reconcile the seemingly opposite actions of PTH on the two arms of the bone remodeling process (i.e., bone formation and bone resorption), it appears that prolonged exposure to high concentrations of the hormone causes bone resorption to prevail, whereas short-term, perhaps pulsatile, stimulation of osteoblasts by PTH may induce anabolic effects resulting in stimulation of bone formation.

PTHrP. Because the circulating concentrations of PTHrP in normal individuals are very low, if not undetectable, and because PTHrP production does not seem to be regulated by circulating calcium levels, PTHrP has no major role in normal mineral homeostasis. When abnormally produced by tumors, the hormone causes hypercalcemia by activating the common PTH/PTHrP receptor in target cells (see Section II). Therefore, its action in bone can be assumed to be identical to that of PTH. However, as the biologic actions of PTHrP remain ill-defined, we cannot exclude that the hormone, or some of its fragments, may be active in skeletal tissue via mechanisms yet to be determined.

Calcitonin. The physiologic action of calcitonin in bone is opposite that of PTH.[221,333] Calcitonin inhibits bone resorption by directly inhibiting osteoclast function.[314,334] Direct regulation of osteoclast activity is an uncommon mechanism of action for factors active on bone turnover. In addition to calcitonin, only PGE_2[335] and IL-4,[336] two other inhibitors of osteoclast function, directly modulate osteoclast activity. Calcitonin affects osteoclasts by interfering with activities that are essential for bone resorption, including cell motility and enzyme activity.[337,338] Although both cAMP and $[Ca^{2+}]_i$ are thought to be involved in mediating the biologic action of calcitonin, it has been proposed that each of the two second messenger pathways may serve a specific function. According to this model, production of cAMP via activation of G_s inhibits cell motility, bringing the osteoclast to a quiescent state (the Q effect), whereas an increase of $[Ca^{2+}]_i$, probably via a G_i-dependent mechanism, induces cell contraction or retraction (the R effect), which is invariably observed when disaggregated mature osteoclasts are exposed to calcitonin.[293,294] These concerted actions of calcitonin on cell motility and shape result in inhibition of osteoclast activity.

1,25(OH)$_2$D$_3$. The action of 1,25(OH)$_2$D$_3$ on bone cells is pleiotropic and complex, reflecting the broad spectrum of biologic effects observed *in vivo*. Vitamin D metabolites are essential for bone formation because hypovitaminosis D leads to rickets or osteomalacia, which can be corrected by exogenous administration of the vitamin.[123,151] However, if administered at high doses and for sufficiently long periods, 1,25(OH)$_2$D$_3$ induces bone resorption.[339] Accordingly, 1,25(OH)$_2$D$_3$ affects both osteoblastic and osteoclastic phases of the bone remodeling process.

Osteoblasts are probably the primary target cell for 1,25(OH)$_2$D$_3$ in bone because they bear abundant vitamin D receptors.[340-342] *In vitro* studies with osteoblast model systems have revealed that 1,25(OH)$_2$D$_3$ stimulates the synthesis of a variety of noncollagenic proteins such as osteocalcin,[297,298,343] matrix Gla protein,[344] osteopontin,[345,346] and fibronectin,[347] as well as alkaline phosphatase activity.[348-351] Although in-depth studies have been performed only for the osteocalcin gene (as noted above), it is believed that stimulation of matrix proteins by 1,25(OH)$_2$D$_3$ is transcriptional. While the exact physiologic roles of osteocalcin, matrix Gla protein, osteopontin, and even alkaline phosphatase are still uncertain, they are believed to be involved in cell adhesion and matrix calcification. Nevertheless, the regulatory action of 1,25(OH)$_2$D$_3$ on all these important components of bone matrix implies an important role of the hormone on bone matrix formation.

The action of 1,25(OH)$_2$D$_3$ on collagen synthesis is more controversial. In several osteoblastic cell systems, 1,25(OH)$_2$D$_3$ inhibits type I collagen synthesis.[330,352,353] However, when examined in primary human osteoblasts[350] or in some human or mouse cell lines,[354,355] the hormone stimulated collagen production. These inconsistencies may reflect a dual action of 1,25(OH)$_2$D$_3$ on the differentiation and activity of cells of the osteoblastic lineage. Recent work in primary cultures of rat calvaria demonstrate that when cultures are exposed to 1,25(OH)$_2$D$_3$ in the early proliferative stage of osteoblast precursors, type I collagen and alkaline phosphatase are suppressed, cell proliferation inhibited, and calcified nodule formation blocked, while genes that are normally expressed at a later stage of osteoblast differentiation, such as osteocalcin and osteopontin, are not turned on.[356,357] These results suggest that 1,25(OH)$_2$D$_3$ may inhibit the differentiation of osteoblast precursors but stimulate the metabolic activity of existing mature osteoblasts. The identification of promoter sequences of genes encoding for bone matrix proteins should help elucidate the regulatory actions of the secosterol on the bone formative process.

Despite the lack of biologic effect and receptors on differentiated osteoclasts, 1,25(OH)$_2$D$_3$ has a potent stimulatory action on osteoclast-mediated bone resorption. The steroid both stimulates the differentiation of mononucleated precursors and enhances the activity of existing osteoclasts.[358,359] Several reports have demonstrated the stimulatory activity of 1,25(OH)$_2$D$_3$ in cells of the monocytic-macrophage lineage, which can be induced to differentiate toward a phenotype with bone resorptive activity.[360,361] Although these cells did not exhibit all the features of an osteoclast, subsequent studies have provided convincing evidence that bone marrow cells contain osteoclast precursors, which can be induced to differentiate into mature osteoclasts by 1,25(OH)$_2$D$_3$ as well as other factors.[362,363] The osteoclastic nature of cells produced in these conditions has been validated using more stringent methodology.

The mechanism(s) that control osteoclast differentiation in marrow cultures is still controversial. The process appears to require the presence of both stromal and hemopoietic cells in the cultures.[364] Osteoblast-like cells derived from bone marrow can substitute for stromal cells as inducers of osteoclast formation.[365] Although the target cell for $1,25(OH)_2D_3$ in these systems is currently unknown, there is reason to believe that the hormone may act through the stromal/osteoblastic cells, which bear receptors for vitamin D. A hypothesis suggesting that osteoblasts, or another marrow-residing cell, mediate the osteoclast-stimulatory activity of $1,25(OH)_2D_3$ was also proposed.[314] In experiments similar to those designed to explore the action of PTH and other bone resorptive factors, stimulation of pit formation by disaggregated osteoclasts on dentine slices was observed using medium conditioned by osteoblastic cells treated with $1,25(OH)_2D_3$.[313] The hormone had no effect when used on osteoclast directly, thus implying the existence of a soluble coupling factor whose nature remains unknown. This represents a fundamental difference with the marrow culture systems, in which physical contact between cells of the two types is required, thus implying the intervention of cell adhesion molecules in the transmission of the resorptive signal to the osteoclast precursors.

The requirement of an intermediate cell for the osteoclast-stimulating action of $1,25(OH)_2D_3$ may not universally apply. Human marrow cultures enriched in osteoclast precursors can progressively differentiate into mature osteoclasts when incubated with $1,25(OH)_2D_3$.[366] In these experiments no osteoblast or stromal cells were required, thus reinforcing the alternative hypothesis that osteoclast precursors are target cells for $1,25(OH)_2D_3$.

2. Kidney

PTH and PTHrP. In the kidney, PTH increases the resorption of filtered calcium and causes phosphaturia by inhibition the tubular resorption of phosphate. The latter effect is mediated by PTH inhibition of the Na^+/P_i cotransport,[367,368] a mechanism driven by the Na^+ electrochemical gradient generated by the Na^+ pump. This action is only partially dependent on cAMP stimulation, and it has been associated with activation of the phospholipase C pathway.[255,256] Presumably, PTH has a similar effect on the distal tubule. In the distal tubule, PTH increases calcium resorption by stimulating the Na^+/Ca^{2+} exchanger on the brush-border membrane,[369] also a mechanism dependent on the transmembrane Na^+ gradient. Perhaps one of the most important actions of PTH on the kidney is its stimulation of the 1α-hydroxylase, which converts 25-OHD to $1,25(OH)_2D_3$, the hormonal form of vitamin D. At the same time, PTH inhibits the alternative pathway that leads to the inactive metabolite, $24,25(OH)_2D_3$, by inhibiting the 24-hydroxylase. Both actions are antagonized by $1,25(OH)_2D_3$, thus providing a tightly controlled feedback loop.[370,371] Although cAMP is the second messenger mediating this effect of PTH, the phospholipase C pathway is also involved, although in a direction opposite that of PTH. The exact molecular mechanism of regulation of the two hydroxylases is still under investigation.[372] Although PTHrP can bind to the renal receptor and mimic all the actions of PTH on the kidney, including stimulation of $1,25(OH)_2D_3$ production,[1,275,373] the circulating levels of $1,25(OH)_2D_3$ are usually lower in hypercalcemia of malignancy than in primary hyperparathyroidism.[49] The biologic bases of this phenomenon are still unknown. In addition to these more classic actions, PTH probably also modulates acid-base balance by regulating renal bicarbonate reabsorption[374,375] as well as renin release by a direct stimulatory action on the myoepitheloid cells of the preglomerular arterioles.[376]

Calcitonin. Although the kidney is clearly a target for calcitonin, the hormone appears to have a minor physiologic role in regulating renal function.[221,333] Calcitonin is probably involved in the transport of ions such as Na^+, K^+, Cl^-, Mg^{2+}, and Ca^{2+} in the thick ascending limb,[377] and it produces natriuresis.[378] A phosphaturic effect has also been reported, but it is unclear whether it has any physiological significance.[379] More recent observations indicate that in fact renal tubule cells transfected with the cloned calcitonin receptor respond to the hormone with an increase of cAMP and associated inhibition of phosphate transport in a manner similar to that reported for PTH.[380] An important action is represented by the stimulation of 1α-hydroxylation of 25(OH)D, an effect that seems independent of cAMP production.[291,381] The potential role of the Ca^{2+}/PKC system in mediating some of the extraskeletal actions of the hormone has also emerged from studies indicating opposite effects of calcitonin on the Na^+/K^+ pump of a renal tubule cell line, depending on the cell cycle.[201]

1,25(OH)$_2$D$_3$. The action of 1,25(OH)$_2$D$_3$ on the kidney has not been studied as well as it has been in other target tissues, but it is believed to be involved in calcium and phosphate transport.[123,124] Stimulation of phosphate transport has been shown in proximal tubule brush-border membranes,[382] in which 1,25(OH)$_2$D$_3$ alters the fluidity of plasma membranes.[234] However, the mechanism by which this effect is translated into the antiphosphaturic action of the secosterol is not known.[123] Perhaps even more important is the feedback inhibition of 1,25(OH)$_2$D$_3$ on 1α-hydroxylase activity[370] and the associated stimulation of the 24-hydroxylase,[371] the first step in the inactivating pathway of vitamin D metabolites. This mechanism ensures not only control of hormone synthesis, but also a rapid inactivation of the circulating metabolite.

3. Intestine

1,25(OH)$_2$D$_3$. The stimulatory action of 1,25(OH)$_2$D$_3$ on lumen-plasma calcium and phosphate transport in enterocytes[341] provides the best example of a function linked to both genomic and nongenomic actions. Extensive evidence demonstrates that 1,25(OH)$_2$D$_3$ stimulates the transcription of the gene encoding for calbindin D,[383,384] a Ca^{2+}-binding protein that mediates Ca^{2+} transport through the intestinal epithelium.[385] While the exact role of calbindin D in this process has not been entirely elucidated, a good correlation between the amount of this protein in the intestinal mucosa and the rate of transepithelial Ca^{2+} transport has been found. As detailed previously, 1,25(OH)$_2$D$_3$ also induces rapid, nongenomic changes in Ca^{2+} transport in intestinal cells. These changes include stimulation of Ca^{2+} uptake in intestinal epithelium,[302] increased net Ca^{2+} transport in perfused duodenal loops,[184,301] and release of lysosomal enzymes.[302] These rapid, nongenomic effects are mediated by changes in cytoplasmic Ca^{2+} homeostasis, a phenomenon also called "transcaltachia".[229] The mechanisms by which 1,25(OH)$_2$D$_3$ alters $[Ca^{2+}]_i$ have been defined with more precision in other target cells, mainly the osteoblasts, but indirect evidence suggests that in fact transcaltachia involves Ca^{2+} channel opening[386,387] and perhaps PKC-dependent phosphorylation.[308] The relationships between the effect on gene transcription and the rapid nongenomic action remain to be established. One scenario considers the activation of Ca^{2+} transport as an initial event, which initiates the transepithelial flux and may also serve as the signal transduction mechanism for other physiological effects. The increased rate of gene transcription and resultant protein synthesis may be responsible for sustaining Ca^{2+} translocation. Thus, the final biological response to 1,25(OH)$_2$D$_3$ results from concurrent genomic and nongenomic actions.

Other, not less important, actions of 1,25(OH)$_2$D$_3$ in intestinal cells include stimulation of phosphate transport[388] and the induction of enterocyte growth and differentiation.[389,390] The latter effect, observed in the early 1970s as the elongation of intestinal villi in vitamin D-deficient rats and chicks,[389,390] was linked recently to modulation of the polyamine pathway.[359,391] The ability of 1,25(OH)$_2$D$_3$ to interfere with the differentiation of intestinal cells reflects the ability of the secosterol to induce differentiation of immature cells into phenotypically more characterized cells, which has been demonstrated in a variety of tissues, in addition to bone and intestine.

B. Functions in Nonclassic Target Cells

1. PTH

Besides its action on cardiovascular tissue, which is discussed at length in other chapters, the effects of PTH have been observed in a number of nonclassical target tissues, although the physiological relevance of PTH action in these tissues is uncertain. PTH and its fragments have been implicated as biologically effective in hematopoietic[392,393] and neural tissues.[191,394-396] In addition, the hormone stimulates hepatic glycogenolysis and gluconeogenesis[397] and inhibits smooth muscle contraction in the gastrointestinal tract, trachea, uterus, and vas deferens.[183] The most studied effects of PTH in nonclassic target cells are regulation of mitogenesis and cell differentiation. The hormone is able to stimulate the proliferation of thymic lymphocytes[187] and chondrocytes.[188] As detailed earlier, the proliferative effect of PTH is almost totally independent of cAMP production and is linked to a domain of the polypeptide chain that can stimulate the phospholipase C system.[188] In fact, the cAMP response may be absent in keratinocytes,[398] where the hormone induces cell differentiation. The accumulated data support the hypothesis that the mitogenic and anabolic actions of PTH may be mediated by activation of the Ca^{2+}/phospholipase C messenger system.

2. PTHrP

Because PTHrP production by breast tissue can be induced by lactation,[399] it has been suggested that this so-called milk protein serves to condition the gastrointestinal absorption of calcium during breast feeding.[71] More recent studies demonstrate that endogenous PTHrP is essential for optimal differentiation of keratinocytes.[400,401] Analogous results have emerged from studies in malignant squamous cells.[64] Because of the wide distribution of and documented biological responses to PTHrP in nonclassic PTH target organs,[402] it has been suggested that the PTHrP family of peptides may utilize novel (non-PTH) signal transduction system(s) in autocrine and paracrine fashions in the process of exerting control over normal physiological processes.[61,263,403,404] None of the cellular mechanisms at the basis of such pleiotropic actions of PTHrP are well understood. If specific receptors which can bind specific PTHrP fragments are indeed identified in different tissue, then PTHrP may truly represent a multifunctional precursor molecule, in analogy to proopiomelanocortin, and in keeping with the PTH/PTHrP polyhormone hypothesis.[286]

3. Calcitonin

Although a precise role for calcitonin the CNS has not been defined, calcitonin or a related peptide is present in the brain,[405] and binding sites for calcitonin have been demonstrated in some areas of the brain and in the pituitary.[219,220] In the CNS calcitonin may be involved in nociception and the modulation of prolactin secretion.[406] Peripherally injected calcitonin has been reported to induce analgesia in humans, but despite the relatively large accumulated literature, the biologic basis of this phenomenon remains unclear, and the role of the hormone in neural physiology uncertain.[221] Likewise, the evidence for a physiological role of calcitonin in the gastrointestinal tract is only circumstantial. For example, several gastrointestinal hormones are potent calcitonin secretagogues, and parenterally administered calcitonin induces gastrointestinal side effects. In addition, calcitonin has been used experimentally in pancreatitis, resulting in the reduction of enzyme secretion and pain relief.[221] However, no documented evidence proves direct modulation of normal gastrointestinal function by calcitonin. It is conceivable that some of the reported actions of exogenously administered calcitonin may be secondary to cross-reaction with receptors of structurally related peptides, mostly CGRPs and amylin, which are abundantly present in the brain and the gut, respectively.[115,222]

4. 1,25(OH)$_2$D$_3$

The spectrum of the biologic actions of 1,25(OH)$_2$D$_3$ and the broad distribution of vitamin D receptors have expanded the role of the hormone well beyond the borders of bone metabolism.

$1,25(OH)_2D_3$ is now recognized as an important regulator of cell development and proliferation in many tissues, as well as in some neoplasias. Space limitations preclude an in-depth analysis of the effects of $1,25(OH)_2D_3$ on tissues other than those regarded as classical targets, and the reader is referred to a recent review on this subject[124] and to other chapters in this book.

As a part of the PTH/vitamin D axis, $1,25(OH)_2D_3$ inhibits the release of PTH by both direct and indirect mechanisms. On the one hand, the increased circulating calcium levels produced by the $1,25(OH)_2D_3$-induced stimulation of intestinal calcium absorption provides an inhibitory signal for PTH synthesis and secretion (see above), while on the other, $1,25(OH)_2D_3$ directly inhibits PTH synthesis by interfering with gene transcription in the parathyroid cells.[47] This action, therefore, provides an essential loop for the feedback control of circulating calcium levels. The feedback control is partly lost in chronic renal failure and expression of vitamin D receptors is reduced, which may contribute to the secondary hyperparathyroidism that is characteristic of the syndrome.[407]

The effect of $1,25(OH)_2D_3$ on cell proliferation and differentiation is a general biologic effect of the hormone. Besides its important role in skeletal maturation and growth, $1,25(OH)_2D_3$ has regulatory actions on differentiation and growth of many other tissues, including the intestine, the hematopoietic and lymphoid systems, and the epidermis. Evidence for a role in differentiation of hemopoietic stem cells has initially come from studies in leukemic cells. $1,25(OH)_2D_3$ reduces the proliferation of these cells, and increases the expression of monocyte/macrophage antigens and phagocytic activity.[408] Although a similar effect has been demonstrated in normal hematopoietic precursors, the concentrations required for this action are supraphysiologic, thus questioning the role of $1,25(OH)_2D_3$ in normal hematopoiesis.[409] There is a growing body of evidence suggesting that $1,25(OH)_2D_3$ interferes with the function of the immune systems by such a wide range of actions that the hormone is considered an immunomodulator. In general, $1,25(OH)_2D_3$ actually function as an immunosuppressant by inhibiting cytokine and antibody production, and decreasing the sensitivity of activated lymphocytes to cytokines. However, in other cases, the hormone appears to enhance the immune response. In-depth analyses of these effects can be found in recent reviews.[410-412] Inhibition of cell growth has been observed in other nonleukemic cancer cells, including melanomas, lung, and colon cancer cells.[123,124] The antiproliferative action of the hormone has generated interest in its potential use in the treatment of malignancies, in particular, leukemias, lymphomas, and breast and colon cancers.[123,413] Because $1,25(OH)_2D_3$ inhibits keratinocyte proliferation and stimulates terminal differentiation toward nonadherent squamous cells in the skin,[414] the hormone has been used as a remedy for psoriasis.[415] Biological responses to $1,25(OH)_2D_3$ have been observed in the reproductive system, pituitary and thyroid glands, pancreas, cartilage, skeletal muscle, liver, and lungs, and range from interference with cell replication and differentiation to regulation of hormonal secretion and release.[124]

REFERENCES

1. Orloff, J. J., Wu, T. L., and Stewart, A. F., Parathyroid hormone-like proteins: biochemical responses and receptor interactions, *Endocrinol. Rev.*, 10, 476, 1989.
2. Gardella, T. J., Wilson, A. K., Keutmann, H. T., Oberstein, R., Potts, J. T., Jr., Kronenberg, H. M., and Nussbaum, S. R., Analysis of parathyroid hormone's principal receptor-binding region by site-directed mutagenesis and analog design, *Endocrinology*, 132, 2024, 1993.
3. Segre, G. V., Niall, H. D., and Habener, J. F., Metabolism of parathyroid hormone: physiological and clinical significance, *Am. J. Med.*, 56, 774, 1974.
4. Goltzman, D., Henderson, B., and Loveridge, M., Cytochemical bioassay of parathyroid hormone. Characteristics of the assay and analysis of circulating hormonal forms, *J. Clin. Invest.*, 65, 1309, 1980.

5. Grunbaum, D., Wexler, M., Antos, M., Gascon-Barre, M., and Goltzman, D., Bioactive parathyroid hormone in canine progressive renal insufficiency, *Am. J. Physiol.*, 247, E442, 1984.
6. MacGregor, R. R., Jilka, R. L., and Hamilton, J. W., Formation and secretion of fragments of parathormone. Identification of cleavage sites, *J. Biol. Chem.*, 261, 1929, 1986.
7. Martin, K. J., Hruska, K. A., and Greenwalt, A., Selective uptake of intact parathyroid hormone by the liver: differences between hepatic and renal uptake, *J. Clin. Invest.*, 58, 781, 1976.
8. D'Amour, P., Huet, P., Segre, G. V., and Rosenblatt, M., Characteristics of bovine parathyroid hormone extraction by dog liver in vitro, *Am. J. Physiol.*, 241, E208, 1981.
9. Segre, G. V., D'Amour, P., Hultman, A., and Potts, J. T., Jr., Effects of hepatectomy, nephrectomy and nephrectomy/uremia on the metabolism of parathyroid hormone in the rat, *J. Clin. Invest.*, 67, 439, 1981.
10. Hanley, D. A., Takatsuki, K., and Sultan, J. M., Direct release of parathyroid hormone fragments from functioning bovine parathyroid glands, *J. Clin. Invest.*, 60, 1367, 1977.
11. Hruska, K. A., Korkor, A., Martin, K., and Slatopolsky, E., Peripheral metabolism of intact parathyroid hormone: role of liver and kidney and the effect of chronic renal failure, *J. Clin. Invest.*, 67, 885, 1981.
12. Hruska, K. A., Martin, K. J., Mennes, P., Greenwalt, A., Anderson, C., Klahr, S., and Slatopolsky, E., Degradation of parathyroid hormone and fragment production by the isolated perfused dog kidney. The effect of glomerular filtration rate and perfusate Ca^{2+} concentrations, *J. Clin. Invest.*, 60, 501, 1977.
13. Daugaard, H., Egfjord, M., Lewin, E., and Olgaard, K., Metabolism of N-terminal and C-terminal parathyroid hormone fragments by isolated perfused rat kidney and liver, *Endocrinology*, 134, 1373, 1994.
14. Segre, G. V., Advances in techniques for measurement of parathyroid hormone, *Trends Endocrinol. Metab.*, 20, 243, 1990.
15. Habener, J. F. and Potts, J. T., Jr., Relative effectiveness of magnesium and calcium on the secretion and biosynthesis of parathyroid hormone in vitro, *Endocrinology*, 98, 197, 1976.
16. Harms, H. M., Neubauer, O., Kayser, C., Wustermann, P. R., Horn, R., Brosa, U., Schlinke, E., Kulpmann, W. R., VonZurMuhlen, A., and Hesch, R. D., Pulse amplitude and frequency modulation of parathyroid hormone in early postmenopausal women before and on hormone replacement therapy, *J. Clin. Endocrinol. Metab.*, 78, 48, 1994.
17. Jubiz, W., Canterbury, J. M., and Reiss, E., Circadian rhythm in serum parathyroid hormone concentration in human subjects: correlation with serum calcium, phosphate, albumin, and growth hormone levels, *J. Clin. Invest.*, 51, 2040, 1972.
18. Calvo, M. S., Eastell, R., Offord, K. P., Bergstralh, E. J., and Burritt, M. F., Circadian variation in ionized calcium and intact parathyroid hormone: evidence for sex differences in calcium homeostasis, *J. Clin. Endocrinol. Metab.*, 72, 69, 1991.
19. Harms, H. M., Schlinke, E., Neubauer, O., Kayser, C., Wustermann, P. R., Horn, R., Kulpmann, W. R., VonZurMuhlen, A., and Hesch, R. D., Pulse amplitude and frequency modulation of parathyroid hormone in primary hyperparathyroidism, *J. Clin. Endocrinol. Metab.*, 78, 53, 1994.
20. Birge, S. J., Peck, W. A., and Whedon, G. D., Study of calcium absorption in man: a kinetic analysis and physiologic model, *J. Clin. Invest.*, 48, 1705, 1969.
21. Arnaud, C. D., Rasmussen, H., and Anast, C., Further studies on the interrelationship between parathyroid hormone and vitamin D, *J. Clin. Invest.*, 45, 1955, 1966.
22. Ney, R. L., Kelly, G., and Bartter, F. C., Actions of vitamin D independent of the parathyroid glands, *Endocrinology*, 82, 760, 1968.
23. Rasmussen, H., DeLuca, H. F., and Arnaud, C. D., The relationship between vitamin D and parathyroid hormone, *J. Clin. Invest.*, 42, 1940, 1963.
24. Au, W. Y. W. and Raisz, L. G., Restoration of parathyroid responsiveness in vitamin D-deficient rats by parenteral calcium or dietary lactose, *J. Clin. Invest.*, 46, 1572, 1967.
25. Estep, H., Shaw, W. A., and Watlington, C., Hypocalcemia due to hypomagnesemia and reversible parathyroid hormone unresponsiveness, *J. Clin. Endocrinol. Metab.*, 29, 842, 1969.
26. Muldowney, F. P., McKenna, T. J., and Kyle, L. H., Parathormone-like effect of magnesium replenishment in steatorrhea, *N. Engl. J. Med.*, 218, 61, 1970.

27. Heath, H., III, Biogenic amines and the secretion of parathyroid hormone and calcitonin, *Endocr. Rev.,* 1, 319, 1980.
28. Brown, E. M., Thatcher, J. G., Watson, E. J., and Leombruno, R., Extracellular calcium potentiates the inhibitory effects of magnesium on parathyroid function in dispersed bovine parathyroid cells, *Metabolism,* 33, 171, 1984.
29. Morrissey, J. and Slatopolsky, E., Effect of aluminum on parathyroid hormone secretion, *Kidney Int.,* 29, S41, 1986.
30. Dietel, M., Dorn, G., Montz, R., and Altenahr, E., Influence of vitamin D_3 1,25-dihydroxyvitamin D_3, and 24,25-dihydroxyvitamin D_3 on parathyroid hormone secretion, adenosine $3',5'$-monophosphate release, and ultrastructure of parathyroid glands in organ culture, *Endocrinology,* 105, 237, 1979.
31. Chertow, B. S., Baker, G. R., Henry, H. L., and Norman, A. W., Effects of vitamin D metabolites on bovine parathyroid hormone release in vitro, *Am. J. Physiol.,* 238, E384, 1980.
32. Windeck, R., Brown, E. M., Gardner, G. D., and Aurbach, G. E., Effect of gastrointestinal hormones on isolated bovine parathyroid cells, *Endocrinology,* 103, 2020, 1978.
33. Au, W. Y. W., Cortisol stimulation of parathyroid hormone secretion by rat parathyroid glands in organ culture, *Science,* 193, 1015, 1976.
34. Fischer, J. A., Oldham, S. B., Sizemore, G. W., and Arnaud, C. D., Calcitonin stimulation of parathyroid hormone secretion in vitro, *Horm. Metab. Res.,* 3, 223, 1971.
35. Brown, E. M., Histamine receptors on dispersed parathyroid cells from pathological human parathyroid tissue, *J. Clin. Endocrinol. Metab.,* 51, 1325, 1980.
36. William, G. A., Longley, R. S., and Bowser, E. N., Parathyroid hormone secretion in normal man and in primary hyperparathyroidism: role of histamine H2 receptors, *J. Clin. Endocrinol. Metab.,* 52, 122, 1981.
37. Brown, E. M., PTH secretion in vivo and in vitro, *Min. Electrolyte Metab.,* 177, 606, 1972.
38. Boucher, A., D'Amour, P., Hamel, L., Fugere, P., Gascon-Barre, M., Lepage, R., and Ste. Marie, J. G., Estrogen replacement decreases the set point of parathyroid hormone stimulation by calcium in normal postmenopausal women, *J. Clin. Endocrinol. Metab.,* 68, 831, 1989.
39. MacDonald, P. N., Ritter, C., Brown, A. J., and Slatopolsky, E., Retinoic acid suppresses parathyroid hormone (PTH) secretion and preproPTH mRNA levels in bovine parathyroid cell culture, *J. Clin. Invest.,* 93, 725, 1994.
40. Mayer, G. P. and Hurst, J. G., Sigmoidal relationship between parathyroid hormone secretion rate and plasma calcium concentration in calves, *Endocrinology,* 102, 1036, 1978.
41. Ramirez, J. A., Goodman, W. G., Gornbein, J. G., Menezes, C., Moulton, L., Segre, G. V., and Salusky, I. B., Direct in vivo comparison of calcium-regulated parathyroid hormone secretion in normal volunteers and patients with secondary hyperparathyroidism, *J. Clin. Endocrinol. Metab.,* 1993.
42. Nemeth, E. F., Regulation of cytosolic calcium by extracellular divalent cations in C-cells and parathyroid cells, *Cell. Calcium,* 11, 323, 1990.
43. Brown, E. M., Extracellular calcium sensing, regulation of parathyroid cell function and the role of calcium and other ions as extracellular (first) messengers, *Physiol. Rev.,* 71, 371, 1991.
44. Brown, E. M., Gamba, G., Riccardi, D., Lombardi, M., Butters, R., Kifor, O., Sun, A., Hediger, M. A., Lytton, J., and Hebert, S. C., Cloning and characterization of an extracellular Ca^{2+}-sensing receptor from bovine parathyroid. *Nature,* 366, 575, 1993.
45. Pollak, M. R., Brown, E. M., Wu Chou, Y., Hebert, S. C., Marx, S. J., Steinmann, B., Levi, T., and Seldman, J. G., Mutations in the human Ca^{2+}-sensing receptor gene cause familial hypocalciuric hypercalcemia and neonatal severe hyperparathyroidism, *Cell,* 75, 1297, 1993.
46. Silver, J., Russell, J., and Sherwood, L. M., Regulation by vitamin D metabolites of messenger ribonucleic acid for preproparathyroid hormone gene transcription in vivo in the rat, *Proc. Natl. Acad. Sci. U.S.A.,* 82, 4270, 1985.
47. Russell, J., Lettieri, D., and Sherwood, L. M., Suppression by $1,25(OH)_2D_3$ of transcription of the pre-proparathyroid hormone gene, *Endocrinology,* 119, 2864, 1986.
48. Okazaki, T., Igarashi, T., and Kronenberg, H. M., $5'$-Flanking region of the parathyroid hormone gene mediates negative regulation by $1,25(OH)_2$ vitamin D_3, *J. Biol. Chem.,* 263, 2203, 1988.

49. Stewart, A. F., Horst, R., Deftos, L. J., Cadman, E. C., Lang, R., and Broadus, A. E., Biochemical evaluation of patients with cancer-associated hypercalcemia, *N. Engl. J. Med.,* 303, 1377, 1980.

50. Budayr, A. A., Nissenson, R. A., Klein, R. F., Pun, K. K., Clark, O. H., Diep, D., Arnaud, C. D., and Strewler, G. J., Increased serum levels of a parathyroid hormone-like protein in malignancy-associated hypercalcemia, *Ann. Intern. Med.,* 111, 807, 1989.

51. Burtis, W. J., Brady, T. G., Orloff, J. J., Ersbak, J. B., Warrell, R. P., Olson, B. R., Wu, T. L., Mitnick, M. E., Broadus, A. E., and Stewart, A. F., Immunochemical characterization of circulating parathyroid hormone-related peptide in patients with humoral hypercalcemia of cancer, *N. Engl. J. Med.,* 322, 1106, 1990.

52. Stewart, A. F. and Broadus, A. E., Clinical review 16: parathyroid hormone-related proteins: coming of age in the 1990s, *J. Clin. Endocrinol. Metab.,* 71, 1410, 1990.

53. Bilezikian, J. P., Parathyroid hormone-related peptide in sickness and health, *N. Engl. J. Med.,* 322, 1151, 1990.

54. Burtis, W. J., Brady, T. G., Orloff, J. J., Ersbak, J. B., Warrell, R. P., Olson, B. R., Wu, T. L., Mitnick, M. E., Broadus, A. E., and Stewart, A. F., Immunochemical characterization of circulating parathyroid hormone-related protein in patients with humoral hypercalcemia of cancer, *N. Engl. J. Med.,* 322, 1106, 1990.

55. Soifer, N. E., Dee, K. E., and Insogna, K. L., Parathyroid hormone-related protein: secretion of a novel mid-region fragment by three different cell lines in culture, *J. Biol. Chem.,* 267, 18236, 1992.

56. Goltzman, D., Hendy, G. N., and Banville, D., Parathyroid hormone-like peptide: molecular characterization and biological properties, *Trends Endocrinol. Metab.,* 20, 39, 1989.

57. Fukayama, S., Bosma, T. J., Goad, D. L., Voelkel, E. F., and Tashjian, A. H., Jr., Human parathyroid hormone (PTH)-related protein and human PTH: comparative biological activities on human bone cells and bone resorption, *Endocrinology,* 123, 2841, 1988.

58. Torres, R., DeLaPiedra, C., and Rapado, A., Effects of the (1-34) fragment of synthetic parathyroid hormone-related protein on tartrate-resistant acid phosphatase and alkaline phosphatase activities, and on osteocalcin synthesis, in cultured fetal rat calvaria, *Min. Electrolyte Metab.,* 19, 64, 1993.

59. Civitelli, R., Martin, T. J., Fausto, A., Gunsten, S. L., Hruska, K. A., and Avioli, L. V., Parathyroid hormone-related peptide transiently increases cytosolic calcium in osteoblast-like cells. Comparison with PTH, *Endocrinology,* 125, 1204, 1989.

60. Schipani, E., Karga, H., Karaplis, A. C., Potts, J. T., Jr., Kronenberg, H. M., Segre, G. V., Abou-Samra, A. B., and Jüppner, H., Identical complementary deoxyribonucleic acids encode a human renal and bone parathyroid hormone (PTH)/PTH-related peptide receptor, *Endocrinology,* 132, 2157, 1993.

61. Orloff, J. J., Reddy, D., DePapp, A. E., Yang, K. H., Soifer, N. E., and Stewart, A. F., Parathyroid hormone-related protein as a prohormone: posttranslational processing and receptor interactions, *Endocr. Rev.,* 15, 40, 1994.

62. Fenton, A. J., Kemp, B. E., Hammonds, R. G., Mitchelhill, K., Moseley, J. M., Martin, T. J., and Nicholson, G. C., A potent inhibitor of osteoclastic bone resorption within a highly conserved petapeptide region of parathyroid hormone-related protein; PTHrP[107-111], *Endocrinology,* 129, 3424, 1991.

63. Orloff, J. J., Soifer, N., Dann, P., and Burtis, W. J., Accumulation of carboxy-terminal fragments of parathyroid hormone-related protein in renal failure, *Kidney Int.,* 43, 1371, 1993.

64. Orloff, J. J., Ganz, M. B., Ribaudo, A. E., Burtis, W. J., Reiss, M., Milstone, L. M., and Stewart, A. F., Analysis of parathyroid hormone-related protein binding and signal transduction mechanisms in benign and malignant squamous cells, *Am. J. Physiol.,* 262, E599, 1992.

65. Bilezikian, J. P., Clinical utility of assays for parathyroid hormone-related protein, *Clin. Chem.,* 38, 179, 1992.

66. Weir, E. C., Brines, M. L., Ikeda, K., Burtis, W. J., Broadus, A. E., and Robbins, R. J., Parathyroid hormone-related peptide gene is expressed in the mammalian central nervous system, *Proc. Natl. Acad. Sci. U.S.A.,* 87, 108, 1990.

67. Thiede, M. A., Daifotis, A. G., Weir, E. C., Brines, M. L., Burtis, W. J., Ikeda, K., Dreyer, B. E., Gardield, R. E., and Broadus, A. E., Intrauterine occupancy controls expression of the parathyroid hormone-related peptide gene in preterm rat myometrium, *Proc. Natl. Acad. Sci. U.S.A.*, 87, 6969, 1990.

68. Hongo, T., Kupfer, J., Enomoto, H., Sharifi, B., Giannella-Neto, D., Forrester, J. S., Singer, F. R., Goltzman, D., Hendy, G. N., Pirola, C., Fagin, J. A., and Clemens, T. L., Abundant expression of parathyroid hormone-related protein in primary rat aortic smooth muscle cells accompanies serum-induced proliferation, *J. Clin. Invest.*, 88, 1841, 1991.

70. Drucker, D. J., Asa, S. L., Henderson, J., and Goltzman, D., The parathyroid hormone-like peptide gene is expressed in the normal and neoplastic human endocrine pancreas, *Mol. Endocrinol.*, 3, 1589, 1989.

71. Budayr, A. A., Halloran, B. P., King, J. C., Diep, D., Nissenson, R. A., and Strewler, G. J., High levels of parathyroid hormone-like protein in milk, *Proc. Natl. Acad. Sci. U.S.A.*, 86, 7183, 1989.

72. Deftos, L. J., Calcitonin and medullary thyroid carcinoma, in *Cecil Textbook of Medicine,* Wyngaarden, J. B., Smith, L. H., Jr., and Bennett, J. C., Eds., W. B. Saunders, Philadelphia, 1991, 1420.

73. Deftos, L. J., *Medullary Thyroid Carcinoma,* S. Karger, New York, 1983.

74. Marx, S. J., Woodward, C. J., and Aurbach, G. D., Calcitonin receptors of kidney and bone, *Science,* 178, 999, 1972.

75. Bell, N. H., Further studies on the regulation of calcitonin release in vitro, *Horm. Metab. Res.,* 7, 77, 1975.

76. Care, A. D., Bates, R. F. L., and Bruce, J. B., Stimulation of calcitonin secretion by gastrointestinal hormones, *J. Endocrinol.,* 52, 27, 1972.

77. Care, A. D., Bates, R. F. L., and Swaminathan, R., The role of gastrin as a calcitonin secretagogue, *J. Endocrinol.,* 51, 735, 1971.

78. Cooper, C. W., Schwesinger, W. H., and Ontjes, D. A., Stimulation of secretion of pig thyrocalcitonin by gastrin and related hormonal peptides, *Endocrinology,* 91, 1079, 1972.

79. Hennessy, J. F., Wells, S. A., Jr., and Ontjes, D. A., A comparison of pentagastrin injection and calcium infusion as provocative agents for the detection of medullary carcinoma of the thyroid, *J. Clin. Endocrinol. Metab.,* 39, 487, 1974.

80. Deftos, L. J., Pituitary cells secrete calcitonin in the reverse hemolytic plaque assay, *Biochem. Biophys. Res. Commun.,* 146, 1350, 1987.

81. Becker, K. L., Monaghan, K. G., and Silva, O. L., Immunocytochemical localization of calcitonin in Kulchitsky cells of human lung, *Arch. Pathol. Lab. Med.,* 104, 196, 1980.

82. Gray, R., Boyle, I., and DeLuca, H. F., Vitamin D metabolism: the role of kidney tissue, *Science,* 172, 1232, 1971.

83. Kaludn, D. N., Hadji-Georgopoulos, A., and Foster, G. V., Evidence for physiological importance of calcitonin in the regulation of plasma calcium in rats, *J. Clin. Invest.,* 55, 722, 1975.

84. Kikuchi, A., Ikeda, K., Kozawa, O., and Takai, Y., Modes of inhibitory action of protein kinase C in the chemotactic peptide-induced formation of inositol phosphates in differentiated human leukemic (HL-60) cells, *J. Biol. Chem.,* 262, 6766, 1987.

85. Singer, F. R., Habener, J. F., and Greene, E., Inactivation of calcitonin by specific organs, *Nature,* 237, 269, 1972.

86. Deftos, L. J., and Roos, B., Medullar thyroid carcinoma and calcitonin gene expression, in *Bone and Mineral Research,* Peck, W. A., Ed., Excerpta Medica, Amsterdam, 1989, 267.

87. Reginster, J. Y., Deroisy, R., Albert, A., Denis, D., Lecart, M. P., Collette, J., and Franchimont, P., Relationship between whole plasma calcitonin levels, calcitonin secretory capacity, and plasma levels of estrone in healthy women and postmenopausal osteoporotics, *J. Clin. Invest.,* 83, 1073, 1989.

88. Deftos, L. J., Weisman, M. H., Williams, G. H., Karpf, D. B., Frumar, A. M., Davidson, B. H., Parthemore, J. G., and Judd, H. L., Influence of age and sex on plasma calcitonin in human beings, *N. Engl. J. Med.,* 302, 1351, 1980.

89. Tiegs, R. D., Body, J., Barta, J. M., and Heath, H., III, Secretion and metabolism of monomeric human calcitonin: effects of age, sex, and thyroid damage, *J. Bone Min. Res.,* 1, 339, 1986.

90. Foresta, C., Scanelli, G., Zanatta, G. P., Busnardo, B., and Scandellari, X., Reduced calcitonin reserve in young hypogonadic osteoporotic men, *Horm. Metab. Res.,* 19, 275, 1987.

91. Tashjian, A. H., Jr., Calcitonin 1976: a review of some recent advances, in *Proc. 5th Int. Congr. Endocrinology,* James, V. H. T., Ed., Excerpta Medica, Amsterdam, 1976, 256.

92. Ivey, J. J., Roos, B. A., Shen, F. H., and Baylink, D. J., Increased immunoreactive calcitonin in idiopathic hypercalciuria, *Metab. Bone Dis. Relat. Res.,* 3, 29, 1981.

93. Taggart, H. M., Ivey, J. J., Sisom, K., Chesnut, C. H., III, Baylink, D. J., and Huber, M. B., Deficient calcitonin response to calcium stimulation in postmenopausal osteoporosis, *Lancet,* 1, 475, 1982.

94. Carter, W. B. and Heath, H., III, Clinically useful calcitonin assays, *Trends Endocrinol. Metab.,* 1, 288, 1990.

95. Elders, M. J., Winfield, B. S., and McNatt, M. L., Glucocorticoid therapy in children, *Am. J. Dis. Child.,* 129, 1393, 1975.

96. Tiegs, R. D., Body, J. J., Wahner, H. W., Barta, J., Riggs, B. L., and Heath, H., III, Calcitonin secretion in postmenopausal osteoporosis, *N. Engl. J. Med.,* 312, 1097, 1985.

97. LoCascio, V., Adami, S., Avioli, L. V., Cominacini, L., Galvanni, G., and Gennari, C., Suppressive effect of chronic glucocorticoid treatment on circulating calcitonin in man, *Calcif. Tissue Int.,* 34, 309, 1982.

98. Murphy, W. A., Whyte, M. P., and Haddad, J. G., Jr., Paget bone disease: radiologic documentation of healing with human calcitonin therapy, *Radiology,* 136, 1, 1980.

99. Avioli, L. V., Calcitonin therapy in osteoporotic syndromes, *South. Med. J.,* 85, 17, 1992.

100. MacIntyre, I., The calcitonin family of peptides, *Ann. N.Y. Acad. Sci.,* 657, 117, 1992.

101. Amara, S. G., Arriza, J. L., Leff, S. E., Swanson, L. W., Evans, R. M., and Rosenfeld, M. G., Expression in brain of a messenger RNA encoding a novel neuropeptide homologous to calcitonin gene-related peptide, *Science,* 229, 1094, 1985.

102. Petermann, J. B., Born, W., Chang, J., and Fischer, J. A., Identification in the human central nervous system, pituitary, and the thyroid of a novel calcitonin gene-related peptide, and partial amino acid sequence in the spinal cord, *J. Biol. Chem.,* 262, 542, 1987.

103. Wimalawansa, S. J., Morris, H. R., and MacIntyre, I., Both α and β calcitonin gene-related peptides are present in plasma, cerebrospinal fluid and spinal cord in man, *Mol. Endocrinol.,* 3, 247, 1990.

104. Lu, B., Fu, W. M., Greengard, P., and Poo, M. M., Calcitonin gene-related peptide potentiates synaptic responses at developing neuromuscular junction, *Nature,* 363, 76, 1993.

105. Brain, S. D., Williams, T. J., Tippins, J. R., Morris, J. R., and MacIntyre, I., Calcitonin gene-related peptide is a potent vasodilator, *Nature,* 313, 54, 1985.

106. Emeson, R. B., Hedjran, F., Yeakley, J. M., Guise, J. W., and Rosenfeld, M. G., Alternative production of calcitonin and CGRP mRNA is regulated at the calcitonin-specific splice acceptor, *Nature,* 341, 76, 1989.

107. Ramana, C. V., DiPette, D. J., and Supowit, S. C., Localization and characterization of calcitonin gene-related peptide mRNA in rat heart, *Am. J. Med. Sci.,* 304, 339, 1992.

108. Kawai, Y., Takami, K., Shiosaka, S., Emson, P. C., Hillyard, C. J., Girgis, S. I., MacIntyre, I., and Tohyama, M., Topographic localization of calcitonin gene-related peptide in rat brain, *Neuroscience,* 15, 747, 1985.

109. Struthers, A. D., Brown, M. J., MacDonald, D. W. R., Beacham, J. L., Stevenson, J. C., Morris, H. R., and MacIntyre, I., Human calcitonin gene related peptide: a potent endogenous vasodilator in man, *Clin. Sci.,* 70, 389, 1986.

110. Bunker, C. B., Reavley, C., O'Shaughnessy, D. J., and Dowd, P. M., Calcitonin gene-related peptide in treatment of severe peripheral vascular insufficiency in Raynaud's phenomenon, *Lancet,* 342, 80, 1993.

111. Bunker, C. B., Terenghi, G., Springall, D. R., Polak, J. M., and Dowd, P. M., Deficiency of calcitonin gene-related peptide in Raynaud's phenomenon, *Lancet,* 336, 1530, 1990.

112. Hirata, Y., Takagi, Y., Takata, S., Fukuda, Y., Yoshimi, H., and Fujita, T., Calcitonin gene-related peptide receptor in cultured vascular smooth muscle and endothelial cells, *Biochem. Biophys. Res. Commun.,* 151, 1113, 1988.

113. Bukoski, R. D. and Kremer, D., Calcium-regulating hormones in hypertension: vascular actions, *Am. J. Clin. Nutr.,* 54, 220S, 1991.
114. DePette, D. J., Schwarzenberger, K., Kerr, N., and Holland, O. B., Dose-dependent systemic and regional hemodynamic effects of calcitonin gene-related peptide, *Am. J. Med. Sci.,* 297, 65, 1989.
115. Goltzman, D., Interactions of calcitonin and calcitonin gene-related peptide at receptor sites in target tissues, *Science,* 227, 1343, 1985.
116. Yamaguchi, A., Chiba, T., Okimura, Y., Yamatani, T., Morishita, T., Nakamura, A., Inui, T., Noda, T., and Fujita, T., Receptors for calcitonin gene-related peptide on the rat liver plasma membranes, *Biochem. Biophys. Res. Commun.,* 152, 376, 1988.
117. Krahn, D. D., Gosnell, B. A., Levine, A. S., and Morley, J. E., Effects of calcitonin gene-related peptide on feeding in the rat, *Peptides,* 5, 861, 1984.
118. Nong, Y. H., Titus, R. G., Ribeiro, J. M. C., and Remold, H. G., Peptides encoded by the calcitonin gene inhibit macrophage's function, *J. Immunol.,* 143, 45, 1989.
119. Lenz, H. J., Rivier, J. E., and Brown, M. R., Biological actions of human and rat calcitonin and calcitonin gene-related peptide, *Reg. Peptides,* 12, 81, 1985.
120. Laufer, R. and Changeux, J. P., Calcitonin gene-related peptide elevates cyclic AMP levels in chick skeletal muscle: possible neurotrophic role for a coexisting neuronal messenger, *EMBO J.,* 6, 901, 1987.
121. Webb, A. R. and Holick, M. F., The role of sunlight in the cutaneous production of vitamin D3, *Annu. Rev. Nutr.,* 8, 375, 1988.
122. Chesney, R. W., Metabolic bone disease, *Pediatr. Rev.,* 5, 227, 1984.
123. Reichel, H., Koeffler, P., and Norman, A. W., The role of the vitamin D endocrine system in health and disease, *N. Engl. J. Med.,* 320, 980, 1989.
124. Walters, M. R., Newly identified actions of the vitamin D endocrine system, *Endocr. Rev.,* 13, 719, 1992.
125. DeLuca, H. F., The vitamin D system in the regulation of calcium and phosphorus metabolism. W. O. Atwater memorial lecture, *Nutr. Rev.,* 37, 161, 1979.
126. Bijvoet, O. L. M., VanderSluysVeer, J., and DeVries, H. R., Natriuretic effect of calcitonin in man, *N. Engl. J. Med.,* 284, 681, 1971.
127. Haddad, J. G., Jr. and Rojanasathit, S., Acute administration of 25-hydroxycholecalciferol in man, *J. Clin. Endocrinol. Metab.,* 42, 284, 1976.
128. Haddad, J. G., Jr., and Chyu, K. J., Competitive protein-binding radioassay for 25-hydroxycholecalciferol, *J. Clin. Endocrinol. Metab.,* 33, 992, 1971.
129. Imawari, M., Kida, K., and Goodman, D. S., The transport of vitamin D and its 25-hydroxy metabolite in human plasma, *J. Clin. Invest.,* 58, 514, 1976.
130. Avioli, L. V. and Haddad, J. G., Jr., Vitamin D: current concepts, *Metabolism,* 22, 507, 1973.
131. Horsting, M. and DeLuca, H. F., In vitro production of 25-hydroxycholecalciferol, *Biochem. Biophys. Res. Commun.,* 36, 251, 1969.
132. Olson, E. B., Jr., Knutson, J. C., and Bhattacharyya, M. H., The effect of hepatectomy on the synthesis of 25-hydroxyvitamin D_3, *J. Clin. Invest.,* 57, 1213, 1976.
133. Baxter, L. A. and DeLuca, H. F., Stimulation of 25-hydroxyvitamin D_3-1α-hydroxylase by phosphate depletion, *J. Biol. Chem.,* 254, 3158, 1976.
134. Preece, M. A., Tomlinson, S., and Ribot, C. A., Studies of vitamin D deficiency in man, *Q. J. Med.,* 44, 575, 1975.
135. McLaughlin, M., Fairney, A., and Lester, E., Seasonal variations in serum 25-hydroxycholecalciferol in healthy people, *Lancet,* 1, 536, 1974.
136. Dent, C. E. and Gupta, M. M., Plasma 25-hydroxyvitamin D levels during pregnancy in Caucasians and in vegetarian and nonvegetarian Asians, *Lancet,* 2, 1057, 1975.
137. Wezeman, F. H., 25-Hydroxyvitamin D_3: autoradiographic evidence of sites of action in epiphyseal cartilage and bone, *Lancet,* 2, 1069, 1976.
138. Raisz, L. G., Trummel, C. L., and Simmons, H., Induction of bone resorption in tissue culture: prolonged response after brief exposure to parathyroid hormone on 25-hydroxycholecalciferol, *Endocrinology,* 90, 744, 1972.
139. Raisz, L. G., Trummel, C. L., and Holick, M. F., 1,25-Dihydroxycholecalciferol: a potent stimulator of bone resorption in tissue culture, *Science,* 175, 768, 1972.

140. Popovtzer, M. M., Robinette, J. B., and DeLuca, H. F., The acute effect of 25-hydroxy-cholecalciferol on renal handling of phosphorus, *J. Clin. Invest.*, 53, 913, 1974.

141. Puschett, J. B., Fernandez, P. C., and Boyle, I. T., The acute tubular effects of 1,25-dihydroxy-cholecalciferol, *Proc. Soc. Exp. Biol. Med.*, 51, 373, 1972.

142. Bikle, D. D., Murphy, E. W., and Rasmussen, H., The ionic control of 1,25-dihydroxyvitamin D_3 synthesis in isolated chick renal mitochondria, *J. Clin. Invest.*, 55, 299, 1975.

143. Bikle, D. D. and Rasmussen, H., The metabolism of 25-hydroxycholecalciferol by isolated renal tubules in vitro as studied by new chromatographic technique, *Biochim. Biophys. Acta*, 362, 425, 1974.

144. Bikle, D. D. and Rasmussen, H., The ionic control of 1,25-dihydroxyvitamin D_3 production in isolated chick renal tubules, *J. Clin. Invest.*, 55, 292, 1975.

145. DiBella, F. P., Dousa, T. P., and Miller, S. S., Parathyroid hormone receptors of renal cortex: specific binding of biologically active ^{125}I-labeled hormone and relationship to adenylate cyclase activation, *Proc. Natl. Acad. Sci. U.S.A.*, 71, 723, 1974.

146. Fournier, A. E., Johnson, W. J., and Taves, D. R., Etiology of hyperparathyroidism and bone disease during chronic hemodialysis. I. Association of bone disease with potentially etiologic factors, *J. Clin. Invest.*, 50, 592, 1971.

147. Portale, A. A., Halloran, B. P., and Morris, R. C., Jr., Physiologic regulation of the serum concentration of 1,25-dihydroxyvitamin D by phosphorus in normal men, *J. Clin. Invest.*, 83, 1494, 1989.

148. Kawashima, H. and Kurokawa, K., Metabolism and sites of action of vitamin D in the kidney, *Kidney Int.*, 29, 98, 1986.

149. Tanaka, Y. and DeLuca, H. F., Stimulation of the 24,25-hydroxyvitamin D_3 production of 1,25-dihydroxyvitamin D_3, *Science*, 183, 1198, 1974.

150. Taylor, C. M., Hughes, S. E., and DeSilva, P., Competitive protein binding assay for 24,25-dihydroxycholecalciferol, *Biochem. Biophys. Res. Commun.*, 70, 1243, 1976.

151. Holick, M. F. and Adams, J. S., Vitamin D metabolism and biological function, in *Metabolic Bone Disease and Clinically Related Disorders*, Avioli, L. V. and Krane, S. M., Eds., W. B. Saunders, Philadelphia, 1990, 155.

152. Klein, G. L., Horst, R. L., and Norman, A. W., Reduced serum levels of 1,25-dihydroxyvitamin D during long-term total parenteral nutrition, *Ann. Intern. Med.*, 94, 638, 1981.

153. Taylor, C. M., Mawer, E. B., and Wallace, J. E., The absence of 24,25-dihydroxycholecalciferol in anephric patients, *Clin. Sci. Mol. Med.*, 55, 541, 1978.

154. Holick, M. F., Kleiner-Bossaller, A., and Schnoes, H. K., 1,24,25-Trihydroxyvitamin D_3, *J. Biol. Chem.*, 248, 6691, 1973.

155. Peacock, M., Taylor, G. A., and Redel, J., The action of two metabolites of vitamin D_3: 25,26-dihydroxycholecalciferol and 24,25-dihydroxycholecalciferol on bone resorption, *FASEB J.*, 62, 248, 1976.

156. Lam, H., Schnoes, H. K., and DeLuca, H. F., 24,25-Dihydroxyvitamin D_3: synthesis and biological activity, *Biochemistry*, 12, 4851, 1973.

157. Eisman, J. A., Hamstra, A. J., and Kream, B. E., A sensitive, precise and convenient method for determination of 1,25-dihydroxyvitamin D in human plasma, *Arch. Biochem. Biophys.*, 176, 235, 1976.

158. Haussler, M. R., Baylink, D. J., and Hughes, M. R., The assay of 1α,25-dihydroxyvitamin D_3: physiologic and pathologic modulation of circulating hormone levels, *Clin. Endocrinol.*, 5, 151S, 1976.

159. Hughes, M. R., Baylink, D. J., and Jones, P. G., Radioligand receptor assay for 25-hydroxyvitamin D_2/D_3 and 1α,25-dihydroxyvitamin D_2/D_3: application to hypervitaminosis D, *J. Clin. Invest.*, 58, 61, 1976.

160. Bikle, D. D., Clinical counterpoint: vitamin D: new actions, new analogs, new therapeutic potential, *Endocr. Rev.*, 13, 765, 1992.

161. Norman, A. W., Nemere, I., Zhou, L., Bishop, J. E., Lowe, K. E., Maiyar, A. C., Collins, E. D., Taoka, T., Sergeev, I., and Farach-Carson, M. C., 1,25($OH)_2$-vitamin D_3, a steroid hormone that produces biologic effects via both genomic and nongenomic pathways, *J. Steroid Biochem. Mol. Biol.*, 41, 231, 1992.

162. Jüppner, H., Abou-Samra, A. B., Uneno, S., Gu, W. X., Potts, J. T., Jr., and Segre, G. V., The parathyroid hormone-like peptide associated with humoral hypercalcemia of malignancy and parathyroid hormone bind to the same receptor on the plasma membrane of ROS 17/2.8 cells, *J. Biol. Chem.,* 263, 8557, 1988.

163. Jüppner, H., Abou-Samra, A. B., Freeman, M., Kong, X. F., Schipani, E., Richards, J., Kolakowski, L. F., Jr., Hock, J. M., Potts, J. T., Jr., Kronenberg, H. M., and Segre, G. V., A G protein-linked receptor for parathyroid hormone and parathyroid hormone-related peptide, *Science,* 254, 1024, 1991.

164. Lin, H. Y., Harris, T. L., Flannery, M. R., Aruffo, A., Kaji, E. H., Gorn, A. H., Kolakowski, L. F., Jr., Lodish, H. F., and Goldring, S. R., Expression cloning of an adenylate cyclase-coupled calcitonin receptor, *Science,* 254, 1022, 1991.

165. Gorn, A. H., Lin, H. Y., Yamin, M., Auron, P. E., Flannery, M. R., Tapp, D. R., Manning, C. A., Lodish, H. F., Krane, S. M., and Goldring, S. R., Cloning, characterization, and expression of a human calcitonin receptor from an ovarian carcinoma cell line, *J. Clin. Invest.,* 90, 1726, 1992.

166. Ishihara, T., Nakamura, S., Kaziro, Y., Takahashi, T., Takahashi, K., and Nagata, S., Molecular cloning and expression of a cDNA encoding the secretin receptor, *EMBO J.,* 10, 1635, 1991.

167. Ishihara, T., Shigemoto, R., Mori, K., Takahashi, K., and Nagata, S., Functional expression and tissue distribution of a novel receptor for vasoactive intestinal polypeptide, *Neuron,* 8, 811, 1993.

168. Thorens, B., Expression cloning of the pancreatic β cell receptor for the glucoincretin hormone glucagon-like peptide, *Proc. Natl. Acad. Sci. U.S.A.,* 89, 8641, 1992.

169. Mayo, K., Molecular cloning and expression of a pituitary-specific receptor for growth hormone-releasing hormone, *Mol. Endocrinol.,* 6, 1734, 1992.

170. Chorev, M., Goodman, M. E., McKee, R. L., Roubini, E., Levy, J. J., Gay, C. T., Reagan, J. E., Fisher, J. E., Caporale, L. H., Golub, E. E., Caulfield, M. P., Nutt, R. F., and Rosenblatt, M., Modifications of position 12 in parathyroid hormone and parathyroid hormone related protein: toward the design of highly potent antagonists, *Biochemistry,* 29, 1580, 1990.

171. Demay, M., Mitchell, J., and Goltzman, D., Comparison of renal and osseous binding of parathyroid hormone and hormonal fragments, *Am. J. Physiol.,* 249, E437, 1985.

172. Orloff, J. J., Wu, T. L., Heath, H., III, Brady, T. G., Brines, M. L., and Stewart, A. F., Characterization of canine renal receptors for the parathyroid hormone-like protein associated with humoral hypercalcemia of malignancy, *J. Biol. Chem.,* 264, 6097, 1989.

173. Shigeno, C., Yamamoto, I., Kitamura, N., Noda, T., Lee, K., Sone, T., Shiomi, K., Ohtaka, A., Fuji, N., Yajima, H., and Konishi, J., Interaction of human parathyroid hormone-related peptide with parathyroid hormone receptors in clonal rat osteosarcoma cells, *J. Biol. Chem.,* 263, 18369, 1988.

174. Abou-Samra, A. B., Jüppner, H., Force, T., Freeman, M., Kong, X. F., Schipani, E., Urena, P., Richards, J., Bonventre, J. V., Potts, J. T., Jr., Kronenberg, H. M., and Segre, G. V., Expression cloning of a common receptor for parathyroid hormone and parathyroid hormone-related peptide from rat osteoblast-like cells: a single receptor stimulates intracellular accumulation of both cAMP and inositol triphosphates and increases in intracellular free calcium, *Proc. Natl. Acad. Sci. U.S.A.,* 89, 2732, 1992.

175. Chabre, O., Conklin, B. R., Lin, H. Y., Lodish, H. F., Wilson, E., Ives, H. E., Catanzariti, L., Hemmings, B. A., and Bourne, H. R., A recombinant calcitonin receptor independently stimulates 3′-5′-cyclic adenosine monophosphate and Ca^{2+}/inositol phosphate signaling pathways, *Mol. Endocrinol.,* 6, 551, 1992.

176. Löwik, C. W. G. M., van Leeuwen, J. P. T. M., van der Meer, J. M., van Zeeland, J. K., Scheven, B. A. A., and Herrmann-Erlee, M. P. M., A two-receptor model for the action of parathyroid hormone on osteoblasts: a role for intracellular free calcium and cAMP, *Cell. Calcium,* 6, 311, 1985.

177. Bringhurst, F. R., Jüppner, H., Guo, J., Urena, P., Potts, J. T., Jr., Kronenberg, H. M., Abou-Samra, A. B., and Segre, G. V., Cloned, stably expressed parathyroid hormone (PTH)/PTH-related peptide receptors activate multiple messenger signals and biological responses in LLC-PK$_1$ kidney cells, *Endocrinology,* 132, 2090, 1993.

178. Trimble, E. R., Bruzzone, R., Biden, T. J., Meechan, C. J., Andreu, D., and Merrifield, R. B., Secretin stimulates cyclic AMP and inositol triphosphate production in rat pancreatic acinar tissue by two fully independent mechanisms, *Proc. Natl. Acad. Sci. U.S.A.*, 84, 3146, 1987.

179. Rao, L. G. and Murray, T. M., Binding of intact parathyroid hormone to rat osteosarcoma cells: major contribution of binding sites for the carboxyl-terminal region of the hormone, *Endocrinology*, 117, 1632, 1985.

180. Murray, T. M., Rao, L. G., Muzaffar, S. A., and Ly, H., Human parathyroid hormone carboxyterminal peptide (53-84) stimulates alkaline phosphatase activity in dexamethasone-treated rat osteosarcoma cells in vitro, *Endocrinology*, 124, 1097, 1989.

181. Fenton, A. J., Kemp, B. E., Kent, G. N., Moseley, J. M., Zheng, M. H., Rowe, D. J., Britto, J. M., Martin, T. J., and Nicholson, G. C., A carboxyl-terminal peptide from the parathyroid hormone-related protein inhibits bone resorption by osteoclasts, *Endocrinology*, 129, 1762, 1991.

182. Fenton, A. J., Martin, T. J., and Nicholson, G. C., Long-term culture of disaggregated rat osteoclasts: inhibition of bone resorption and reduction of osteoclast-like cell number by calcitonin and PTHrP[107-139], *J. Cell Physiol.*, 155, 1, 1993.

183. Mok, L. L. S., Nickols, G. A., Thompson, J. C., and Cooper, C. W., Parathyroid hormone as smooth muscle relaxant, *Endocr. Rev.*, 10, 420, 1989.

184. Nemere, I. and Norman, A. W., Parathyroid hormone stimulates calcium transport in perfused duodena from normal chicks: comparison with the rapid (transcaltachic) effect of 1,25-dihydroxyvitamin D_3, *Endocrinology*, 119, 1406, 1986.

185. Yamamoto, I., Potts, J. T., Jr., and Segre, G. V., Circulating bovine lymphocytes contain receptors for parathyroid hormone, *J. Clin. Invest.*, 71, 404, 1983.

186. Perry, H. M., III, Chappel, J. C., and Bellorin-Font, E., Parathyroid hormone receptors in circulating human mononuclear leukocytes, *J. Biol. Chem.*, 259, 5531, 1984.

187. Atkinson, M. J., Hesch, R., Cade, C., Wadwah, M., and Perris, A. D., Parathyroid hormone stimulation of mitosis in rat thymic lymphocytes is independent of cyclic AMP, *J. Bone Min. Res.*, 2, 303, 1987.

188. Schlüter, K. D., Hellestern, H., Wingender, E., and Mayer, H., The central part of parathyroid hormone stimulates thymidine incorporation of chondrocytes, *J. Biol. Chem.*, 264, 11087, 1989.

189. Pun, K. K., Arnaud, C. D., and Nissenson, R. A., Parathyroid hormone receptors in human dermal fibroblasts: structural and functional characterization, *J. Bone Min. Res.*, 3, 453, 1988.

190. Henderson, J. E., Kremer, R., Rhim, J. S., and Goltzman, D., Identification and functional characterization of adenylate cyclase-linked receptors for parathyroid hormone-like peptides on immortalized human keratinocytes, *Endocrinology*, 130, 449, 1992.

191. Pang, P. K. T., Kaneko, T., and Harvey, S., Immunocytochemical distribution of PTH immunoreactivity in vertebrate brains, *Am. J. Physiol.*, 255, R643, 1988.

192. Löffler, F., vanCalker, D., and Hamprecht, B., Parathyrin and calcitonin stimulate cyclic AMP accumulation in cultured murine brain cells, *EMBO J.*, 1, 297, 1982.

193. Rafferty, B., Zanelli, J. M., Rosenblatt, M., and Schulster, D., Corticosteroidogenesis and adenosine 3'-5'-monophosphate production by the amino-terminal (1-34) fragment of human parathyroid hormone in rat adrenocortical cells, *Endocrinology*, 113, 1036, 1983.

194. Silve, C. M., Hradek, G. T., Jones, A. L., and Arnaud, C. D., Parathyroid hormone receptor in intact embryonic chicken bones: characterization and cellular localization, *J. Cell Biol.*, 94, 379, 1982.

195. Rouleau, M. F., Warshawsky, H., and Goltzman, D., Parathyroid hormone binding in vivo to renal, hepatic, and skeletal tissues of the rat using a radioautoradiographic approach, *Endocrinology*, 118, 919, 1986.

196. Rouleau, M. F., Mitchell, J., and Goltzman, D., In vivo distribution of parathyroid hormone receptors in bone: evidence that a predominant osseous target cell is not the mature osteoblast, *Endocrinology*, 123, 187, 1988.

197. Mitchell, J., Rouleau, M. F., and Goltzman, D., Biochemical and morphological characterization of parathyroid hormone receptor binding to the rat osteosarcoma cell line UMR-106, *Endocrinology*, 126, 2327, 1990.

198. Civitelli, R., Fujimori, A., Bernier, S., Warlow, P. M., Goltzman, D., Hruska, K. A., and Avioli, L. V., Heterogeneous [Ca^{2+}]$_i$ response to parathyroid hormone correlates with morphology and receptor distribution in osteoblastic cells, *Endocrinology*, 130, 2392, 1992.

199. Klein, P. S., Sun, T. J., Saxe, C. L., III, Kimmel, A. R., Johnson, R. L., and Devreotes, P. N., A chemoattractant receptor controls development in *Dictyostelium discoideum, Science*, 241, 1467, 1988.

200. Attwood, T. K., Eliopuolos, E. E., and Findlay, J. B. C., Multiple sequence alignment of protein families showing low sequence homology: a methodological approach to using database pattern-matching discriminators for G-protein-linked receptors, *Gene*, 98, 153, 1991.

201. Chakraborty, M., Chatterjee, D., Kellokumpu, S., Rasmussen, H., and Baron, R., Cell cycle-dependent coupling of the calcitonin receptor to different G proteins, *Science*, 251, 1078, 1991.

202. Bizzarri, C. and Civitelli, R., Activation of the Ca^{2+} message system by parathyroid hormone is dependent on the cell cycle, *Endocrinology*, 134, 133, 1994.

203. Warshawsky, H., Goltzman, D., Rouleau, M. F., and Bergeron, J. J. M., Direct in vivo demonstration by radioautography of specific binding sites for calcitonin in skeletal and renal tissues of the rat, *J. Cell Biol.*, 85, 682, 1980.

204. Heersche, J. N. M., Marcus, R., and Aurbach, G. D., Calcitonin and the formation of 3′,5′-AMP in bone and kidney, *Endocrinology*, 94, 251, 1974.

205. Nicholson, G. C., Moseley, J. M., Sexton, P. M., Mendelshon, F. A., and Martin, T. J., Abundant calcitonin receptors in isolated rat osteoclasts, *J. Clin. Invest.*, 78, 355, 1986.

206. Marx, S. J., Woodward, C. J., Aurbach, G. D., Glassman, H., and Keutmann, H. J., Renal receptors for calcitonin: binding and degradation of the hormone, *J. Biol. Chem.*, 248, 4797, 1973.

207. Forrest, S. M., Ng, K. W., Findlay, D. M., Michelangeli, V. P., Livesey, S. A., Partridge, N. C., Zajac, J. D., and Martin, T. J., Characterization of an osteoblast-like clonal cell line which responds to both parathyroid hormone and calcitonin, *Calcif. Tissue Int.*, 37, 51, 1985.

208. Ito, N., Yamazaki, H., Miyahara, T., Kozuka, H., and Sudo, H., Response of osteoblastic clonal cell line (MC3T3-E1) to eel calcitonin at a specific cell density or differentiation stage, *Calcif. Tissue Int.*, 40, 200, 1987.

209. Farley, J. R., Tarbaux, N. M., Hall, S. L., Lainkhart, T. A., and Baylink, D. J., The antibone-resorptive agent calcitonin also acts in vitro to directly increase bone formation and bone cell proliferation, *Endocrinology*, 123, 159, 1988.

210. Chausmer, A. and Stevens, M., Autoradiographic evidence for calcitonin receptors on testicular Leydig cells, *Science*, 216, 735, 1982.

211. Chausmer, A., Stuart, C., and Stevens, M., Identification of testicular cell plasma membrane receptors for calcitonin, *J. Lab. Clin. Med.*, 96, 933, 1980.

212. Silvestroni, L., Menditto, A., Frajese, G., and Ghessi, L., Identification of calcitonin receptors in human spermatozoa, *J. Clin. Endocrinol. Metab.*, 65, 742, 1987.

213. Nicholson, G. C., D'Santos, C. S., Evans, T., Moseley, J. M., Kemp, B. E., and Michelangeli, V. P., Human placental calcitonin receptors, *Biochem. J.*, 250, 877, 1988.

214. Fouchereau-Peron, M., Moukhtar, M. S., Benson, A. A., and Milhaud, G., Characterization of specific receptors for calcitonin in porcine lung, *Proc. Natl. Acad. Sci. U.S.A.*, 78, 3973, 1981.

215. Findlay, D. M., DeLuise, M., Michelangeli, V. P., Ellison, M., and Martin, T. J., Properties of a calcitonin receptor and adenylate cyclase in BEN cells, a human cancer cell line, *Cancer Res.*, 40, 1311, 1980.

216. Findlay, D. M., Michelangeli, V. P., Moseley, J. M., and Martin, T. J., Calcitonin binding and deregulation by two cultured human breast cancer cell lines (MCF7 and T47D), *J. Biochem.*, 196, 513, 1981.

217. Marx, A. J., Aurbach, G. D., Gavin, J. R., and Buell, D. W., Calcitonin receptors on cultured human lymphocytes, *J. Biol. Chem.*, 249, 6812, 1974.

218. Body, J. J., Gilbert, F., Nejai, S., Fernandez, G., Van Langendonk, A., and Borkowski, A., Calcitonin receptors on circulating normal human lymphocytes, *J. Clin. Endocrinol. Metab.*, 71, 675, 1990.

219. Fischer, J. A., Tobler, P. H., Kaufmann, M., Born, W., Henke, H., Cooper, P. E., Sagar, S. M., and Martin, J. B., Calcitonin: regional distribution of the hormone and its binding sites in the human brain and pituitary, *Proc. Natl. Acad. Sci. U.S.A.*, 78, 7801, 1981.

220. Maurer, R., Marbach, P., and Mousson, R., Salmon calcitonin binding sites in rat pituitary, *Brain Res.,* 261, 346, 1983.
221. Azria, M., *The Calcitonins. Physiology and Pharmacology,* S. Karger, Basel, 1989.
222. Zhu, G., Dudley, D. T., and Saltiel, A. R., Amylin increases cyclic AMP formation in L6 myocytes through calcitonin gene-related peptide receptors, *Biochem. Biophys. Res. Commun.,* 177, 771, 1991.
223. McDonnell, D. P., Mangelsdorf, D. J., Pike, J. W., Haussler, M. R., and O'Malley, B. W., Molecular cloning of complementary DNA encoding the avian receptor for vitamin D, *Science,* 235, 1214, 1987.
224. Baker, A. R., McDonnell, D. P., Hughes, M., Crisp, T. M., Mangelsdorf, D. J., Haussler, M. R., Pike, J. W., Shine, J., and O'Malley, B. W., Cloning and expression of full-length cDNA encoding human vitamin D receptor, *Proc. Natl. Acad. Sci. U.S.A.,* 85, 3294, 1988.
225. Burmester, J. K., Maeda, N., and DeLuca, H. F., Isolation and expression of rat 1,25-dihydroxyvitamin D_3 receptor cDNA, *Proc. Natl. Acad. Sci. U.S.A.,* 85, 1005, 1988.
226. Evans, R. M., The steroid and thyroid hormone receptor superfamily, *Science,* 240, 889, 1988.
227. Minghetti, P. P. and Norman, A. W., $1,25(OH)_2$-vitamin D_3 receptors: gene regulation and genetic circuitry, *FASEB J.,* 2, 3043, 1988.
228. Pike, J. W., Vitamin D_3 receptors: structure and function in transcription, *Annu. Rev. Nutr.,* 11, 189, 1991.
229. Nemere, I. and Norman, A. W., Steroid hormone actions at the plasma membrane: induced calcium uptake and exocytotic events, *Mol. Cell. Endocrinol.,* 80, C165, 1991.
230. Fontaine, O., Matsumoto, T., Goodman, D. B. P., and Rasmussen, H., Liponomic control of Ca^{2+} transport: relationship to mechanism of action of 1,25-dihydroxyvitamin D_3, *Proc. Natl. Acad. Sci. U.S.A.,* 78, 1751, 1981.
231. Putkey, J. A., Spieloogel, A. M., Sauerheber, R. D., Dumlap, C. S., and Norman, A. W., Vitamin D-mediated intestinal calcium transport. Effects of essential fatty acid deficiency and spin label studies of enterocyte membrane lipid fluidity, *Biochim. Biophys. Acta,* 688, 177, 1982.
232. Bikle, D. D., Whitney, J., and Munson, S., The relationship of membrane fluidity to calcium flux in chick intestinal brush border membranes, *Endocrinology,* 114, 260, 1984.
233. Brasitus, T. A., Dudeja, P. K., Eby, B., and Lau, K., Correction by 1,25-dihydroxy-cholecalciferol of the abnormal fluidity and lipid composition of enterocyte brush-border membranes in vitamin D-deprived rats, *J. Biol. Chem.,* 261, 16404, 1986.
234. Kurnik, B. R. C., Huskey, M., Hagerty, D., and Hruska, K. A., Vitamin D metabolites stimulate phosphatidylcholine transfer to renal brush-border membranes, *Biochim. Biophys. Acta,* 858, 47, 1986.
235. Caffrey, J. M. and Farach-Carson, M. C., Vitamin D_3 metabolites modulate dihydropyridine-sensitive calcium currents in clonal rat osteosarcoma cells, *J. Biol. Chem.,* 264, 20265, 1989.
236. Civitelli, R., Kim, Y. S., Gunsten, S. L., Fujimori, A., Huskey, M., Avioli, L. V., and Hruska, K. A., Nongenomic activation of the Ca^{2+} message system by vitamin D metabolites in osteoblast-like cells, *Endocrinology,* 127, 2253, 1990.
237. Baran, D. T., Sorensen, A. M., Honeyman, T. W., Ray, T. W., and Holick, M. F., $1\alpha,25$-Dihydroxyvitamin D_3-induced increments in hepatocyte cytosolic calcium and lysophosphatidylinositol: inhibition by pertussis toxin and $1\beta,25$-dihydroxyvitamin D_3, *J. Bone Min. Res.,* 5, 517, 1990.
238. Lieberher, M., Grosse, B., Duchambon, P., and Drüeke, T., A functional cell surface type receptor is required for the early action of 1,25-dihydroxyvitamin D_3 on the phosphoinositide metabolism in rat enterocytes, *J. Biol. Chem.,* 264, 20403, 1989.
239. Barsony, J. and Marx, S. J., Receptor-mediated rapid action of $1\alpha,25$-dihydroxycholecalciferol: increase of intracellular cGMP in human skin fibroblasts, *Proc. Natl. Acad. Sci. U.S.A.,* 85, 1223, 1988.
240. Matsumoto, T., Kawanobe, Y., Morita, K., and Ogata, E., Effect of 1,25-dihydroxyvitamin D_3 on phospholipid metabolism in a clonal osteoblast-like rat osteogenic sarcoma cell line, *J. Biol. Chem.,* 260, 13704, 1985.
241. Baran, D. T. and Kelly, A. M., Lysophosphatidylinositol: a potential mediator of 1,25-dihydroxyvitamin D-induced increments in hepatocyte cytosolic calcium, *Endocrinology,* 122, 930, 1988.

242. Baran, D. T., Sorensen, A. M., and Honeyman, T. W., Rapid actions of 1,25-dihydroxyvitamin D$_3$ on hepatocyte phospholipids, *J. Bone Min. Res.*, 3, 593, 1988.

243. Tang, W., Ziboh, V. A., Rivakah Isseroff, R., and Martinez, D., Novel regulatory actions of 1α,25-dihydroxyvitamin D$_3$ on the metabolism of polyphosphoinositides in murine epidermal keratinocytes, *J. Cell. Physiol.*, 132, 131, 1987.

244. Wali, R. K., Baum, C. L., Sitrin, M. D., and Brasitus, T. A., 1,25(OH)$_2$ vitamin D$_3$ stimulates membrane phosphoinositide turnover, activates protein kinase C, and increases cytosolic calcium in rat colonic epithelium, *J. Clin. Invest.*, 85, 1296, 1990.

245. Berridge, M. J., Inositol triphosphate and calcium signalling, *Nature*, 361, 315, 1993.

246. Rosenblatt, M., Goltzman, D., Keutmann, H. T., Tregear, G. W., and Potts, J. T., Jr., Chemical and biological properties of synthetic, sulfur-free analogues of parathyroid hormone, *J. Biol. Chem.*, 251, 159, 1976.

247. Potter, R. L., Tregear, G. W., Keutmann, H. T., Niall, H. D., Sauer, R., Deftos, L. J., Dawson, B. F., Hogan, M. L., and Aurbach, G. D., Synthesis of a biologically active N-terminal tetratriacontapeptide of parathyroid hormone, *Proc. Natl. Acad. Sci. U.S.A.*, 68, 63, 1971.

248. Goltzman, D., Peytremann, A., Callahan, E. A., Tregear, G. W., and Potts, J. T., Jr., Analysis of the requirements of parathyroid hormone action on renal membranes with the use of inhibiting analogues, *J. Biol. Chem.*, 250, 3199, 1975.

249. Tregear, G. W., Rietschoten, J. V., Greene, E., Keutmann, H. T., Niall, H. D., Reit, B., Parsons, J. A., and Potts, J. T., Jr., Bovine parathyroid hormone: minimum chain length of synthetic peptide required for biological activity, *Endocrinology*, 93, 1349, 1973.

250. Klein, D. C. and Raisz, L. G., Role of adenosine-3',5'-monophosphate in the hormonal regulation of bone resorption: studies with cultured fetal bone, *Endocrinology*, 89, 818, 1971.

251. Dziak, R. and Stern, P. H., Responses of fetal rat bone cells and bone organ cultures to the ionophore, A23187, *Calcif. Tissue Res.*, 22, 137, 1976.

252. Lorenzo, J. A. and Raisz, L. G., Divalent cation ionophores stimulate resorption and inhibit DNA synthesis in cultured fetal rat limb bone, *Science*, 212, 1157, 1981.

253. Herrmann-Erlee, M. P. M., Nijweide, P. J., van der Meer, J. M., and Ooms, M. A. C., Action of bPTH and bPTH fragments on embryonic bone in vitro: dissociation of the cyclic AMP and bone resorbing response, *Calcif. Tissue Int.*, 35, 70, 1983.

254. Horiuchi, N., Rosenblatt, M., Keutmann, H. T., Potts, J. T., Jr., and Holick, M. F., A multiresponse parathyroid hormone assay: an inhibitor has agonist properties in vivo, *Am. J. Physiol.*, 244, E589, 1983.

255. Cole, J. A., Forte, L. R., Eber, S. L., Thorne, P. K., and Poelling, R. E., Regulation of sodium-dependent phosphate transport by parathyroid hormone in opossum kidney cells: adenosine 3',5'-monophosphate-dependent and -independent mechanisms, *Endocrinology*, 122, 2981, 1988.

256. Cole, J. A., Carnes, D. L., Forte, L. R., Eber, S. L., Poelling, R. E., and Thorne, P. K., Structure-activity relationship of parathyroid hormone analogs in the opossum kidney cell line, *J. Bone Min. Res.*, 4, 723, 1989.

257. Hruska, K. A., Goligorsky, M., Scoble, J., Tsutsumi, M., Westbrook, S. L., and Moskowitz, D., Effects of parathyroid hormone on cytosolic calcium in renal proximal tubular primary cultures, *Am. J. Physiol.*, 251, F188, 1988.

258. Reid, I. R., Civitelli, R., Halstead, L. R., Avioli, L. V., and Hruska, K. A., Parathyroid hormone acutely elevates intracellular calcium in osteoblast-like cells, *Am. J. Physiol.*, 253, E45, 1987.

259. Yamaguchi, D. T., Hahn, T. J., Iida-Klein, A., Kleeman, C. R., and Muallem, S., Parathyroid hormone activated calcium channels in an osteoblast-like osteosarcoma cell line: cAMP-dependent and -independent calcium channels, *J. Biol. Chem.*, 262, 7711, 1987.

260. Donahue, H. J., Fryer, M. J., Eriksen, E. F., and Heath, H., III, Differential effects of parathyroid hormone and its analogues on cytosolic calcium ion and cAMP levels in cultured rat osteoblast-like cells, *J. Biol. Chem.*, 263, 13522, 1988.

261. Lieberherr, M., Effects of vitamin D$_3$ metabolites on cytosolic free calcium in confluent mouse osteoblasts, *J. Biol. Chem.*, 262, 13168, 1987.

262. Hruska, K. A., Moskowitz, D., Esbrit, P., Civitelli, R., Westbrook, S. L., and Huskey, M., Stimulation of inositol triphosphate and diacylglycerol production in renal tubular cells by parathyroid hormone, *J. Clin. Invest.*, 79, 230, 1987.

263. Civitelli, R., Reid, I. R., Westbrook, S. L., Avioli, L. V., and Hruska, K. A., Parathyroid hormone elevates inositol polyphosphates and diacylglycerol in a rat osteoblast-like cell line, *Am. J. Physiol.*, 255, E660, 1988.

264. Farndale, R. W., Sandy, J. R., Atkinson, S. J., Pennington, S. R., Meghi, S., and Meikle, M. C., Parathyroid hormone and prostaglandin E_2 stimulate both inositol phosphates and cyclic AMP accumulation in mouse osteoblast cultures, *Biochem. J.*, 252, 263, 1988.

265. Iida-Klein, A., Yee, D. C., Brandli, D. W., Mirikitani, E. J. M., and Hahn, T. J., Effects of calcitonin on 3',5'-cyclic adenosine monophosphate and calcium second messenger generation and osteoblast function in UMR 106-06 osteoblast-like cells, *Endocrinology*, 130, 381, 1992.

266. Cosman, F., Morrow, B., Kopal, M., and Bilezikian, J. P., Stimulation of inositol phosphate formation in ROS 17/2.8 cell membranes by guanine nucleotide, calcium, and parathyroid hormone, *J. Bone Min. Res.*, 4, 413, 1989.

267. Partridge, N. C., Kemp, B. E., Veroni, M. C., and Martin, T. J., Activation of adenosine 3',5'-monophosphate-dependent protein kinase in normal and malignant bone cells by parathyroid hormone, prostaglandin E_2, and prostacyclin, *Endocrinology*, 108, 220, 1981.

268. Livesey, S. A., Kemp, B. E., Re, C. A., Partridge, N. C., and Martin, T. J., Selective hormonal activation of cyclic-AMP-dependent protein kinase isoenzymes in normal and malignant osteoblasts, *J. Biol. Chem.*, 257, 14983, 1982.

269. Fujimori, A., Cheng, S., Avioli, L. V., and Civitelli, R., Structure-function relationship of parathyroid hormone: activation of phospholipase C, protein kinase A and C in osteosarcoma cells, *Endocrinology*, 130, 29, 1992.

270. Iida-Klein, A., Varlotta, V., and Hahn, T. J., Protein kinase C activity in UMR-106-01 cells: effects of parathyroid hormone and insulin, *J. Bone Min. Res.*, 4, 767, 1989.

271. Abou-Samra, A. B., Jüppner, H., Westerberg, D., Potts, J. T., Jr., and Segre, G. V., Parathyroid hormone causes translocation of protein kinase-C from cytosol to membranes in rat osteosarcoma cells, *Endocrinology*, 124, 1107, 1989.

272. Jouishomme, H., Whitfield, J. F., Chakravarthy, B. R., Durkin, J. P., Gagnon, L., Isaac, R. J., MacLean, S., Neugebauer, W., Willick, G., and Rixon, R. H., The protein kinase-C activation domain of the parathyroid hormone, *Endocrinology*, 130, 53, 1992.

273. Rodan, S. B., Noda, M., Wesolowski, G., Rosenblatt, M., and Rodan, G. A., Comparison of postreceptor effects of 1-34 human hypercalcemia factor and 1-34 human parathyroid hormone in rat osteosarcoma cells, *J. Clin. Invest.*, 81, 924, 1988.

274. Fukayama, S., Bosma, T. J., Goad, D. L., Voelkel, E. F., and Tashjian, H., Jr., Human parathyroid hormone (PTH)-related protein and human PTH: comparative biological activities on human bone cells and bone resorption, *Endocrinology*, 123, 2841, 1988.

275. Nissenson, R. A., Diep, D., and Strewler, G. J., Synthetic peptides comprising the amino-terminal sequence of a parathyroid hormone-like protein from human malignancies. Binding to parathyroid hormone receptors and activation of adenylate cyclase in bone cells and kidney, *J. Biol. Chem.*, 263, 12866, 1988.

276. Hepler, J. R. and Gilman, A. G., G proteins, *Trends Cell Biol.*, 17, 383, 1992.

277. Ransjö, M. and Lerner, U., Effects of cholera toxin on cyclic AMP accumulation and bone resorption in cultured mouse calvaria, *Biochim. Biophys. Acta*, 930, 4177, 1987.

278. McKee, R. L., Caulfield, M. P., and Rosenblatt, M., Treatment of bone-derived ROS 17/2.8 cells with dexamethasone and pertussis toxin enables detection of partial agonist activity for parathyroid hormone antagonists, *Endocrinology*, 127, 76, 1990.

279. Rizzoli, R. and Bonjour, J. P., Effect of pertussis toxin on parathyroid hormone-stimulated cyclic AMP production in cultured kidney cells, *J. Bone Min. Res.*, 3, 605, 1988.

280. Babich, M., King, K. L., and Nissenson, R. A., G protein-dependent activation of a phosphoinositide-specific phospholipase C in UMR-106 osteosarcoma cell membranes, *J. Bone Min. Res.*, 4, 549, 1989.

281. Rosenblatt, M., Callahan, E. A., Mahaffey, J. E., Port, A., and Potts, J. T., Jr., Parathyroid hormone inhibitors. Design, synthesis and biologic evaluation of hormone analogues, *J. Biol. Chem.*, 252, 5847, 1977.

282. Fujimori, A., Cheng, S., Avioli, L. V., and Civitelli, R., Dissociation of second messenger activation by parathyroid hormone fragments in osteosarcoma cells, *Endocrinology*, 128, 3032, 1991.

283. Partridge, N. C., Opie, A. N., Opie, R. T., and Martin, T. J., Inhibitory effects of parathyroid hormone on growth of osteogenic sarcoma cells, *Calcif. Tissue Int.*, 37, 519, 1985.

284. Reid, I. R., Civitelli, R., Avioli, L. V., and Hruska, K. A., Parathyroid hormone depresses cytosolic pH and DNA synthesis in osteoblast-like cells, *Am. J. Physiol.*, 255, E9, 1988.

285. Herrmann-Erlee, M. P. M., van der Meer, J. M., Löwik, C. W. G. M., van Leeuwen, J. P. T. M., and Bonnekamp, P. M., Different roles for calcium and cyclic AMP in the action of PTH: studies in bone explants and isolated bone cells, *Bone*, 9, 93, 1988.

286. Mallette, L. E., The parathyroid hormone polyhormones: new concepts in the spectrum of peptide hormone action, *Endocr. Rev.*, 12, 110, 1991.

287. Civitelli, R., Bacskai, B. J., Mahaut-Smith, M. P., Adams, S. R., Avioli, L. V., and Tsien, R. Y., Single-cell analysis of cyclic AMP response to parathyroid hormone in osteoblastic cells, *J. Bone Min. Res.*, 9, (in press), 1994.

288. Marx, S. J., Woodward, C. J., and Aurbach, G. D., Calcitonin receptors in kidney and bone, *Science*, 178, 998, 1972.

289. Rizzo, A. J. and Goltzman, D., Calcitonin receptors in the central nervous system of the rat, *Endocrinology*, 108, 1672, 1981.

290. Twery, M. J., Seitz, P. K., Nickols, G. A., Cooper, C. W., Gallagher, J. P., and Orlowski, R. C., Analogue separates biological effects of salmon calcitonin on brain and renal cortical membranes, *Eur. J. Pharmacol.*, 155, 285, 1988.

291. Kawashima, H., Torikai, S., and Kurokawa, K., Calcitonin selectively stimulates 25-hydroxyvitamin D_3-1α-hydroxylase in proximal straight tubule of rat kidney, *Nature*, 301, 337, 1981.

292. Murphy, E., Chamberlin, M. E., and Mandel, L. J., Effects of calcitonin on cytosolic Ca^{2+} in a suspension of rabbit medullary thick ascending limb tubules, *Am. J. Physiol.*, 251, C491, 1986.

293. Zaidi, M., Datta, H. K., Moonga, B. S., and McIntyre, I., Evidence that the action of calcitonin on rat osteoclasts is mediated by two G proteins acting via separate post-receptor pathways, *J. Endocrinol.*, 126, 473, 1990.

294. Moonga, B. S., Towhidul Alam, A. S. M., Bevis, P. J. R., Avaldi, F., Soncini, R., Huang, C. L., and Zaidi, M., Regulation of cytosolic free calcium in isolated rat osteoclasts by calcitonin, *J. Endocrinol.*, 132, 241, 1992.

295. Malgaroli, A., Meldolesi, J., Zambonin-Zallone, A., and Teti, A., Control of cytosolic free calcium in rat and chicken osteoclasts, *J. Biol. Chem.*, 264, 14342, 1989.

296. Miyauchi, A., Hruska, K. A., Greenfield, E. M., Duncan, R. L., Alvarez, J. I., Barattolo, R., Colucci, S., Zambonin-Zallone, A., Teitelbaum, S. L., and Teti, A., Osteoclast cytosolic calcium, regulated by voltage-gated calcium channels and extracellular calcium, controls podosome assembly and bone resorption, *J. Cell Biol.*, 111, 2543, 1990.

297. Yoon, K., Rutledge, S. C., Buenaga, R. F., and Rodan, G. A., Characterization of the rat osteocalcin gene: stimulation of promoter activity by 1,25-dihydroxyvitamin D_3, *Biochemistry*, 27, 8521, 1988.

298. Demay, M. B., Roth, D. A., and Kronenberg, H. M., Regions of the rat osteocalcin gene which mediate the effect of 1,25-dihydroxyvitamin D_3 on gene transcription, *J. Biol. Chem.*, 264, 2279, 1989.

299. Morrison, N. A., Shine, J., Fragonas, J. C., Verkest, V., McMenemy, M. L., and Eisman, J. A., 1,25-Dihydroxyvitamin D-responsive element and glucocorticoid repression in the osteocalcin gene, *Science*, 246, 1158, 1989.

300. Ozono, K., Liao, J., Scott, R. A., Kerner, S. A., and Pike, J. W., The vitamin D response element in the human osteocalcin gene: association with a nuclear proto-oncogene enhancer, *J. Biol. Chem.*, 265, 21881, 1990.

301. Nemere, I., Yoshimoto, Y., and Norman, A. W., Calcium transport in perfused duodena from normal chicks: enhancement within 14 minutes of exposure to 1,25-dihydroxyvitamin D_3, *Endocrinology*, 115, 1476, 1984.

302. Nemere, I. and Szego, C. M., Early actions of parathyroid hormone and 1,25-dihydroxycholecalciferol on isolated epithelial cells from rat intestine. I. Limited lysosomal enzyme release and calcium uptake, *Endocrinology*, 108, 1450, 1981.

303. De Boland, A. R. and Boland, R. L., Rapid changes in skeletal muscle calcium uptake induced in vitro by 1,25-dihydroxyvitamin D₃ are suppressed by calcium channel blockers, *Endocrinology*, 120, 1858, 1987.

304. Oshima, J., Watanabe, M., Hirosumi, J., and Orimo, H., 1,25(OH)₂D₃ increases cytosolic Ca²⁺ concentration of osteoblastic cells, clone MC3T3-E1, *Biochem. Biophys. Res. Commun.*, 145, 956, 1987.

305. Baran, D. T. and Milne, M. L., 1,25-Dihydroxyvitamin D increases hepatocyte cytosolic calcium levels: a potential regulator of vitamin D-25-hydroxylase, *J. Clin. Invest.*, 77, 1622, 1986.

306. Sugimoto, T., Ritter, C., Reid, I. R., Morrissey, J., and Slatopolsky, E., Effect of 1,25-dihydroxyvitamin D₃ on cytosolic calcium in dispersed parathyroid cells, *Kidney Int.*, 33, 850, 1988.

307. Vesely, D. L. and Juan, D., Cation-dependent vitamin D activation of human renal cortical guanylate cyclase, *Am. J. Physiol.*, 246, E115, 1984.

308. De Boland, A. R. and Norman, A. W., Evidence for involvement of protein kinase C and cyclic adenosine 3′,5′ monophosphate-dependent protein kinase in the 1,25-dihydroxy-vitamin D₃-mediated rapid stimulation of intestinal calcium transport, *Endocrinology*, 127, 39, 1990.

309. Kubota, M., Ng, K. W., and Martin, T. J., Effect of 1,25-dihydroxyvitamin D₃ on cyclic AMP responses to hormones in clonal osteogenic sarcoma cells, *Biochem. J.*, 231, 11, 1985.

310. Rodan, G. A. and Martin, T. J., Role of osteoblasts in hormonal control of bone resorption — a hypothesis, *Calcif. Tissue Int.*, 33, 349, 1981.

311. McSheehy, P. M. J. and Chambers, T. J., Osteoblastic cells mediate osteoblastic responsiveness to parathyroid hormone, *Endocrinology*, 118, 824, 1986.

312. McSheehy, P. M. J. and Chambers, T. J., Osteoblast-like cells in the presence of parathyroid hormone release soluble factor that stimulates osteoclastic bone resorption, *Endocrinology*, 119, 1654, 1986.

313. McSheehy, P. M. J. and Chambers, T. J., 1,25-Dihydroxyvitamin D₃ stimulates rat osteoblastic cells to release a soluble factor that increases osteoclastic bone resorption, *J. Clin. Invest.*, 80, 425, 1987.

314. Chambers, T. J., McSheehy, P. M. J., Thomson, B. M., and Fuller, K., The effect of calcium-regulating hormones and prostaglandins on bone resorption by osteoclasts disaggregated from neonatal rabbit bones, *Endocrinology*, 116, 234, 1985.

315. Thomson, B. M., Saklatvala, J., and Chambers, T. J., Osteoblasts mediate interleukin 1 stimulation of bone resorption by rat osteoclasts, *J. Exp. Med.*, 164, 104, 1986.

316. Perry, H. M., III, Skogen, W., Chappel, J. C., Kahn, A. J., Wilner, G., and Teitelbaum, S. L., Partial characterization of a parathyroid hormone-stimulated resorption factor(s) from osteoblast-like cells, *Endocrinology*, 125, 2075, 1989.

317. Morris, C. A., Mitnick, M. E., Weir, E. C., Horowitz, M., Kreider, B. L., and Insogna, K. L., The parathyroid hormone-related protein stimulates human osteoblast-like cells to secrete a 9,000 dalton bone-resorbing protein, *Endocrinology*, 126, 1783, 1990.

318. Civitelli, R., Beyer, E. C., Warlow, P. M., Robertson, A. J., Geist, S. T., and Steinberg, T. H., Connexin43 mediates direct intercellular communication in human osteoblastic cell networks, *J. Clin. Invest.*, 91, 1888, 1993.

319. Schiller, P. C., Mehta, P. P., Roos, B. A., and Howard, G. A., Hormonal regulation of intercellular communication: parathyroid hormone increases connexin43 gene expression and gap-junctional communication in osteoblastic cells, *Mol. Endocrinol.*, 6, 1433, 1992.

320. Tam, C. S., Heersche, J. N. M., Murray, T. M., and Parsons, J. A., Parathyroid hormone stimulates the bone apposition rate independently of its resorptive action: differential effects of intermittent and continuous administration, *Endocrinology*, 110, 506, 1982.

321. Gunness-Hey, M. and Hock, M. M., Increased trabecular bone mass in rats treated with human synthetic parathyroid hormone, *Metab. Bone Dis. Relat. Res.*, 5, 177, 1984.

322. Reeve, J., Meunier, P. J., Parsons, J. A., Bernat, M. Bijvoet, O. L. M., Courpron, P., Edouard, C., Klenerman, L., Neer, R. M., Renier, J. C., Slovick, D. M., Vismans, F. J. F. E., and Potts, J. T., Jr., Anabolic effect of human parathyroid hormone fragment on trabecular bone in involutional osteoporosis: a multicentre trial, *Br. Med. J.*, 280, 1340, 1980.

323. Slovick, D. M., Rosenthal, D. I., Doppelt, S. H., Potts, J. T., Jr., Daly, M. A., Campbell, J. A., and Neer, R. M., Restoration of spinal bone in osteoporotic men by treatment with human parathyroid hormone (1-34) and 1,25-dihydroxyvitamin D, *J. Bone Min. Res.*, 1, 377, 1986.

324. Hodsman, A. B., Steer, B. M., Fraher, L. J., and Drost, D. J., Bone densitometric and histomorphometric responses to sequential human parathyroid hormone (1-38) and salmon calcitonin in osteoporotic patients, *Bone Min.*, 14, 67, 1991.

325. Majeska, R. J. and Rodan, G. A., Alkaline phosphatase inhibition by parathyroid hormone and isoproterenol in a clonal rat osteosarcoma cell line, *Calcif. Tissue Int.*, 34, 59, 1982.

326. Kumegawa, M., Ikeda, E., Tanaka, S., Haneji, T., Yora, T., Sakagishi, Y., Minami, N., and Hiramatsu, M., The effects of prostaglandin E_2, parathyroid hormone, 1,25-dihydroxy-cholecalciferol, and cyclic nucleotide analogs on alkaline phosphatase activity in osteoblastic cells, *Calcif. Tissue Int.*, 36, 72, 1984.

327. Yee, J. A., Stimulation of alkaline phosphatase activity in cultured neonatal mouse calvaria bone cells by parathyroid hormone, *Calcif. Tissue Int.*, 37, 530, 1985.

328. McDonald, B. R., Gallagher, J. A., and Russell, R. G. G., Parathyroid hormone stimulates the proliferation of cells derived from human bone, *Endocrinology*, 118, 2445, 1986.

329. Partridge, N. C., Jeffrey, J. J., Ehlich, L. S., Teitelbaum, S. L., Fliszar, C., Welgus, H. G., and Kahn, A. J., Hormonal regulation of the production of collagenase and a collagenase inhibitor activity by rat osteogenic sarcoma cells, *Endocrinology*, 120, 1956, 1987.

330. Kream, B. E., Rowe, D., Smith, M. D., Maher, V., and Majeska, R. J., Hormonal regulation of collagen synthesis in a clonal rat osteosarcoma cell line, *Endocrinology*, 119, 1922, 1986.

331. Partridge, N. C., Dickson, C. A., Kopp, K., Teitelbaum, S. L., Crouch, E. C., and Kahn, A. J., Parathyroid hormone inhibits collagen synthesis at both ribonucleic acid and protein levels in rat osteogenic sarcoma cells, *Mol. Endocrinol.*, 3, 232, 1989.

332. Bellows, C. G., Ishida, H., Aubin, J. E., and Heersche, J. N. M., Parathyroid hormone reversibly suppresses the differentiation of osteoprogenitor cells into functional osteoblasts, *Endocrinology*, 127, 3111, 1990.

333. Martin, K. J. and Moseley, J. M., Calcitonin, in *Metabolic Bone Disease and Clinically Related Disorders*, Avioli, L. V. and Krane, S. M., Eds., W. B. Saunders, Philadelphia, 1990, 131.

334. Chambers, T. J. and Hall, T. J., Cellular and molecular mechanisms in the regulation and function of osteoclasts, *Vitam. Horm.*, 46, 41, 1991.

335. Chambers, T. J., Fuller, K., and McSheehy, P. M. J., The effects of calcium regulating hormones on bone resorption by isolated human osteoclastoma cells, *J. Pathol.*, 145, 297, 1985.

336. Bizzarri, C., Shioi, A., Teitelbaum, S. L., Ohara, J., Harwalkar, V. A., Erdman, J. M., Lacey, D. L., and Civitelli, R., Interleukin-4 inhibits bone resorption and increases cytosolic calcium $[Ca^{2+}]_i$ in murine osteoclasts, *J. Biol. Chem.*, 269, 13817, 1994.

337. Chambers, T. J., Chambers, J. C., Darby, J. A., and Fuller, K., The effect of human calcitonin on cytoplasmic spreading of rat osteoclasts, *J. Clin. Endocrinol. Metab.*, 63, 1080, 1986.

338. Chambers, T. J., Fuller, K., and Darby, J. A., Hormonal regulation of acid phosphatase release by osteoclasts disaggregated from neonatal rat bones, *J. Cell. Physiol.*, 132, 92, 1987.

339. Stern, P. H., The D vitamins and bone, *Pharmacol. Rev.*, 32, 47, 1980.

340. Manolagas, S. C., Haussler, M. R., and Deftos, L. J., 1,25-Dihydroxyvitamin D_3 receptor-like macromolecule in rat osteogenic sarcoma cell lines, *J. Biol. Chem.*, 255, 4414, 1980.

341. Norman, A. W., Roth, J., and Orci, L., The vitamin D endocrine system: steroid metabolism, hormone receptors, and biologic response (calcium binding proteins), *Endocr. Rev.*, 3, 331, 1982.

342. Narbaitz, R., Stumpf, W. E., Sar, M., Huang, S., and DeLuca, H. F., Autoradiographic localization of target cells for 1,25-dihydroxyvitamin D_3 in bones from fetal rats, *Calcif. Tissue Int.*, 35, 177, 1983.

343. Price, P. A. and Baukol, S. A., 1,25-Dihydroxyvitamin D increases synthesis of the vitamin K-dependent bone protein by osteosarcoma cells, *J. Biol. Chem.*, 255, 11660, 1980.

344. Fraser, J. D., Otawara, Y., and Price, P. A., 1,25-Dihydroxyvitamin D_3 stimulates the synthesis of matrix-carboxyglutamic acid protein by osteosarcoma cells, *J. Biol. Chem.*, 263, 911, 1988.

345. Prince, C. W. and Butler, W. T., 1,25-Dihydroxyvitamin D regulates the biosynthesis of osteopontin, a bone-derived, cell attachment protein, *Collagen Rel. Res.*, 7, 305, 1987.

346. Noda, M., Yoon, K., Prince, C. W., Butler, W. T., and Rodan, G. A., Transcriptional regulation of osteopontin production in rat osteosarcoma cells by type β transforming growth factor, *J. Biol. Chem.*, 263, 13916, 1988.

347. Franceschi, R. T., James, W. M., and Zerlauth, G., 1α,25-Dihydroxyvitamin D specific regulation of growth, morphology, and fibronectin in a human osteosarcoma cell line, *J. Cell. Physiol.*, 123, 401, 1985.

348. Majeska, R. J. and Rodan, G. A., The effect of 1,25-(OH)$_2$D$_3$ on alkaline phosphatase in osteoblastic osteosarcoma cells, *J. Biol. Chem.*, 257, 3362, 1982.

349. Mulkins, M. A., Manolagas, S. C., Deftos, L. J., and Sussman, H. H., 1,25-Dihydroxyvitamin D$_3$ increases bone alkaline phosphatase enzyme levels in human osteogenic sarcoma cells, *J. Biol. Chem.*, 258, 6219, 1983.

350. Beresford, J. N., Gallagher, J. A., and Russell, R. G. G., 1,25-Dihydroxyvitamin D$_3$ and human bone-derived cells in vitro: effects on alkaline phosphatase, type I collagen and proliferation, *Endocrinology*, 119, 1776, 1986.

351. Boyan, B. D., Schwartz, Z., Bonevald, L. F., and Swain, L. D., Localization of 1,25-(OH)$_2$D$_3$-responsive alkaline phosphatase in osteoblast-like (ROS 17/2.8, MG-63, and MC-3T3) and growth cartilage cells in culture, *J. Biol. Chem.*, 264, 11879, 1988.

352. Wong, G. L., Luben, R. A., and Cohn, D. V., 1,25-Dihydroxycholecalciferol and parathormone: effects on isolated osteoclast-like and osteoblast-like cells, *Science*, 197, 663, 1977.

353. Raisz, L. G., Maina, G. M., Gworek, S. C., Dietrich, J. W., and Canalis, E., Hormonal control of bone collagen synthesis in vitro. Inhibitory effect of l-hydroxylated vitamin D metabolites, *Endocrinology*, 102, 731, 1977.

354. Franceschi, R. T., Romano, P. R., and Park, K., Regulation of type I collagen synthesis by 1,25-dihydroxyvitamin D$_3$ in human osteosarcoma cells, *J. Biol. Chem.*, 263, 18938, 1988.

355. Kurihara, N., Ishizuka, S., Kiyoki, M., Haketa, Y., Ikeda, K. et al., Effects of 1,25-dihydroxyvitamin D$_3$ on osteoblastic MC3T3-E1 cells, *Endocrinology*, 118, 940, 1986.

356. Owen, T. A., Aronow, M. S., Barone, L. M., Bettencourt, B., Stein, G. S., and Lian, J. B., Pleiotropic effects of vitamin D on osteoblast gene expression are related to the proliferative and differentiated state of the bone cell phenotype: dependency upon the basal level of gene expression, duration of exposure, and bone matrix competency in normal rat osteoblastic cultures, *Endocrinology*, 128, 1496, 1991.

357. Ishida, H., Bellows, C. G., Aubin, J. E., and Heersche, J. N. M., Characterization of the 1,25-(OH)$_2$D$_3$-induced inhibition of bone nodule formation in long-term cultures of fetal rat calvaria cells, *Endocrinology*, 132, 61, 1993.

358. Suda, T., Takahashi, N., and Martin, T. J., Modulation of osteoclast differentiation, *Endocr. Rev.*, 13, 66, 1992.

359. Suda, T., Shinki, T., and Takahashi, N., The role of vitamin D in bone and intestinal cell differentiation, *Annu. Rev. Nutr.*, 10, 195, 1990.

360. Bar-Shavit, Z., Teitelbaum, S. L., Reitsma, P., Hall, A., Pegg, L. E., Trail, J., and Kahn, A. J., Induction of monocytic differentiation and bone resorption by 1,25-dihydroxyvitamin D$_3$, *Proc. Natl. Acad. Sci. U.S.A.*, 80, 5907, 1983.

361. Shiina, Y., Yamaguchi, A., Yamana, H., Abe, E., Yoshiki, S., and Suda, T., Comparison of the mechanisms of bone resorption induced by 1α,25-dihydroxyvitamin D$_3$ and lipopolysaccharides, *Calcif. Tissue Int.*, 39, 28, 1986.

362. Roodman, G. D., Ibbotson, K. J., McDonald, B. R., Kuehl, T. J., and Mundy, G. R., 1,25-Dihydroxyvitamin D$_3$ causes formation of multinucleated cells with several osteoclast characteristics in cultures of primate marrow, *Proc. Natl. Acad. Sci. U.S.A.*, 82, 8213, 1985.

363. Takahashi, N., Yamana, H., Yoshiki, S., Roodman, G. D., Mundy, G. R., Jones, S. J., Boyde, A., and Suda, T., Osteoclast-like cell formation and its regulation by osteotropic hormones in mouse bone marrow cultures, *Endocrinology*, 122, 1373, 1988.

364. Takahashi, N., Akatsu, T., Udagawa, N., Sasaki, T., Yamaguchi, A., Mosley, J. M., Martin, T. J., and Suda, T., Osteoblastic cells are involved in osteoclast formation, *Endocrinology*, 123, 2600, 1988.

365. Udagawa, N., Takahashi, N., Akatsu, T., Sasaki, T., Yamaguchi, A., Kodama, H., Martin, T. J., and Suda, T., The bone marrow-derived stromal cell lines MC3T3-G2/PA6 and ST2 support osteoclast-like cell differentiation in cocultures with mouse spleen cells, *Endocrinology*, 125, 1805, 1989.

366. Kurihara, N., Chenu, C., Miller, M., Civin, C., and Roodman, G. D., Identification of committed mononuclear precursors for osteoclast-like cells formed in the long term human marrow cultures, *Endocrinology,* 126, 2733, 1990.

367. Cole, J. A., Eber, S. L., Poelling, R. E., Thorne, P. K., and Forte, L. R., A dual mechanism for the regulation of kidney phosphate transport by parathyroid hormone, *Am. J. Physiol.,* 253, E221, 1987.

368. Caverzasio, J., Brown, C. D. A., Biber, J., Bonjour, J. P., and Murer, H., Sodium-dependent phosphate transport inhibited by parathyroid hormone and cyclic AMP stimulation in an opossum kidney cell line, *J. Biol. Chem.,* 261, 3233, 1986.

369. Jayakumar, A., Cheung, L., Liang, C. T., and Sacktor, B., Sodium gradient-dependent calcium uptake in renal basolateral membrane vesicles, *J. Biol. Chem.,* 259, 10827, 1984.

370. Armbrecht, H. J., Wogsurawat, N., Zenser, T. V., and Davis, B. B., Effect of PTH and $1,25(OH)_2D_3$ on renal $25(OH)D_3$ metabolism, adenylate cyclase, and protein kinase, *Am. J. Physiol.,* 246, E102, 1984.

371. Chandler, J. S., Chandler, S. K., Pike, J. W., and Haussler, M. R., 1,25-Dihydroxyvitamin D_3 induces 25-hydroxyvitamin D_3-24-hydroxylase in a culture's monkey kidney cell line (LLC-MK$_2$) apparently deficient in the high affinity receptor for the hormone, *J. Biol. Chem.,* 259, 2214, 1984.

372. Henry, H. L., Vitamin D hydroxylases, *J. Cell. Biochem.,* 49, 4, 1992.

373. Yates, A. J. P., Gutierrez, G. E., Smolens, P., Travis, P. S., Katz, M. S., Aufdemorte, T. B., Boyce, B. F., Hymer, T. K., Poser, J. W., and Mundy, G. R., Effects of a synthetic peptide of a parathyroid hormone-related protein on calcium homeostasis, renal tubular calcium reabsorption, and bone metabolism in vivo and in vitro in rodents, *J. Clin. Invest.,* 81, 932, 1988.

374. Muldowney, F. P., Carroll, D. V., and Donohoe, J. R., Correction of renal bicarbonate wastage by parathyroidectomy, *Q. J. Med.,* 40, a487, 1971.

375. Muldowney, F. P., Donohoe, J. R., and Freaney, R., Parathormone-induced renal bicarbonate wastage in intestinal malabsorption and in chronic renal failure, *Ir. J. Med. Sci.,* 3, 221, 1970.

376. Helwig, J. J., Musso, M. J., Judes, C., and Nickols, G. A., Parathyroid hormone and calcium: interactions in the control of renin secretion in the isolated nonfiltering rat kidney, *Endocrinology,* 129, 1233, 1991.

377. Di Stefano, A., Wittner, M., Nitschke, R., Braitsch, R., Greger, R., Bally, C., Amiel, C., Roinel, N., and deRouffignac, C., Effects of parathyroid hormone and calcitonin on Na^+, Cl^-, K^+, Mg^{2+} and Ca^{2+} transport in cortical and medullary thick ascending limbs of mouse kidney, *Pfluegers Arch.,* 417, 161, 1990.

378. Elaouf, J. M., Roinel, N., and deRouffignac, C., ADH-like effect of calcitonin on electrolyte transport by Henle's loop of rat kidney, *Am. J. Physiol.,* 254, F62, 1984.

379. Martin, T. J. and Melick, R. A., The acute effects of porcine calcitonin in man, *Aust. Med.,* 18, 258, 1969.

380. Muff, R., Kaufmann, M., Born, W., and Fischer, J. A., Calcitonin inhibits phosphate uptake in opossum kidney cells stably transfected with a porcine calcitonin receptor, *Endocrinology,* 134, 1593, 1994.

381. Jaeger, P., Jones, W., Clemens, T. L., and Hayslett, J. P., Evidence that calcitonin stimulates 1,25-dihydroxyvitamin D production and intestinal absorption of calcium in vivo, *J. Clin. Invest.,* 78, 456, 1986.

382. Kurnik, B. R. C., Huskey, M., and Hruska, K. A., 1,25-Dihydroxycholecalciferol stimulates renal phosphate transport by directly altering membrane phosphatidylcholine composition, *Biochim. Biophys. Acta,* 917, 81, 1987.

383. Theofan, G., Nguyen, A. P., and Norman, A. W., Regulation of calbindin-D_{28K} gene expression by 1,25-dihydroxyvitamin D_3 is correlated to receptor occupancy, *J. Biol. Chem.,* 261, 16943, 1986.

384. Dupret, J. M., Brun, P., Perret, C., Lomri, N., Thomasset, M., and Cuisinier-Gleizes, P., Transcriptional and post-transcriptional regulation of vitamin D-dependent calcium-binding protein gene expression in the rat duodenum by 1,25-dihydroxycholecalciferol, *J. Biol. Chem.,* 262, 16553, 1987.

385. Christakos, S., Gabrielides, C., and Rhoten, W. B., Vitamin D-dependent calcium binding proteins: chemistry, distribution, functional considerations, and molecular biology, *Endocr. Rev.,* 10, 3, 1989.

386. De Boland, A. R., Nemere, I., and Norman, A. W., Ca^{2+}-channel agonist BAY K8644 mimics 1,25(OH)$_2$-vitamin D$_3$ rapid enhancement of Ca^{2+} transport in chick perfused duodenum, *Biochem. Biophys. Res. Commun.*, 166, 217, 1990.

387. De Boland, A. R. and Norman, A. W., Influx of extracellular calcium mediates 1,25-dihydroxy-vitamin D$_3$-dependent transcaltachia (the rapid stimulation of duodenal Ca^{2+} transport), *Endocrinology*, 127, 2475, 1990.

388. Karsenty, G., Lacour, B., Ulmann, A., Pierandrei, E., and Drueke, T., Early effects of vitamin D metabolites on phosphate fluxes in isolated rat enterocytes, *Am. J. Physiol.*, 248, G40, 1985.

389. Birge, S. J. and Alpers, D. H., Stimulation of intestinal mucosal cell proliferation by vitamin D, *Gastroenterology*, 64, 977, 1973.

390. Spielvogel, A. M., Farley, R. D., and Norman, A. W., Studies on the mechanism of action of calciferol. V. Turnover time of chick intestinal epithelial cells in relation to the intestinal action of vitamin D, *Exp. Cell Res.*, 74, 359, 1972.

391. Shinki, T., Takahashi, N., Kadofuku, T., Sato, T., and Suda, T., Induction of spermidine N^1-acetyltransferase by 1α,25-dihydroxyvitamin D$_3$ as an early common event in the target tissues of vitamin D, *J. Biol. Chem.*, 260, 2185, 1985.

392. Benigni, A., Livio, M., Dodesini, P., Schieppati, A., Panigada, M., Mecca, G., DeGaetano, G., and Remuzzi, G., Inhibition of human platelet aggregation by parathyroid hormone, *Am. J. Nephrol.*, 5, 243, 1985.

393. Remuzzi, G., Dodesini, P., Livio, M., Mecca, G., Benigni, A., Schieppati, A., Poletti, E., and DeGaetano, G., Parathyroid hormone inhibits human platelet function, *Lancet*, 2, 1321, 1981.

394. Goldstein, D. A., Chui, L. A., and Massry, S. G., Effect of parathyroid hormone and uremia on peripheral nerve calcium and motor nerve conduction velocity, *J. Clin. Invest.*, 62, 88, 1978.

395. Fraser, R. A., Kronenberg, H. M., Pang, P. K. T., and Harvey, S., Parathyroid hormone messenger ribonucleic acid in the rat hypothalamus, *Endocrinology*, 127, 2517, 1990.

396. Kostyuk, P. G., Lukyanetz, E. A., and Ter-Markosyan, A. S., Parathyroid hormone enhances calcium current in snail neurones — simulation of the effect by phorbol esters, *Pfluegers Arch.*, 420, 146, 1992.

397. Moxley, M. A., Bell, N. H., and Wagle, S. R., Parathyroid hormone stimulation of glucose and urea production in isolated liver cells, *Am. J. Physiol.*, 227, 1058, 1974.

398. Whitfield, J. F., Chakravarthy, B. R., Durkin, J. P., Isaacs, R. J., Jouishomme, H., Sikorska, M., Williams, R. E., and Rixon, R. H., Parathyroid hormone stimulates protein kinase C but not adenylate cyclase in mouse epidermal keratinocytes, *J. Cell Physiol.*, 150, 299, 1992.

399. Thiede, M. A. and Rodan, G. A., Expression of a calcium-mobilizing parathyroid hormone-like peptide in lactating mammary tissue, *Science*, 242, 278, 1988.

400. Kaiser, S. M., Sebag, M., Rhim, J. S., Kremer, R., and Goltzman, D., Antisense-mediated inhibition of parathyroid hormone-related peptide production in a keratinocyte cell line impedes differentiation, *Mol. Endocrinol.*, 8, 139, 1994.

401. Kremer, R., Karaplis, A. C., Henderson, J. E., Gulliver, W., Banville, D., Hendy, G., and Goltzman, D., Regulation of parathyroid hormone-like peptide in cultured normal human keratinocytes, *J. Clin. Invest.*, 87, 884, 1991.

402. Halloran, B. P. and Nissenson, R. A., *Parathyroid Hormone-Related Protein: Normal Physiology and Its Role in Cancer*, CRC Press, Boca Raton, FL, 1992.

403. Rodan, S. B. and Rodan, A. R., Dexamethasone effects on b-adrenergic receptors and adenylate cyclase regulatory proteins Gs and Gi in ROS 17/2.8 cells, *Endocrinology*, 118, 2510, 1986.

404. Civitelli, R., Agnusdei, D., Nardi, P., Zacchei, F., Avioli, L. V., and Gennari, C., Effects of one-year treatment with estrogens on bone mass, intestinal calcium absorption and 25-hydroxyvitamin D-1α-hydroxylase reserve in postmenopausal osteoporosis, *Calcif. Tissue Int.*, 42, 77, 1988.

405. Deftos, L. J., Burton, D., Bone, H. G., Catherwood, B. D., Parthermore, J. G., Moore, R. Y., Minick, S., and Guillemin, R., Immunoreactive calcitonin in the intermediate lobe of the pituitary, *Life Sci.*, 23, 743, 1978.

406. Shah, G. V., Wang, W., Grosvernor, C. E., and Crowley, W. R., Calcitonin inhibits basal and thyrotropin-releasing hormone-induced release of prolactin from anterior pituitary cells: evidence for a selective action exerted proximal to segretagogue-induced increases in cytosolic Ca^{2+}, *Endocrinology*, 127, 622, 1990.

407. Korkor, A. B., Reduced binding of [³H]1,25-dihydroxyvitamin D₃ in the parathyroid glands of patients with renal failure, *N. Engl. J. Med.*, 316, 1573, 1987.

408. Abe, E., Miyaura, C., Sagakami, H., Takeda, M., Konno, K., Yamazaki, T., Yoshiki, S., and Suda, T., Differentiation of mouse myeloid leukemia cells induced by 1α,25-dihydroxyvitamin D₃, *Proc. Natl. Acad. Sci. U.S.A.*, 78, 4990, 1981.

409. Munker, R., Norman, A. W., and Koeffler, H. P., Vitamin D compounds: effect on clonal proliferation and differentiation of human myeloid cells, *J. Clin. Invest.*, 78, 424, 1986.

410. Manolagas, S. C., Hustmyer, F. G., and Yu, X., 1,25-Dihydroxyvitamin D₃ and the immune system, *Proc. Soc. Exp. Biol. Med.*, 191, 238, 1989.

411. Reichel, H. and Norman, A. W., Systemic effects of vitamin D, *Annu. Rev. Med.*, 40, 71, 1989.

412. Amento, E. P., Vitamin D and the immune system, *Steroids*, 49, 55, 1987.

413. Eisman, J. A., Koga, M., Sutherland, R. L., Barkla, D. H., and Tutton, P. J. M., 1,25-Dihydroxyvitamin D₃ and the regulation of human cancer cell replication, *Proc. Soc. Exp. Biol. Med.*, 191, 221, 1989.

414. Smith, E. L. and Holick, M. F., The skin: the site of vitamin D₃ synthesis and a target tissue for its metabolite 1,25-dihydroxyvitamin D₃, *Steroids*, 49, 103, 1987.

415. Holick, M. F., 1,25-Dihydroxyvitamin D₃ and the skin: a unique application for the treatment of psoriasis, *Proc. Soc. Exp. Biol. Med.*, 191, 246, 1989.

2

Cardiovascular Actions of Parathyroid Hormone

M. F. Crass, III

CONTENTS

I. INTRODUCTION AND HISTORY

The idea of possible cardiovascular actions of parathyroid hormone (PTH) is not new. The flow chart shown in Figure 1 lists the earliest observations up to 1980. In 1925, Collip and Clark,[1] in their earliest characterization of PTH, showed a transient lowering of blood pressure in dogs. Data from their paper, shown in Figure 2, clearly demonstrate the fall in blood pressure after intravenous or subcutaneous administration of a crude parathyroid extract. Subsequent reports by Handler et al.[2] and Handler and Cohn,[3] who were among the first to demonstrate parathyroid extract-induced phosphaturia, showed that intravenous injection of a crude parathyroid extract resulted in marked increases not only in glomerular filtration rate, but renal plasma flow as well. These findings were accompanied by a fall in mean arterial blood pressure of 8 to 16 mmHg.

Characterization of this hypotensive property of parathyroid extracts was not begun until a series of reports was published by Charbon and colleagues in The Netherlands over the period of 1966 to 1974. Charbon's group[4,5] confirmed the diuretic, phosphaturic, and hypotensive effects observed previously and theorized that the diuretic effects of the parathyroid extracts occurred as a result of a "changed renal circulation". This was confirmed when Charbon, using a partially purified PTH (2000 USP units/mg), showed a small dose-dependent increase in canine renal artery blood flow and a 100% increase in celiac artery flow, accompanied by no change in mesenteric, carotid, or aortic blood flow.[6,7] These selective vasodilatory effects were accompanied, at high doses only, by a decrease in mean arterial blood pressure, but no cardiac contractile effects or changes in heart rate were observed. The increases in renal and celiac blood flow after a single intravenous injection of PTH extract were transient, the maximal vasodilator effects occurring after 1 min with a $T_{1/2}$ of roughly 5 min. However, it was also shown[8,9] that continuous intravenous infusion of PTH caused a sustained augmentation of flow in both renal and celiac circulations. Further experiments using selective organ extirpation and flow probe methodologies showed that the celiac flow response to PTH[6] and PTH-(1-34)[7,10] could be attributed exclusively to an increase in hepatic arterial blood flow. Thus, Charbon and colleagues must be credited with the first direct evidence for PTH-induced vasodilation.

The above studies and others by Berthelot and Gairard,[11] Schleiffer et al.,[12,13] and Lindner et al.[14] set the stage for the vigorous and highly productive research program of Pang and collaborators,[15] beginning with their first published reports with mammals in 1980. These studies showed that bolus injections of a variety of amino terminal PTH-(1-34) preparations elicited a precipitous decline in blood pressure in dogs and rats. In this context it was shown that the dog was ten times more sensitive to the hypotensive actions of PTH as compared to rats. Pang and co-workers also showed in this study that it was PTH per se, and not a contaminant, that was vasoactive and that hypotensive doses were not accompanied by calcemia. Finally, this early study confirmed and extended specificity studies of Charbon et al.[6] by showing that α-adrenergic, β-adrenergic, histaminergic, or cholinergic blockade did not diminish PTH-induced hypotension. These initial studies in mammals by Pang and colleagues, more than those of any other laboratory, provided the foundation and impetus for their continuing investigations and those of numerous other investigators.

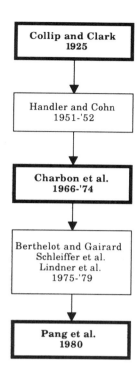

FIGURE 1   Cardiovascular actions of parathyroid hormone to 1980. Dates and investigators providing pivotal developments during this period are outlined in bold.

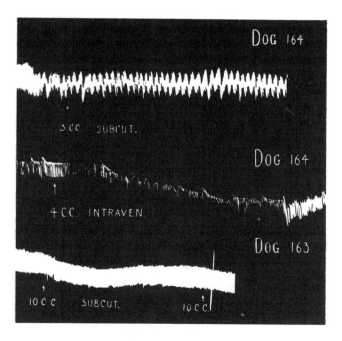

FIGURE 2   Early observations in dogs by Collip and Clark showing hypotensive responses following subcutaneous or intravenous administration of a partially purified parathyroid extract. (From Collip, J. B. and Clark, E. P., *J. Biol. Chem.*, 64, 485, 1925, © The American Society for Biochemistry and Molecular Biology. With permission.)

II. SYSTEMIC AND REGIONAL BLOOD FLOW RESPONSES TO PARATHYROID HORMONE: *IN VIVO* STUDIES

The hypotensive action in concert with demonstrations by Charbon et al.[7,10] that parathyroid extract and PTH-(1-34) elicited regional gastrointestinal blood flow responses, and those by Schleiffer et al.[13] that PTH directly relaxed isolated blood vessels led to a series of studies to assess specific cardiodynamic effects of the hormone. The first of the major studies was done by Pang and colleagues,[16] who examined regional vascular responses to the hormone in dogs using radiolabeled microspheres. In these experiments the responses were quantitatively different in 14 different vascular beds, and regional blood flows in pancreas, stomach, and liver increased by large percentages. Coronary, renal, and adrenal circulations also showed substantial flow responses to PTH. Later, Wang et al.[17] showed dose-related increases in coronary, celiac, and renal blood flow, but mesenteric and skeletal blood flows were not stimulated; in fact, these beds constricted, which was a likely result of the fall in observed mean blood pressure and the triggering of reflex adrenergic vasoconstriction. In these dog studies blood flow in coronary, celiac, and renal circulations was shown to increase after intravenous doses of PTH, which would have yielded physiological plasma concentrations as low as 1 pM. Further studies to assess regional vasodilation by PTH in dogs confirmed that sensitivity to PTH varied markedly in different vascular beds.[18] Intraarterial injections of PTH-(1-34) resulted in dose-related increases in blood flow of 178 and 162% in coronary and celiac circulations, respectively, and an increase of 30% or less in the renal circulation.[18] As before, these experiments showed that the mesenteric circulation vasoconstricted at low doses of PTH, indicating that vasoconstriction of the splanchnic or mesenteric bed following PTH-(1-34) is probably not due entirely to the adrenergic reflex activity, an interpretation supported by the experiments of Charbon and Hulstaert.[10] Evidence for direct PTH-induced vasodilation of the pulmonary bed was not obtained.[18] The studies of Charbon[7,8] suggested that the hormonal response in the celiac circulation may have been limited to the hepatic circulation. Indeed, more recent experiments by Moore and others,[19] in which PTH-(1-34) was directly administered into the dog hepatic artery, showed that hepatic arterial blood flow was increased by 55%. Insofar as other regional circulations are concerned, bone blood flow was not altered by exogenous administration of PTH.[20] A thorough and comprehensive study of systemic and regional effects of PTH on blood flow was recently reported by Roca-Cusachs et al.[21] using microsphere methodology in conscious, unanesthetized, and unrestrained rats. Their results showed that the PTH-(1-34)-induced blood flow responses in rats were similar to those reported[16,18] previously in anesthetized dogs. However, of great importance, Roca-Cusachs and colleagues[21] showed that (1) systemic and regional vascular effects of PTH-(1-34) are not appreciably altered by anesthesia per se, (2) vascular resistance and blood flow in the brain, an organ not previously studied in terms of PTH effects *in vivo*, is not directly affected by PTH, and (3) the coronary circulation of the component structures of the heart showed the greatest sensitivity to the vascular effects of PTH relative to other regional circulations.

A. Blood Flow Responses to Parathyroid Hormone in the Coronary Circulation

The *in vivo* studies discussed above were designed primarily to compare blood flow responses to PTH in different regional circulations rather than to examine the detailed characteristics of the flow response in a representative vascular bed *in vivo*. Consistent with the reportedly high sensitivity of the coronary arteries to the vascular actions of PTH, detailed studies of PTH effects in this regional vascular bed have been reported in instrumented open-chest anesthetized dogs *in vivo*. Thus, the following discussion of data obtained in the coronary circulation serves perhaps as a representative responsive regional circulation for the purpose of characterizing the flow response to PTH.

In these studies, blood flow was monitored with an electromagnetic flow probe on the left circumflex coronary artery, unless indicated otherwise, and PTH in several forms (or vehicle) were administered by bolus or infusion via an angiocath needle in the left circumflex artery. A dose-related increase in coronary blood flow was observed up to a near-maximum of 160% above vehicle control values, the near-maximum response being obtained at 25 pmol/kg.[22] No significant hypotension was seen at this dose when administered by the intracoronary route. Bolus injection of PTH-(1-34) elicited a flow response duration of approximately 8 min, but infusion of the polypeptide caused a sustained hyperemia.[23] Again, no sustained hypotension was observed during or after intracoronary infusion, due to hemodilution or loss of activity in the systemic circulation, or both. Additional studies were carried out to determine specific regional and transmural (endocardium/epicardium) blood flow responses to the hormone fragment. The anesthetized, instrumented, open-chest dog model was used as before. PTH-(1-34) was infused into the left circumflex artery (0.008 nmol/kg/min). Using the reference withdrawal method, radionuclide-labeled (^{51}Cr, ^{85}Sr, ^{141}Ce) microspheres were injected before (basal or "PRE" flow), during (8 min after new steady-state or "PEAK" flow), and after (restoration of basal or "POST" flow) a 20-min infusion of PTH-(1-34). The heart was then sectioned and subsectioned (Figure 3A). No statistically significant changes in mean arterial pressure, left ventricular dynamics, or heart rate were observed during the three phases of the study (data not shown). Data on regional blood flows are shown in Figures 3B and C. During infusion of PTH-(1-34), mean left ventricular myocardial blood flow increased from 76 ± 2 to 152 ± 4 ml/min/100 g and calculated coronary resistance decreased from 1.61 ± 0.08 to 0.67 ± 0.06 mmHg/ml/min/100 g (Figure 3B). No regional differences in coronary flow were detected. Similarly, no differences in left ventricular endocardium/epicardium blood flow ratios were seen (Figure 3C). Furthermore, similar PTH-(1-34) flow responses and resistance changes were evident in terms of total and regional flows in the right ventricle and the interventricular septum (data not shown). These studies confirmed the potent coronary vasodilator effect of PTH-(1-34). The results also indicated that intracoronary infusions of PTH-(1-34) resulted in uniform regional and transmural increases in coronary blood flow and that the increased flow was probably not the result of a shunting or "steal" phenomenon.

Pang et al.[15] showed that the hypotensive effect of PTH was specific to other receptor-operated vasoactive mechanisms. A similar study[23] was carried out with four receptor systems which were well characterized in terms of the coronary flow response. Using blocking drugs and measuring the coronary blood flow response to the appropriate agonist before and after the blocking agent, it was shown in independent experiments that α-adrenergic, β-adrenergic, muscarinic, and histaminergic blockade had no statistically significant effect on the vasodilator action of PTH. Thus, at least in terms of the aforementioned receptor systems, the PTH-induced vasodilation resulted from a specific and direct interaction with a vascular receptor site. This study did not assess a possible role of vasodilator prostaglandins in PTH-induced vasodilation, but Wang et al.[17] have reported that inhibition of prostaglandin synthesis with indomethacin did not alter stimulation of renal blood flow by PTH-(1-34). Other reports[24,25] using different vascular preparations have clearly indicated that inhibition of prostaglandin synthesis with indomethacin did not alter the blood flow, hypotensive, or *in vitro* vasorelaxant responses to PTH-(1-34). Conversely, two groups have reported[26,27] that indomethacin pretreatment of intact rats or a perfused rat hind limb preparation appeared to antagonize the vascular actions of PTH. A simple resolution of these apparently conflicting findings is not readily apparent.

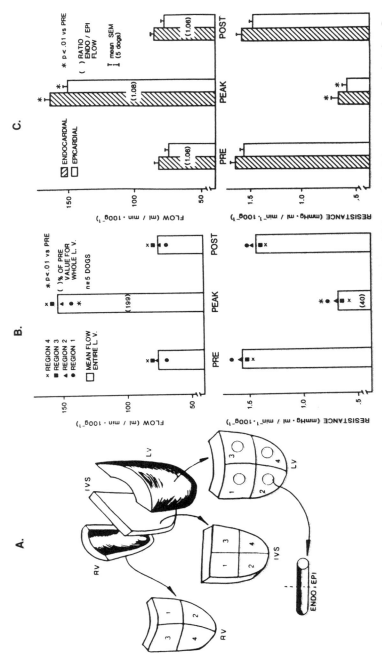

FIGURE 3 Regional myocardial blood flow responses to intracoronary administration of PTH-(1-34) in anesthetized, instrumented, open-chest dogs. In (A) the method for sectioning and subsectioning the ventricles is shown. Subsectional regions for the left ventricle, interventricular septum, and right ventricle are numbered. The flow data (upper panel) and calculated resistance data (lower panel) for each of the numbered regions in the left ventricle are shown in (B). In (C), left ventricular endocardial and epicardial blood flows and calculated endocardial/epicardial flow ratios are shown in the upper panel, and values for calculated resistance in endocardial and epicardial regions are presented in the lower panel. Data for the interventricular septum and the right ventricle are not shown (see text). This study was performed with the collaboration of Dr. R. M. Lust, Division of Cardiac Surgery, East Carolina University School of Medicine, Greenville, North Carolina.

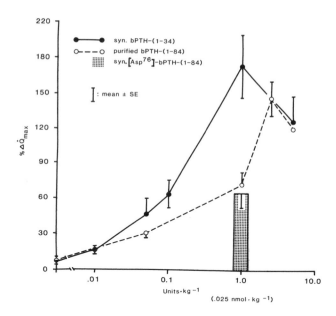

FIGURE 4 Comparison of coronary blood flow responses after intracoronary administration of bovine PTH-(1-34) and two different preparations of bovine PTH-(1-84) in the left circumflex coronary artery of anesthetized, instrumented, open-chest dogs. The vasodilator response to the synthetic [Asp76]-bPTH-(1-84) was observed at only one dose (0.025 nmol/kg) due to the limited availability of the hormone. $\%\Delta\dot{Q}_{max}$ = maximum percent change in blood flow. Doses of the various PTH preparations are shown on the horizontal axis. Each point or bar represents the mean ± S.E. for 4 to 6 dogs.

Pang and colleagues have examined structure-activity relationships in terms of the hypotensive effects of PTH. In studies of structure-hypotensive activity relationships, Pang et al.[28,29] and McCarron et al.[30] confirmed that the hypotensive action of the native hormone resides in the 1 to 34 amino terminal fragment. Furthermore, substitution of the methionyl residues at positions 8 and 18 of PTH-(1-34) with a hydrophobic, sterically similar synthetic amino acid (i.e., norleucine), thus forming an oxidation-resistant analogue,[31] did not result in loss of hypotensive activity.

Following the above-mentioned findings of others, similar structure-activity relationships were focused specifically on blood flow in the PTH-sensitive coronary circulation. Initially, vasodilator activity of two preparations of the parent hormone, PTH-(1-84), were compared with that of the amino terminal fragment, PTH-(1-34), in acute instrumented dogs. As can be seen in Figure 4, potency of PTH-(1-34) exceeded that of the parent hormone, but efficacies of PTH-(1-84) and PTH-(1-34) were comparable. In addition, synthetically pure fragments of the entire human PTH molecule were tested over a broad dose range for coronary vasodilator and other cardiovascular effects. As shown in Figure 5, only the amino terminal PTH-(1-34) fragment showed vasodilator activity. Furthermore, with the exception of PTH-(1-34), no other fragment of the parent molecule altered blood pressure, left ventricular pressures, dP/dt$_{max}$, or heart rate at any of the doses tested (data not shown).

In another set of experiments on structure-coronary artery vasodilator activity, analogues of PTH-(1-34), with the methionines at positions 8 and 18 replaced by norleucines — [Nle8,Nle18,Tyr34]-bPTH-(1-34) amide — or additionally with positions 1 and 2 or 1 to 6 omitted — [Nle8, Nle18, Tyr34]-bPTH-(3-34) amide or [Tyr34]-bPTH-(7-34) — were tested for vasodilator activity. Both compounds (3-34 and 7-34) bind to the PTH receptor[32-34] and have little or no agonist activity, thus they have been used widely as competitive antagonists in

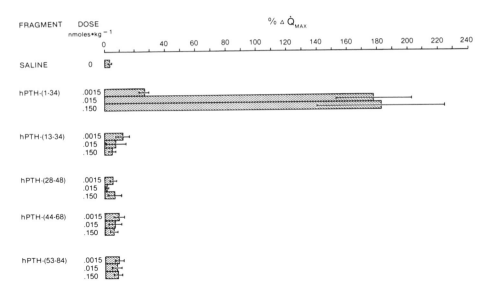

FIGURE 5 Coronary blood flow responses to synthetic fragments of the entire human PTH molecule. Each PTH peptide fragment or vehicle was administered individually by intracoronary injection into the left circumflex coronary artery of anesthetized, instrumented, open-chest dogs. $\%\Delta\dot{Q}_{max}$ = maximum percent change in blood flow. Each bar represents the mean ± S.E. for 5 to 10 dogs.

classical PTH target tissues. It also should be noted that the phenylalanine residue at the 34 position having the C-terminal carboxyl group can be substituted with a tyrosine amide without loss of activity,[35] indicating that it is out of the critical region that determines biological activity. Only the 1-34 analogue with the 8 and 18 methionines substituted by norleucine residues showed essentially full vasodilator activity as compared to bPTH-(1-34) (Figure 6). These findings were consistent with the structure-hypotensive activity data of Ellison and McCarron[36] and Pang et al.[28] Pang and colleagues[29] have shown further that oxidation of the two methionyl residues of unsubstituted bPTH-(1-34) with H_2O_2 resulted in the loss of hypotensive activity, but did not destroy the hypercalcemic action of the 1-34 peptide fragment. Only the methionyl residues were oxidized (to methionyl sulfoxide or sulfone) and no other parts of the molecule were affected. This observation was of considerable interest as it clearly separated the hypercalcemic and hypotensive functions of the hormone. Subsequent studies by Hong et al.[37] indicated that loss of vasorelaxant activity by H_2O_2-induced methionine oxidation may be attributed to conformational changes, perhaps induced by oxidatively generated negative charges. Furthermore, because the norleucine-substituted analogue of bPTH-(1-34), which was not affected by H_2O_2 treatment, was fully active in terms of vasodilation and thus hypotensive activity, it is clear that the methionyl residues are not required. Further evidence[38] suggested that amino acids at positions 25-27 may be important for vascular or hypotensive activity or both, perhaps even binding of the hormone. This would be consistent with the similarly observed binding region for the hormone at other target sites.[39,40] In the present study, omission of amino acids at positions 1 and 2, and therefore, expectedly, omission of positions 1-6, resulted in complete loss of coronary artery vasodilation (Figure 6).

Thus, essentially total vasodilator activity resides in the amino terminal 1-34 fragment, and there is an absolute requirement for positions 1 and 2, but not the methionines at positions 8 and 18, to elicit the blood flow and hypotensive responses.

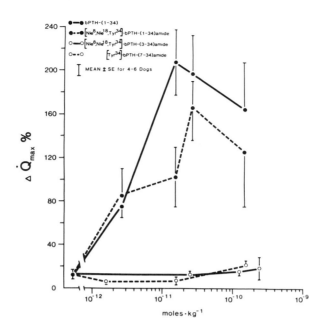

FIGURE 6   Coronary blood flow responses to PTH-(1-34) or different substituted analogues (see key). Varying doses of the peptides were administered by intracoronary injection into the left circumflex coronary artery of anesthetized, instrumented, open-chest dogs. $\Delta\dot{Q}_{max}\%$ = maximum percent of change in blood flow.

B.   Comparison of Regional Blood Flow Responses to PTH-(1-34) with Those of Other Vasodilator Substances: The Coronary Circulation

Several potent hypotensive peptide substances have been identified and characterized. The characteristics of some of these peptides have been compared with those of PTH-(1-34) in terms of hypotensive activity in anesthetized dogs.[41] These studies showed that intravenously administered PTH-(1-34) was somewhat less potent, but tended to have greater efficacy and duration of hypotensive action as compared to certain of the other peptides tested, which included substance P, vasoactive intestinal peptide (VIP), neurotensin, and bradykinin. However, regional flow responses to these peptides have not been systematically compared to those of PTH-(1-34) in the same animal model over a broad dose range. Using the anesthetized, instrumented dog model, the coronary flow response and other cardiovascular effects of PTH-(1-34) were compared to those of VIP, substance P, bradykinin, and neurotensin. The peptides were administered by intracoronary injection over a dose range of 10^{-15} to 10^{-8} mol/kg. The results for coronary blood flow are shown in Figure 7. It can be seen that all peptides, with the exception of neurotensin, increased coronary blood flow in a dose-dependent fashion. In terms of vasodilator potency (geometric mean ED_{50} values in moles per kilogram) substance P ranked first (7.0×10^{-15}), and bradykinin (2.0×10^{-12}), PTH-(1-34) (3.4×10^{-12}), and VIP (6.0×10^{-12}) were approximately equipotent. However, the efficacy of substance P was only half that of PTH-(1-34), VIP, and bradykinin; the latter three peptides were approximately equal. Similarly, the duration of the substance P-induced coronary vasodilation was short relative to that of the other vasodilatory peptides (Table 1). Duration of the flow responses to the various peptides ranked as PTH-(1-34) >> bradykinin = VIP > substance P. All of the peptides, including neurotensin, displayed hypotensive activity. Thus, these findings indicated that other than substance P and neurotensin, PTH-(1-34) had a potency and efficacy

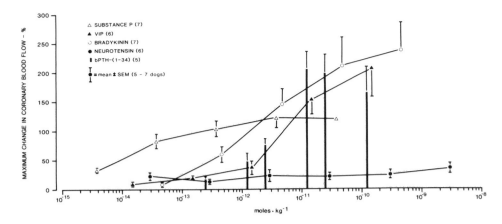

FIGURE 7   Comparison of the coronary blood flow response to PTH-(1-34) with those of several other vasodilator/
hypotensive peptides (see key). Varying doses of each peptide were administered by intracoronary
injection into the left circumflex coronary artery of anesthetized, instrumented, open-chest dogs. The
dose-related PTH-(1-34) responses are shown by the vertical bars.

TABLE 1   Duration of coronary blood flow
response to PTH-(1-34) and other
hypotensive peptides in the dog

Peptide[a]	No. of dogs	Duration of response, coronary blood flow $(s \pm S.E.)$
PTH-(1-34)	5	370 ± 60
VIP	6	173 ± 76
Substance P	7	95 ± 32
Bradykinin	7	205 ± 56
Neurotensin	6	108 ± 57

[a] At approximate ED_{50} doses for each response; all values represent mean $\pm$ S.E. (standard error) for the number of dogs indicated.

comparable to the other peptides in terms of coronary vasodilation, but had substantially
greater duration of action as compared to the other peptides. In general, these results in the
coronary circulation resemble those of the hypotension study of Tenner et al.,[41] although the
peptides as a whole appeared to be considerably more potent as coronary vasodilators than as
hypotensive agents.

The coronary flow response to PTH-(1-34) also has been compared with the flow responses
of nonpeptide vasodilators such as adenosine[42] and certain calcium channel blockers.[43] These
comparative studies also were performed in the anesthetized instrumented open-chest dog. In
the first of these experiments adenosine was administered into the left anterior descending
coronary artery, and the flow response compared to that following a similar administration of
PTH-(1-34). PTH-(1-34) was substantially more potent than adenosine based on geometric
mean ED_{50} values of approximately 4×10^{-12} and 2×10^{-10} mol/kg for PTH-(1-34) and
adenosine, respectively. The two vasodilators showed comparable effectiveness (maximum
flow responses), but predictably, the duration of the adenosine flow response was much less
than that of PTH-(1-34) in view of the rapid disappearance or enzymatic conversion of
adenosine.[44] In a second group of experiments[43] comparing the PTH flow responses to those

of the calcium antagonist compounds nifedipine, verapamil, and diltiazem, the vasodilators were administered by intracoronary (left circumflex artery) injection over a dose range of 10^{-13} to 10^{-7} mol/kg. Figure 8 shows the relative flow responses. Although the plateau of the flow response to nifedipine was not obtained, PTH-(1-34) appeared to be approximately 100-fold more potent as a vasodilator. As compared to diltiazem, the PTH fragment was 1000-fold more potent, and compared to verapamil, PTH-(1-34) appeared some 5000-fold more potent in terms of coronary vasodilation. Thus, these three structurally diverse and well-characterized nonpeptide calcium antagonist compounds, in addition to exogenously administered adenosine, were considerably less potent as compared to PTH-(1-34) in terms of their respective blood flow responses in the coronary circulation.

C. Other Cardiodynamic Effects of Parathyroid Hormone

In addition to the strong vascular effects of PTH, several reports have suggested that PTH may have effects on cardiac contractile function and heart rate in the intact animal. Crass and Pang[22] initially reported that in the anesthetized, instrumented open-chest dog, the marked coronary vasodilation following intracoronary PTH-(1-34) bolus injection was accompanied at higher doses of the peptide by an increase in left ventricular contractile force of approximately 46% relative to isotonic saline control values. No alteration in heart rate was observed, however. In a later report[23] that used the same dog model, the increase in contractile force at high doses was confirmed, but a small chronotropic effect of <20 beats per minute also was observed. Conversely, when a low dose of PTH was infused (vs. bolus injection), no heart rate effect was seen, although the contractile response was clearly evident. No hypotensive effect was observed in the studies involving intracoronary infusion of PTH-(1-34). Because of the absence of hypotension and thus reflex adrenergic stimulation of the heart, the increase in left ventricular contractile force with low dose infusion of PTH-(1-34) could have been due either to an increase in coronary perfusion (and hence cardiac myocyte oxygenation) or to a direct inotropic action of the peptide. With high doses of the peptide eliciting a marked dose-related hypotension, it is reasonably safe to predict that the dose-related increase in left ventricular contractile force and heart rate was, at least in part, a manifestation of reflex adrenergic actions. Wang et al.[17] reported a small (<12%) increase in heart rate in anesthetized instrumented dogs in which PTH-(1-34) was administered intravenously. The modest increase in heart rate did not appear to be statistically significant. This group also reported a 25% augmentation in cardiac output at the highest dose tested, occurring in concert with a substantial decline in arterial blood pressure. Taking this into account, the postulated increase in venous return secondary to observed peripheral vasoconstriction and increase in stroke volume and an apparent increase in heart rate (all expected manifestations of reflex adrenergic activity) probably accounted for the reported increase in cardiac output.

Additional reports[21,45-47] in unanesthetized, conscious animals provided important support for cardiodynamic effects of PTH. These papers followed a 1975 report by Berthelot and Gairard[11] which showed a transient decline in mean arterial pressure in unanesthetized rats, with no change in cardiac output (no data shown) following intravenous administration of a crude parathyroid extract. Daugirdas et al.[45] used instrumented unanesthetized dogs to assess the effects of PTH-(1-34) on mean arterial, pulmonary artery, and central venous pressures. Heart rate also was measured, as was cardiac output by thermodilution methodology. PTH-(1-34) was administered into the right atrium. At doses of PTH-(1-34) eliciting profound hypotension (decline of 34 mmHg in mean arterial pressure), heart rate increased commensurately by 20 to 30%, while apparent transient increases in central venous pressure and pulmonary pressure were observed. These pressure and heart rate changes were accompanied by a 20% increase in cardiac output, which was statistically significant. These findings were

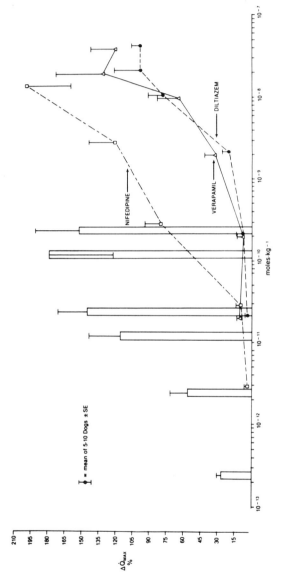

FIGURE 8   Comparison of the coronary blood flow response to PTH-(1-34) with those of several calcium antagonist compounds. Varying doses of PTH-(1-34) or each calcium antagonist were administered by intracoronary injection into the left circumflex coronary artery of anesthetized, instrumented, open-chest dogs. The dose-related PTH-(1-34) responses are shown by the vertical bars. $\Delta\dot{Q}_{max}\%$ = maximum percent change in blood flow.

consistent with reflex stimulation of cardiac pump function. In a more recent study by Jordan and co-workers,[46] the actions of PTH-(1-34) on cardiovascular function were tested in conscious sheep. The ewes were infused with low doses of PTH-(1-34) via the left jugular vein. Mean arterial blood pressure and heart rate were measured and cardiac output was calculated. Several new and interesting observations were reported in this study, which employed infusion doses of PTH-(1-34) that resulted in near-physiological plasma concentrations of 10^{-10} to $10^{-9}M$. A relatively slight fall in mean arterial blood pressure was observed, amounting to only 10 mmHg at the highest dose infused. Despite this small decline in blood pressure, heart rate in the ewes increased by 75%. Furthermore, these workers observed a 176% increase in calculated cardiac output during PTH-(1-34) infusion. As implied by Jordan and colleagues,[46] the marked increase in cardiac output cannot be attributed entirely, if at all, to adrenergic reflex activity, and thus may represent a direct effect of PTH-(1-34) on the ventricular myocytes and pacemaker cells of this species. Another interesting feature of these studies was the observed increase in plasma renin activity and decreased renal vascular resistance (increased renal plasma flow) following PTH-(1-34) infusion. Others[14,16,48] have reported similar findings in anesthetized and unanesthetized dogs. Thus, PTH-(1-34) can elicit at least three mechanisms to account for its cardiodynamic effects, e.g., direct effects on cardiac myocytes and perhaps also pacemaker cells, or indirectly via hypotension-induced reflex adrenergic activity and/or stimulation of the renin-angiotensin system. Finally, in the recent study in conscious and unrestrained rats by Roca-Cusachs et al.,[21] bolus intravenous injections of PTH-(1-34) were shown to produce dose-related increases in heart rate and cardiac output (but with no change in stroke volume) in the presence of similarly dose-related decreases in total peripheral resistance and, thus, mean arterial pressure. A more recent study in conscious rats by Kishimoto et al.[47] showed very similar results. Collectively, these careful and interesting studies in unanesthetized and unrestrained animals by Roca-Cusachs et al.,[21] Daugirdas et al.,[45] Jordan et al.,[46] and Kishimoto et al.[47] provided data that are in good agreement with results from earlier assessments in anesthetized animals, thus enhancing the physiological importance of the cardiovascular actions of PTH.

Summarizing to this point, *in vivo* evidence for possible direct contractile and heart rate effects of PTH-(1-34) is somewhat uncertain, as direct effects on these parameters of cardiac function could be masked by strong reflex responses to the potent hypotensive action of the peptide, as well as by effects of PTH-(1-34)-induced activation of the renin-angiotensin system. It remains for *in vitro* studies to elucidate the nature of possible direct inotropic, chronotropic, and, of course, vascular effects of PTH. The following sections present *in vitro* evidence for such direct effects.

III. CHARACTERIZATION OF THE VASODILATOR (VASORELAXANT) EFFECTS OF PARATHYROID HORMONE: *IN VITRO* STUDIES

A. Parathyroid Hormone Effects on Vasorelaxation

The potent and efficacious blood flow and hypotensive actions of PTH or its 1-34 amino terminal fragment in the intact animal have been confirmed by a large body of data obtained *in vitro* using vessels from different vascular beds in a variety of animal species. Within 1 year of the last paper by Charbon and Hulstaert[10] on the cardiovascular effects of PTH *in vivo*, the first *in vitro* demonstrations of the vasorelaxant effects of PTH were reported by the French group of Berthelot, Gairard, and Schleiffer.[11-13] Using helical strips of rat thoracic aorta, these workers demonstrated that a relatively crude parathyroid extract diminished phenylephrine- and norepinephrine-induced contractions by roughly 50%. This loss of contractile tension was observed chiefly during the slow phase of contraction. The inhibition of tension development was not evident when inactivated PTH was employed. Pang et al.[15] confirmed PTH-induced vasorelaxation *in vitro* by demonstrating a significant reduction in methoxamine-induced tension in helical strips of rabbit thoracic aorta following administration of PTH-(1-34). Subsequent to these initial reports, vasorelaxation following administration of PTH-(1-34), PTH-(1-84), or other analogues to (1) precontracted helical strips or cylindrical segments of rat[11] or rabbit[49] aorta, porcine, bovine and human cerebral vessels,[50] porcine coronary arteries,[51] rat tail artery,[52] and rabbit renal artery;[53] (2) superfused afferent and efferent renal arterioles;[54] (3) isolated perfused organs such as rat heart[55] and rat[56] and dog[15] kidneys; (4) *in situ* perfused rat hind limb;[15] (5) dog heart-lung preparation;[57] and (6) isolated perfused rat aorta[25] and rat mesenteric artery arcade[58] has been reported.

B. Determining Endothelium Dependency for the Vascular Response to Parathyroid Hormone

It is accepted that the endothelium mediates the vasodilator actions of a host of vasoactive peptide and nonpeptide substances,[59] and that the mode of mediation involves the synthesis of an endothelium-dependent relaxing factor identified as nitric oxide, the precursor of which is arginine.[60] Pang and colleagues[52] were probably the first to address the question of endothelium dependency in terms of the vasorelaxant effect of PTH-(1-34). Because of their contention that conductance-type arteries are less responsive to PTH, they employed the resistance-like rat tail artery. Helical strips of arteries which had been denuded (via scraping) of endothelial cells were compared to strips with intact endothelium in terms of PTH-(1-34)-induced vasorelaxations. Following precontraction with arginine vasopressin, PTH-(1-34) produced concentration-dependent relaxations that were similar in potency and efficacy with or without endothelium. This result led to the conclusion that the PTH-(1-34)-induced vasorelaxant effect was not endothelium dependent. Using a different vessel (rat aortic strips), Nickols et al.[61] confirmed that the vasodilator action of PTH-(1-34) occurred independently of endothelium in studies of vessels with mechanically disrupted endothelium and those treated with the inhibitor of endothelium-relaxing factor synthesis, nordihydroguaiaretic acid. Additional support for this thesis was provided by Crass et al.[25] using a perfused rat thoracic aorta preparation. Saponin, a surfactant, was used to ensure the complete removal of endothelium from the vessel lumen and stumps of the intercostal arteries. Loss of the vasorelaxant action of acetylcholine was used to assess deendothelialization. Again, PTH-(1-34)-induced vasorelaxation was shown to be independent of an intact endothelium. All of the studies cited above documented endothelium removal by ultrastructural analyses. These findings strongly suggest that the PTH receptor is primarily located on the vascular smooth muscle cell and that vasorelaxation in response to PTH is not a result of the actions of an endothelium-generated relaxing substance.

C. Characterization of the Vascular Parathyroid Hormone Receptor

Pharmacological evidence for the presence of PTH receptors on blood vessels has been obtained from *in vivo* studies in which substituted analogues of PTH-(1-34) were employed. *In vitro* experiments using these analogues in several different blood vessel preparations have provided similar evidence. In addition, these analogues have been useful in interpreting possible adensoine 3′:5′−cyclic phosphate (cAMP) mediation of the vascular response,[50,56,58,62] a topic discussed in Section IIID.

Unlike the PTH receptor of kidney and bone, the receptor on vascular smooth muscle cells has received relatively little attention in terms of its detailed characterization by workers in the field. Orloff and colleagues[63,64] performed covalent labeling of PTH receptors on cultured rat aorta and bovine aorta smooth muscle cells and membranes using a ^{125}I-labeled norleucine derivative of human PTH-(1-34) and cross-linking with disuccinimidyl-suberate. Autoradiography showed that the radioligand labeled a 50 kDa binding form as well as two smaller forms of 25 and 14 kDa. Nickols et al.[65] compared binding of ^{125}I-labeled rat PTH-(1-34) in renal microvessels and tubules. Although density of receptor sites (B_{max}) was slightly greater in tubules, K_D values or affinities were similar (approximately 0.5 nM) in the arteriole-like vessels and tubules. Hill coefficients suggested a one-site model for both. The affinity values were similar to those reported by the Nickols group for the vasorelaxant response to PTH-(1-34) in a perfused rat mesenteric artery preparation.[58] Furthermore, specificity was high in that rat and human calcitonins, calcitonin gene-related peptide (CGRP), rat atrial natriuretic factor (ANF), and vasopressin did not compete. Finally, a more recent study by Ureña et al.[66] examined the tissue distribution of a parathyroid hormone/parathyroid hormone-related protein (PTH/PTHrP) receptor messenger RNA (mRNA). Rat PTH/PTHrP receptor cDNA was used to probe for expression of the receptor employing Northern blot analysis. The receptor transcript was visible in aorta and heart as well as a variety of other tissues, being 2.3 to 2.5 kb in length. Thus, evidence from binding studies and receptor mRNA identification on vascular tissues, coupled with earlier pharmacological and structure-activity relationships, helps to confirm the physiological significance of PTH-induced blood flow changes and related actions on blood pressure regulation.

D. Signal Transduction Mechanisms Involved in the Blood Flow and Hypotensive Actions of Parathyroid Hormone

The documented blood flow and hypotensive effects of PTH *in vivo* and vasorelaxant effects *in vitro*, in concert with the findings of inhibition of inward calcium fluxes by receptor-operated pathways and presence of vascular PTH receptors, lead logically to a discussion of mechanisms involved in transducing receptor activation to vascular smooth muscle contraction. Fruitful research into this question was based on early observations that adenylate cyclase activation and cAMP production in smooth muscle, including vascular (coronary artery) tissue, led to vasodilation[67-69] and mediated bone[70] and kidney[71] effects of PTH.

Lindner et al.[14] were probably the first to provide indirect evidence for the involvement of cAMP in the vasorelaxant effects of PTH. In unanesthetized dogs, these workers observed a 60 to 70% increase in mean renal blood flow after bolus injection of a purified PTH extract and a 40 to 50% increase after injection of PTH-(1-34). By comparison, similar injections of dibutyryl cAMP (dbcAMP) elicited a 75% increase in renal blood flow. Neither PTH nor dbcAMP caused a change in blood pressure, thus the effects appeared to be confined to the renal circulation. Based on their data, a correlation between the cAMP effect and mediation of PTH-induced vasodilation was only speculative. Rambausek et al.[26] demonstrated that PTH-(1-34) increased cAMP production in smooth muscle cells cultured from explants of newborn rabbit aortic media. These workers also noted an increase in cyclic guanosine monophosphate (cGMP) following PTH-(1-34) administration, but from a quantitative standpoint the importance of this cyclic nucleotide in mediating PTH-(1-34)-induced vasorelaxation could be questioned.[72] Using rat cerebral cortex microvessels, Huang et al.[73] reported the first study of PTH effects in brain vessels. Their work demonstrated that a purified parathyroid extract such as PTH-(1-84), PTH-(1-34), and the norleucine-substituted amide form of PTH-(1-34) all stimulated adenylate cyclase activity and cAMP production in the cerebral microvessels. On the other hand, the Nle-substituted amide of bPTH-(3-34) and human PTH-(3-34) did not stimulate adenylate cyclase. bPTH-(3-34), a known competitive antagonist of the hypotensive actions of PTH, reduced stimulation of adenylate cyclase by 36% at equimolar concentrations. PTH-(1-34)-induced cAMP production was markedly enhanced by the addition of guanosine triphosphate (GTP), not inhibited by α- or β-adrenergic blockade, additive with cAMP production by co-present isoproterenol and thus occurred via a separate pathway, and of comparable potency ($ED_{50} = 10$ nM) to that observed with renal cortical membranes.[74] A preliminary note[75] and a later report by Nickols[49] showed that PTH increased cAMP production by as much as tenfold in cultured rat aorta vascular smooth muscle cells, and that the PTH response was potentiated by forskolin and the cAMP phosphodiesterase inhibitor, methylisobutylxanthine. In addition, Nickols demonstrated PTH stimulation of aortic vascular smooth muscle membrane adenylate cyclase activity. Confirming previous findings by Suzuki et al.,[50] Nickols and colleagues[61] demonstrated that isoproterenol, added in the presence of PTH, produced an additive effect on cAMP production, again suggesting that the two cAMP agonists were acting via separate receptor mechanisms. Two groups[53,76] reported no increase in cAMP. Stanton et al.[76] obtained interesting data on PTH-(1-34) effects in cultured bovine aortic vascular smooth muscle cells which showed a decrease in vascular cAMP production within 30 s of PTH(1-34) addition lasting at least 5 min. The duration of the depressed cAMP production was concentration dependent, i.e., the higher the concentration of PTH, the longer the depression of cAMP. Conversely, Nickols[49] reported responses in rat, rabbit, and bovine cultured vascular smooth muscle cells in which tissue cAMP levels increased, in a concentration-dependent fashion, three- to sixfold within 1 min of PTH addition, and continued to increase up to 10 min after the administration of PTH.

Subsequently, the studies of Pang et al.[77] added much credibility to the role of cAMP as a mediator of PTH-induced vasorelaxation in studies using the rat tail artery. These workers showed that PTH fulfilled three of the criteria developed by Sutherland et al.[78] for cAMP involvement as a second messenger by demonstrating, in the arginine vasopressin-contracted tail artery, that dbcAMP produced relaxation; PTH-(1-34)-induced relaxation was potentiated by the phosphodiesterase inhibitor, methylisobutylxanthine; and PTH-(1-34) increased cAMP. The fourth key criterion, that PTH stimulated adenylate cyclase in vascular smooth muscle cell membranes, was demonstrated by others.[49,73] Furthermore, Nickols et al.[61] showed that PTH-(1-34) activated adenylate cyclase of membranes from rat aortas with or without an intact endothelium.

Correlations between vasorelaxation and cAMP concentrations in vascular smooth muscle following PTH addition were performed by Nickols.[49] He showed that methylisobutylxanthine, forskolin, or papaverine, in doses singularly insufficient to elicit vasorelaxation, acted synergistically with PTH to relax rabbit aortic strips. Temporal correlations were also reported[72] in rabbit aortic strips that were quick-frozen in liquid nitrogen at various time intervals after exposure to PTH-(1-34). Within 30 s of the addition of PTH-(1-34), a threefold increase in cAMP was observed which was accompanied by a 10% relaxation. Five minutes after addition of PTH-(1-34), tissue cAMP was increased twofold over basal levels, accompanied by vasorelaxation amounting to 36%. Because the peak cAMP response occurred within 30 s, coupled with a slower onset of relaxation and a time to maximal relaxation of 3 min after PTH-(1-34) addition, an argument could be made that PTH increased cAMP production prior to or coincident with onset of relaxation. Furthermore, neither of the two competitive PTH antagonists, [Nle^8, Nle^{18}, Tyr^{34}]-bPTH-(3-34) or [Nle^8, Nle^{18},Tyr^{34}]-bPTH-(7-34), stimulated cAMP production or vasorelaxation. Others[79,80] have also provided evidence, although not as direct, for correlations between vasorelaxation and cAMP production in response to PTH. The aforementioned evidence strongly supports postreceptor transduction of the vasorelaxant effect by a mechanism involving adenylate cyclase activation and cAMP production. Although GTP, or an analogue thereof, enhanced PTH-induced vasorelaxation,[49,73] little is known of the possible role of postreceptor membrane-bound guanine nucleotide binding proteins (or G proteins). Nevertheless, one can speculate on several possibilities for the mode of action of PTH-induced increments in cAMP concentration in the vascular smooth muscle cell. For example, PTH stimulation of cAMP production could lead to activation of cAMP-dependent protein kinase, which in turn would phosphorylate myosin light chain kinase

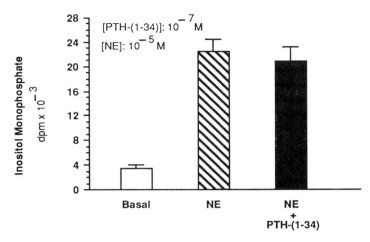

FIGURE 9   Effects of PTH-(1-34) on inositol monophosphate production in rat aorta. Each bar represents the mean ± S.E. (6 segments). See text for details.

(MLCK).[81] By phosphorylating a serine residue in the calmodulin-binding domain of MLCK, the affinity of MLCK for calmodulin is diminished. Another possibility would involve cAMP-mediated stimulation of Ca^{2+} uptake by sarcoplasmic reticulum,[82] perhaps via phosphorylation of the sarcoplasmic reticulum protein, phospholamban.[83] Because norepinephrine-stimulated vascular smooth muscle contractions can be initiated by α_1-adrenoceptor stimulation of both transmembrane Ca^{2+} influx and translocation of bound intracellular Ca^{2+},[84,85] (the latter process involves inositol 1,4,5-trisphosphate [InsP$_3$] formation), and because cAMP reportedly inhibits this process in other types of cells,[86] it is possible that PTH could inhibit this process by virtue of its inhibition of norepinephrine contractions and stimulation of cAMP production in vascular smooth muscle. This possibility was assessed in a preliminary fashion in rat thoracic aorta ring segments. In brief, weighed aortic segments from Sprague-Dawley rats were incubated with ^{3}H-inositol in oxygenated Krebs-Ringer buffer for 90 min. The ring segments were washed repeatedly and individual segments were transferred to tubes containing $10^{-2}\,M$ LiCl with or without $10^{-7}\,M$ PTH-(1-34) in oxygenated buffer for 10 min. The rings were then incubated with or without $10^{-5}\,M$ norepinephrine for 60 min at 37°C and turnover was terminated by addition of 1:2 CHCl$_3$:methanol. Water followed by CHCl$_3$ was added to the tubes and the tubes were centrifuged. An aliquot of upper phase was applied to anion exchange columns containing Dowex 1X anion exchange resin (formate form). Water-soluble ^{3}H-inositol-containing compounds were eluted from these columns with solutions containing increasing concentrations of ammonium formate as described by Berridge et al.[87] The results are shown in Figure 9. As expected, basal inositol monophosphate was increased 6.6-fold in the presence of norepinephrine. In the presence of PTH-(1-34), inositol monophosphate stimulation by norepinephrine was decreased slightly, but the decrease relative to values obtained in the absence of PTH was not statistically significant. Although concentration-response curves would have been appropriate and helpful in the interpretation of these preliminary experiments, the one PTH-(1-34) concentration tested, $10^{-7}\,M$, was selected because it yielded near-maximal vasorelaxation in the rat thoracic aorta.[25] In lieu of additional data present indications are that PTH-(1-34), acting via cAMP or another as yet unidentified pathway(s), may not exert its vasorelaxant effect through inhibition of InsP$_3$ stimulation of internal Ca^{2+} release.

Aside from the ability of norepinephrine to increase intracellular Ca^{2+} concentration, the catecholamine also increased Ca^{2+} sensitivity of the contractile elements.[88-90] Calcium sensitivity of vascular smooth muscle contractile proteins is decreased by dbcAMP.[91] Thus, defining the mechanism of PTH-induced vasorelaxation, a possible role of PTH in decreasing Ca^{2+} sensitivity of the contractile apparatus via cAMP production may be a fruitful area of investigation.

Other studies have provided insight into preferential sites of action of PTH in the inhibition of vascular smooth muscle contraction. Suzuki et al.[50] studied the vasorelaxant action of PTH-(1-34) and a preparation of PTH-(1-84) in helical strips of human and bovine middle cerebral arteries and bovine and porcine basilar arteries, which had been precontracted with prostaglandin $F_{2\alpha}$ ($PGF_{2\alpha}$) or KCl (15 to 20 mM). Their results with bovine cerebral and basilar arteries showed that both PTH-(1-34) and PTH-(1-84) elicited more potent inhibitions of $PGF_{2\alpha}$ contractions than contractions induced by KCl, and only at the highest PTH concentration tested (10^{-7} M) were greater than 10% inhibition of K^+-induced contractions observed in bovine middle cerebral arteries. More recent experiments[25] in the perfused intact rat thoracic aorta showed that PTH-(1-34), in concentrations up to 6×10^{-8} M, did not inhibit 35 mM KCl-induced contractions, but did inhibit contractions induced by norepinephrine, phenylephrine, and arginine vasopressin in a concentration-dependent fashion. Crass and co-workers[25] stated, however, that a substantially higher concentration (6.5×10^{-7} M) of PTH-(1-34) inhibited 35 mM KCl-induced contractions by roughly 50%. In a preliminary report,[92] the vasorelaxant potential of PTH-(1-34) over the concentration range of 10^{-10} to 10^{-7} M was assessed in porcine coronary artery ring segments precontracted with high KCl or $PGF_{2\alpha}$. PTH-(1-34) did not inhibit developed tension induced with high K^+, but readily relaxed $PGF_{2\alpha}$ precontracted segments in a concentration-dependent fashion. Pang and colleagues,[93] studying the actions of PTH-(1-34) in strips of rat tail artery, observed substantially more potent inhibition of arginine vasopressin-induced contractions than those elicited by 60 mM KCl. The above observations with PTH are consistent with other reports[91,94,95] that have shown that vasorelaxation agonists with actions mediated by adenylate cyclase activation and cAMP production inhibit high K^+- or electromechanically induced contractions with less potency as compared to α_1-adrenoceptor- and other pharmacomechanically induced contractions. The reasons for these differences in inhibitory potency of PTH-(1-34) or cAMP relative to high K^+-stimulated vs. agonist-stimulated contractions are not clear, but may relate to the resulting quantitative changes in intracellular Ca^{2+} concentration following stimulation. Abe and Karaki[91] examined a possible correlation between intracellular Ca^{2+} concentrations of rat aorta and inhibition of norepinephrine-induced and high K^+-induced contractions by cAMP. This team noted that inhibition by cAMP was greater when the stimulated intracellular Ca^{2+} concentration was lower, as in the case of norepinephrine.

Finally, another possible site of action of PTH via cAMP could involve the Ca^{2+}-activated K^+ channel (K_{Ca}), with resulting hyperpolarization and vasorelaxation. Recent findings[96] in cultured porcine coronary artery smooth muscle cells provided evidence for the activation of K_{Ca} by direct cAMP activation and indirectly by phosphorylation of the K_{Ca} channel by cAMP-dependent protein kinase. Activation by both direct and indirect modes required the presence of intracellular Ca^{2+}. Direct cAMP activation of K_{Ca} was observed at a physiologically significant intracellular Ca^{2+} concentration of 10^{-6} M, and was specific in that activation was not mimicked by adenosine monophosphate (AMP), adenosine diphosphate (ADP), or adenosine triphosphate (ATP). In a related but slightly different context it is conceivable that operation of the K_{Ca} channel could help to explain why PTH and cAMP exhibit less inhibitory potency on high K^+-induced as compared to agonist-induced vascular contractions. In the high extracellular [K^+]-induced contraction setting the K^+ channels may be kept open, opposing cAMP stimulation of the K_{Ca} channels, and thus depolarization would be maintained. Conversely, normal extracellular K^+ concentrations in the agonist-induced contraction setting would facilitate the hyperpolarizing effect of K_{Ca} channel activation by cAMP.

Thus, although still quite speculative, it would appear that the vascular PTH receptor may be linked, via adenylate cyclase activation and cAMP production, to the inhibition of events at multiple sites which modulate membrane Ca^{2+} channels and perhaps intracellular Ca^{2+} mobilization. Indeed, direct evidence for the inhibition of transmembrane $^{45}Ca^{2+}$ influx in vascular smooth muscle is presented in the next section, and evidence for the direct inhibition of L-type Ca^{2+} channel currents by PTH and cAMP is presented and discussed by other authors in this volume.

E. Actions of Parathyroid Hormone on Calcium Fluxes in Vascular Smooth Muscle

The first experiments to assess possible effects of PTH on vascular Ca^{2+} movements were reported by Schleiffer, Berthelot, and Gairard.[12,13] These workers showed that the incubation of parathyroid extracts with strips of rat aorta resulted in a concentration-related biphasic stimulation of transmembrane $^{45}Ca^{2+}$ flux. Measuring $^{45}Ca^{2+}$ in the lanthanum-resistant fraction of the strips, they showed that low doses of PTH extract stimulated an influx of Ca^{2+} into the cell without enhancing Ca^{2+} efflux, but showed that a tenfold higher dose of PTH decreased influx and stimulated efflux. They viewed the results at the higher dose of PTH which inhibited influx and enhanced efflux of Ca^{2+}, as a correlate with their concomitant assessments of vasorelaxation, in which PTH reduced the slow or tonic phase of norepinephrine-induced contraction without affecting the phasic or rapid initial phase of contraction. This view would be consistent with partial dependence of the tonic phase of tension development on extracellular Ca^{2+}.[97] More recently, Schleiffer and co-workers,[98] using 10^{-10} to $10^{-7} M$ PTH-(1-34) instead of a crude parathyroid extract, demonstrated inhibition of basal Ca^{2+} uptake and a concentration-related inhibition of both high potassium-stimulated uptake (100 mM) and norepinephrine-stimulated $^{45}Ca^{2+}$ uptake. Furthermore, these workers did not observe stimulation of Ca^{2+} efflux by PTH-(1-34) in either aortic strips or cultured aortic myocytes. Pang and colleagues[93] also confirmed PTH-induced inhibition of transmembrane $^{45}Ca^{2+}$ influx using rat tail artery strips stimulated by three different vasoconstrictor agonists: 60 mM KCl, arginine vasopressin, and Bay K-8644. Thus, PTH-(1-34) inhibited Ca^{2+} entry via calcium channels opened by depolarization, receptor-operated mechanisms, or by a mechanism that allowed prolonged opening of the channels (i.e., Bay K-8644). Kawashima,[99] using cultured fetal rat aorta smooth muscle cells, has offered the only conflicting evidence regarding the actions of PTH-(1-34) on Ca^{2+} fluxes in vascular tissue. This study reported that human PTH-(1-34), over the range of 5 to 80 nM, actually increased the cytosular Ca^{2+} concentration and that the increase was abolished in zero calcium media, increased in proportion to the Ca^{2+} concentration of the incubation media, and blocked in the presence of nisoldipine, a Ca^{2+} channel blocker. The nature of these results would seem to suggest that the cultured fetal rat aorta cell line employed did not express the PTH receptor, or that the receptor was otherwise phenotypically changed. Thus, these results do not easily compare with those of others that were obtained using intact vessel segments or cultured vascular smooth muscle cells from other sources, and which uniformly demonstrated inhibition of $^{45}Ca^{2+}$ uptake at similar PTH-(1-34) concentrations. In this context, Bukoski and colleagues[100] did not demonstrate stimulation of $^{45}Ca^{2+}$ uptake in cultured rat mesenteric vascular smooth muscle cells exposed to near-physiological concentrations of PTH (i.e., 200 pM). Furthermore, Pang et al.[101,102] have recently reported quantitative assessments of L-type voltage-dependent Ca^{2+} channels in cultured rat tail artery vascular smooth muscle cells. Although the amount of data using vascular smooth muscle cells reported so far is somewhat limited, they reported 40% or more inhibition of L-type channel activity by bovine PTH-(1-34) in the range of 10^{-7} to $10^{-6} M$. This group[103] also has provided evidence that PTH-(1-34)-induced inhibition of L-type Ca^{2+}

currents may be mediated by cAMP. This work and related studies are described in a separate chapter of this volume.

Thus, the bulk of the evidence cited above and to date clearly indicates PTH-related direct or indirect (or both) inhibition of inward transmembrane Ca^{2+} fluxes which, in concert with other possible cAMP-mediated perturbations of internal Ca^{2+} movements, may help to explain the vasorelaxant effects of the hormone.

IV. CHARACTERIZATION OF THE CARDIAC EFFECTS OF PARATHYROID HORMONE: *IN VITRO* STUDIES

A. Actions of Parathyroid Hormone on Contractile Function

Although evidence for a direct effect of PTH on myocardial contraction in the intact animal is limited, *in vitro* studies have provided further evidence for such effects. The first study was presented in a preliminary report by Tuma et al.[104] that showed that low doses of several different parathyroid extracts produced an increase in contractile force and elicited a positive inotropic effect in isometrically contracting right ventricular papillary muscles of the cat. The effect appeared to be biphasic, as higher doses caused a marked negative inotropism. Using a similar right ventricular papillary muscle preparation from the rat, Katoh and co-workers[105] confirmed this positive inotropic effect at physiological concentrations of PTH-(1-34). The positive inotropic response was concentration-related over the dose range 10^{-12} to $10^{-10} M$ and also tended to be biphasic, because contractility decreased at higher doses of 10^{-9} to $10^{-8} M$. The contractility effect was not evident in the presence of an H_2O_2-denatured parathyroid peptide. Several additional observations in these early studies were of particular interest. For example, the inotropic effect of PTH was partially blocked by propranolol and markedly decreased by prior reserpinization of the donor rats. Interpretation of these combined results indicated that the PTH-(1-34)-induced positive inotropism was in part mediated by endogenous norepinephrine acting via the β-adrenergic receptor. Because no stimulation of adenylate cyclase was observed, it was concluded that PTH per se did not exert its contractile effects directly via the β-adrenoceptor. Finally, Katoh et al.[105] demonstrated that the inotropic effect of PTH was blocked by a Ca^{2+} channel antagonist, indicating the dependence of the contractile effect upon transmembrane Ca^{2+} influx. Kondo et al.[106] reported inotropic effects of PTH-(1-34) in right ventricular papillary muscles from the guinea pig and also examined associated electrophysiological parameters. In electrically driven papillary muscles, the inotropic effect was inhibited by verapamil, and the presence of a β-adrenoceptor blocker had no effect on the contractile response to PTH-(1-34). Voltage-clamp experiments showed that PTH-(1-34) significantly increased the slow inward current, suggesting a stimulatory action on Ca^{2+} flux. Dog ventricular papillary muscles also elicited an increase in contractile tension in response to PTH-(1-34), but ventricular strips of rats, snakes, pigeons, and quail did not, nor did atria from a variety of lower vertebrates.[107] Guinea pig atria have been used as well to assess a possible interaction of PTH with the β-adrenergic-mediated contractile functions in heart.[108] Although PTH-(1-34) was shown to have no inotropic effect in atria of this species per se, it antagonized the effects of agents that inhibit extracellular Ca^{2+} influx and effectively inhibited the cardiodepressant actions of verapamil, a well-known Ca^{2+} antagonist. Tenner and Pang[109] did not observe an effect on atrial or ventricular contractility in isolated rat preparations *in vitro*. Although these findings were similar to those in guinea pig atria,[108] they did not agree with published reports of effects in rat ventricular papillary muscles[104,105] and guinea pig papillary muscles.[106] Sham et al.[110] reported positive inotropic effects in frog atria. Thus, based on data in rats, guinea pigs and frogs, atrial contractile effects of PTH appeared to be species specific, and PTH showed regional ventricular effects, at least for rat and guinea pig.

Hashimoto et al.[57] employed a donor-supported dog heart-lung preparation to assess, among other parameters, possible contractile effects of PTH-(1-34) and an impure PTH-(1-84). PTH-(1-34) or PTH-(1-84) were administered into the left atrium and contractile effects were determined by changes in right atrial pressure and left ventricular dP/dt. Both forms of PTH elicited significantly decreased right atrial pressure development and increased left ventricular dP/dt, each indicative of positive inotropism. Because the β-adrenoceptor blocker, pindolol, did not block the inotropic effect, it appeared that the contractility effect was direct with respect to ventricular myocytes. Accompanying effects included a markedly increased coronary flow without a change in myocardial oxygen consumption. Using an isolated perfused rat heart preparation, Nickols et al.[55] examined changes in left ventricular dP/dt following bolus intraarterial injections of PTH-(1-34). These workers did not observe a statistically significant change in left ventricular contractility after PTH-(1-34) in this isolated denervated rat heart preparation. Thus, the results in rats reported by Nickols et al.[55] and Tenner and Pang[109] are not in agreement with the observations in rat papillary muscles by Tuma et al.[104] and Katoh et al.[105] Hence, a definitive conclusion regarding PTH-(1-34)-induced positive inotropism in rat is not possible with the data available. It should be noted, however, that different strains of rats were used in the studies and, further, that right ventricular papillary muscle responses to PTH in the rat were not indicative of similar responses in the intact rat left ventricle. The results from dog papillary and ventricular muscles[57,107] present a more consistent set of *in vitro* data, suggesting the possibility that the density and/or affinity of PTH receptors on dog ventricular myocytes may be greater as compared to myocytes of other species. Furthermore, *in vitro* findings in dog models were in close agreement with data obtained from dogs *in vivo*.[23]

B. Actions of Parathyroid Hormone on Heart Rate

The data suggesting a direct effect of PTH on cardiac pacemaker function are more consistent in terms of results from a variety of animal species. Probably the first studies designed to assess a possible effect of PTH on heart rate were performed by Larno and colleagues[111] in 1980. Noting the similarity of actions of PTH on heart rate to those of β-adrenoceptor agonists and high Ca^{2+} concentrations, particularly the effects on cAMP production and Ca^{2+} uptake in noncardiovascular tissues, these workers investigated the effects of these stimulatory conditions alone and in concert on beat rate in spontaneously contracting neonatal rat cultured cardiac myocytes. PTH-(1-34) increased beat rate by as much as 40 to 50% over a concentration range of 6×10^{-10} to $1.2 \times 10^{-8} M$. The observed response to PTH was reduced in the presence of a β-adrenoceptor blocker, but because the latter did not abolish the effect of PTH on beat rate, it was concluded that PTH was not interacting directly with the β-adrenoceptor. Indeed, Bogin et al.[112] showed that the PTH effect on beat rate in cultured heart cells was not mediated through β-adrenoceptor activation. It was observed that both PTH-(1-34) and an impure form of PTH-(1-84) stimulated beat rate in dose-related fashion in cultured neonatal rat heart cells. The increase in beat rate was greater with the crude PTH-(1-84) when compared to high doses of PTH-(1-34), and neither form of PTH was active after H_2O_2 treatment. In characterizing this action on the heart cells further Bogin and colleagues observed that PTH-(1-34) transiently stimulated cAMP, a finding which differed from that of Katoh et al.,[105] who observed no stimulation of adenylate cyclase by PTH-(1-34) in a membrane fraction of ventricular homogenates from young rats. In addition, Bogin and co-workers[112] showed that the presence of extracellular Ca^{2+} enhanced PTH-(1-34)-induced stimulation, and, interestingly, the greatest enhancement of beat rate by PTH-(1-34) occurred at the lowest Ca^{2+} concentration tested (0.2 mM). This result suggested that PTH may act to increase Ca^{2+} availability to the cardiac pacemaker. In this context, verapamil essentially abolished the PTH effect on beat rate, and in terms of receptor specificity neither α-adrenergic blockade with phenoxybenzamine nor β-adrenergic blockade with propranolol inhibited PTH stimulation of beat rate. Hashimoto et al.[57] found that the donor-supported dog heart-lung preparation also responded to both PTH-(1-34) and a crude PTH-(1-84) with an increase in heart rate and, like Bogin and associates,[112] these workers observed no effect of β-adrenergic blockade with pindolol on the heart rate response.

Likewise, Tenner et al.[113] showed a marked positive chronotropic effect of PTH-(1-34) in isolated spontaneously beating rat right atria, which was concentration-dependent over a range of 2.5×10^{-9} to 5×10^{-8} M. These *in vitro* experiments showed that the PTH-induced chronotropic response was not significantly reduced in the presence of β-adrenergic blockade with propranolol, and they observed a small increase in atrial cAMP, which appeared to precede onset of the PTH-induced chronotropic response. A further and interesting feature of this study was carried out in the intact anesthetized rat, in which Tenner and co-workers, like others,[17,23,46,47] observed an increased heart rate in conjunction with the hypotension induced by intravenous PTH-(1-34). Using propranolol pretreatment to determine if this change in heart rate was due entirely to reflex adrenergic activity, the results of Tenner and colleagues[113] showed that a portion of the PTH-induced chronotropic response remained, thus providing new and helpful evidence in the intact animal setting that PTH does indeed directly stimulate pacemaker function in rat heart. The positive chronotropic action of PTH-(1-34) has been confirmed in a variety of terrestrial vertebrates by Sham and co-workers.[107,110] Kondo et al.[106] used electrophysiological techniques to analyze the positive chronotropic action of PTH-(1-34) in spontaneously beating rabbit sinus node cells. PTH-(1-34), at 10^{-7} M, increased the spontaneous firing rate, which was accompanied by an increase in the maximum upstroke velocity of the sinus node cell action potential. These effects on firing rate and maximum upstroke velocity were abolished by pretreatment with verapamil, but neither rate function parameter was affected by pretreatment with a β-adrenoceptor blocker at doses that completely blocked similar actions of isoprenaline, a β-adrenoceptor agonist. Finally, Nickols et al.[55] confirmed the validity of the chronotropic effect of PTH by demonstrating a stimulation of heart rate in isolated perfused rat hearts. Their results in a denervated preparation, along with those of Tenner et al.[113] in propranolol-pretreated intact rats, seem to provide clear support for a direct action of PTH on pacemaker function.

With the evidence that PTH has demonstrable effects on cardiac muscle, an obvious necessity arises to characterize the presumed presence of PTH receptors as well as postreceptor signaling mechanisms in this tissue. Unfortunately, little information on these subjects is available, although evidence for PTH receptors in heart has been reported by Ureña et al.[66] in 1993. As discussed in the section on the vascular PTH receptor, these investigators identified a PTH/PTHrP receptor mRNA in rat heart. The receptor transcript was visible in heart, being 2.3 to 2.5 kb in length. The mechanism(s) which may lead to expression of the receptor in heart and the related function(s) of these mRNAs remain to be elucidated. That stimulation of Ca^{2+} entry into cardiac myocytes or pacemaker cells may in part define the mechanism of PTH action in heart muscle has been implied in previously discussed work.[105,106,108,112]

The actions of PTH-(1-34) on L-type Ca^{2+} channel activity in neonatal rat ventricular cells were studied using whole cell voltage-clamp techniques.[114,115] The L-type Ca^{2+} channel in heart may be a principal route for Ca^{2+} entry into cardiac myocytes, and thus is a mechanism for increasing the intracellular Ca^{2+} concentration associated with activating the contractile apparatus. Wang and colleagues[114] have shown marked enhancement of L-type Ca^{2+} channel activity by PTH-(1-34) and demonstrated inhibition of this activity using the Ca^{2+} channel blocker, nifedipine. Another report by this group[103] examined a possible key role for cAMP in mediating the stimulatory actions of PTH-(1-34) on the L-type Ca^{2+} channel. Using the patch-clamp technique with cultured neonatal rat ventricular myocytes, these workers showed that 10^{-6} M dbcAMP, like PTH-(1-34), increased L-type channel currents, and that these effects individually were additive. Rampe et al.[115] also reported activation of L-type Ca^{2+} channels at somewhat lower, near-physiologic concentrations of PTH. They observed enhanced Ca^{2+} uptake, which was statistically significant at 300 pM and, as in Wang's studies, inhibited by nifedipine. Of further interest, PTH-(1-34) increased ventricular myocyte cAMP levels, albeit slightly, again suggesting the possibility of cAMP modulation of PTH-(1-34) actions on L-type Ca^{2+} channel activity. These exciting studies on the L-type Ca^{2+} channel are discussed in detail in Chapter 3 of this volume.

V. POSSIBLE MODULATING ROLE OF CALCITONIN ON THE CARDIOVASCULAR ACTIONS OF PARATHYROID HORMONE

The role of calcitonin in calcium homeostasis and balance has been widely recognized;[116] its actions on classical target sites in kidney, bone, and small intestine are generally opposite those of PTH. On the other hand, solid evidence for direct cardiovascular actions of calcitonin per se is lacking, but a variety of reports, albeit conflicting, nevertheless have suggested effects of the hormone on cardiac function as well as possible vascular and blood pressure effects. For example, reports have variously indicated positive, negative, or no inotropic effects,[19,117,118] and conflicting data have been reported for effects on heart rate.[19,117,119] Most reports indicate no chronotropic effects. Although chronic salmon calcitonin administration reportedly[120] decreased blood pressure in deoxycorticosterone/saline hypertensive rats, more recent studies by Wegener and McCarron,[121] using SHR and WKY rats, and Peguero-Rivera and Corder,[119] using WKY rats, indicated no statistically significant effects (using $p < 0.05$ as level of significance) of calcitonin on blood pressure under conditions ranging from chronic vs. acute administration of the hormone, to anesthetized vs. awake animals, and to various sources of calcitonin including those of the human and salmon types. Of interest, however, was the observation[122] that salmon calcitonin inhibited basal renin release from rat kidney slices, and because verapamil restored renin secretion it was inferred that inhibition of renin release was dependent on stimulation of transmembrane Ca^{2+} influx. Some earlier evidence exists that supports this contention.[123]

Despite the essentially negative findings in direct cardiac and systemic cardiovascular effects of calcitonin, the possibility of local hemodynamic effects of the hormone cannot be excluded. Indeed, Driessens and Vanhoutte[20] demonstrated a potent vasoconstrictor effect of calcitonin in a perfused dog tibial preparation *in vitro*. In 1972, Charbon and Pieper[124] reported that calcitonin from various sources partially inhibited PTH extract-induced celiac/hepatic and renal arterial vasodilation in dogs. As these workers did not observe effects of intravenously administered calcitonin on celiac/hepatic or renal blood flows, they postulated that calcitonin may have exerted a type of noncompetitive antagonism on the mechanism of PTH-induced vasodilation. One exception to the above was that synthetic human calcitonin did not inhibit but actually stimulated PTH-induced blood flow in both regional vascular beds. Subsequently, Moore et al.[19] examined the effects of salmon calcitonin on coronary and hepatic blood flow in the dog. These experiments showed that salmon calcitonin was highly vasoactive in the two regional circulations. Calcitonin elicited a dose-related vasoconstriction and calculated increase in vascular resistance of the coronary circulation with or without propranolol pretreatment. In propranolol-treated dogs, the calcitonin-elicited vasoconstriction was quantitatively similar to that induced by norepinephrine. Contrary to the findings of Charbon and Pieper,[124] Moore and co-workers observed a dose-related increase in directly measured hepatic arterial blood flow by calcitonin. Furthermore, pretreatment of the dogs with calcitonin resulted in an augmentation of PTH-(1-34)-induced coronary vasodilation as well as a similar augmentation of PTH-(1-34)-stimulated hepatic arterial vasodilation. The latter observation seemed to be consistent with data presented by Charbon and Pieper[124] specific to their experiments with synthetic human calcitonin, but not with calcitonin from other sources. The mechanisms involved in calcitonin-induced coronary vasoconstriction and, conversely, hepatic vasodilation have not been elucidated but strongly imply regional differences in the effects of calcitonin on vascular smooth muscle Ca^{2+} fluxes. The nature of the regional augmentation effects of calcitonin on PTH-induced vasodilation remains to be studied.

VI. PARATHYROID HORMONE IN CARDIOVASCULAR PATHOPHYSIOLOGY

A. Possible Cardioprotective Actions of Parathyroid Hormone in Acute Cardiac Failure and Cardiogenic Shock and in Experimental Myocardial Ischemia

Based on the cardiovascular actions of PTH discussed previously, including coronary vasodilation and dilation of other regional vascular beds leading to a decreased peripheral vascular resistance and hypotension, several studies have been performed with the intent of assessing possible cardioprotective actions of the hormone in ischemic dog models.

In the first of these studies[125], two groups of instrumented, open-chest, pharmacologically sympathectomized dogs were studied. A control group of animals, in which a stepwise occlusion of the left anterior descending coronary artery (LAD) was performed, was observed for 4 h, during which the dogs developed acute myocardial ischemia, leading to symptoms of left ventricular failure and cardiogenic shock. A 72% decline in cardiac index, a 68% decline in mean arterial blood pressure, and an increase in mean left atrial pressure >200% were indicative of left ventricular failure and shock. In a second group of dogs, an intravenous infusion of PTH-(1-34) was begun 30 min after onset of ischemia and continued for the remaining 4-h experimental period. PTH-(1-34) infusion resulted in a marked improvement in cardiac index, stabilization of mean arterial pressure, and a substantial reduction in left atrial pressure. Furthermore, no change in blood lactate was observed in the PTH-(1-34)-treated group, whereas lactate was increased up to threefold in the control group during the last 2 h of the ischemic period. These reported improvements in cardiodynamics in the PTH-(1-34)-treated group were associated with substantial reductions in ischemia-induced damage to the myocardium. Methylene blue was used to delineate the area at risk of infarction, and incubation of myocardial tissue with triphenyl tetrazolium chloride was employed to distinguish between viable myocardium and infarcted tissue. PTH-(1-34) appeared capable, under the conditions cited, of eliciting a substantial reduction in infarction size, an apparent result of significant improvements in cardiodynamics and avoidance of cardiogenic shock.

In a related study performed by Feola and Crass,[126] a different experimental design was used to assess possible effects of PTH-(1-34) in acute myocardial ischemia. As before, pentobarbital-anesthetized, instrumented, open-chest dogs were used. The LAD artery was permanently ligated. Two randomly assigned groups were formed in which one group received a low dose intracoronary (left circumflex artery) infusion of PTH-(1-34) for 10 min at 30-min intervals beginning 30 min post-LAD occlusion and continuing in this pattern for 5 h. The second, control group did not receive PTH-(1-34) under otherwise identical conditions. Using techniques for assessing myocardial mass at risk and mass of infarction similar to those of the Feola et al.[125] study, it was reported that PTH-(1-34) treatment resulted in a reduction in the percentage of the area at risk which infarcted from 75% in controls to 25% in the treated group. Caution in interpreting both of the above-mentioned studies seems warranted in light of a more recent report by Conway et al.[127] Although they did not precisely reproduce the conditions of the earlier studies,[125,126] confirmatory evidence that PTH-(1-34) possessed cardioprotective action when administered in the ischemic setting in pentobarbital-anesthetized dogs was provided. Their data, although lacking statistical significance due to variability in the groups, showed that PTH-(1-34) elicited an apparent decrease of approximately 36% in infarcted risk area. Of considerable interest is that Conway and co-workers[127] showed that the same experimental design in dogs anesthetized with α-chloralose did not display a PTH-(1-34)-related reduction in infarct size — indeed, infarct size in treated animals appeared greater than that of controls. They proposed that the different anesthetics may have partially accounted for the discrepant results, suggesting greater retention of sympathetic activity in α-chloralose animals and, further, that PTH-(1-34), when administered in the ischemic setting in α-chloralose dogs, may have induced a steal phenomenon favoring nonischemic zones at the expense of ischemic regions. The results of this study, without negating the potential cardioprotective actions of PTH, suggested that the model of experimental myocardial ischemia is critical in assessing cardioprotective actions of vasodilator peptides and other agents. Additional studies in chronic awake animals and in the isolated perfused ischemic heart preparation would be helpful in clarifying the existing observations.

B. Possible Role of Parathyroid Hormone in the Cardiovascular Manifestations of Renal Failure

Secondary hyperparathyroidism is a common feature of patients with renal failure.[128,129] A variety of cardiovascular abnormalities are also associated with renal failure,[130] which can include ischemic heart disease, hypertension, and increases in afterload and preload. Indeed, uremic cardiomyopathy with associated disorders of ventricular function is probably the leading cause of mortality in patients with end-stage renal disease. Although the origin of uremic cardiomyopathy may be multifaceted,[131,132] it has been argued that the increased blood levels of PTH together with PTH-mediated changes in myocardial Ca^{2+} handling, heart rate, and myocardial metabolism may be key toxic factors in uremia.[133,134] Some studies[135] have shown that myocardial function in uremic patients improved following parathyroidectomy. Indirect and direct evidence for PTH-enhanced myocardial Ca^{2+} uptake in animals has been reported in References 105, 106, 108, 112, 114, and 115 and discussed previously in this chapter. That this effect of PTH could lead directly to myocardial calcification in renal failure with attending secondary hyperparathyroidism has not been shown, at least in certain patient studies.[136] However, Rostand et al.[136] did support the concept of generally poor control of calcium and phosphorus as a precipitating factor in the myocardial calcification of renal failure.

Several recent studies have not supported the idea of a direct role for PTH in the induction of the depressed cardiovascular function associated with renal disease. For example, in patients with end-stage renal disease, Gafter et al.[137] concluded that secondary hyperparathyroidism had little effect on cardiac function, and parathyroidectomy did not ameliorate cardiac performance over the long term. In a 1993 review of factors that depress cardiac function in various stages of renal disease, Hörl and Riegel[138] said, "Secondary hyperparathyroidism appears not to be a clinically relevant myocardial depressant factor (MDF) in uremia." Finally, Fellner et al.[139] studied a group of hemodialysis patients before and after parathyroidectomy and concluded that PTH did not have direct effects on cardiac contractile function in these patients.

Thus, despite early evidence to the contrary, recent and mostly clinical studies are not very supportive of the concept that the cardiotoxicity of uremia is a manifestation of altered parathyroid physiology as regards direct effects of PTH on the heart.

C. Areas of Possible Parathyroid Hormone Involvement in Cardiovascular Pathophysiology Not Covered in this Chapter

Subject areas closely related to the cardiovascular effects of PTH include the actions of PTH in experimental and clinical forms of hypertension and the occurrence and characterization of a parathyroid hypertensive factor. These topics have been intentionally omitted from the present chapter because they are discussed in detail and with considerable expertise by authors of other chapters in this volume.

VII. SUMMARY AND CONCLUSIONS

Parathyroid hormone, in a variety of forms ranging from crude parathyroid extracts to synthetically pure forms of the hormone, has potent and efficacious vasodilator effects which have been observed in numerous animal species and in different regional circulations. Thus, it follows that PTH is a strong hypotensive agent. In addition, the hormone has direct actions on the heart. These varied cardiovascular actions were shown to be specific and were observed at doses or concentrations which were not calcemic. The synthetically pure amino terminal 1-34 peptide fragment of the parent 84-amino acid polypeptide hormone, which contains all of the biological activity of the hormone, has been available commercially for many years and is widely used in characterization studies.

In vivo the coronary and hepatic circulations were shown to be the most sensitive and responsive to the vasodilator actions of PTH, although blood flow responses were observed in renal, mesenteric, and other circulations. The coronary vasodilator response was uniform in transmural (endocardium/epicardium) blood flow, and the regional blood flow response and hypotensive action occurred independent of other agonist-mediated vasodilator systems. Structure-activity studies have shown that the parent hormone, or PTH-(1-84), and PTH-(1-34) were roughly comparable in terms of vasodilator potency and efficacy, that the amino acids at positions 1 and 2 were required, but that the methionyl residues at positions 8 and 18 and the phenylalanyl residue at position 34 were not required for full vasodilator and hypotensive activity. The amino acids at positions 25 to 27 may be critical sites for binding of the hormone. Comparison of PTH with substance P, VIP, and bradykinin in vasodilator action in the coronary circulation of the dog indicated that PTH-(1-34) had comparable potency and efficacy with respect to VIP and bradykinin but was less potent, although more efficacious, than substance P. Duration of the PTH-induced coronary vasodilation and hypotensive actions tended to be greater than that of the other vasodilator/hypotensive peptides. PTH-(1-34) was also more potent as a coronary vasodilator than adenosine, nifedipine, diltiazem, and verapamil. Studies in the intact animal suggested that PTH increased myocardial contractile function, heart rate, and, in some reports, cardiac output. These studies in both anesthetized and unanesthetized animals did not indicate clearly whether the actions on the heart were of a direct nature or were adrenergically mediated events occurring in secondary fashion to PTH-induced hypotension.

Vasorelaxation studies *in vitro* confirmed the vasodilator actions of PTH *in vivo*. The vasorelaxant effect was not endothelium-dependent, indicating a probable location of the PTH receptor on the vascular smooth muscle cell. Characterization of the PTH receptor of vascular smooth muscle has received relatively little attention. Covalent labeling of vascular PTH receptors with a labeled PTH(1-34) analogue and binding studies in renal microvessels have documented the presence of the receptor and its specificity. Also, PTH/PTHrP receptor transcripts have been identified in rat aorta. The principal mode of postreceptor transduction following PTH receptor activation involves adenylate cyclase activation with resulting cAMP production. Interaction of PTH with its receptor may result in a more potent inhibition of pharmacomechanically induced contractions as compared to contractions induced by depolarization. Available data indicate that the inhibition of $InsP_3$ production is not a major pathway of action of PTH in terms of vasorelaxation. PTH-(1-34) clearly inhibits inward transmembrane Ca^{2+} fluxes, and recent evidence demonstrates inhibition of L-type Ca^{2+} channels in vascular smooth muscle cells.

In vitro experiments have not consistently shown direct positive inotropic effects of PTH, but convincing evidence for positive chronotropic actions of PTH-(1-34) has been obtained, thus clarifying results from *in vivo* studies. The cardiac muscle PTH receptor has not been characterized with appropriate binding studies, but a PTH/PTHrP receptor mRNA has been identified in rat heart. Similarly, postreceptor transduction systems have not been thoroughly studied, although a few reports indicated mediation via cAMP production. It is clear that PTH stimulates inward transmembrane Ca^{2+} flux in cardiac muscle. Recent evidence shows stimulation of L-type Ca^{2+} channel activity by PTH-(1-34).

Experimental evidence for a cardioprotective action in the ischemic myocardium has been presented, but must be interpreted with caution. Also, the purported role of PTH as a uremic toxin has been discussed in light of recent findings.

The reader is referred to a comprehensive review, published in 1989 by Mok et al.,[140] which includes a helpful discussion of research developments on PTH effects in uterine, tracheal, and gastrointestinal smooth muscle.

Finally, I have noted the exciting emergence of literature on PTHrP, which possesses cardiovascular actions similar to those of PTH. The reader is referred to the detailed chapter on PTHrP in this volume.

REFERENCES

1. Collip, J. B. and Clark, E. P., Further studies on the physiological action of a parathyroid hormone, *J. Biol. Chem.*, 64, 485, 1925.
2. Handler, P., Cohn, D. V., and DeMaria, W. J. A., Effect of parathyroid extract on renal excretion of phosphate, *Am. J. Physiol.*, 165, 434, 1951.
3. Handler, P. and Cohn, D. V., Effect of parathyroid extract on renal function, *Am. J. Physiol.*, 169, 188, 1952.
4. Charbon, G. A. and Hoekstra, M. H., The influence of parathyroid extract on the sodium excretion, *Arch. Int. Pharmacodyn.*, 141, 1, 1963.
5. Charbon, G. A., A diuretic and hypotensive action of a parathyroid extract, *Acta Physiol. Pharmacol. Neerl.*, 14, 1, 1963.
6. Charbon, G. A., Brummer, F., and Reneman, R. S., Diuretic and vascular action of parathyroid extracts in animals and man, *Arch. Int. Pharmacodyn.*, 171, 1, 1968.
7. Charbon, G. A., Parathormone — a selective vasodilator, in *Parathyroid Hormone and Thyrocalcitonin (Calcitonin)*, Int. Congr. Ser. No. 159, Talmadge, R. V. and Belanger, L. F., Eds., Exerpta Medica, Amsterdam, 1968, 475.
8. Charbon, G. A., A rapid and selective vasodilator effect of parathyroid hormone, *Eur. J. Pharmacol.*, 3, 275, 1968.
9. Charbon, G. A., Vasodilator action of parathyroid hormone used as bioassay, *Arch. Int. Pharmacodyn.*, 178, 296, 1969.
10. Charbon, G. A. and Hulstaert, P. F., Augmentation of arterial hepatic and renal flow by extracted and synthetic parathyroid hormone, *Endocrinology*, 95, 621, 1974.
11. Berthelot, A. and Gairard, A., Effet de la parathormone sur la pression arterielle et la contraction de l'aorte isolee de rat, *Experientia*, 31, 457, 1975.
12. Schleiffer, R., Berthelot, A., and Gairard, A., Effects of parathyroid extract on blood pressure and arterial contraction and on ^{45}Ca exchange in isolated aorta in the rat, *Blood Vessels*, 16, 220, 1979.
13. Schleiffer, R., Berthelot, A., and Gairard, A., Action of parathyroid extract on arterial blood pressure and on contraction and ^{45}Ca exchange in isolated aorta of the rat, *Eur. J. Pharmacol.*, 58, 163, 1979.
14. Lindner, A., Tremann, J. A., Plantier, J., Chapman, W., Forrey, A. W., Haines, G., and Palmieri, G. M., Effects of parathyroid hormone on the renal circulation and renin secretion in unanesthetized dogs, *Min. Elect. Metab.*, 1, 155, 1978.

15. Pang, P. K. T., Tenner, T. E., Yee, J. A., Yang, M., and Janssen, H. F., Hypotensive action of parathyroid hormone preparations on rats and dogs, *Proc. Natl. Acad. Sci. U.S.A.*, 77, 675, 1980.

16. Pang, P. K. T., Janssen, H. F., and Yee, J. A., Effects of synthetic parathyroid hormone on vascular beds of dogs, *Pharmacology*, 21, 213, 1980.

17. Wang, H.-H., Drugge, E. D., Yen, Y.-C., Blumenthal, M. R., and Pang, P. K. T., Effects of synthetic parathyroid hormone on hemodynamics and regional blood flows, *Eur. J. Pharmacol.*, 97, 209, 1984.

18. Crass, M. F., III, Jayaseelan, C. L., and Darter, T. C., Effects of parathyroid hormone on blood flow in different regional circulations, *Am. J. Physiol.*, 253(Reg. Integrative Comp. Physiol. 22), R634, 1987.

19. Moore, P. L., Strickland, M. L., and Crass, M. F., III, Vasoactive characteristics of calcitonin in coronary and hepatic circulations, *J. Hypertens.*, 4(Suppl. 5), S186, 1986.

20. Driessens, M. and Vanhoutte, P. M., Effect of calcitonin, hydrocortisone, and parathyroid hormone on canine blood vessels, *Am. J. Physiol.*, 241(Heart Circ. Physiol. 10), H91, 1981.

21. Roca-Cusachs, A., DiPette, D. J., and Nickols, G. A., Regional and systemic hemodynamic effects of parathyroid hormone-related protein: preservation of cardiac function and coronary and renal flow with reduced blood pressure, *J. Pharmacol. Exp. Ther.*, 256, 110, 1991.

22. Crass, M. F., III and Pang, P. K. T., Parathyroid hormone: a coronary artery vasodilator, *Science*, 207, 1087, 1980.

23. Crass, M. F., III, Moore, P. L., Strickland, M. L., Pang, P. K. T., and Citak, M. S., Cardiovascular responses to parathyroid hormone, *Am. J. Physiol.*, 249(Endocrinol. Metab. 12), E187, 1985.

24. Yang, M. C. M. and Pang, P. K. T., Vascular actions of parathyroid hormone, in *Comparative Endocrinology of Calcium Regulation*, Oguro, C. and Pang, P. K. T., Eds., Japan Scientific Society Press, Tokyo, 19, 219, 1982.

25. Crass, M. F., III, Hulsey, S. M and Bulkley, T. J., Use of a new pulsatile perfused rat aorta preparation to study the characteristics of the vasodilator effect of parathyroid hormone, *J. Pharmacol. Exp. Ther.*, 245, 723, 1988.

26. Rambausek, M., Ritz, E., Rascher, W., Kreusser, W., Mann, J. F., Kreye, V. A., and Mehls, O., Vascular effects of parathyroid hormone (PTH), *Adv. Exp. Med. Biol.*, 151, 619, 1982.

27. Saglikes, Y., Massry, S. G., Iseki, K., Nadler, J. L., and Campese, V. M., Effect of PTH on blood pressure and response to vasoconstrictor agonists, *Am. J. Physiol.*, 248(Renal Fluid Electrolyte Physiol. 17), F674, 1985.

28. Pang, P. K. T., Wang, M. C. M., Kenny, A. D., and Tenner, T. E., Structure and vascular activity relationships of parathyroid hormone and some hypotensive peptides, *Clin. Exp. Hyper. Theor. Pract.*, A4(1–2), 189, 1982.

29. Pang, P. K. T., Yang, M. C. M., Keutmann, H. T., and Kenny, A. D., Structure activity relationship of parathyroid hormone: separation of the hypotensive and the hypercalcemic properties, *Endocrinology*, 112, 284, 1983.

30. McCarron, D. A., Ellison, D. H., and Anderson, S., Vasodilation mediated by human PTH (1-34) in the spontaneously hypertensive rat, *Am. J. Physiol.*, 246(Renal Fluid Electrolyte Physiol. 15), F96, 1984.

31. Rosenblatt, M., Goltzman, D., Keutmann, H. T., Tregear, G. W., and Potts, J. T., Chemical and biological properties of synthetic sulfur-free analogues of parathyroid hormone, *J. Biol. Chem.*, 251, 159, 1976.

32. Rosenblatt, M., Peptide hormone antagonists that are effective in vivo — lessons from parathyroid hormone, *N. Engl. J. Med.*, 315, 1004, 1986.

33. Horiuchi, N. and Rosenblatt, M., Evaluation of a parathyroid hormone antagonist in an in vivo multiparameter bioassay, *Am. J. Physiol.*, 253(Endocrinol. Metab. 16), E187, 1987.

34. Segre, G. V., Rosenblatt, M., Tully, G. L., III, Laugharn, J., Reit, B., and Potts, J. T., Evaluation of an in vitro parathyroid hormone antagonist in vivo in dogs, *Endocrinology*, 116, 1024, 1985.

35. Rosenblatt, M. and Potts, J. T., Design and synthesis of parathyroid hormone analogues of enhanced biological activity, *Endocr. Res. Commun.*, 4, 115, 1977.

36. Ellison, D. and McCarron, D. A., Structural pre-requisites for the hypotensive action of parathyroid hormone, *Am. J. Physiol.*, 246(Renal Fluid Electrolyte Physiol. 15), F551, 1984.

37. Hong, B.-S., Yang, M. C. M., Liang, J. N., and Pang, P. K. T., Correlation of structured changes in parathyroid hormone with its vascular action, *Peptides*, 7(6), 1131, 1986.

38. Pang, P. K. T., Yang, M. C. M., Tenner, T. E., Chang, J. K., and Shimizu, M., Hypotensive action of synthetic fragments of parathyroid hormone, *J. Pharmacol. Exp. Ther.*, 216, 567, 1981.

39. Rosenblatt, M., Segre, G. V., Tyler, G. A., Shepard, G. L., Nussbaum, S. R., and Potts, J. R., Identification of a receptor-binding region in parathyroid hormone, *Endocrinology*, 107, 545, 1980.

40. Draper, M. W., The structure of parathyroid hormone: its effects on biological action, *Min. Electrolyte Metab.*, 8, 159, 1982.

41. Tenner, T. E., Yang, C. M., Chang, J. K., Schimizu, M., and Pang, P. K. T., Pharmacological comparison of bPTH-(1-34) and other hypotensive peptides in the dog, *Peptides*, 1(4), 285, 1980.

42. Crass, M. F., III, Citak, M. S., Strickland, M.L., and Moore, P. L., Cardiovascular effects of parathyroid hormone in the dog: a comparison with adenosine, *Proc. West. Pharmacol. Soc.*, 29, 5, 1986.

43. Crass, M. F., III, Comparison of the cardiovascular effects of parathyroid hormone with those of nifedipine, verapamil and diltiazem, *Fed. Proc.*, 44(Abstr.), 1643, 1985.

44. Rubio, R., Berne, R. M., and Katori, M., Release of adenosine in reactive hyperemia of the dog heart, *Am. J. Physiol.*, 216, 56, 1969.

45. Daugirdas, J. T., Al-Kudsi, R. R., Ing, T. S., Yang, M. C. M., Leehey, D. J., and Pang, P. K. T., Hemodynamic effects of bPTH (1-34) and its analogue Nle^{8,18} Tyr^{34}bPTH (3-34) amide, *Min. Electrolyte Metab.*, 13, 33, 1987.

46. Jordan, L. R., Dallemagne, C. R., and Cross, R. B., Cardiovascular effects of parathyroid hormone in conscious sheep, *Exp. Physiol.*, 76, 251, 1991.

47. Kishimoto, H., Tsumura, K., Fujioka, S., Uchimoto, S., Yamashita, N., Suzuki, R., Yoshimaru, K., Shimura, M., Sasakawa, O., and Morii, H., Effects of parathyroid hormone-related protein on systemic and regional hemodynamics in conscious rats. A comparison with human parathyroid hormone, in *Calcium-Regulating Hormones, Part I, Role in Disease and Aging*, Morii, H., Ed., S. Karger, Basel, 1991, 72.

48. Smith, J. M., Mouw, D. R., and Vander, A. J., Effect of parathyroid hormone on plasma renin activity and sodium excretion, *Am. J. Physiol.*, 236(Fluid Electrolyte Physiol. 3), F311, 1979.

49. Nickols, G. A., Increased cyclic AMP in cultured vascular smooth muscle cells and relaxation of aortic strips by parathyroid hormone, *Eur. J. Pharmacol.*, 116, 137, 1985.

50. Suzuki, Y., Lederis, K., Huang, M., LeBlanc, F. E., and Rorstad, O. P., Relaxation of bovine, porcine and human brain arteries by parathyroid hormone, *Life Sci.*, 33, 2497, 1983.

51. Crass, M. F., III and Brewer, K. S., Vasorelaxant effect of parathyroid hormone on isolated segments of porcine coronary artery, *Artery*, 15(2), 61, 1988.

52. Pang, P. K. T., Yang, M. C. M., Shew, R., and Tenner, T. E., The vasorelaxant action of parathyroid hormone fragments on isolated rat tail artery, *Blood Vessels*, 22, 57, 1985.

53. Winquist, R. J., Baskin, E. P., and Vlasuk, G. P., Synthetic tumor- derived human hypercalcemic factor exhibits parathyroid hormone-like vasorelaxation in renal arteries, *Biochem. Biophys. Res. Commun.*, 149, 227, 1987.

54. Trizna, W. and Edwards, R. M., Relaxation of renal arterioles by parathyroid hormone and parathyroid hormone-related protein, *Pharmacology*, 42, 91, 1991.

55. Nickols, G. A., Nana, A. D., Nickols, M. A., DiPette, D. J., and Asimakis, G. K., Hypotension and cardiac stimulation due to the parathyroid hormone-related protein, humeral hypercalcemia of malignancy factor, *Endocrinology*, 125, 834, 1989.

56. Musso, M.-J., Barthelmebs, M., Imbs, J.-L., Plante, M., Bollack, C., and Helwig, J.-J., The vasodilator action of parathyroid hormone fragments on isolated perfused rat kidney, *Naunyn-Schmiedeberg's Arch. Pharmacol.*, 340, 246, 1989.

57. Hashimoto, K., Nakagawa, Y., Shibuya, T., Satoh, H., Ushijima, T., and Imai, S., Effects of parathyroid hormone and related polypeptides on the heart and coronary circulation of dogs, *J. Cardiovasc. Pharmacol.*, 3, 668, 1981.

58. Nickols, G. A., Metz, M. A., and Cline, W. H., Jr., Vasodilation of the rat mesenteric vasculature by parathyroid hormone, *J. Pharmacol. Exp. Ther.*, 236, 419, 1986.

59. Furchgott, R. F. and Zawadski, J. V., The obligatory role of endothelial cells in the relaxation of arterial smooth muscle by acetylcholine, *Nature*, 288, 373, 1980.

60. Sakuma, I., Stuehr, D. J., Gross, S., Nathan, C., and Levi, R., Identification of arginine as a precursor of endothelium-derived relaxing factor, *Proc. Natl. Acad. Sci. U.S.A.*, 85, 8664, 1988.

61. Nickols, G. A., Metz, M. A., and Cline, W. H., Jr., Endothelium-independent linkage of parathyroid hormone receptors of rat vascular tissue with increased adenosine 3′,5′-monophosphate and relaxation of vascular smooth muscle, *Endocrinology*, 119, 349, 1986.

62. Helwig, J.-J., Yang, M. C. M., Bollack, C., Judes, C., and Pang, P. K. T., Structure-activity relationship of parathyroid hormone: relative sensitivity of rabbit renal microvessel and tubule adenylate cyclases to oxidized PTH and PTH inhibitors, *Eur. J. Pharmacol.*, 140, 247, 1987.

63. Orloff, J. J., Wu, T. L., Goumas, D., and Stewart, A. F., Receptors for parathyroid hormone-like peptide in vascular smooth muscle, *Clin. Res.*, 37(Abstr.), 457a, 1989.

64. Orloff, J. J., Wu, T. L., and Stewart, A. F., Parathyroid hormone-like proteins: biochemical responses and receptor interactions, *Endocrinol. Rev.*, 10, 476, 1989.

65. Nickols, G. A., Nickols, M. A., and Helwig, J.-J., Binding of parathyroid hormone and parathyroid hormone-related protein to vascular smooth muscle of rabbit renal microvessels, *Endocrinology*, 126, 721, 1990.

66. Ureña, P., Kong, X.-F., Abou-samra, A.-B., Jüppner, H., Kronenberg, H. M., Potts, J. T., and Segre, G. V., Parathyroid hormone PTH/PTH-related peptide receptor messenger ribonucleic acids are widely distributed in rat tissues, *Endocrinology*, 133, 617, 1993.

67. Vegesna, R. V. K. and Diamond, J., Effects of isoproterenal and forskolin on tension, cyclic AMP levels, and cyclic AMP dependent protein kinase activity in bovine coronary artery, *Can. J. Physiol. Pharmacol.*, 62, 1116, 1984.

68. Hardman, J. G., Cyclic nucleotides and smooth muscle contraction: some conceptual and experimental considerations, in *Smooth Muscle: An Assessment of Current Knowledge*, Bulbring, E., Brading, A. F., Jones, A. W., and Tomita, T., Eds., University of Texas Press, Austin, 1981, 249.

69. Adelstein, R. S., Conti, M. A., Hathaway, D. R., and Klee, C. B., Phosphorylation of smooth muscle myosin light chain kinase by the catalytic subunit of adnosine 3′:5′-monophosphate-dependent protein kinase, *J. Biol. Chem.*, 253, 8347, 1978.

70. Chase, L. R., Fedak, S. A., and Aurbach, G. D., Activation of skeletal adenyl cyclase by parathyroid hormone in vitro, *Endocrinology*, 84, 761, 1969.

71. Chase, L. R. and Aurbach, G. D., Renal adenyl cyclase: anatomically separate sites for parathyroid hormone and vasopressin, *Science*, 15, 545, 1968.

72. Nickols, G. A. and Cline, W. H., Jr., Parathyroid hormone-induced changes in cyclic nucleotide levels during relaxation of the rat aorta, *Life Sci.*, 40, 2351, 1987.

73. Huang, M., Hanley, D. A., and Rorstad, O. P., Parathyroid hormone stimulates adenylate cyclase in rat cerebral microvessels, *Life Sci.*, 32, 1009, 1983.

74. Goltzman, D., Callahan, E. N., Tregear, G. W., and Potts, J. J., Jr., Influence of guanyl nucleotides on parathyroid hormone-stimulated adenylyl cyclase activity in renal cortical membranes, *Endocrinology*, 103, 1352, 1978.

75. Nickols, G. A., Metz, M. A., and Cline, W. H., Jr., Characteristics of parathyroid homone action in rat vascular tissue, *Fed. Proc.*, 42, 652, 1983.

76. Stanton, R. C., Plant, S. B., and McCarron, D. A., cAMP response of vascular smooth muscle cells to bovine parathyroid hormone, *Am. J. Physiol.*, 247(Endocrinol. Metab. 10), E822, 1985.

77. Pang, P. K. T., Yang, M. C. M., Tenner, T. E., Jr., Kenny, A. D., and Cooper, C. W., Cyclic AMP and the vascular action of parathyroid hormone, *Can. J. Physiol. Pharmacol.*, 64, 1543, 1986.

78. Sutherland, E. W., Robison, G. A., and Butcher, R. W., Some aspects of the biological role of adenosine 3′,5′-monophosphate (cyclic AMP), *Circulation*, 37, 279, 1968.

79. Bergman, C., Schoeffter, P., Stoclet, J. C. and Gairard, A., Effect of parathyroid hormone and antagonist on cAMP levels, *Can. J. Physiol. Pharmacol.*, 65, 2349, 1987.

80. Crass, M. F., III and Scarpace, P. J., Vasoactive properties of a parathyroid hormone-related protein in the rat aorta, *Peptides*, 14, 179, 1993.

81. Payne, M. E., Elzinga, M., and Adelstein, R. A., Smooth muscle myosin light chain kinase. Amino acid sequence at the site phosphorylated by adenosine cyclic-3′,5′ phosphate dependent protein kinase whether or not calmodulin is bound, *J. Biol. Chem.*, 261, 16346, 1986.

82. Bulbring, E. and Tomita, T., Catecholamine action on smooth muscle, *Pharmacol. Rev.*, 39, 49, 1987.

83. Raeymaekers, L. and Jones, L. R., Evidence for the presence of phospholamban in the endoplasmic reticulum of smooth muscle, *Biochim. Biophys. Acta*, 882, 258, 1986.

84. Chiu, A. T., McCall, D. E., Thoolen, M. J. M. C., and Timmermans, P. B. M. W. M., Ca^{++} utilization in the constriction of rat aorta to full and partial alpha-1 adrenoceptor agonists, *J. Pharmcol. Exp. Ther.*, 238, 224, 1986.

85. Chiu, A. T., Bozarth, J. M., and Timmermans, P. B. M. W. M., Relationship between phosphatidylinositol turnover and Ca^{++} mobilization induced by alpha-1 adrenoceptor stimulation in the rat aorta, *J. Pharmacol. Exp. Ther.*, 240, 123, 1987.

86. Campbell, M. D., Subramaniam, S., Kotlikoff, M. I., Williamson, J. R., and Fluharty, S. J., Cyclic AMP inhibits inositol polyphosphate production and calcium mobilization in neuroblastoma x glioma NG-108-15 cells, *Mol. Pharmacol.*, 36, 282, 1990.

87. Berridge, M. J., Dawson, R. M. C., Downes, C. P., Heslop, J. P., and Irvine, R. F., Changes in the levels of inositol phosphates after agonist-dependent hydrolysis of membrane phosphoinositides, *Biochem. J.*, 212, 473, 1983.

88. Sato, K., Ozaki, H., and Karaki, H., Changes in cytosolic calcium level in vascular smooth muscle strip measured simultaneously with contraction using fluorescent Ca^{++} indicator fura 2, *J. Pharmacol. Exp. Ther.*, 246, 294, 1988.

89. Ozaki, H., Ohyama, T., Sato, K., and Karaki, H., Ca^{2+}-dependent and independent mechanisms of sustained contraction in vascular smooth muscle of rat aorta, *Jpn. J. Pharmacol.*, 52, 509, 1990.

90. Karaki, H., Sato, K., and Ozaki, H., Different effects of norepinephrine and KCl on cytosolic Ca^{2+}-tension relationship in vascular smooth muscle of rat aorta, *Eur. J. Pharmacol.*, 151, 325, 1988.

91. Abe, A. and Karaki, H., Mechanisms underlying the inhibitory effect of dibutyryl cyclic AMP in vascular smooth muscle, *Eur. J. Pharmacol.*, 211, 305, 1992.

92. Neufeld, M. D. and Crass, M. F., III, Vasorelaxant effect of parathyroid hormone (PTH) in porcine coronary arteries, *Proc. Soc. Exp. Biol. Med.*, 191(Abstr.), 98, 1989.

93. Pang, P. K. T., Yang, M. C. M., and Sham, J. S. K., Parathyroid hormone and calcium entry blockade in a vascular tissue, *Life Sci.*, 42, 1395, 1988.

94. Abe, A. and Karaki, H., Effect of forskolin on cytosolic Ca^{++} level and contraction in vascular smooth muscle, *J. Pharmacol. Exp. Ther.*, 249, 895, 1989.

95. Lincoln, T. M. and Fisher-Simpson, V., A comparison of the effects of forskolin and nitroprusside on cyclic nucleotides and relaxation in rat aorta, *Eur. J. Pharmacol.*, 101, 17, 1983.

96. Minami, K., Fukuzawa, K., Nakaya, Y., Zeng, X.-R., and Inoue, I., Mechanism of activation of the Ca^{2+}-activated K$^+$ channel by cyclic AMP in cultured porcine coronary artery smooth muscle cells, *Life Sci.*, 53, 1129, 1993.

97. Van Breeman, C., Farinas, B. R., Gerba, P., and McNaughton, E. D., Excitation-contraction coupling in rabbit aorta studied by the lanthanum method for measuring cellular calcium influx, *Circ. Res.*, 30, 44, 1972.

98. Schleiffer, R., Bergmann, C., Pernot, F., and Gairard, A., Parathyroid hormone acute vascular effect is mediated by decreased Ca^{2+} uptake and enhanced cAMP level, *Mol. Cell. Endocrinol.*, 67, 63, 1989.

99. Kawashima, H., Parathyroid hormone causes a transient rise in intracellular ionized calcium in vascular smooth muscle cells, *Biochem. Biophys. Res. Commun.*, 166, 709, 1990.

100. Bukoski, R. D., Xue, H., and McCarron, D. A., Effect of 1,25(OH)$_2$ vitamin D$_3$ and ionized Ca^{2+} on ^{45}Ca uptake by primary cultures of aortic myocytes of spontaneously hypertensive and Wistar Kyoto normotensive rats, *Biochem. Biophys. Res. Commun.*, 146, 1330, 1987.

101. Pang, P. K. T., Wang, R., Shan, J., Karpinski, E., and Benishin, C. G., Specific inhibition of long-lasting, L-type calcium channels by synthetic parathyroid hormone, *Proc. Natl. Acad. Sci. U.S.A.*, 87, 623, 1990.

102. Wang, R., Karpinski, E., and Pang, P. K. T., Parathyroid hormone selectively inhibits L-type calcium channels in single vascular smooth muscle cells of the rat, *J. Physiol.*, 441, 325, 1991.

103. Wang, R., Wu, L., Karpinski, E., and Pang, P. K. T., The effects of parathyroid hormone on L-type voltage-dependent calcium channel currents in vascular smooth muscle cells and ventricular myocytes are mediated by a cyclic AMP dependent mechanism, *FEBS Lett.*, 282, 331, 1991.

104. Tuma, S. N., Michael, L. H., and Entman, M. L., Effect of parathyroid hormone on cardiac muscle, *Clin. Res.*, 27(Abstr.), 735A, 1979.

105. Katoh, Y., Klein, K. L., Kaplan, R. A., Sanborn, W. G., and Kurokawa, K., Parathyroid hormone has a positive inotropic action in the rat, *Endocrinology*, 109, 2252, 1981.

106. Kondo, N., Shibata, S., Tenner, T. E., and Pang, P. K. T., Electromechanical effects of bPTH-(1-34) on rabbit sinus node cells and guinea pig papillary muscles, *J. Cardiovasc. Pharmacol.*, 11, 619, 1988.

107. Sham, J. S. K., Wong, V. C. K., Chiu, K. W., and Pang, P. K. T., Comparative study on the cardiac actions of bovine parathyroid hormone (1-34), *Gen. Comp. Endocrinol.*, 61, 148, 1986.

108. Lhoste, F., Drüeke, T., Larno, S., and Boissier, J. R., Cardiac interaction between parathyroid hormone, β-adrenoceptor agents, and verapamil in the guinea pig in vitro, *Clin. Exp. Pharmacol. Physiol.*, 7, 119, 1980.

109. Tenner, T. E. and Pang, P. K. T., Cardiac actions of parathyroid hormone, *Proc. West. Pharmacol. Soc.*, 25, 263, 1982.

110. Sham, J. S. K., Kenny, A. D., and Pang, P. K. T., Cardiac actions and structural-activity relationship of parathyroid hormone on isolated frog atrium, *Gen. Comp. Endocrinol.*, 55, 373, 1984.

111. Larno, S., Lhoste, F., Auclair, M.-C., and Lechat, P., Interaction between parathyroid hormone and the β-adrenoceptor system in cultured rat myocardial cells, *J. Mol. Cell. Cardiol.*, 12, 955, 1980.

112. Bogin, E., Massry, S. G., and Harary, I., Effect of parathyroid hormone on rat heart cells, *J. Clin. Invest.*, 67, 1215, 1981.

113. Tenner, T. E., Jr., Ramanadham, S., Yang, M. C. M. and Pang, P. K. T., Chronotropic actions of bPTH-(1-34) in the right atrium of the rat, *Can. J. Physiol. Pharmacol.*, 61, 1162, 1983.

114. Wang, R., Karpinski, E., and Pang, P. K. T., Two types of voltage-dependent calcium channel currents and their modulation by parathyroid hormone in neonatal rat ventricular cells, *J. Cardiovasc. Pharmacol.*, 17, 990, 1991.

115. Rampe, D., Lacerda, A. E., Dage, R. C., and Brown, A. M., Parathyroid hormone: an endogenous modulator of cardiac calcium channels, *Am. J. Physiol.*, 261(Heart Circ. Physiol. 30), H1945, 1991.

116. Austin, L. A. and Heath, H., Calcitonin: physiology and pathophysiology, *N. Engl. J. Med.*, 304, 269, 1981.

117. Chiba, S. and Himori, B. S., Effects of salmon calcitonin on SA nodal pacemaker activity and contractility in isolated, blood-perfused atrial and papillary muscle preparations of dogs, *Jpn. Heart J.*, 18, 214, 1977.

118. Fiore, C. E., Carnemolla, G., Grillo, S., Grimaldi, D. R., and Petralito, A., Inotropic effects of calcitonin in man, *Acta Cardiol.*, 33, 155, 1978.

119. Peguero-Rivera, A. M. and Corder, C. N., Hemodynamic effects of calcitonin in the normal rat, *Peptides*, 13, 571, 1992.

120. Aldred, J. P., Luna, P. D., Zeedyk, R. A., and Bastian, J. W., Inhibition by salmon calcitonin of deoxycorticosterone acetate (DOCA)-induced hypertension in the rat, *Proc. Soc. Exp. Biol. Med.*, 152, 557, 1976.

121. Wegener, L. L. and McCarron, D. A., Acute intravenous calcitonin: failure to modify systemic blood pressure, *Peptides*, 9, 1191, 1988.

122. Resnick, L. M., Churchill, M. C., Churchill, P. C., Laragh, J. H., and Orlowski, R., Effects of calcitonin, calcitonin analogues, and calcitonin gene-related peptide on basal in vitro renin secretion, *Am. J. Hypertens.*, 2, 453, 1989.

123. Schleiffer, R., Helwig, J. J., Pernot, F., and Gairard, A., Vascular effects of calcitonin and parathyroid hormone, in *Calcitonin 1984*, Doepfner, W., Ed., Exerpta Medica, Amsterdam, 1986, 15.

124. Charbon, G. A. and Pieper, E. E., Effect of calcitonin on parathyroid hormone-induced vasodilation, *Endocrinology*, 91, 828, 1972.

125. Feola, M., Gonzalez, H., and Canizaro, P. C., Vasoactive parathyroid hormone in the treatment of acute ischemic left ventricular failure and the prevention of cardiogenic shock, *Circ. Shock*, 17, 163, 1985.

126. Feola, M. and Crass, M. F., III, Parathyroid hormone reduces acute ischemic injury of the myocardium, *Surg. Gynecol. Obstet.*, 163, 523, 1986.

127. Conway, D. R., Kim, D., Djuricin, G., VanDenburgh, A., Jacobs, H. K., Rosel, T. J., and Prinz, R. A., The effect of parathyroid hormone on the acutely ischemic myocardium, *Am. Surg.*, 56, 463, 1990.

128. Arnaud, C. D., Hyperparathyroidism and renal failure, *Kidney Int.*, 4, 89, 1973.

129. Llach, F. and Massry, S. G., On the mechanism of secondary hyperparathyroidism in moderate renal insufficiency, *J. Clin. Endocrinol. Metab.*, 61, 601, 1985.

130. Ayus, J. C., Frommer, J. P., and Young, J. B., Cardiac and circulatory abnormalities in chronic renal failure, *Semin. Nephrol.*, 1, 112, 1981.

131. Drüeke, T., LePailleur, C., Sigal-Saglier, M., Zingraff, J., Crosnier, J., and DiMatteo, J., Left ventricular function in hemodialysis patients with cardiomyopathy, *Nephron*, 28, 80, 1981.

132. Drüeke, T. and LePailleur, C., Cardiomyopathy in patients on maintenance hemodialysis, *Contrib. Nephrol.*, 52, 27, 1984.

133. Massry, S. G., Is parathyroid hormone a uremic toxin?, *Nephron*, 19, 125, 1977.

134. Massry, S. G., Parathyroid hormone and uremic myocardiopathy, *Contrib. Nephrol.*, 41, 231, 1984.

135. Drüeke, T., Fauchet, M., Fleury, J., Lesourd, P., Toury, Y., LePailleur, C., Devernejoul, P., and Crosnier, J., Effect of parathyroidectomy on left ventricular function in hemodialysis patients, *Lancet*, 1, 112, 1980.

136. Rostand, S. G., Sanders, C., Kirk, K. A., and Rutsky, E. A., Myocardial calcification and cardiac dysfunction in chronic renal failure, *Am. J. Med.*, 85, 651, 1988.

137. Gafter, U., Battler, A., Eldar, M., Zevin, D., Neufeld, H. N., and Levi, J., Effect of hyperparathyroidism on cardiac function in patients with end-stage renal disease, *Nephron*, 41, 30, 1985.

138. Hörl, W. H. and Riegel, W., Cardiac depressant factors in renal disease, *Circulation*, 87(Suppl. IV), IV77, 1993.

139. Fellner, S. K., Lang, R. M., Neumann, A., Bushinsky, D. A., and Borow, K. M., Parathyroid hormone and myocardial performance in dialysis patients, *Am. J. Kidney Dis.*, 18, 320, 1991.

140. Mok, L. L. S., Nickols, G. A., Thompson, J. C., and Cooper, C. W., Parathyroid hormone as a smooth muscle relaxant, *Endocr. Rev.*, 10, 420, 1989.

3

Modulation of Voltage-Dependent Ca^{2+} Channels in Vascular Smooth Muscle Cells and Ventricular Myocytes by Parathyroid Hormone

Edward Karpinski

CONTENTS

I. INTRODUCTION

The concentration of cytosolic free Ca^{2+} is important for the control of many essential cellular functions. Typically, the concentration of cytosolic free Ca^{2+} in quiescent cells is 50 to 200 nM, while the Ca^{2+} concentration in the extracellular fluid is approximately 1 to 2 mM. Hence, there is a large concentration gradient of Ca^{2+} across the cell membrane. Electrical or chemical stimulation of the cell will increase the intracellular Ca^{2+} and this increase is in part due to the influx of Ca^{2+} across the cell membrane. Ca^{2+} moves down its concentration gradient through membrane pores which are selective for this ion. These pores are part of the more complex structures that are Ca^{2+} channels. The best-described class of Ca^{2+} channels are the time- and voltage-dependent Ca^{2+} channels. Some evidence also exists that ligand-gated or receptor-operated Ca^{2+} channels are expressed in some cells.[1] The activation of voltage-dependent Ca^{2+} channels requires depolarization of the cell membrane. Voltage-dependent Ca^{2+} channels however, can be modulated by hormones, neurotransmitters, and drugs.[2] Most hormones and transmitters modulate voltage-dependent Ca^{2+} channels through transmembrane transducers which are guanine nucleotide binding proteins (G proteins).

There are many examples of Ca^{2+} channel modulation by hormones and neurotransmitters. In an early report, Reuter[3] demonstrated that the plateau of the action potential in sheep Purkinje fibers was shifted toward more positive potentials by increasing extracellular Ca^{2+} or by the addition of adrenaline. Later studies have shown that activation of β-adrenergic receptors increases the Ca^{2+} channel current in cardiac muscle cells,[3] and this effect is directly involved in the increased rate and force of contraction of the heart that are produced by sympathetic activation. In a more recent study, isoproterenol, a β-adrenergic agonist, has been reported to enhance both the high and low threshold Ca^{2+} channel currents in guinea pig ventricular myocytes.[4] The binding of the β-agonist to the β-receptor activates a G protein (G_s) which in turn activates adenylate cyclase. This increases adenosine 3':5'-cyclic phosphate (cAMP) levels and results in the phosphorylation of a channel protein through a cAMP-dependent kinase (protein kinase A, or PKA).[5] Ono et al.[6] reported that calcitonin gene-related peptide (CGRP) increased the Ca^{2+} channel currents in frog and rabbit atrial myocytes. This effect was reversible and also mediated by cAMP.

II. PARATHYROID HORMONE

In addition to its classical hypercalcemic effect, parathyroid hormone (PTH) has cardiovascular effects. These actions of PTH were described extensively in Chapter 2 and are only briefly discussed in this chapter. Vasorelaxation induced by the active synthetic fragment of bovine PTH (bPTH-(1-34)) has been reported in both *in vivo* and *in vitro* experiments.[7] The amino acids of PTH in position 1 (serine/alanine for human/bovine) and 2 (valine) are essential for the vascular action of PTH.[8] Additional studies have demonstrated that PTH could act as a Ca^{2+} entry blocker in vascular tissues.[9] The conclusion that PTH blocked Ca^{2+} entry in vascular tissues was based on the observations that rat tail artery helical strips contracted with KCl or arginine vasopressin could be relaxed by bPTH-(1-34). In addition, bPTH-(1-34) was able to inhibit the calcium uptake caused by KCl or arginine vasopressin, and this inhibition was concentration dependent.

The cardiac actions of PTH also have been studied extensively. Evidence exists that PTH has positive chronotropic and inotropic actions.[10,11] Bogin et al.[12] showed that bPTH-(1-34) and bPTH-(1-84) produced an immediate and sustained increase in the beating rate of cultured rat heart cells. Verapamil, a Ca^{2+} channel antagonist, blocked the PTH effect. This suggests that the positive chronotropic effect of PTH is due to the influx of Ca^{2+} into the cell through Ca^{2+} channels. It has also been reported that the positive inotropic effect of bPTH-(1-34) can be abolished by verapamil,[13] methoxyverapamil,[14] or a low Ca^{2+} medium (0.12 mM).[13] The study of Kondo et al.[13] using the single sucrose gap technique also showed that bPTH-(1-34) increased the slow, inward current.

It is clear that the cardiovascular actions of PTH involve the modulation of Ca^{2+} influx. This may not be the only action of PTH, but this modulation may explain much of the cardiovascular action of this hormone. Although it is apparent that the major part of the cardiovascular action of PTH involves the modulation of Ca^{2+} influx, most evidence is indirect. The study by Kondo et al.[13] is the only exception. This study provides preliminary evidence that PTH increased the slow, inward current in papillary muscle; however, problems are inherent in the single sucrose gap technique when applied to whole tissue preparations, such as accumulation of ions in the extracellular space. In addition, it is difficult to eliminate effects mediated by nerves and local reflexes. In subsequent sections, evidence from two laboratories is presented supporting the hypothesis that PTH has a direct action on Ca^{2+} influx in vascular smooth muscle cells and ventricular myocytes. These studies identify the specific Ca^{2+} channels and, in part, the intracellular mechanisms involved.

III. Ca^{2+} CHANNELS

Voltage-operated or -gated Ca^{2+} channels are widespread in their distribution. All excitable and secretory cells express Ca^{2+} channels. Activation of Ca^{2+} channels via changes in membrane voltage creates a net inward depolarizing current (inward Ca^{2+} current), and the resulting increase in intracellular Ca^{2+} can act as a chemical trigger for secretion, muscle contraction, and other Ca^{2+}-sensitive events. Comparing the Ca^{2+} channel to other ion channels shows that it is unique in its dual properties, and hence allows the Ca^{2+} channel to play a variety of roles in coupling excitation to secretion or to contraction. It is now clear that the diversity of Ca^{2+} channel functions is reflected by the diversity of Ca^{2+} channel types.[15] Based on various parameters, such as single-channel conductances, selectivity, single-channel kinetics, and sensitivity to organic antagonists and agonists (dihydropyridines), three different subtypes of voltage-dependent Ca^{2+} channels have been identified in chick dorsal root ganglion neurons.[15] They are called T-, N-, and L-Ca^{2+} channels.[16] One or more of the channel subtypes have been identified in various cell preparations.[17] The T-, or transient, channel has a single-channel conductance of 8 to 10 ps, reaches a maximum at –10 mV (holding potential of –100 mV), and is inactivated rapidly and completely. The L-, or long-lasting, channel has a single-channel conductance of 25 ps, is activated at more positive voltages, does not inactivate (or inactivates very slowly), and is sensitive to dihydropyridines. The N-, or neuronal, channel has a single-channel conductance of 13 ps and is activated in the same range as the L-channel but inactivates. In summary, the subtypes of Ca^{2+} channels, based on their electrophysiological properties, are low threshold inactivating (T), high threshold noninactivating (L), and high threshold inactivating (N).

IV. Ca²⁺ CHANNELS IN VASCULAR SMOOTH MUSCLE CELLS

In various types of smooth muscle cells the inward movement of Ca^{2+} through Ca^{2+} channels plays an important role in excitation coupling. The electrophysiological characteristics of Ca^{2+} channels were unknown until the development of two techniques, the enzymatic isolation of single vascular smooth muscle cells and the Giga seal single electrode voltage clamp.[18] Largely as a result of these developments, it has become clear that at least two types of Ca^{2+} channels are expressed in vascular smooth muscle cells.[19]

Hirst et al.[20] described two types of Ca^{2+}-dependent currents (Ca^{2+} channels) in voltage-clamped segments of proximal rat middle cerebral arterioles. In their studies, one current was activated at low membrane depolarization, while the other current was activated at higher depolarization. The low threshold current (negative activation range) did not inactivate substantially, whereas the high threshold current inactivated rapidly (<200 ms). In cultures of azygous venous muscle from neonatal rats, Sturek and Hermsmeyer[21] also described two types of Ca^{2+} channel currents. One current was activated by small depolarizations in the range of −40 mV and the peak inward current occurred at −10 mV. This Ca^{2+} channel current inactivated rapidly. The other Ca^{2+} channel current was activated at more positive voltages with a maximum at 4 mV and did not inactivate appreciably. Since then, other reports have identified two types of time- and voltage-dependent Ca^{2+} channel currents in arterial smooth muscle cells, including those from rat mesenteric artery,[22] guinea pig aorta,[23] rabbit ear artery,[24] and rat tail artery.[25] Based on the characteristics of the inward currents generated, the two types of currents are the T-channel and L-channel currents. The currents are generated by the activation of the T- and L-channels. The T-channels, which activate quickly and then inactivate, may contribute to the generation of smooth muscle action potentials. The L-channels, which display little or no inactivation, are thought to be important for excitation-contraction coupling. The distribution of these Ca^{2+} channels in the various parts of arterial systems may be related to the different functional roles of those arteries.

Figure 1 shows the inward Ca^{2+} channel current from a vascular smooth muscle cell. This was a primary culture of rat tail artery vascular smooth muscle. Ba^{2+} (20 mM) was the charge carrier and 11 mM EGTA was included in the pipette solution. The cell was voltage clamped at −80 mV. Depolarization to more positive potentials activated a time- and voltage-dependent inward current. The current was activated at −50 mV and the peak inward current occurred at 0 mV. The inward current shown in Figure 1 consists of two components of inward current: the T component and the L component. Shifting the holding potential to −50 or −40 mV inactivates most of the T component of inward Ca^{2+} current.[25] Figure 2 shows a characteristic L-channel current from a vascular smooth muscle cell (rat tail artery). The holding potential was −50 mV. The current activates at −30 mV and the peak inward L-channel current occurs at +20 mV.

V. Ca²⁺ CHANNELS IN CARDIAC MYOCYTES

The first description of an L-type calcium channel current in cardiac tissue was made by Reuter[3] in 1967. Because the sucrose gap method was the best available technique at that time, the calcium conductance in cardiac tissue was simply described as a single population of channels. In 1985, Nilius and co-workers[26] reported that in addition to the L-channel, a T-channel was also present in cardiac cells. Based on experiments that used the whole cell

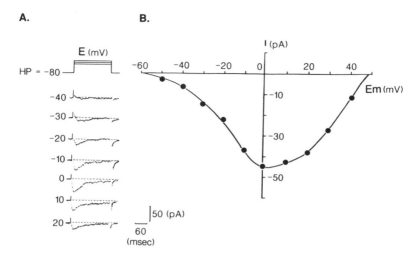

FIGURE 1 Inward Ca^{2+} channel currents obtained from a rat tail artery vascular smooth muscle cell. Ba^{2+} was used as a charge carrier and the pipette solution contained 11 mM EGTA. The inward current contains a large T-channel component but some L-channel current is also present. (A) Original current records obtained 8 min after the cell was voltage clamped. The currents were activated by depolarizing the cell from −80 mV to various test potentials as indicated next to the current records. Leakage and capacitive currents have been subtracted but capacitive subtraction was imperfect. (B) The current voltage relationship obtained from the cell described in A. The peak inward current occurred at 0 mV. (From Wang, R. et al., *Am. J. Physiol.*, 256(25), H1361, 1989. With permission.)

version of the patch clamp technique,[4,27] T- and L-channel currents were separated and identified.

T- and L-channels are expressed in different densities in various cardiac tissues. L-channels are the predominant channels in adult cardiac myocytes and are sensitive to dihydropyridines. T-channels are expressed at lower densities than L-channels in most cardiac tissues. T-channels, from cardiac cells, are not sensitive to dihydropyridines, but are sensitive to nickel and tetramethrin.[28] The relative magnitude of the T-channel current is small in adult ventricular cells, larger in atrial cells, and largest in natural pacemaker cells.[29,30] In contrast, it has been reported that the density of T-channels is greater than L-channels in embryonic chick ventricular myocytes.[31]

Differences are also found in the characteristics of cardiac Ca^{2+} channels. For example, the L-channel steady-state inactivation characteristics are different in cardiac muscle cells when compared to smooth muscle cells. When the membrane potential is shifted from −80 to −40 mV, the L-channel current is inactivated by approximately 50% in smooth muscle cells but less than 10% in atrial cells.[17,32] The dihydropyridine sensitivity of L-channels is also different in cardiac cells from that in neurons, and neuron L-channels are more insensitive. In addition, the peak of the I-V relationship of the L-channel current is shifted toward more negative potentials by Bay K-8644 (dihydropyridine agonist) in cardiac cells but not in neurons.[33] The shift in the I-V relationship reflects a change in the channel gating mode.[16]

A third type of calcium channel was reported by Rosenberg and Tsien[34] in cardiac sarcolemmal membranes. This channel opened at the normal resting potential. Later, this background calcium conductance, or B-channel, was confirmed using the single-channel recording technique in adult rat ventricular myocytes.[35] B-channel currents were detected only at negative potentials. This channel was not sensitive to inorganic blockers, such as cobalt, cadmium, or nickel. Bay K-8644 increased B-channel currents.

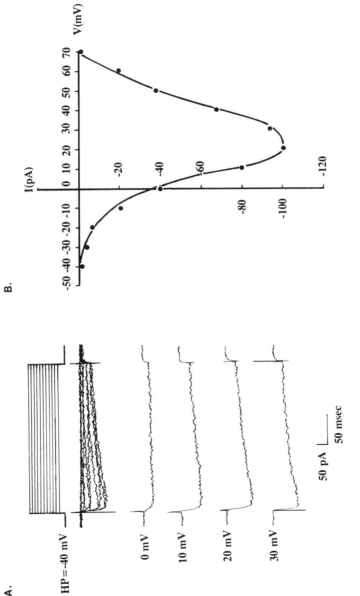

FIGURE 2   L-Ca²⁺ channel current in a vascular smooth muscle cell from the rat tail artery. Ba²⁺ was used as the charge carrier and the pipette solution contained 11 m*M* EGTA. (A) Original current records obtained 5 min after the cell was voltage clamped. The currents were activated by depolarizing the cell from a holding potential of −40 mV to the test potentials as indicated next to the current records. Leakage and capacitive currents were subtracted on line. (B) The current voltage relationship obtained from the cell described in A. The peak inward current occurred at +20 mV. (From Li, B., Liu, Q., and Karpinski, E., unpublished data.)

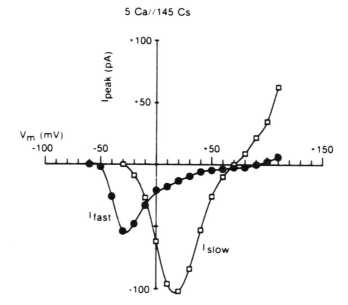

FIGURE 3 Two components of inward Ca^{2+} currents in a canine atrial cell. The two components I_{fast} and I_{slow} were separated using holding potentials of –80 and –30 mV as described in the text. The charge carrier was 5 mM Ca^{2+}, and 145 mM Cs was included in the pipette solution. (Reproduced from Bean, B., *J. Gen. Physiol.*, 86, 1, 1985. With permission of the Rockefeller University Press.)

In addition to the above electrophysiological and pharmacological characteristics of cardiac T- and L-channels, the distribution, characteristics, and functional importance of calcium channels vary during the developmental stages of cardiac myocytes. Although the existence of L-channels in neonatal rat ventricular cells has been established,[5] typical T-channels were not fully described or characterized until reports by Rampe et al.[36] and Wang et al.[37]

Figure 3 shows the two components of inward Ca^{2+} currents from a canine atrial cell. The charge carrier was 5 mM Ca^{2+}. These two components (I_{fast} and I_{slow}) were separated using holding potentials of –80 and –30 mV. The component of current that rapidly activates and inactivates I_{fast} was separated from the slower maintained component I_{slow} by subtracting the current activated from a holding potential of –30 mV from the current activated from –80 mV. A similar separation of inward current in a neonatal ventricular myocyte is shown in Figure 4. The charge carrier in this case was 20 mM Ba^{2+} and the two holding potentials used were –80 and –40 mV. This manipulation resulted in the separation of the T and L components of the inward current in neonatal ventricular cells.

VI. EFFECT OF PARATHYROID HORMONE ON Ca^{2+} CHANNELS IN VASCULAR SMOOTH MUSCLE CELLS (RAT TAIL ARTERY)

A. Effect of bPTH-(1-34) on the T-Channel Current

T- and L-channel currents in most cell types may be approximately separated as described in the text (see Figure 3) by measuring the inward currents at two holding potentials. To obtain an inward current that is primarily a T-channel current, the L component of the inward current can be inhibited using an L-channel antagonist. The effects of agents on T-channels can then be studied.[38] Figure 5 shows such an experiment. A vascular smooth muscle cell was pretreated with nifedipine (5 μM). This concentration of nifedipine completely inhibited the

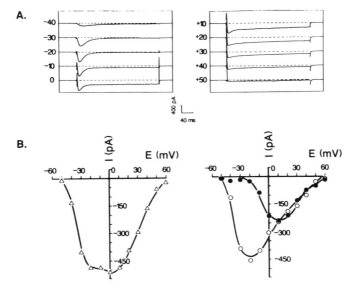

FIGURE 4   Ca²⁺ channel currents from neonatal rat ventricular cells. (A) The inward currents were activated from a holding potential of –80 mV to the test potentials (mV) indicated next to each record. (B) The current voltage relationships were obtained from the same cell as in A. The current voltage relationship (open triangles) was constructed using the peak current values in A. Separation of the T and L components using the current at 200 ms as an index of the L-channel component is shown in B. The L-channel component of current is plotted using solid circles and the T-channel component of current is plotted using open circles. (From Wang, R. et al., *J. Cardiovas. Pharmacol.*, 17, 990, 1991. With permission.)

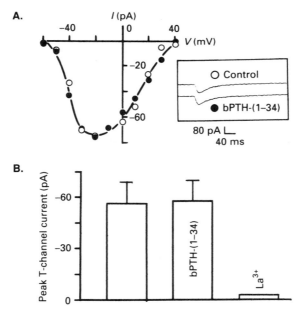

FIGURE 5   The effect of bPTH-(1-34) on T-channel currents in vascular smooth muscle cells dissociated from rat tail artery. These cells were pretreated with nifedipine (5 μ*M*) to block the L-channel current. (A) The I-V relationship before (open circles) and after (closed circles) 1 μ*M* bPTH-(1-34). The current records shown in the insert were obtained from the same cell and were activated by depolarizing the cell to –20 V from a holding potential of –80 mV. (B) The effect of bPTH-(1-34) on the peak T-channel current in a group of cells (*n* = 5). bPTH-(1-34) (1 μ*M*) did not change the peak amplitude of T-channel currents. T-channel currents were completely inhibited by 2 m*M* La³⁺. (From Wang, R. et al., *J. Physiol.*, 44, 325, 1991. With permission.)

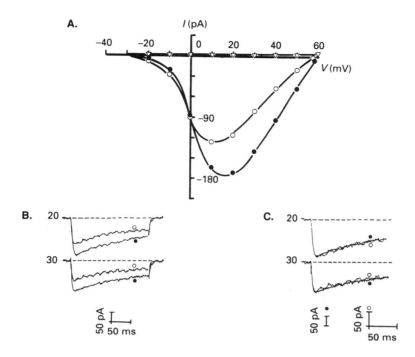

FIGURE 6 The effect of bPTH-(1-34) on the L-channel currents in a smooth muscle cell dissociated from rat tail artery. (A) The I-V relationships before (closed circles) and after (open circles) 1 μM bPTH-(1-34) and after 2 mM La^{3+} (open triangles). bPTH-(1-34) (1 μM) inhibited the peak L-channel current by 26.3% and La^{3+} completely blocked the L-channel current. (B) The original current records before and after the addition of bPTH-(1-34). Test potentials shown are in millivolts. (C) The current records in the presence of bPTH-(1-34) were rescaled and superimposed on the control current records using the same scale as in B. The superimposed currents show that bPTH-(1-34) did not alter the kinetics of inactivation of the L-channel currents. In all records, leakage and capacitative currents have been subtracted and the holding potential was –40 mV. (From Wang, R. et al., *J. Physiol.*, 44, 325, 1991. With permission.)

L-channel current leaving the T component of the inward current. bPTH-(1-34) at a concentration of 1 μM did not affect the T-channel current. This is shown in the current records and the current voltage relationship of Figure 5. The subsequent application of La^{3+} completely eliminated the transient inward current (T-channel current). Figure 5B shows the combined results from a group of cells.

B. Effect of bPTH-(1-34) on the L-Channel Current

The magnitude of the dihydropyridine-sensitive current (L-channel) was reduced by bPTH-(1-34). The addition of bPTH-(1-34) to a static bath decreased the current within 2 to 3 min and this decrease reached a steady state within 5 min. Figure 6 shows the effect of bPTH-(1-34) (1 μM) on the L-channel current in one vascular smooth muscle cell. The inhibitory effect of bPTH-(1-34) was most evident at positive potentials. To observe the effect of bPTH-(1-34) on the kinetics of the L-channel current, the inward currents at two test potentials were compared. When reduced current records obtained in the presence of bPTH-(1-34) (Figure 6B) were scaled and superimposed on the inward current records before bPTH-(1-34), no difference was noted in the time course of activation or inactivation. This shows that bPTH-(1-34) has no effect on L-channel kinetics. In addition, the potential at which the currents were activated, the voltage at which the peak inward current occurred, and the apparent reversal potential were not affected by bPTH-(1-34). The inhibitory effect of bPTH-(1-34) may be

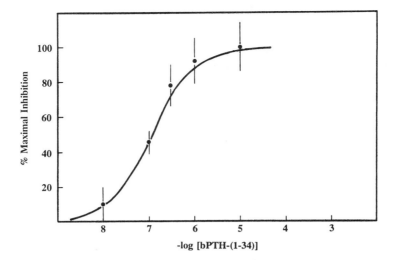

FIGURE 7   The effect of different concentrations of bPTH-(1-34) on the L-channel current in vascular smooth muscle cells dissociated from rat tail artery. PTH inhibited the L-channel current. The solid curve is the least-squares fit to the Hill function of the data, which is plotted as the mean ± SEM. The Hill function was of the form: % of maximal inhibition = 100% maximal inhibition $x(1 + (K/X)^n)^{-1}$ where K is the concentration at which one half maximal inhibition occurs, X is the concentration of the agent, and n is the power of the function. The inhibition at $10^{-5} M$, which was 40.4 ± 6%, was taken to be the maximal inhibition. K calculated from the Hill function was $1.2 \times 10^{-7} M$ and n = 1. (From Lui, B., Li, Q., and Karpinski, E., unpublished data.)

reversed by solution exchange (wash out). The inhibitory effect of bPTH-(1-34) on the L-channel current is concentration dependent. At a concentration of $10^{-5} M$, the L-channel current was inhibited by 40.4 ± 6%. Figure 7 shows the effect of concentration on the inhibitory effect of bPTH-(1-34). The solid curve is the least-squares fit of the Hill function to the experimental data. The inhibition of the L-channel current by 10 μM bPTH-(1-34) of 40.4% was defined as the maximal inhibition. The concentration at which half-maximal inhibition occurred was calculated from the best fit Hill function to be $1.2 \pm 0.1 \times 10^{-7} M$.

C.   Summary and Discussion

The conclusion which may be drawn from the data presented in this section is that the active N-terminal fragment of bovine PTH, bPTH-(1-34), exerts its vasorelaxing effect on vascular smooth muscle through its action on the L-channel. This confirms earlier results obtained from tension and flux studies by Pang et al.[9] and the suggestion that PTH may exert its action on blood vessels by inhibiting Ca²⁺ channels. It is also clear that PTH does not affect the T-channel.

The presence of PTH receptors on vascular smooth muscle cells has been demonstrated.[39,40] Parathyroid hormone is not lipid-soluble because it is a charged protein. It is likely that PTH exerts its effect on L-channels by binding to its receptors and activating cytoplasmic second messengers which modify the L-channel current. This, in part, can be confirmed by the use of antagonists. The 3-34 amino acid fragment of PTH can act as an antagonist of bPTH-(1-34).[8,41] The study of Wang et al.[38] shows that a concentration of 1 μM bPTH-(3-34) completely inhibited the effect of 1 μM bPTH-(1-34) on the L-channel current. The same concentration of bPTH-(3-34) had no effect on the L-channel current. No change occurred in either the magnitude or kinetics of the L-channel current after the addition of 1 μM bPTH-(3-34). A

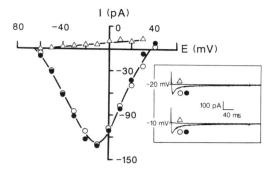

FIGURE 8   The effect of bPTH-(1-34) on the T-channel current in a neonatal rat ventricular myocyte. The I-V relationships of the T-channel current in a ventricular myocyte before and after 1 μ*M* bPTH-(1-34) are shown along with the current records at two test potentials. The T-channel currents were activated by depolarizing the cell from a holding potential of –80 mV. bPTH-(1-34) at this concentration had no effect on the T-channel current. The charge carrier was 20 m*M* Ba^{2+} and intracellular Ca^{2+} was buffered using 10 m*M* EGTA. (From Wang, R. et al., *J. Cardiovasc. Pharmacol.*, 17, 990, 1991. With permission.)

plausible explanation for this result is that bPTH-(3-34) occupies the same binding sites as bPTH-(1-34) and hence decreased bPTH-(1-34) binding below effective levels. The complete inhibition of the bPTH-(1-34) effect by an equimolar concentration of bPTH-(3-34) is difficult to explain because in most reports in which bPTH-(3-34) is used, much higher concentrations of bPTH-(3-34) are required to produce complete inhibition of bPTH-(1-34). However, all of the other reports measure effects such as tension.[41] The contraction of vascular smooth muscle involves multiple factors which include the inward movement of Ca^{2+} via Ca^{2+} channels. Wang et al.[38] measured the effect of bPTH-(3-34) and bPTH-(1-34) only on the L-channel current, and hence the complete inhibition of bPTH-(1-34) by an equimolar concentration bPTH-(3-34) is plausible.

A potential mediator of the bPTH-induced modulation of L-channels is cAMP. cAMP is a potent relaxant of many smooth muscles.[42] Using cultured vascular smooth muscle cells, a 1-min treatment with bPTH-(1-34) causes five- to tenfold increases in cAMP concentrations.[43] Several studies have suggested that the hypotensive action of bPTH-(1-34) may involve cAMP.[44,45] Pang et al.[45] reported that bPTH-(1-34) increased cAMP levels in rat tail strips and that the vasodilatatory action of bPTH-(1-34) was potentiated by isobutylmethylxanthine (IBMX, a phosphodiesterase inhibitor) and decreased by imidazole (a phosphodiesterase stimulator). Further evidence supporting the role of cAMP in the PTH modulation of L-channels in vascular smooth muscle is presented in Section VIII.

VII.   EFFECT OF PARATHYROID HORMONE ON Ca^{2+} CHANNELS IN CARDIAC MYOCYTES

A.   Effect of Parathyroid Hormone on the T-Channel Current

An experiment in which the L-channel was inhibited by nifedipine leaving primarily the T component is shown in Figure 8. The cell was a neonatal ventricular myocyte and 20 m*M* Ba^{2+} was the charge carrier. The cell was pretreated with 10 μ*M* nifedipine and the T-channel component elicited by depolarizing the cell from a holding potential of –80 mV. Addition of 1 μ*M* bPTH-(1-34) had no effect on the T component of the inward Ca^{2+} channel current. This current was completely blocked by 2 m*M* La^{3+}.

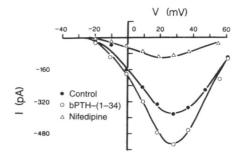

FIGURE 9   The effect of bPTH-(1-34) (1 μ*M*) on the L-channel current in a neonatal ventricular myocyte. The I-V relationship before and after bPTH-(1-34) is shown. Subsequent addition of 10 μ*M* nifedipine almost blocked the L-channel current. bPTH-(1-34) increased the L-channel current. The charge carrier was 20 m*M* Ba²⁺ and the intracellular Ca²⁺ was buffered using 10 m*M* EGTA. (From Wang, R. et al., *J. Cardiovasc. Pharmacol.*, 17, 990, 1991. With permission.)

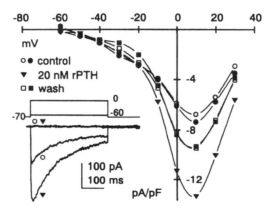

FIGURE 10   The effect of 20 n*M* rPTH-(1-34) on the L-channel current in a neonatal ventricular myocyte. The L-channel currents were activated by depolarizing the cell from a holding potential of –70 mV to the various test potentials. The control and wash I-V relationships with open symbols were obtained first. Control I-Vs were separated by 10 min and the rPTH-(1-34) I-V was obtained 15 min after the addition of rPTH-(1-34); wash I-Vs were obtained at 20 and 26 min after the start of washing. The inset shows the current records at the indicated potentials from the I-V relationships with the corresponding symbols. The currents have been normalized to cell capacitance. The charge carrier was 40 m*M* Ba²⁺ and the intracellular Ca²⁺ was buffered to 135 n*M*. (From Rampe, D. et al., *Am. J. Physiol.*, 261(6), H1945, 1991. With permission.)

B.   Effect of Parathyroid Hormone on the L-Channel Current

The effect of bPTH-(1-34) (1 m*M*) on the L-channel current in neonatal rat ventricular myocytes is shown in Figure 9. The intracellular solution in this experiment contained 10 m*M* EGTA, which buffered the intracellular Ca²⁺ below physiological levels. bPTH-(1-34) increased the L-channel current by about 30% and nifedipine (10 μ*M*) almost completely inhibited the current. A similar experiment in which the intracellular Ca²⁺ was buffered to physiological levels (135 n*M* calculated) is shown in Figure 10. The figure illustrates the effect of 20 n*M* of the active 1-34 amino acid fragment of rat parathyroid hormone (rPTH) on the L-channel current in neonatal rat ventricular cells. The holding potential in this experiment was –70 mV, and a small T-channel component is apparent in the I-V relationship. rPTH (20 n*M*) almost doubled the inward current. Data from both studies[37,46] suggest that the PTH effect

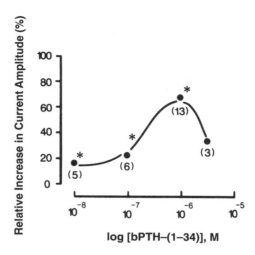

FIGURE 11 The effect of different concentrations of bPTH-(1-34) on the L-channel current in neonatal rat ventricular myocytes. PTH increased the L-channel current. The data are plotted as the mean ± SEM. The increase of the L-channel current at a concentration of 1 μM bPTH-(1-34) was taken as the maximal effect, which was an increase of $73 \pm 13\%$. The concentration at which half the maximal effect occurred was calculated from a fitted Hill function and was $1.4 \times 10^{-7} M$. (From Wang, R. et al., *J. Cardiovasc. Pharmacol.*, 17, 990, 1991. With permission.)

on cardiac myocytes was not completely reversible, at least during the time frame of the experiment.

The effect of the concentration of bPTH-(1-34) and the L-channel response is shown in Figure 11. This is an experiment in which bPTH-(1-34) was used on cells having the intracellular Ca^{2+} buffered by 10 mM EGTA. As the concentration of bPTH-(1-34) was increased from 10 nM to 1 μM, the magnitude of the L-channel current also increased. At higher concentrations of bPTH-(1-34) fewer cells responded to the peptide, and at a concentration of 10 μM the effect was less than that at 1 μM, suggesting some type of desensitization. The effect of bPTH-(1-34) concentration on the L-channel current in ventricular myocytes is shown in Figure 11. The Hill function was fitted to the data using the effect at a concentration of 1 μM as the maximal effect. The concentration of bPTH-(1-34) at which 50% of the maximal effect occurred was calculated to be $1.4 \times 10^{-7} M$.

C. Analysis of the Parathyroid Hormone Effect at the Single L-Channel Level

The study by Rampe et al.[46] used cell-attached patches to show that rPTH-(1-34) (10 nM) increased the mean open time of single-channel currents. Figure 12 shows consecutive current records in the absence or presence of rPTH-(1-34) (10 nM). The number of channel openings was increased as was the integral of the Ca^{2+} channel current during step depolarizations. Figure 13 shows the effect of rPTH-(1-34) (10 nM) on the mean open times of the L-Ca^{2+} channels. There is a small, significant increase in the channel opening time after the addition of 10 nM rPTH-(1-34).

D. Summary and Discussion

The data presented in this section[37,46] show that PTH exerts its inotropic effects on ventricular tissue by increasing the L-channel current. This is supported by experiments using the whole cell and the cell-attached version of the patch clamp technique, and was also confirmed using flux studies.[46] The differences in the effective concentrations of PTH used by the two groups are likely due to the differences in the intracellular Ca^{2+} concentrations. Wang et al.[37] buffered

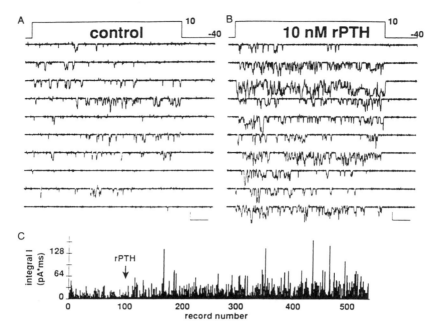

FIGURE 12 The effects of rPTH on single Ca^{2+} channel currents in rat ventricular myocytes. Consecutive records from a cell-attached patch control (No. 10–19) and after addition of 10 nM rPTH-(1-34) (No. 251–260) are shown in A and B, respectively. Records were obtained at 36°C and a frequency of 1 Hz. Ba^{2+} (115 mM) was the charge carrier. The holding and pulse protocols are shown at the top and the 10 ms and 2 pA calibration at the bottom. The data were analogue filtered at 2.4 KHz (-3 dB) using an 8-pole Bessel filter before digitization at 20 KHz. The data were idealized and the integral of idealized single channel currents is shown in C. Data acquisition was halted at record 100 for about 30 s to add rPTH as indicated by the arrow and after every 100 records for about 10 s. At least two channels were present in this patch. (From Rampe, D. et al., *Am. J. Physiol.*, 261(6), H1945, 1991. With permission.)

intracellular Ca^{2+} concentrations to $<10^{-8}$ M. This level of intracellular Ca^{2+} would reduce the activity of any Ca^{2+}-dependent mechanisms. Rampe et al.[46] buffered intracellular Ca^{2+} to physiological levels (135 nM) and hence the concentrations of PTH required were much lower. However, the conclusions of the two studies were similar, i.e., PTH modulates/increases L-Ca^{2+} channel current in neonatal rat ventricular myocytes. This mechanism is mediated by G_s and cAMP and evidence to support this hypothesis is presented in Section IX.

VIII. ROLE OF ADENOSINE 3':5'-CYCLIC PHOSPHATE IN THE PARATHYROID HORMONE MODULATION OF L-Ca²⁺ CHANNELS IN VASCULAR SMOOTH MUSCLE CELLS

There is much evidence that PTH regulates Ca^{2+} homeostasis by activating kidney and bone adenylate cyclase. A study by Helwig et al.[44] has shown that bPTH-(1-34) increased cAMP accumulation in isolated renal cortex microvessels and glomeruli. The increase in cAMP accumulation caused by bPTH-(1-34) was potentiated by guanosine triphosphate (GTP) in microvessels, but not in glomeruli. The effect of bPTH-(1-34) on microvessels could be inhibited by the sulfur-free PTH analogue, [Nle⁸,¹⁸, Tyr³⁴] bPTH-(1-34) NH₂, and oxidized PTH.[47] In vascular smooth muscle, using cultured cells and vascular strips, it has been demonstrated that PTH increases cAMP levels,[41,43] and that this increase in cAMP plays an important role in the vascular effect of PTH. The relaxation of vascular strips by PTH precontracted by KCl was rapid, but the maximal effect did not develop for 5 to 6 min.[43] This

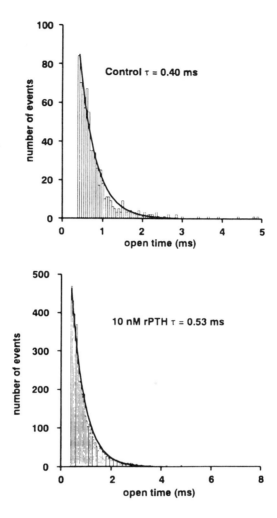

FIGURE 13 Open time histograms calculated from the patch shown in Figure 12. The control open time distribution is shown at the top and the open time distribution after rPTH is shown at the bottom. There is an increase in open time after 10 nM rPTH-(1-34). (From Rampe, D. et al., *Am. J. Physiol.*, 261(6), H1945, 1991. With permission.)

is in agreement with the study of Wang et al.,[37] who reported that a period of 5 min was required to establish the inhibitory effect of bPTH-(1-34) on L-channel currents in rat tail artery vascular smooth muscle cells. The time course of cAMP accumulation in vascular smooth muscle induced by bPTH-(1-34) is similar. For example, in isolated vascular smooth muscle cells the increase in cAMP occurred within 1 min and was maximal at 5 to 10 min after treatment with bPTH-(1-34).[43]

Experiments by Wang et al.[48] have demonstrated that dibutyryl cAMP (dbcAMP) mimics the effect of PTH on L-channel currents. The L-channel current was decreased by $26 \pm 11\%$ after dbcAMP was added to the bath. The concentration of dbcAMP in the bath solution was 1 mM, and the decrease in current was measured 10 min after addition of dbcAMP to a static bath. In another series of experiments,[48] imidazole, a phosphodiesterase stimulator, was used. Vascular smooth muscle cells were pretreated with 1 mM imidazole for 20 min. At a concentration of 1 μM, bPTH-(1-34) produced a small decrease in L-channel current. The magnitude of the decrease was approximately 8%. In cells not pretreated with imidazole,

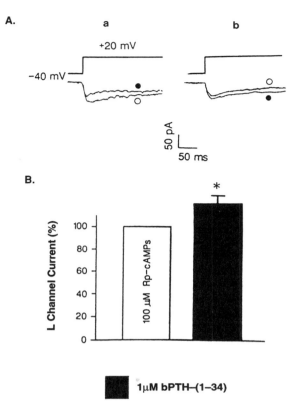

FIGURE 14 The inhibition of the bPTH-(1-34) effect on L-channel currents in vascular smooth muscle by the intracellular application of Rp-cAMPs. (A) Current records in the absence (open circles) and presence (filled circles) of 1 μ*M* bPTH-(1-34). The currents shown at left were obtained from a cell without intracellular Rp-cAMPs. The currents shown at right were obtained from a cell with intracellular Rp-cAMPs (100 μ*M*). (B) The effect of bPTH-(1-34) on the L-channel current in vascular smooth muscle cells is reversed by intracellular Rp-cAMPs ($p < 0.05$, $n = 5$). (From Wang, R. et al., *FEBS Lett.*, 282, 331, 1991. With permission.)

bPTH-(1-34) at a similar concentration decreased the L-channel current by about 36%. This suggests that cAMP accumulation mediates the effect of PTH.

A more direct experiment involves the use of Rp-cAMPs, a cAMP antagonist. Rp-cAMPs is a cAMP analogue with a sulfur atom substitution in the equatorial exocyclic oxygen position, which binds to the cAMP-binding sites on the cAMP-dependent protein kinase. Rp-cAMPs has a much greater binding affinity than does cAMP (90-fold greater).[49] The binding of Rp-cAMPs to the regulatory subunits does not induce dissociation of the holoenzyme and hence competitively inhibits the cAMP-induced activation of cAMP-dependent protein kinase. The results of experiments in which Rp-cAMPs (100 μ*M*) was included in the pipette solution are shown in Figure 14. Figure 14A shows the effects of the intracellular application of Rp-cAMPs in two cells. The current records shown in Figure 14A(left panel) were obtained from a cell without intracellular Rp-cAMPs. The application of 1 μM bPTH-(1-34) decreased the L-channel currents. When 100 μM Rp-cAMPs was included in the pipette solution, subsequent application of bPTH-(1-34) (1 μ*M*) caused a small increase in the L-channel current. Data from two groups of cells are shown in Figure 14B. Two interesting points arise from these experiments. The most obvious observation from the results shown in Figure 14B is that inhibition of PKA abolished the decrease in L-channel current caused by bPTH-(1-34).

Another probably significant observation is that after the intracellular application of Rp-cAMPs, bPTH-(1-34) caused a small but significant increase in the L-channel current. This then suggests that the modulatory effect of bPTH-(1-34) on L-channel currents is in part mediated by PKA. Further analysis of the results with Rp-cAMPs suggests that PTH may have a cAMP-independent effect on the L-channel current in vascular smooth muscle cells. This effect is opposite to that of the cAMP-dependent effect (i.e., an increase in the L-channel current instead of a decrease). Unfortunately, this is only speculation at this time due to a lack of experimental data.

IX. ROLE OF ADENOSINE 3′:5′-CYCLIC PHOSPHATE IN THE PARATHYROID HORMONE MODULATION OF L-Ca^{2+} CHANNELS IN VENTRICULAR MYOCYTES

Parathyroid hormone has been shown to increase cAMP levels in target organs such as the kidney.[50] In addition, Bogin et al.[12] have reported that PTH increased cAMP levels in cardiac tissue. This observation has been confirmed and extended in neonatal rat ventricular myocytes and is shown in Figure 15. bPTH-(1-34) increased cAMP accumulation in neonatal rat ventricular cells with an EC$_{50}$ of $1.1 \pm 0.06 \times 10^{-9}M$ (Figure 15A). In the same study, Rampe et al.[46] demonstrated that pretreatment of neonatal rat ventricular myocytes with cholera toxin increased the stimulated Ca^{2+} uptake and blocked any further increases by bPTH-(1-34) (10 μM) (Figure 15B). Also shown is the effect of bPTH-(3-34), a nonactive peptide fragment of bPTH, on Ca^{2+} uptake. The 3-34 amino acid sequence of bPTH-(3-34) was used to help show that the PTH effect was mediated specifically via a PTH receptor. Fragments of PTH such as bPTH-(3-34) act as antagonists of bPTH-(1-34) in some systems.[8,38,41] These results and the results from Section VII suggest that the modulation of L-channels in ventricular myocytes by PTH is mediated by a G-protein (G$_s$) and cAMP. This is similar to the β-adrenergic modulation of L-channels in the same tissue.

The role of the cAMP cascade in the mediation of the PTH effect in cardiac myocytes has also been demonstrated by Wang et al.[48] This study confirms many of the other observations which suggest the involvement of the cAMP second messenger cascade in the modulation of L-channel current in cardiac cells. An important observation is the effect of bPTH-(1-34) on the L-channel current in cells dialyzed with 100 μM Rp-cAMPs, a PKA inhibitor. The results of this experiment are shown in Figure 16. Rp-cAMPs inhibited the increase in L-channel current caused by bPTH. Another interesting observation is that in cells dialyzed with 100 μM Rp-cAMPs, 1 μM of bPTH-(1-34) caused a small decrease in L-channel current (see Figure 16A). In neonatal ventricular myocytes dialyzed with 100 μM Rp-cAMPs the peak amplitude of the L-channel current was decreased by bPTH-(1-34) (1 μM). This decrease was approximately $14 \pm 4\%$ and is shown in Figure 16B. This suggests that, as was the case for vascular smooth muscle cells, PTH activates other second messenger cascades or that Rp-cAMPs has additional intracellular actions. If this is a real effect of PTH, the inhibitory effect may then be overshadowed by the cAMP-dependent effect.

X. GENERAL SUMMARY AND DISCUSSION

A. Summary

Based on the data presented in this and previous chapters, several conclusions may be drawn:

1. PTH decreases the L-channel current in vascular smooth muscle cells.
2. PTH increases the L-channel current in neonatal ventricular myocytes.

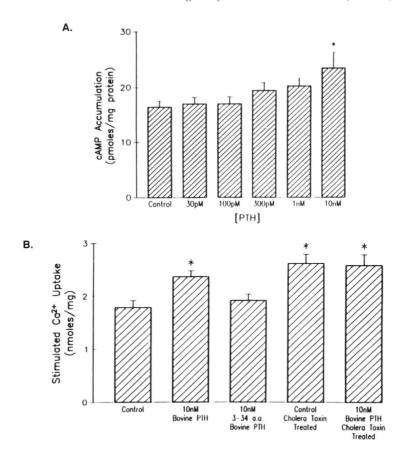

FIGURE 15 (A) The effects of PTH on cAMP accumulation and Ca^{2+} influx in cardiac myocytes. Cells were incubated with various concentrations of rPTH-(1-34) for 10 min prior to measuring cAMP accumulation. Bars indicate SEM, * indicates significantly greater than control ($p < 0.05$ ANOVA, least significant difference, $n = 5$). (B) Stimulated Ca^{2+} uptake in response to bPTH-(1-34) and bPTH-(3-34) and cholera toxin pretreatment (2 µg/ml, 18 to 20 h) * indicates significantly greater than control ($p < 0.05$ ANOVA, least significant difference). Error bars represent SEM, $n = 9$. (From Rampe, D. et al., *Am. J. Physiol.*, 261(6), H1945, 1991. With permission.)

3. The PTH modulation of the channels in both cell types, which is the basis for the changes in the currents, is at least in part cAMP-dependent.

B. Effect of Parathyroid Hormone on L-Channels in Vascular Smooth Muscle

Parathyroid hormone has been implicated in the modulation of voltage-dependent calcium channels in many cell types. The potent vasodilator PTH-(1-34) inhibited KCl-stimulated vasoconstriction and ⁴⁵Ca^{2+} uptake in rat tail artery strips.[8,9] In neuroblastoma and vascular smooth muscle cells, bPTH-(1-34) inhibited L-channel currents.[51] This effect of PTH on voltage-dependent Ca^{2+} channels provides an explanation for PTH-induced vasorelaxation. Hence, the data in the chapter support the view proposed by Pang et al.[9] that PTH inhibits Ca^{2+} channels in vascular smooth muscle cells. This view was based on tension and flux studies. The rat tail artery has contractile properties similar to those of small resistance vessels.[52] The activation of L-calcium channels in these cells is likely the link between excitation and contraction of these cells. Consequently, the inhibition of L-channels reduces the amount of

A.

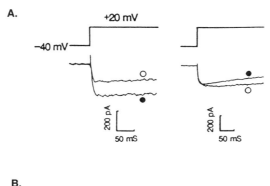

B.

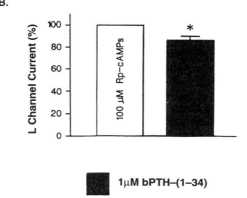

1μM bPTH–(1–34)

FIGURE 16 The inhibition of the bPTH-(1-34) effect on L-channel currents in neonatal rat ventricular myocytes by the intracellular application of Rp-cAMPs. (A) Current records in the absence (open circles) or presence (filled circles) of 1 μM bPTH-(1-34). The currents shown at left were obtained from a cell without intracellular Rp-cAMPs. The currents shown at right were obtained from a cell with intracellular Rp-cAMPs (100 μM). (B) The effect of bPTH-(1-34) on L-channel currents in neonatal ventricular myocytes is reversed by intracellular Rp-cAMPs (100 μM) ($p < 0.05$, $n = 7$). (From Wang, R. et al., *FEBS Lett.*, 282, 331, 1991. With permission.)

Ca^{2+} that enters the cell and this is most likely part of the PTH-induced vasorelaxation mechanism. Because PTH has different roles in various target organs and Ca^{2+} channels behave differently in various tissues,[22] it is reasonable to suggest that PTH regulates Ca^{2+} channels differently in other tissues, i.e., heart.

The normal circulating concentration of PTH is about 10^{-10} M.[53,54] The threshold concentration of bPTH-(1-34) for relaxing the rat tail artery strips precontracted by KCl was approximately 10^{-8} M.[9] In the experiments presented in this chapter which used single vascular smooth muscle cells, the EC_{50} of bPTH-(1-34) was 1.2×10^{-7} M. A possible explanation for this difference is the experimental approach which uses a high concentration of EGTA in the intracellular solution. As a result, the intracellular free Ca^{2+} concentration is estimated to be $<10^{-9}$ M.[55] The low concentration of intracellular calcium will reduce the calcium-induced inactivation of Ca^{2+} channel currents, but the activity of some intracellular-dependent enzymes will be decreased. If the effect of bPTH-(1-34) on the L-channel current in vascular smooth muscle cells is mediated by a calcium-dependent step, a higher concentration of bPTH-(1-34) may be required. Additionally, in studies using single cells, enzymatic treatment may cause damage to membrane proteins. It has been reported that in cell dialysis experiments, the concentrations of agents used to block or mimic hormonal responses were much higher than those used in biochemical studies (i.e., 10^{-6} M instead of 10^{-9} M).[56]

C. Effect of Parathyroid Hormone on L-Channels in Ventricular Myocytes

Several studies have shown that PTH causes positive inotropic and chronotropic effects in cardiac muscle.[10-14] It has been suggested that the cardiac actions of PTH may be due to the modulation of Ca^{2+} entry into the cell via Ca^{2+} channels. PTH increases stimulated (high K^+) Ca^{2+} influx in neonatal rat ventricular myocytes with an EC_{50} of $4.3 \pm 0.05 \times 10^{-11}$ M.[46] This influx was nifedipine sensitive. In experiments using an intracellular solution with an intracellular free Ca^{2+} concentration of 135 nM, Rampe et al.[46] showed that 20 nM rPTH-(1-34) increased the L-channel current by a factor of nearly 2. In addition, rPTH increased the single channel mean open time. In a parallel study using the same cell preparation Wang et al.[37] also demonstrated that bPTH-(1-34) increased the L-current. In this study, a high concentration of EGTA was used to ensure an intracellular free Ca^{2+} concentration of $<10^{-9}$ M, and the threshold concentration was approximately 10^{-8}. The concentration at which half the maximal effect occurred was about 1.4×10^{-7} M. The response of the cells was related to the concentration of the peptide. When the concentration of the peptide was increased beyond a critical value, the effect of PTH was decreased rather than continuously increased or saturated. It has been postulated[57] that the tissue became rapidly resistant to PTH and the response to higher concentrations then decreased.

PTH has opposite effects on L-Ca^{2+} channels in various cell types. This hormone inhibited L-channel currents in neuroblastoma and vascular smooth muscle cells and activated L-channel currents in neonatal ventricular cells. These selective actions of PTH may be partially explained if the PTH receptor is coupled to the L-channel by other second messenger pathways. However, Sections VIII and IX presented evidence that the effects of PTH on L-channel current in vascular smooth muscle cells and ventricular myocytes are mediated at least in part by cAMP. Alternatively, PTH receptors could be tissue specific, resulting in different effects of PTH on L-channels in various tissues.

D. Effect of Parathyroid Hormone on L-Channels in Vascular Smooth Muscle Cells and Ventricular Myocytes is Mediated by an Adenosine 3′:5′-Cyclic Phosphate-Dependent Mechanism

The effect of PTH on ventricular myocytes is mediated by cAMP. From the evidence presented in Section IX and in other chapters, it is likely that activation of the PTH receptor activates G_s, which in turn increases accumulation of cAMP. cAMP activates PKA, which in turn phosphorylates the L-Ca^{2+} channels. It is well documented that L-Ca^{2+} channel activity is increased by PKA phosphorylation.[5,58] Further analysis at the single channel level[46] shows that PTH causes a small increase in Ca^{2+} channel mean open time and an increase in the integral of the Ca^{2+} channel current (single-channel currents). This is consistent with the hypothesis that the primary effect resulting from PKA phosphorylation of the L-Ca^{2+} channel is an increase in the probability of the Ca^{2+} channel being open. This mechanism is similar to that seen with β-agonists in cardiac tissue. In addition, although it has not been demonstrated for PTH, it is not possible to rule out direct activation of the L-channel by G_s or the contribution of other second messenger pathways.

The mechanism by which PTH modulates L-channels in vascular smooth muscle (rat tail artery) is different. PTH increases cAMP accumulation and decreases the L-channel current in vascular smooth muscle cells. A PKA inhibitor (Rp-cAMPs) blocks the PTH-induced inhibition of L-channel current. Experiments using dbcAMP showed that dbcAMP also inhibited the L-channel current. The L-channel current in vascular smooth muscle cells which were pretreated with imidazole, a phosphodiesterase stimulator, did not respond to PTH. An explanation of the potential mechanism is difficult because there are many unknowns. A tempting conclusion would be to suggest that PTH activates a receptor which in turn activates G_s, and subsequently the cAMP cascade. The final part is difficult to describe. It is possible that PKA activates a phosphatase (undocumented), which results in the dephosphorylation of the L-Ca^{2+} channels and reduces the probability of the channels being open. The activation of protein kinase C (PKC) by cAMP is unlikely, even though PKC has been shown to inhibit Ca^{2+} channels.[59] Lincoln et al.[60] give evidence that cAMP can activate the cyclic guanosine monophosphate (cGMP) -dependent protein kinase in vascular smooth muscle cells. In this potential mechanism, the final stage leading to L-Ca^{2+} channel dephosphorylation is unknown.

An increase in intracellular cGMP is also known to relax vascular smooth muscle. However, it has been reported that bPTH-(1-34) caused very small changes in cGMP accumulation in rabbit aorta.[41] Much larger changes occurred in cAMP accumulation, and it is unlikely that cGMP mediates the PTH modulation of the L-channel in vascular smooth muscle cells. Another possibility is that PTH activates two different PTH receptors that are coupled to different second messenger cascades. Although evidence exists for more than one type of PTH receptor, the details of the G protein coupling and potential second messenger pathways are not well documented. A recent report[61] shows that in addition to the well-documented effect of PTH, the activation of adenylate cyclase, PTH also causes phosphoinositide breakdown and the generation of diacylglycerol, which in turn activates PKC. The cells used in this study were ROS 17/2 rat osteosarcoma cells. Human parathyroid hormone (hPTH-(1-84)) increased PKC activity at two widely separated concentrations. Maximal PKC activity occurred at about 10 pM and 10 nM and the maximal cAMP accumulation occurred at about 10 nM. This shows that PTH can activate two separate intracellular second messenger pathways. The general conclusion of this study[61] is that ROS 17/2 cells have both high and low affinity PTH receptors coupled to PKC. The low affinity receptors are also coupled to adenylate cyclase and when activated by PTH cause an increase in cAMP. On the basis of this report[61], it is tempting to speculate that PTH decreases the L-channel current in vascular smooth muscle cells by activating low affinity PTH receptors, which in turn activate protein kinase, causing a decrease in the L-channel current. The increase in cAMP would not be important if that were the case.

Several good arguments explain why the above scheme is not likely. First, osteosarcoma cells are a primary target cell for PTH, a calcium-regulating hormone, whereas vascular smooth muscle cells are not likely primary target cells, and therefore their response to PTH would not be similar. A second point, which strongly supports the involvement of the cAMP second messenger cascade, comes from experiments using Rp-cAMPs.[48] Rp-cAMPs is an inhibitor of PKA, and the intracellular application of Rp-cAMPs completely inhibited the PTH effect on the L-channel current. Finally, a study using bPTH-(3-34),[62] which is known to be a bPTH-(1-34) antagonist, shows that bPTH-(3-34) increases PKC activity but does not increase cAMP accumulation in rat osteosarcoma and murine T lymphoma cells. An earlier report by Wang et al.[48] very clearly shows that bPTH-(3-34) has no effect on the L-channel current in vascular smooth muscle cells. Hence, as suggested earlier in this chapter, it is likely that the inhibitory effect of PTH on the L-channel is mediated by cAMP and PKA. The final mechanism, however, remains to be determined.

ACKNOWLEDGMENTS

The author would like to thank Dr. P. K. T. Pang for his helpful discussions and critical comments during the preparation of this manuscript, and Dr. Rosemary Pang for her editorial assistance. The author is also grateful to Doreen Eichenlaub for typing the manuscript.

REFERENCES

1. Benham, C. D. and Tsien, R. W., A novel receptor-operated Ca^{2+} permeable channel activated by ATP in smooth muscle, *Nature,* 328, 275, 1987.
2. Reuter, H., Calcium channel modulation by neurotransmitters, enzymes and drugs, *Nature,* 301, 569, 1983.
3. Reuter, H., The dependence of slow inward current in Purkinje fibers on the extracellular calcium-concentration, *J. Physiol.,* 192, 479, 1967.
4. Mitra, R. and Morad, M., Two types of calcium channels in guinea pig ventricular myocytes, *Proc. Natl. Acad. Sci. U.S.A.,* 93, 5340, 1986.
5. Tsien, R. W., Bean, B. P., Hess, P., Lansman, J. B., and Nowycky, M. C., Mechanisms of calcium channel modulation by β-adrenergic agents and dihydropyridine calcium agonist, *J. Mol. Cell Cardiol.,* 18, 691, 1986.
6. Ono, K., Dely, M., Nakijima, T., Irisawa, H., and Giles, W., Calcitonin gene-related peptide regulates calcium current in heart muscle, *Nature,* 340(31), 721, 1989.
7. Pang, P. K. T., Tenner, T. E., Jr., Yee, J. A., and Janssen, H. F., Hypotensive action of parathyroid hormone preparations on rats and dogs, *Proc. Natl. Acad. Sci. U.S.A.,* 77, 675, 1980.
8. Daugirdas, J. T., Al Kudsi, R. R., Ing, T. S., Yang, M. C. M., Leehey, D. J., and Pang, P. K. T., Hemodynamic effects of bPTH(1-34) and its analogue Nle[8,18] Tyr[34] bPTH(3-34) amide, *Min. Electrolyte Metab.,* 13, 33, 1987.
9. Pang, P. K. T., Yang, M. C. M., and Sham, J. S. K., Parathyroid hormone and calcium entry blockade in a vascular tissue, *Life Sci.,* 42, 1395, 1988.
10. Hashimoto, K., Nakagawa, Y., Shibuya, T., Satoh, H., Ushijima, T., and Imai, S., Effects of parathyroid hormone and related polypeptides on the heart and coronary circulation of dogs, *J. Cardiovasc. Pharmacol.,* 3, 668, 1981.
11. Tenner, T. E., Jr., Ramanadham, S., Yang, M. C., and Pang, P. K. T., Chronotropic actions of bPTH-(1-34) in the right atrium of the rat, *Can. J. Physiol. Pharmacol.,* 61(10), 1162, 1983.
12. Bogin, E., Massry, S. G., and Harvey, I., Effect of parathyroid hormone on rat heart cells, *J. Clin. Invest.,* 67, 1215, 1981.
13. Kondo, N., Shibata, S., Tenner, T. E., Jr., and Pang, P. K. T., Electromechanical effects of bPTH-(1-34) on rabbit sinus node cells and guinea pig papillary muscles, *J. Cardiovasc. Pharmacol.,* 11, 619, 1988.
14. Katoh, Y., Klein, K. L., Kaplan, R. A., Sanborn, W. G., and Kurokawa, K., Parathyroid hormone has a positive inotropic action in the rat, *Endocrinology,* 109(6), 2252, 1981.
15. McCleskey, E. W., Fox, A. P., Feldman, D., and Tsien, R. W., Different types of calcium channels, *J. Exp. Biol.,* 124, 177, 1986.
16. Nowycky, M. C., Fox, A. P., and Tsien, R. W., Three types of neuronal calcium channels with different calcium agonist sensitivity, *Nature,* 316, 440, 1985.
17. Bean, B. P., Multiple types of calcium channels in heart muscle and neurons, *Ann. N.Y. Acad. Sci.,* 560, 334, 1989.
18. Hamill, O. P., Marty, A., Neher, E., Sakmann, B., and Sigworth, F. J., Improved patch-clamp techniques for high resolution current recording from cells and cell-free membrane patches, *Pfluegers Arch.,* 39, 85, 1981.
19. Reuter, H., A variety of calcium channels, *Nature,* 316, 391, 1985.
20. Hirst, G. D. S., Silverbery, G. D., and Van Helden, D. F., The action potential and underlying ionic currents in proximal rat middle cerebral arterioles, *J. Physiol.,* 371, 289, 1986.
21. Sturek, M. and Hermsmeyer, K., Calcium and sodium channels in spontaneously contracting vascular muscle cells, *Science,* 233, 475, 1986.
22. Bean, B. P., Sturek, M., Puga, A., and Hermsmeyer, K., Calcium channels in muscle cells isolated from rat mesenteric arteries: modulation by dihydropyridine drugs, *Circ. Res.,* 59(2), 229, 1986.
23. Caffrey, J. M., Josephson, I. R., and Brown, A. M., Calcium channels of amphibian stomach and mammalian aorta smooth muscle cells, *Biophys. J.,* 49, 1237, 1986.

24. Benham, C. D., Hess, P., and Tsien, R. W., Two types of calcium channels in single smooth muscle cells from rabbit ear artery studied with whole-cell and single-channel recordings, *Circ. Res.,* 61(Suppl. 1), I10, 1987.

25. Wang, R., Karpinski, E., and Pang, P. K. T., Two types of calcium channels in isolated smooth muscle cells from rat tail artery, *Am. J. Physiol.,* 256(25), H1361, 1989.

26. Nilius, B., Hess, P., Lansman, J. B., and Tsien, R. W., A novel type of cardiac calcium channel in ventricular cells, *Nature,* 316, 443, 1985.

27. Bean, B., Two kinds of calcium channels in canine atrial cells: differences in kinetics, selectivity, and pharmacology, *J. Gen. Physiol.,* 86, 1, 1985.

28. Hagiwara, N., Irisawa, H., and Kameyama, M., Contribution of two types of calcium currents to the pacemaker potentials of rabbit sino-atrial node cells, *J. Physiol.,* 395, 233, 1988.

29. Tsien, R. W., Hess, P., and Nilius, B., Cardiac calcium currents at the level of single channels, *Experientia,* 43, 1169, 1987.

30. Tsien, R. W., Hess, P., McCleskey, E. W., and Rosenberg, R. L., Calcium channels: mechanisms of selectivity, permeation, and block, *Annu. Rev. Biophys. Biophys. Chem.,* 16, 265, 1987.

31. Kawano, S. and DeHaan, R. L., Analysis of the T-type calcium channel in embryonic chick ventricular myocytes, *J. Membr. Biol.,* 116, 9, 1990.

32. Bean, B. P., Classes of calcium channels in vertebrate cells, *Ann. Rev. Physiol.,* 51, 367, 1989.

33. Wang, R., Karpinski, E., Wu, L., and Pang, P. K. T., Flunarizine selectively blocks transient calcium channel currents in N1E-115 cells, *J. Pharmacol. Exp. Ther.,* 254(3), 1006, 1990.

34. Rosenberg, R. L. and Tsien, R. W., Calcium-permeable channels from cardiac sarcolemma open at resting membrane potentials, *Biophys. J.,* 51(Abstr.), 29, 1987.

35. Coulombe, A., Lefevre, I. A., Baro, I., and Coraboeuf, E., Barium- and calcium-permeable channels open at negative membrane potentials in rat ventricular myocytes, *J. Membr. Biol.,* 111, 57, 1989.

36. Rampe, D., Skattebol, A., Triggle, D. J., and Brown, A. M., Effects of McN-6186 on voltage-dependent Ca^{2+} channels in heart and pituitary cells, *J. Pharmacol. Exp. Ther.,* 248(1), 164, 1989.

37. Wang, R., Karpinski, E., and Pang, P. K. T., Two types of voltage-dependent calcium channel currents and their modulation by parathyroid hormone in neonatal rat ventricular cells, *J. Cardiovasc. Pharmacol.,* 17, 990, 1991.

38. Wang, R., Karpinski, E., and Pang, P. K. T., Parathyroid hormone selectively inhibits L-type calcium channels in single vascular smooth cells of the rat, *J. Physiol.,* 441, 325, 1991.

39. Nickols, G. A., Nickols, M. A., and Helwig, J. J., Binding of parathyroid hormone (PTH) and parathyroid hormone-related protein (PTHrp) to rabbit renal microvessels and tubules, *FASEB J.,* 3(Abstr.), A283 1989.

40. Nickols, G. A., Nickols, M. A., and Helwig, J. J., Binding of parathyroid hormone and parathyroid hormone-related protein to vascular smooth muscle of rabbit renal microvessels, *Endocrinology,* 126(2), 721, 1990.

41. Nickols, G. A. and Cline, W. H. Jr., Parathyroid hormone-induced changes in cyclic nucleotide levels during relaxation of the rat aorta, *Life Sci.,* 40(24), 2351, 1987.

42. Hardman, J. G., Cyclic nucleotides and smooth muscle contraction: some conceptual and experimental considerations, in *Smooth Muscle: An Assessment of Current Knowledge,* Bulbring, E., Brading, A. F., Jones, A. W., and Tomita, T., Eds., University of Texas Press, Austin, 1981, 249.

43. Nickols, G. A., Increased cyclic AMP in cultured vascular smooth muscle cells and relaxation of aortic strips by parathyroid hormone, *Eur. J. Pharmacol.,* 116, 137, 1985.

44. Helwig, J. J., Schleiffer, R., Judes, C., and Gairard, A., Distribution of parathyroid hormone-sensitive adenylate cyclase in isolated rabbit renal cortex microvessels and glomeruli, *Life Sci.,* 35, 2649, 1984.

45. Pang, P. K. T., Yang, M. C. M., Tenner, T. E., Jr., Kenny, A. D., and Cooper, C. W., Cyclic AMP and the vascular action of parathyroid hormone, *Can. J. Physiol. Pharmacol.,* 64, 1543, 1986.

46. Rampe, D., Lacerda, A. E., Dage, R. C., and Brown, A. M., Parathyroid hormone: an endogenous modulator of cardiac calcium channels, *Am. J. Physiol.,* 261(6), H1945, 1991.

47. Helwig, J. J., Yang, M. C. M., Bollack, C., Judes, C., and Pang, P. K. T., Structure-activity relationship of parathyroid hormone: relative sensitivity of rabbit renal microvessel and tubule adenylate cyclases to oxidized PTH and PTH inhibitors, *Eur. J. Pharmacol.*, 140, 247, 1987.
48. Wang, R., Wu, L. Y., Karpinski, E., and Pang, P. K. T., The effects of parathyroid hormone on L-type voltage-dependent calcium channel currents in vascular smooth muscle cells and ventricular myocytes are mediated by a cAMP dependent mechanism, *FEBS Lett.*, 282, 331, 1991.
49. Rothermel, J. D. and Botelho, L. H. P., A mechanistic and kinetic analysis of the interactions of the diastereoisomers of adenosine 3',5'-(cyclic) phosphorothioate with purified cyclic AMP-dependent protein kinase, *Biochem. J.*, 251, 757, 1988.
50. Potts, J. T., Kronenberg, H. M., and Rosenblatt, M., Parathyroid hormone: chemistry, biosynthesis and mode of action, *Adv. Protein. Chem.*, 35, 323, 1982.
51. Pang, P. K. T., Wang, R., Shan, J., Karpinski, E., and Benishin, C. G., Specific inhibition of long lasting, L-type calcium channels by synthetic parathyroid hormone, *Proc. Natl. Acad. Sci. U.S.A.*, 87, 623, 1990.
52. Frost, B. R., Gerke, D. C., and Frewin, D. D., The effect of 2-phenylalanine-8-lysine vasopressin (octapressin) on blood vessels in the rat tail, *Aust. J. Exp. Biol. Med. Sci.*, 54, 403, 1976.
53. Fischer, J. A., Binswanger, U., and Dietrich, F. M., Human parathyroid hormone. Immunological characterization of antibodies against a glandular extract and the synthetic amino-terminal fragments 1-12 and 1-34 and their use in the determination of immunoreactive hormone in human sera, *J. Clin. Invest.*, 54, 1382, 1974.
54. Carnes, D. L., Anast, C. S., and Forte, L. R., Renal parathyroid hormone-dependent adenylate cyclase activity after repletion of vitamin D-deficient rats with vitamin D₂, *Biochim. Biophys. Acta*, 629, 546, 1980.
55. Sada, H., Kojima, M., and Sperelakis, N., Fast inward current properties of voltage-dependent ventricular cells of embryonic chick heart, *Am. J. Physiol.*, 255(24), H540, 1988.
56. Hescheler, J., Tang, M., Jastorff, B., and Trautwein, W., On the mechanism of histamine induced enhancement of the cardiac Ca²⁺ current, *Pfluegers Arch.*, 410, 23, 1987.
57. Musso, M.-J., Barthelmebs, M., Imbs, J.-L., Plante, M., and Bollack, C., The vasodilator action of parathyroid hormone fragments on isolated perfused rat kidney, *Naunyn-Schmiedeberg's Arch. Pharmacol.*, 34, 246, 1989.
58. Trautwein, W. and Heschler, J., Regulation of cardiac L-type calcium current by phosphorylation and G proteins, *Ann. Rev. Physiol.*, 52, 257, 1990.
59. Galizzi, J.-P., Qar, J., Fosset, M., van Renterghem, C., and Lazunski, M., Regulation of calcium channels in aortic muscle cells by protein kinase C activators (diacylglycerol and phorbol esters) and by peptides (vasopressin and bombesin) that stimulate phosphoinositide breakdown, *J. Biol. Chem.*, 262, 6947, 1987.
60. Lincoln, T. M., Cornwell, T. L., and Taylor, A. E., cGMP-dependent protein kinase mediates the reduction of Ca⁺⁺ by cAMP in vascular smooth muscle cells, *Am. J. Physiol.*, 258, C399, 1990.
61. Jouishomme, H., Whitfield, J. F., Chakravarthy, B., Durkin, J. P., Gagnon, L., Isaacs, R. J., MacLean, S., Neugenbauer, W., Willick, G., and Rixon, R. H., The protein kinase-C activation domain of the parathyroid hormone, *Endocrinology*, 130, 53, 1992.
62. Chakravarthy, B. R., Durkin, J. P., Rixon, R. H., and Whitfield, J. F., Parathyroid hormone fragment [3-34] stimulates protein kinase-C (PKC) activity in rat osteosarcoma and murine T-lymphoma cells, *Biochem. Biophys. Res. Commun.*, 171, 1105, 1990.

4

Role of the Parathyroid Gland in Experimental Hypertension

Alexis Gairard, Nadji Boulebda, Fanny Pernot, and Bruno Van Overloop

CONTENTS

I. INTRODUCTION

Bone, kidney, and intestine are the main targets for parathyroid hormone (PTH), a peptide hormone produced by the parathyroid glands.[1] In addition, cardiovascular effects of the hormone, including vasodilation and hypotension, have been described, initially with parathyroid extracts and then with the synthetic hormone bovine PTH-(1-84) [bPTH-(1-84)] and fragments [rat, bovine, and human PTH-(1-34)]. Recently, high affinity binding sites for PTH fragments have been described on vessels such as rabbit renal microvessels.[2] More recently, a PTH-related protein (PTHrP) and its messenger RNA transcripts were described in normal tissues, including heart and vessels. Vasodilatory properties of PTHrP have been established in normotensive and genetically hypertensive rats (SHR),[3] and vasorelaxant properties were shown in isolated perfused aortas.[4] The above involved acute effects, and were observed mainly at pharmacological doses.

In humans primary hyperparathyroidism has been associated with hypertension,[5] and numerous reports indicating an involvement of parathyroid function in blood pressure regulation have appeared during the last decade. Clinical observations have shown that primary hyperparathyroidism is frequently associated with elevated serum calcium and systolic blood pressure.[6] Similarly, young mild-to-moderate hypertensives displayed enhanced serum PTH levels.[7,8] Moreover, chronic PTH infusion has been shown to elicit hypertension in normal subjects.[9] Finally, relationships among dietary calcium, sodium intake, and blood pressure,[10] as well as between calcium metabolic indices and blood pressure,[11-13] have been described in patients with essential hypertension.

This chapter examines both acute and chronic effects of parathyroidectomy and of cross-transplantation of parathyroids on cardiovascular reactivity in rats. These effects involve alterations in myocardial and vascular smooth muscle calcium function as well as hormonal and neuronal activities, suggesting multifactorial mechanisms which probably compete at different levels.

II. PARATHYROID, CALCIUM, AND HYPERTENSION

Parathyroidectomy performed in young SHR delays the development of and attenuates the level of hypertension. The necessity for the presence of parathyroid glands in the development of hypertension was first described in mineralocorticoid hypertensive rats[14] and then in SHR.[15] These data were confirmed and extended in SHR[16-18] and stroke-prone SHR (SHR-SP).[19,20] It appears that genetically hypertensive rats from the Lyon (LH) and Milan (MHS) strains are also sensitive to bilateral parathyroidectomy performed in young (5-week-old) rats[21] (Figure 1).

A novel cell type was described recently in the parathyroid glands of SHR,[22] and transplantation of SHR parathyroid glands into previously parathyroidectomized Sprague-Dawley rats resulted in a chronic increase in blood pressure.[18] Development of hypertension was also observed in WKY rats after transplantation of parathyroid glands from SHR-SP.[23] Similarly, in young Lyon (LH) and Milan (MNS) normotensive rats, cross-transplantation with parathyroid glands from a young animal of the corresponding hypertensive strain chronically enhanced blood pressure[24,25] (Figure 2). Moreover, a circulating hypertensive factor in SHR, which enhances blood pressure and tail artery calcium uptake in normotensive rats,[26] disappears after parathyroidectomy.[18] Thus, parathyroid glands produce a factor (PHF) which is involved in the development of hypertension and obviously differs from PTH.[27] Clinical results obtained in humans after parathyroidectomy are less clear cut, i.e., parathyroidectomy corrected hypertension in some studies with primary hyperparathyroidism,[28] but not in others.[29] Parathyroidectomy caused a fall in the blood pressures of uremic patients exhibiting secondary hyperparathyroidism. Whether existing pressures were normal or increased, the magnitude of the hypotensive effect was correlated with the preexisting systolic blood pressure.[30] As shown mainly in normotensive and hypertensive rats, secretion of the parathyroid glands was modulated and blood pressures modified by calcium-enriched or calcium-deficient diets. Calcium-enriched (two- to fourfold, mainly with $CaCO_3$) diets lowered blood pressures in experimental models of hypertension in the rat, including mineralocorticoid,[31] Dahl salt-sensitive,[32] renal,[33] and genetic (SHR[34-36] and LH[37]) models.

When normal values for serum calcium were reestablished with a calcium-fortified diet after parathyroidectomy, hypertension was still decreased in SHR[19] and LH[37] rats (Figure 1). The lack of a chronic hormonal secretion from parathyroids (PTH, PHF, or both) is thus able to impair the increase of blood pressure. Administration of parathyroid extract in DOCA + NaCl-treated parathyroidectomized rats elevated arterial blood pressure,[38] and chronic PTH administration reversed the antihypertensive effect of calcium loading in young hypertensive rats.[39] As expected, a low calcium diet enhanced the development of hypertension in SHR[40,41] and LH rats.[40]

III. PARATHYROID AND CARDIOVASCULAR REACTIVITY

Cardiovascular reactivity was studied in order to elucidate the mechanisms by which parathyroidectomy delays the development and attenuates the level of hypertension. The blood pressure response to bolus noradrenaline administration was measured in anesthetized

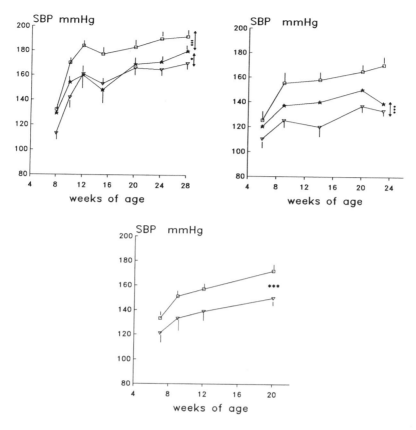

FIGURE 1 Parathyroidectomy and evolution of systolic blood pressure (SBP) in SHR (top left panel), LH (top right panel) and MHS (bottom panel) male rats. Controls: open squares; parathyroidectomy: open triangles; parathyroidectomy fed a calcium-enriched diet: stars. Parathyroidectomy was performed at 4 to 5 weeks of age. Statistical significance determined by ANOVA; * p <0.05, ** p <0.01, *** p <0.001. (Redrawn from Reference 15 for SHR and from Reference 21 for LH.)

parathyroidectomized rats whose blood pressure regulation was suppressed by vagotomy and atropine treatment, or in conscious rats with intact nerve functions. *In vivo*, cardiovascular reactivity to norepinephrine in parathyroidectomized rats from both SHR and WKY controls was decreased, as was calcium content in aortic and heart fragments.[42] These results also were observed in awake parathyroidectomized LH hypertensive rats[21] as well as in normotensive parathyroidectomized Wistar rats.[42] A change in the hind limb vascular reactivity to norepinephrine and vasopressin was not observed in parathyroidectomized SHR or WKY rats;[20] other regional circulations have not been studied.

It is well known that secretion of hormones is calcium dependent. Thus, it is possible that parathyroidectomy could impair the development of hypertension by inducing variations in vasoactive hormones. However, the plasma levels of norepinephrine and angiotensin II did not change in parathyroidectomized SHR-SP.[19] In addition, plasma atrial natriuretic peptide (ANP) did not change in parathyroidectomized SHR.[17]

Vascular reactivity can be measured *in vitro* using conduit vessels such as the aorta, or resistance vessels such as mesenteric arteries. With parathyroidectomized SHR and normotensive parathyroidectomized Wistar rats, Schleiffer and Gairard[43] observed an unexpected result in terms of aortic contraction; i.e., an enhanced response to norepinephrine in which extracellular calcium concentrations played a key role. A similar result was obtained in parathyroidectomized LH rats. The presence of endothelium was mandatory in the aortas of

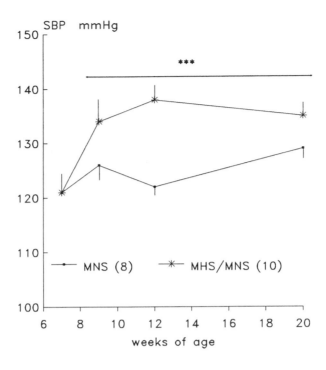

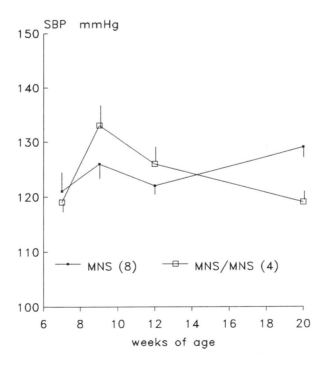

FIGURE 2 Evolution of systolic blood pressure (SBP) after cross-transplantation of one parathyroid gland from 5-week-old MHS donor rat (top panel) and in 5-week-old normotensive parathyroidectomized MNS recipients (bottom panel). MHS/MNS vs. MNS: *** $p < 0.001$ by ANOVA for weeks 9 to 20. (Redrawn from Reference 24.)

both SHR and LH rats.[21,43] It appeared also that endothelium-dependent contractile responses to norepinephrine and serotonin were enhanced in SHR mesenteric resistance vessels after parathyroidectomy, without any change in vascular smooth muscle intracellular calcium, as measured by the fura 2 technique.[44] Similarly, intracellular calcium concentrations in platelets of parathyroidectomized SHR were not lowered despite a reduction in blood pressure.[45] Moreover, this hyperreactivity was also observed in aortas from normotensive strains of parathyroidectomized Wistar and WKY rats.[43,46] Depolarization with KCl also induced an enhanced response in the aorta of the parathyroidectomized SHR[46] and parathyroidectomized SHR mesenteric vessels.[44] Thus, it appears that both voltage- and receptor-operated mechanisms are involved. In the presence of indomethacin, the potentiating effect of parathyroidectomy on norepinephrine-induced contraction was still observed, ruling out a specific production of vasoconstrictors from the arachidonic cascade in endothelium of the parathyroidectomized rat.[47] Hyperactivity of rat aortas that occurs after parathyroidectomy is not linked to hypertension because it is observed in normotensive Wistar and WKY rats, but probably is related to a decrease in endothelial nitric oxide release or activity. It would appear evident that enhanced vascular force generation does not participate directly in the attenuated hypertension in SHR observed after parathyroidectomy.

In conclusion, parathyroid gland activity can modulate vascular contractililty and cellular calcium turnover. Parathyroidectomy ameliorates vascular lesions induced by 11-deoxycorticosterone in heart and kidney despite inducing a small depression in blood pressure.[48] Parathyroidectomy also induces a protective effect against the tissue damage observed in salt-loaded SHR-SP.[49] Vascular and cardiac muscle are considered to be target organs for the parathyroid secretions, PTH and PHF, and these factors may play a role in normal and pathophysiologic cardiovascular control. Their contribution to growth, multiplication, and pathological modifications of vascular and cardiac cells during hypertension remains to be delineated further.

IV. SUMMARY

Several reports in the 1980s suggested an involvement of parathyroid function in blood pressure regulation in animals and humans. Moreover, enriched calcium diets lowered blood pressure in experimental hypertension (mineralocorticoid in Sprague-Dawley rats and genetic in SHR, Dahl, and LH rats). Removal of parathyroid glands (parathyroidectomy) in weanling rats attenuated and delayed the development of mineralocorticoid and genetic hypertension in the rat and cured hypertension in the great majority of primary hyperparathyroid subjects. More recently, experiments have been performed to better delineate the role of the parathyroid glands in blood pressure regulation. *In vivo* cardiovascular reactivity to norepinephrine and calcium content in aortic and heart fragments were all decreased in parathyroidectomized rats from both SHR and LH strains. On the other hand, *in vitro* aortic contractions from parathyroidectomized SHR and LH rats displayed unexpectedly enhanced responses to norepinephrine which were endothelium-dependent and linked to decreased endothelium derived relaxing factor (EDRF) production during chronic hypocalcemia. Because a hypertensive factor (PHF) is produced by the parathyroid glands in genetic hypertensive rats from SHR, Dahl, LH, and MHS strains, and because PHF is also found in human hypertensives, it appears that relationships exist between parathyroids and the regulation of arterial blood pressure, and that these relationships are certainly of great clinical importance.

ACKNOWLEDGMENT

The authors thank Dr. Richard Bukoski for critically reading the manuscript.

REFERENCES

1. Habener, J. F., Rosenblatt, M., and Potts, J., Parathyroid hormone: biochemical aspects of biosynthesis, secretion, action and metabolism, *Physiol. Rev.*, 64, 985, 1984.
2. Nickols, G. A., Nickols, M. A., and Helwig, J. J., Binding of parathyroid hormone and parathyroid hormone-related protein to vascular smooth muscle of rabbit renal microvessels, *Endocrinology*, 126, 721, 1990.
3. DiPette, D. J., Christenson, W., Nickols, M. A., and Nickols, G. A., Cardiovascular responsiveness to parathyroid hormone (PTH) and PTH-related protein in genetic hypertension, *Endocrinology*, 130, 2045, 1992.
4. Crass, M. F., III and Scarpace, P. J., Vasoactive properties of parathyroid hormone-related protein in the rat aorta, *Peptides*, 14, 179, 1993.
5. Rosenthal, F. D. and Roy, S., Hypertension in hyperparathyroidism, *Br. Med. J.*, 4, 396, 1972.
6. Christensson, T., Helstrom, K., and Wengle, B., Blood pressure in subjects with hypercalcaemia and primary hyperparathyroidism detected in a health screening programme, *Eur. J. Clin. Invest.*, 7, 109, 1977.
7. Grobbee, D. E., Hackeng, W. H. L., Berkenhagen, J. C., and Hofman, A., Raised plasma intact parathyroid hormone concentrations in young people with mildly raised blood pressure, *Br. Med. J.*, 296, 8145, 1988.
8. Brickman, A. S., Nybi, M. D., Von Hungen, K., Eggena, P., and Tuck, M. L., Calcitropic hormones, platelet calcium, and blood pressure in essential hypertension, *Hypertension*, 16, 515, 1990.
9. Hulter, H. N., Melby, J. C., Peterson, J. C., and Cooke, C. R., Chronic continuous PTH infusion results in hypertension in normal subjects, *J. Clin. Hypertens.*, 4, 360, 1986.
10. Resnick, L. M., Di Fabio, B., Marion, R. M., James, G. D., and Laragh, J. H., Dietary calcium modifies the pressor effects of dietary salt intake in essential hypertension, *J. Hypertens.*, 4(Suppl. 6), S679, 1986.
11. Van Hooft, I. M., Grobbee, D. E., Frölich, M., Pols, H. A., and Hofman, A., Alterations in calcium metabolism in young people at risk for primary hypertension. The Dutch Hypertension and Offspring Study, *Hypertension*, 21, 267, 1993.
12. Hvarfner, A., Bergström, R., Mörlin, C., Wide, L., and Ljunghall, S., Relationships between calcium metabolic indices and blood pressure in patients with essential hypertension as compared with a healthy population, *J. Hypertens.*, 5, 451, 1987.
13. Zachariah, P., Schwartz, G. L., Strong, C. G., and Ritter, S., Parathyroid hormone and calcium: a relationship in hypertension, *Am. J. Hypertens.*, 1, 79S, 1988.
14. Berthelot, A., Schleiffer, R., and Gairard, A., Parathyroïde et hypertension arterielle à l'acétate de désoxycorticostérone chez le rat, *Can. J. Physiol. Pharmacol.*, 57, 157, 1979.
15. Schleiffer, R., Berthelot, A., Pernot, F., and Gairard, A., Parathyroids, thyroids and development of hypertension in SHR, *Jpn. Circ. J.*, 45, 1272, 1981.
16. Baksi, S. N., Hypotensive action of parathyroid hormone in hypoparathyroid and hyperparathyroid rat, *Hypertension*, 11, 509, 1988.
17. Geiger, H., Bahner, U., Palkovits, M., Seewaldt, B., and Heidland, A., Is the effect of calcium diet or parathyroidectomy on the development of hypertension in spontaneously hypertensive rats mediated by atrial natriuretic peptide?, *Kidney Int.*, 34 (Suppl. 25), S93, 1988.
18. Pang, P. K. T. and Lewanczuk, R. Z., Parathyroid origin of a new circulating hypertensive factor in spontaneously hypertensive rats, *Am. J. Hypertens.*, 2, 898, 1989.
19. Mann, J. E. F., Wiecek, A., Bommer, J., Ganten, U., and Ritz, E., Effects of parathyroidectomy on blood pressure in spontaneously hypertensive rats, *Nephron*, 45, 46, 1987.
20. Wiecek, A., Kuczera, M., Ganten, U., Ritz, E., and Mann, J. F. E., Influence of parathyroidectomy on blood pressure and vascular reactivity in spontaneously hypertensive rats, *Clin. Exp. Hypertens.*, 11, 1525, 1989.
21. Pernot, F., Schleiffer, R., Berthelot, A., Vincent, M., Sassard, J., and Gairard, A., Parathyroidectomy in the Lyon hypertensive rat: cardiovascular reactivity and aortic responsiveness, *J. Hypertens.*, 8, 1111, 1990.

22. Kaneko, T., Ohtani, R., Lewanczuk, R. Z., and Pang, P. K. T., A novel cell type in the parathyroid glands of spontaneously hypertensive rats, *Am. J. Hypertens.*, 2, 549, 1989.

23. Neuser, D., Schulte-Brinckmann, R., and Kazda, S., Development of hypertension in WKY rats after transplantation of parathyroid glands from SHR/SP, *J. Cardiovasc. Pharmacol.*, 16, 971, 1990.

24. Pernot, F., Burkard, C., and Gairard, A., Parathyroid cross-transplantation and development of high blood pressure in rats, *J. Cardiovasc. Pharmacol.*, 23(Suppl 2), 518, 1994.

25. Burkard, C., Vincent, M., Ferrari, P., Sassard, J., and Gairard, A., Parathyroid transplantation in Lyon and Milan rat strain: preliminary results on blood pressure, in *Genetic Hypertension*, Sassard, J., Ed., John Libbey Eurotext, 1992, 577.

26. Lewanczuk, R. Z., Wang, J., Zhang, Z., and Pang, P. K. T., Effects of spontaneously hypertensive rat plasma on blood pressure and tail artery calcium uptake in normotensive rats, *Am. J. Hypertens.*, 2, 26, 1989.

27. Pang, P. K. T. et al., this volume.

28. Broulik, P. D., Horky, K., and Pacovsky, V., Blood pressure in patients with primary hyperparathyroidism before and after parathyroidectomy, *Exp. Clin. Endocrinol.*, 86, 346, 1985.

29. Lafferty, F. W., Primary hyperparathyroidism: changing clinical spectrum, prevalence of hypertension and discriminant analysis of laboratory test, *Arch. Intern. Med.*, 141, 1761, 1981.

30. Pizzarelli, F., Fabrizi, F., Postorino, M., Curatola, G., Zoccali, C., and Maggiore, Q., Parathyroidectomy and blood pressure in hemodialysis patients, *Nephron*, 63, 384, 1993.

31. Berthelot, A., Gairard, A., Goyault, M., and Pernot, F., Relation between calcium and cardiovascular reactivity in mineralocorticoid induced hypertension in the rat, *Br. J. Pharmacol.*, 70, 301, 1980.

32. Peuler, J. D., Morgan, D. A., and Mark, A. L., High calcium diet reduces blood pressure in Dahl sodium-sensitive rats by neural mechanism, *Hypertension*, 9, 159, 1987.

33. Kageyama, Y., Suzuki, H., and Arima, K., Oral calcium treatment lowers blood pressure in renovascular hypertensive rats by suppressing the renin angiotensin system, *Hypertension*, 10, 375, 1987.

34. Ayachi, S., Increased dietary calcium lowers blood pressure in the spontaneously hypertensive rat, *Metabolism*, 28, 1234, 1979.

35. McCarron, D. A., Yung, N. H., Ugoretz, B. A., and Krutzik, S., Disturbances in calcium metabolism in the spontaneously hypertensive rat, *Hypertension*, 3(Suppl. I), I161, 1981.

36. Bukoski, R. D. and McCarron, D. A., Altered aortic reactivity and lowered blood pressure associated with high calcium intake, *Am. J. Physiol.*, 251, H976, 1986.

37. Pernot, F., Schleiffer, R., Bergmann, C., Vincent, M., Sassard, J., and Gairard, A., Dietary calcium, vascular reactivity and genetic hypertension in the Lyon rat strain, *Am. J. Hypertens.*, 3, 846, 1990.

38. Berthelot, A. and Gairard, A., Parathyroid hormone- and deoxycorticosterone acetate-induced hypertension in the rat, *Clin. Sci.*, 58, 365, 1980.

39. Kishimoto, H., Tsumura, K., Fujioka, S., Uchimoto, S., and Morii, H., Chronic parathyroid hormone administration reverse the antihypertensive effect of calcium loading in young spontaneously hypertensive rats, *Am. J. Hypertens.*, 6, 234, 1993.

40. Schleiffer, R., Pernot, F., Berthelot, A., and Gairard, A., Low calcium diet enhances development of hypertension in the spontaneously hypertensive rat, *Clin. Exp. Hypertens.*, 6, 783, 1984.

41. Togari, A., Arai, M., Shamoto, T., Matsumoto, S., and Nagatsu, T., Elevation of blood pressure in young rats fed a low calcium diet, *Biochem. Pharmacol.*, 38, 889, 1989.

42. Schleiffer, R., Pernot, F., and Gairard, A., Parathyroidectomy, cardiovascular reactivity and calcium distribution in aorta and heart of spontaneously hypertensive rats, *Clin. Sci.*, 71, 505, 1986.

43. Schleiffer, R. and Gairard, A., Influence of parathyroidectomy on aortic responsiveness to noradrenaline in spontaneously hypertensive rats, *Arch. Int. Pharmacodyn. Ther.*, 292, 189, 1988.

44. Schleiffer, R., Xue, H., McCarron, D. A., and Bukoski, R.D., Effect of chronic and subacute parathyroidectomy on blood pressure and resistance artery in the spontaneously hypertensive rat, *J. Hypertens.*, 11, 709, 1993.

45. Oshima, T., Schleiffer, R., Young, E.W., McCarron, D.A., and Bukoski, R.D., Effect of parathyroidectomy on platelet calcium in spontaneusly hypertensive rats, *J. Hypertens.*, 9, 155, 1991.

46. Boulebda, N., Van Overloop, B., and Gairard, A., Endothelium-derived relaxing factor, hypertension and chronic parathyroidectomy in SHR and WKY rats, *Clin. Exp. Pharmacol. Physiol.*, 20, 773, 1993.

47. Boulebda, N. and Gairard, A., Characterization of endothelium-derived relaxing factor involvement in the potentiating effect of parathyroidectomy on norepinephrine-induced rat aortic contraction, *Fund. Clin. Pharmacol.*, 8, 93, 1994.

48. Yang, F. and Nickerson, P. A., Effect of parathyroidectomy on arterial hypertrophy, vascular lesions, and calcium content in deoxycorticosterone-induced hypertension, *Res. Exp. Med.*, 188, 289, 1988.

49. Kazda, S., Garthof, B., Hirth, C., Preiss, W., and Stasch, J. P., Parathyroidectomy mimicks the protective effect of calcium antagonist nimodipine in salt loaded stroke-prone spontaneously hypertensive rats, *J. Hypertens.*, 4(Suppl. 3), S483, 1986.

5

Parathyroid Hypertensive Factor — A New Hypertensive Hormone from the Parathyroid Gland

P. K. T. Pang, C. G. Benishin, J. Shan, and R. Z. Lewanczuk

CONTENTS

I. INTRODUCTION

A. The Parathyroid Gland and Vascular Actions

Since the first description of the hypotensive actions of parathyroid gland extracts by Collip and Clark,[1] the parathyroid gland has been associated with vascular actions. As early as 1928, parathyroid extracts were reported to be useful in the treatment of congestive heart failure, where they were associated with a reduction in blood pressure in hypertensive patients.[2] Years later, in 1951, the hypotensive action of parathyroid hormone (PTH) was rediscovered.[3] It was not until the early 1980s, however, that the vascular actions of PTH were studied in detail. In 1980, Pang et al. reported a vasodilatory action of PTH on the coronary arteries of dogs.[4] Subsequent studies showed that PTH possessed hypotensive properties when injected into rats or dogs.[5] These observations were ultimately extended to include a wide variety of vertebrates.[6] Structure-function studies of PTH have since demonstrated that the vascular actions of the hormone reside in the 34 amino acid N-terminal portion, with the C-terminal portion being devoid of vascular effects.[7-10] In addition, it has been shown that the first two N-terminal amino acids are particularly related to the vascular effects of PTH, as are the amino acids in positions 24-28.[7-10]

The mechanism of the vascular effects of PTH has been well studied in the past. PTH has been shown to have a direct vasorelaxant effect on vascular smooth muscle both *in vivo* and *in vitro*.[5,11-15] This action is endothelium independent.[15] In terms of cardiac effects, PTH has a positive chronotropic and inotropic effect.[4,11,12,16-19] Thus, hemodynamically, the hypotensive actions of PTH would seem to be due solely to vasodilation and not to any suppressive effect on cardiac output. Coincidental with the vasorelaxant effect of PTH is a decrease in intracellular calcium, as measured indirectly by calcium-45 uptake.[12,20,21] A further extension of this work has shown that PTH acts as an endogenous calcium channel blocker, albeit at levels significantly greater than those present in the circulation.[22,23] This, however, is not to negate the fact that pathologically elevated levels of PTH, as seen in primary or secondary hyperparathyroidism, might not have some hypotensive actions by virtue of increased tissue levels. The vasorelaxant action of PTH appears to be linked to its ability to stimulate adenylate cyclase and, hence, the formation of cyclic adenosine monophosphate (cAMP).[15,24-26] Indeed, factors that potentiate adenylate cyclase-mediated effects also potentiate the vasodilatory actions of PTH.[15,24,26] Although PTH does have direct calcium channel blocking activity, some of the calcium channel blocking activity is also cAMP-dependent.[27] Interestingly, the action of PTH in decreasing intracellular calcium in vascular smooth muscle is in opposition to its actions on other tissues. In red blood cells,[28] cardiac myocytes,[29] and liver cells,[30] PTH has been reported to increase intracellular calcium levels. What the physiological role of PTH is in these tissues is not known. Indeed, the physiological role of PTH, if any, on the vasculature is also not understood. Recently, however, the discovery of PTH-related peptide (PTH-rP) has offered a possible explanation for the vascular actions of PTH. PTH-rP, it turns out, is at least three- to tenfold more potent than PTH is in causing vasorelaxation.[31-33] The local production of PTH-rP in vascular tissue and sites adjacent to the vasculature has thus led to the suggestion that PTH-rP might serve a paracrine role in regulating vascular tone. As with PTH, the vascular actions of PTH-rP involve a decrease in intracellular calcium and the stimulation of adenylate cyclase.[33] Thus, it may be that PTH-rP is the natural ligand for PTH-related receptors on the vasculature and that PTH has effects in only supraphysiological concentrations or in pathological conditions.

B. PTH and Hypertension

With the hypotensive, vasorelaxant actions of PTH apparently so completely defined, it is somewhat surprising that PTH has been suggested to be a "hypertensive" hormone. Such a suggestion would appear to be utterly paradoxical — how can a hormone that is vasorelaxant and hypotensive cause hypertension? A closer examination of the evidence, however, reveals that it is the parathyroid gland, not PTH, which is linked to hypertension.

The first evidence for the involvement of the parathyroid gland in hypertension came from the experiments of Schleiffer et al., who demonstrated in 1981 that parathyroidectomy in spontaneously hypertensive rats (SHRs) led to a reduction in blood pressure.[34] As PTH was the only known product of the parathyroid gland at that time, the presumption was that PTH must play a role in hypertension — at least in SHRs. Further work showed that SHR rats did indeed have increased circulating levels of PTH,[35,36] apparently supporting the premise that PTH was somehow involved in hypertension. In human studies, increased levels of PTH also were found in a proportion of hypertensive patients.[37] This finding, together with the known effects of PTH in increasing intracellular calcium in some tissues, led to the hypothesis that

PTH caused an increase in blood pressure by increasing intracellular calcium in vascular smooth muscle. Studies on the direct actions of PTH, however, consistently showed that it was a vasodilator and that under no circumstances could it cause vasoconstriction.

The role of PTH in hypertension was further confused by studies in patients with primary hyperparathyroidism. In 1958, Hellstrom et al. described the hypotensive actions of parathyroidectomy in human patients.[38] Since then, it has been realized that a significantly increased proportion of primary hyperparathyroid patients are hypertensive.[39-44] Parathyroidectomy in such hypertensive primary hyperparathyroid patients often resulted in a decrease in blood pressure,[38,39,42,43] again apparently supporting a hypertensive role for PTH. In some series, however, the hypotensive effect of parathyroidectomy was less consistent, with some patients even showing an increase in blood pressure postparathyroidectomy.[38,39,41-44] In fact, upon a review of the literature, it would appear that in terms of blood pressure, some hypertensive hyperparathyroid patients benefit from parathyroidectomy, some patients are unchanged, and some patients develop worsened hypertension. On this basis it is difficult to assign a hypertensive role to PTH. Yet such attempts are still made. One cited explanation for the apparent inconsistency between the direct vascular actions of PTH and its circumstantial implication in hypertension is that chronic exposure to PTH increases blood pressure, whereas acute exposure decreases blood pressure. Thus, studies have been carried out examining the effects of chronic PTH administration on blood pressure.[45,46] These studies, by and large, have shown an increase in blood pressure or in the rate of development of hypertension in response to PTH. Unfortunately, the apparent hypertensive effects of PTH could not be separated from the hypercalcemic actions of PTH. Because hypercalcemia, regardless of cause, can raise blood pressure, these studies provided no further information on the putative hypertensive actions of PTH.

II. RATIONALE FOR A SECOND VASOACTIVE SUBSTANCE IN THE PARATHYROID GLAND

By 1986, a number of researchers had reported increased levels of PTH in various forms or models of hypertension.[35-37,47,48] For the most part, opinion was that PTH was somehow primarily involved in the genesis of hypertension in these cases. In 1986, however, a solution to the apparent PTH-hypertension paradox was offered by data published by Resnick et al.[37] In this study, Resnick and co-workers classified hypertensive patients according to their renin profiles. Calcium and calcium-regulating hormones were then characterized in the resulting three groups of low-, normal-, and high-renin profile patients. This analysis showed that the low-renin group of hypertensive patients, representing approximately 30 to 40% of all essential hypertensive patients, behaved as if they were calcium deficient. That is, compared to patients in the other two renin categories, they had higher PTH and 1,25-dihydroxy-cholecalciferol-vitamin D [1,25 $(OH)_2$ D] levels but lower calcitonin levels. The converse was true for the high-renin group. Although there was no difference in total serum calcium between groups, when ionized calcium (i.e., unbound calcium) was measured, it was found to be lower in the low-renin group. In other words, the low-renin patients with elevated PTH levels actually did seem to be relatively hypocalcemic! If PTH elevation was primary in these patients, they should have been hypercalcemic, if anything. On the other hand, if the patients were relatively calcium deficient, an elevation in PTH would be an entirely normal and appropriate endocrine response. Moreover, because PTH was elevated in the face of a low ionized calcium, this suggested that somehow the action of PTH was being inhibited or antagonized. If this were not the case, PTH would be elevated but the ionized calcium would be normal, in accordance with a reset calcium homeostatic mechanism. This raises the question, therefore, as to whether PTH actions are inhibited in low-renin hypertension. Indeed,

TABLE 1   Reasons for suspecting the presence of a second vasoactive factor in the parathyroid gland

- PTH is hypotensive, but increased parathyroid gland activity has been associated with hypertension.
- Suppression of PTH levels by dietary calcium decreased blood pressure in SHRs.
- Parathyroidectomy decreased blood pressure in SHRs.
- In human primary hyperparathyroidism, parathyroidectomy often decreased blood pressure.
- PTH levels were increased in hypertension, but end-organ effects were inhibited.
- An increase in dietary salt could increase both blood pressure and PTH.

if one examines the noncalcemic effects of PTH in hypertensive animals or subjects, it is evident that these effects are also attenuated. Examples include reductions in urinary calcium resorption, urinary cAMP generation, and intestinal calcium absorption. In order to explain this reduction in end-organ sensitivity to the actions of PTH a number of possibilities were postulated. First, it was thought that a circulating inhibitor of PTH might exist. Second, it was hypothesized that PTH receptors might somehow be reduced in number or sensitivity. Finally, it was possible that postreceptor defects might be responsible for the reduction in PTH sensitivity. Because humans and SHRs which also have increased PTH levels, are not born hypertensive, it was thought that a genetic structural defect leading to hypertension and PTH resistance was unlikely. On the other hand, the presence of an inducible circulating inhibitor of PTH with hypertensive actions was not inconsistent with existing observations. Finding the source of secretion of such an inhibitor was an even greater puzzle. Recalling, however, that parathyroidectomy could reduce blood pressure in both hypertensive rats and primary hyperparathyroid hypertensive humans, the parathyroid gland was thought to be a candidate for the site of secretion of this putative combination PTH inhibitor/pressor substance. Indeed, the secretion of a second vasoactive, hypertensive substance from the parathyroid gland had the potential to resolve the paradox whereby the parathyroid gland was known to be important in hypertension, yet its only known product, PTH, was hypotensive. A summary of evidence for the origin of a second vasoactive substance from the parathyroid gland is given in Table 1.

III. THE DISCOVERY OF PARATHYROID HYPERTENSIVE FACTOR

In accordance with the above reasoning, it was hypothesized that a circulating inhibitor of the actions of PTH might exist in low-renin hypertensive human subjects and certain animal models. The spontaneously hypertensive rat was known to be hypertensive and have increased levels of PTH. It was therefore thought that plasma from this rat should contain PTH-inhibitory circulating factor. Thus, in an initial set of experiments, plasma obtained from SHRs, dialyzed at 1000 mol wt cutoff to remove vasoactive ions such as calcium and small known pressors such as epinephrine, was infused into normotensive rats. PTH was then injected in the presence or absence of the dialyzed SHR plasma. When SHR plasma was present, the vascular actions of PTH were inhibited. When control normotensive rat plasma was infused, no inhibition was seen.[49] To confirm these observations, dialyzed SHR or normotensive control plasma was injected into normotensive rats in a bolus manner. PTH was again injected repetitively. Results of these studies showed an early (within 5 min) inhibition of the hypotensive effects of PTH which lasted for approximately 60 min (Figure 1). Thus, the presence of a circulating inhibitor of at least the vascular actions of PTH was seemingly confirmed.

During these plasma infusion experiments, however, an even more intriguing phenomenon was noted. When SHR plasma was infused or injected, the blood pressure of the anesthetized, normotensive assay animal increased. Such a response was not seen with normotensive plasma. What was more interesting was that this effect was delayed, not beginning until

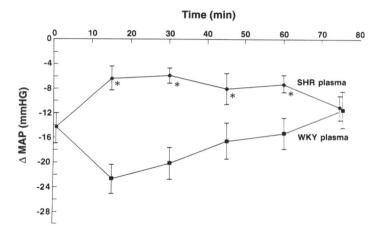

FIGURE 1   Inhibitory effect of PHF-containing SHR plasma on the hypotensive effect of PTH in anesthetized rats. PHF-containing SHR plasma or normotensive WKY plasma was injected into anesthetized rats followed by repetitive doses of PTH. The depressor effect of PTH following plasma injection was compared to the effect prior to plasma injection. PHF-containing SHR plasma is seen to inhibit the hypotensive actions of PTH. * $p < 0.05$ vs. time 0 value. (Reprinted by permission of Elsevier Science Publishing Co., Inc., from Vascular and calcemic effects of plasma from spontaneously hypertensive rats, by Lewanczuk, R. Z. and Pang, P. K. T., *American Journal of Hypertension*, 3, 189S–194S, © 1990 by the American Journal of Hypertension, Inc.)

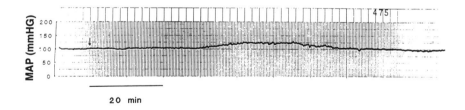

FIGURE 2   Representative physiographic tracing of PHF effect on mean arterial pressure. PHF-containing sample was injected into an anesthetized rat at the time indicated by the arrow. An increase in mean arterial pressure began approximately 30 min after injection with the peak pressure occurring about 50 min after injection. (Reprinted by permission of Elsevier Science Publishing Co., Inc., from The occurrence of parathyroid hypertensive factor (PHF) in Dahl rats, by Lewanczuk, R. Z. and Pang, P. K. T., *American Journal of Hypertension*, 6, 758–762, © 1993 by the American Journal of Hypertension, Inc.)

approximately 30 min after bolus injection or intravenous infusion. At first it was thought that this effect was volume related. However, when saline or normotensive rat plasma was infused or injected in a similar manner, no hypertensive effect was seen. Thus, the presence of a circulating hypertensive factor in SHR plasma was also suggested.[50] This "factor," however, had novel properties. First, it had a delayed onset of action — approximately 30 min following bolus injection. Second, it had a prolonged action, with peak effects on blood pressure not being seen until 45 to 60 min after injection and persisting until approximately 75 min postinjection. This pattern of pressor effect was, and still is, unique. "Traditional" pressors such as epinephrine, angiotensin II, and vasopressin all have a rapid onset and short duration of action. It is this unique effect on blood pressure which has evolved into a bioassay for this hypertensive factor, now termed parathyroid hypertensive factor (PHF). A sample tracing of this delayed, prolonged pressor effect is shown in Figure 2. Because of the inherent variability of a bioassay of this nature, individual samples are usually assayed in replicates of six, the

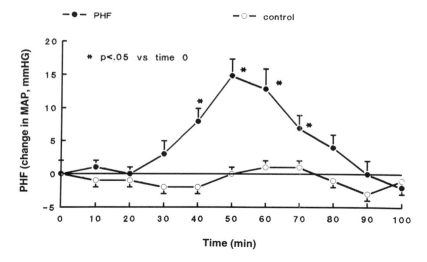

FIGURE 3   Mean effect of repetitive individual PHF bioassays. PHF containing SHR plasma or normotensive WKY plasma was injected into six anesthetized rats. Results represent the average change in mean arterial pressure at regular time intervals following injection.

mean representing a PHF "level." Results from such a bioassay of an individual sample are shown in Figure 3.

IV. COMPARISON OF PTH AND PHF

A. Site of Origin

Circumstantial evidence suggested a parathyroid origin for PHF in the SHR. Nevertheless, other tissues also have been implicated as sources of hypertensive "factors." Most notable amongst these tissues is the kidney. It was through the early work of Dahl that evidence for the involvement of circulating factors in hypertension first came to light.[51] In these original experiments it was shown that a normotensive rat connected in parabiosis with a hypertensive rat soon developed hypertension. Subsequent studies suggested that at least one of these putative circulating factors was of renal origin.[52,53] Other tissue sites implicated in the secretion of hypertensive "factors" in the SHR include the adrenal glands[54,55] and the spleen.[56] Thus, the parathyroid gland was by no means the only possible site of secretion of PHF.

In order to test the hypothesis that the parathyroid gland was the site of PHF secretion, a number of studies were carried out. First, parathyroidectomy of SHR was shown to result in the disappearance of PHF activity from the plasma and in a significant decrease in blood pressure.[57] This, of course, did not prove that the parathyroid gland was the source of PHF, merely that PHF detection was parathyroid dependent. In a second set of experiments, parathyroid cross-transplantation was carried out between normotensive and SHRs.[57] First, rats were parathyroidectomized. Then parathyroid glands from SHRs were cross-transplanted into normotensive rats, and normotensive rat parathyroid glands were transplanted into SHRs. As a control, normotensive parathyroid glands were also transplanted into normotensive rats. Results of this experiment revealed no change in blood pressure in the normotensive rats receiving normotensive parathyroid glands. Normotensive rats receiving SHR parathyroid glands, however, demonstrated an increase in blood pressure, and PHF-like activity became detectable in their plasma. SHRs receiving the normotensive parathyroids showed a marked drop in blood pressure, and PHF could no longer be detected in their plasma. While these results supported a parathyroid origin for PHF, they were by no means definitive. Again, they

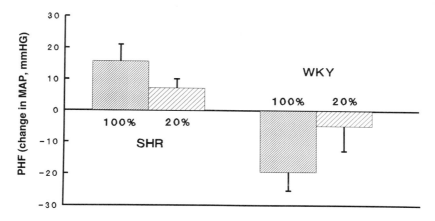

FIGURE 4   PHF content of parathyroid cell culture media as measured by PHF bioassay. Aliquots of SHR and WKY parathyroid cell culture media were assayed according to the usual PHF bioassay procedure. SHR cell culture media demonstrated PHF-like activity, whereas WKY media actually caused a decrease in blood pressure in the assay system, possibly because of the effects of PTH. 100% refers to aliquot calculated to contain the PHF equivalent of 1 ml of SHR plasma; 20% refers to an aliquot containing 20% of the amount of PHF as found in 1 ml of SHR plasma.

merely proved that the parathyroid gland was necessary for PHF secretion or activation. In order to establish the parathyroid origin of PHF, therefore, a more direct experiment was carried out. In this experiment, parathyroid glands from SHR and their normotensive genetic control Wistar-Kyoto (WKY) rats were grown in organ culture under conditions of varying calcium concentration.[58] Media from these cultures were then dialyzed and assayed for PHF. Results showed that SHR but not WKY cultures had PHF detectable in the culture medium. Such secretion was stimulated by a low ambient calcium concentration, as is the case for PTH. In fact, media from WKY cultures did actually induce a dose-dependent decrease in blood pressure when injected into assay rats (Figure 4). Such a finding could be consistent with a depressor effect of PTH presumably present in the culture media.

Further evidence for the parathyroid origin of PHF was provided by antibody studies. In these studies, PHF purified from parathyroid cell culture media was used to generate a polyclonal antibody.[59] This antibody was subsequently shown to cross-react with PHF purified from the plasma, strongly suggesting that parathyroid PHF and plasma PHF were the same substance. In addition, injection of the PHF antibody, but not naive mouse serum, induced dose-dependent decreases in blood pressure in SHRs.

If PHF was therefore truly secreted by the parathyroid gland, its cellular site of secretion needed to be established. Interestingly, despite the number of parathyroidectomy studies carried out on hypertensive rats, only one study had been reported on parathyroid histology in the SHR.[60] This study showed that SHR parathyroid glands were hyperplastic compared with normotensive WKY glands. Unfortunately, this study did not concentrate on individual cellular morphology. When SHR parathyroid glands were histologically studied by our group, the presence of a darkly staining cell type was noted.[61] These cells occurred in clusters in the parathyroid gland, usually near the surface of the gland. Such cells, by electron microscopy, had vacuolated cytoplasm and pyknotic nuclei, yet they did not seem to be degenerating or dying cells. By carrying out serial sectioning of SHR parathyroid glands, these cells were shown to comprise up to 15% of the total cells in some parathyroid glands. Such cells were totally absent in WKY parathyroid glands. When these cells were enumerated, the cell number correlated both with the mean arterial pressure and the PHF level in the respective animal. This, of course, did not prove that these cells secrete PHF. Recently, however, immunohistochemical staining of SHR and WKY parathyroid cells with a different antibody indicated that these cells likely do secrete PHF (Pang et al., unpublished observations). The PTH secreting cells of the rat parathyroid, however, did not stain with this antibody.

In humans, evidence for a parathyroid origin of PHF is more tentative. Unlike rats, one cannot carry out parathyroidectomy and cross-transplantation studies in humans. Luckily there is a circumstance that does afford access to parathyroid tissue. That is at the time of surgery for hyperparathyroidism. As discussed earlier, many primary hyperparathyroid patients are hypertensive. When PHF levels were assayed in hypertensive and normotensive primary hyperparathyroid patients, it was found that almost all hypertensive but no normotensive patients had significant PHF levels.[62] These patients were then followed postoperatively. In those patients who had significant PHF levels preoperatively, parathyroidectomy (parathyroid adenomas in all cases) led to a decrease in blood pressure and, more importantly, PHF-like activity became undetectable in their plasma. In those patients who did not have significant PHF levels, parathyroidectomy had no effect on blood pressure. Thus, circumstantial evidence was obtained for a parathyroid origin of PHF in humans. Unfortunately, actual parathyroid tissue has not yet been cultured from human patients. This, of course, would provide more direct evidence for a parathyroid origin of PHF in humans. Such studies are planned in the near future, however.

To summarize, the parathyroid gland appears to be the major source of secretion of PHF in the rat, where such secretion is associated with a novel cell type. Circumstantial evidence also now exists for a parathyroid origin for PHF in humans. Whether the parathyroid gland is the sole site of secretion of PHF is not known. PTH is also secreted by the parathyroid gland by the well-described light and dark cells in the rat, and by the chief cells in humans. Thus, both PHF and PTH are secreted by the parathyroid gland, yet their interrelationship is not well understood.

B. Control of Secretion

Even though PTH has been known to exist for almost 80 years, little is known about the factors that control its secretion from the parathyroid gland. Certainly it is known that an increase in extracellular calcium can suppress PTH secretion.[63-66] How this signal is detected and transduced in the parathyroid gland is not well understood. Moreover, even the rate or direction of change in serum calcium may affect PTH secretion.[67] How this calcium signal is perceived by the parathyroid gland also is not known. Chromogranin A, which is co-secreted with PTH, has recently been shown to have paracrine and even autocrine effects in suppressing PTH secretion.[68] Whether this role is physiologically important or not is unknown. Moreover, it is not known if chromogranin A secretion also directly responds to changes in the ambient calcium milieu.

The control of PHF secretion is even less well-understood than that of PTH. As mentioned above, PHF shares a similarity with PTH such that an increase in ambient calcium concentration or an increase in calcium intake can affect PHF secretion. Evidence for the effects of ambient calcium concentration on PHF secretion comes from SHR parathyroid organ and parathyroid cell cultures, where a low calcium level stimulates and a "normal" calcium level inhibits PHF secretion.[58] Evidence for the effects of calcium feeding on PHF secretion comes from a study of SHRs that were placed on three levels of calcium intake: low, normal, and high. Rats in the high calcium intake group had lower blood pressures and lower PHF levels than did the groups on low or normal calcium (Figure 5).[69] These effects were seen despite no differences in ionized calcium levels between the high and normal calcium groups. Other factors that affect PHF secretion have not yet been well identified. In SHR rats, an increase in salt intake has a nonsignificant effect on PHF level (Lewanczuk and Pang, unpublished

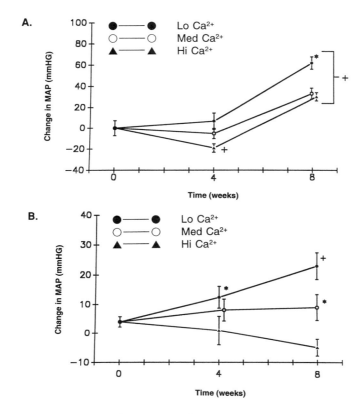

FIGURE 5   (A) Change in mean arterial pressures of SHR rats on various calcium diets. SHR rats were assigned to one of three levels of calcium intake (low, normal, high) and maintained on the respective diet for 8 weeks. Mean arterial pressure and PHF level were measured at 0, 4, and 8 weeks. + = p <0.05 vs. time 0; * = p <0.05 vs. medium and high calcium. (B) PHF levels (denoted as change in MAP in bioassay) in dietary groups. * = p <0.05 vs. baseline; + = p <0.01 vs. baseline. (Reprinted by permission of Elsevier Science Publishing Co., Inc., from The effects of dietary calcium on blood pressure in spontaneously hypertensive rats, by Lewanczuk, R. Z. and Pang, P. K. T., *American Journal of Hypertension*, 3, 349–353, © 1990 by the American Journal of Hypertension, Inc.)

data). In humans, however, a high salt diet tends to increase PHF levels.[70] In another rat model of hypertension, the Dahl salt-sensitive rat, an increase in salt intake increases both PHF levels and blood pressure in a correlated manner.[71] Salt intake has no effect on Dahl salt-resistant rats. Interestingly, an increase in salt intake or saline infusion has been reported to increase PTH levels in humans.[72,73] Thus, as far as is known, both PTH and PHF respond to factors affecting their secretion in a similar manner. Whether this is because of (1) a generalized increase in parathyroid gland activity, (2) resistance to PTH effects with subsequent positive feedback, or (3) compensatory secretion of one hormone to counteract the effects of the other (e.g., secretion of the hypotensive PTH to counteract the hypertensive PHF) is not known. Nevertheless, because of the parallels in the control of secretion of the two substances, information obtained regarding control of secretion of one of these substances will likely contribute information to the understanding of the other.

C. Mechanism of Action

The mechanism of action of PTH is much better understood than is the control of its secretion. PTH, after binding to its cell surface receptor, exerts most of its effects through the stimulation

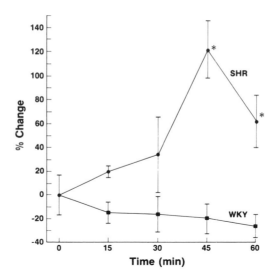

FIGURE 6   Potentiation of norepinephrine effect by PHF-containing SHR plasma. Norepinephrine was given in repetitive bolus doses to anesthetized rats following bolus injection of WKY or PHF-containing SHR plasma. Results are plotted as percentage change in mean arterial pressure response above baseline response. PHF-containing SHR plasma is seen to potentiate norepinephrine pressor effects with a time course similar to that of the pressor effects of the plasma alone.

of adenylate cyclase, leading to the formation of cAMP. This is its mechanism of action in the major target tissues of bone and kidney.[74] Through these actions, PTH promotes bone remodeling and resorption, renal calcium resorption, and natriuresis and stimulates the renal enzyme 1-α-hydroxylase. Stimulation of this latter enzyme increases the production of the active $1,25(OH)_2D$ from inactive 25-OHD. Vitamin D, in turn, exerts its own effects on bone and kidney as well as on gut calcium absorption. In vascular tissue, as discussed above, PTH causes vasorelaxation. This again is linked with its adenylate cyclase stimulating activity.[15,24-26] It should be noted, at this point, that stimulation of cAMP in vascular smooth muscle normally leads to vasorelaxation, regardless of agonist.[75] In addition to its hypotensive actions related to cAMP stimulation, PTH also may have a direct effect on the L-type calcium channels in vascular smooth muscle, further promoting vasorelaxation.[23]

Preliminary studies have been carried out to investigate the mechanism of action of PHF. Despite being secreted by the same gland and apparently being subject to the same regulatory influences, the actions of PHF at a cellular and organ level often appear to be diametrically opposed to those of PTH. First, PTH is hypotensive and a vasodilator. PHF, of course, causes hypertension when injected into normotensive animals. Whether PHF is a direct vasoconstrictor is more questionable. When tested *in vitro*, PHF does not cause direct vasoconstriction. Rather, it potentiates the action of other classical vasoconstrictors such as norepinephrine (Figure 6).[76] This potentiation correlates with *in vivo* findings whereby PHF potentiates the actions of norepinephrine, vasopressin, and angiotensin II by up to 100%.[77] Second, PTH blocks L-type calcium channels in vascular smooth muscle and leads to a reduction in intracellular calcium. PHF, on the other hand, causes an increase in calcium uptake into vascular smooth muscle strips, with a time course paralleling its hypertensive action (Figure 7).[50] This increase in calcium uptake is matched by an observed increase in free intracellular calcium in vascular smooth muscle cells (Figure 8).[76] Such an increase in intracellular calcium also occurs gradually, with no evidence of a hysteresis effect as is seen with "classical" vasoconstrictors. This finding may therefore explain why PHF does not cause vasoconstriction

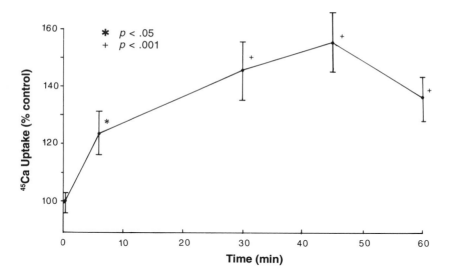

FIGURE 7 Effect of PHF-containing SHR plasma on $^{45}Ca^{2+}$ uptake in vascular smooth muscle. Vascular smooth muscle strips from rat tail arteries were incubated in the presence of PHF-containing SHR plasma and $^{45}Ca^{2+}$. SHR plasma is seen to increase $^{45}Ca^{2+}$ uptake over basal levels with a time course similar to that for the pressor effect. Neither WKY plasma or buffer alone has any effect on $^{45}Ca^{2+}$ uptake (data not shown). (Reprinted by permission of Elsevier Science Publishing Co., Inc., from Effects of spontaneously hypertensive rat plasma on blood and tail artery calcium uptake in normotensive rats, by Lewanczuk, R. Z., et al., *American Journal of Hypertension,* 2, 26–31, © 1989 by American Journal of Hypertension, Inc.)

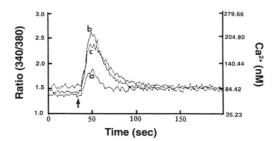

FIGURE 8 Effect of PHF on intracellular calcium in vascular smooth muscle cells as measured by Fura-2. An increase in intracellular calcium was induced by 30 mM KCl alone (a), after incubation with PHF for 45 min (b), and following washes (c). PHF is seen to potentiate the rise in intracellular calcium seen with KCl. (From Shan, J., Benishin, R. Z., Lewanczuk, R. Z., and Pang, P. K. T., The mechanism of the vascular action of parathyroid hypertensive factor, *Journal of Cardiovascular Pharmacology,* in press, 1994. With permission.)

itself but potentiates the actions of other calcium dependent vasoconstrictors. Some of this action of PHF appears to be due to effects on L-type calcium channels in vascular smooth muscle, whereby opening of these channels is promoted by PHF (Figure 9).[76] A third area of difference, related to the second, is the action of PHF on cAMP. Whereas PTH stimulates cAMP formation, PHF leads to an apparent decrease in cAMP levels. This action, it seems, is due to a stimulatory effect of PHF on cAMP phosphodiesterase.[76] Thus, if vascular smooth muscle relaxation is promoted by an increase in cAMP, it is logical to assume that factors that

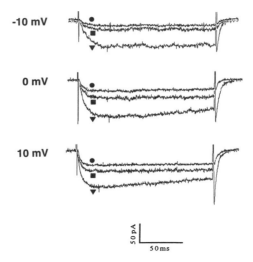

FIGURE 9   Effect of PHF on L-channel activity in vascular smooth muscle cells. Original recordings of three test pulses (–10, 0, and 10 mV) are shown. The control inward current was determined before (circles) and 35 min (squares) and 55 min (triangles) after application of PHF. PHF is seen to enhance L-channel calcium current. (From Shan, J., Benishin, R. Z., Lewanczuk, R. Z., and Pang, P. K. T., The mechanism of the vascular action of parathyroid hypertensive factor, *Journal of Cardiovascular Pharmacology,* in press, 1994. With permission.)

decrease cAMP will inhibit vasorelaxation or even lead to enhanced vasoconstriction. Other possible signal transduction systems also have been studied in relation to PHF. No evidence, however, has been obtained for a direct action of PHF on G-proteins, adenylate cyclase, or protein kinase A. In addition, PHF does not stimulate the phospholipase C pathway, neither in the formation of inositol bisphosphate nor in the activation of protein kinase C.

At an organ level, PTH causes calcium retention and sodium loss in the kidney. The acute effect of PHF, in contrast, is to cause sodium retention.[78] Such an effect may partially explain the sodium retention seen in low-renin hypertension as well as in rat models where PHF has been detected, such as the SHR, Dahl-S, and deoxycorticosterone acetate (DOCA)-salt rats. The acute effects of PHF on renal calcium handling, however, are similar to those of PTH. That is, PHF leads to calcium retention.[78] This is not necessarily surprising, as calcium and sodium both tend to be handled the same way by the kidney. In terms of the chronic effects of PHF on renal calcium handling, nothing is known. Interestingly, SHRs do have increased urinary calcium loss.[35] Whether this may be due to a chronic effect of PHF or an intrinsic abnormality in the SHR kidney, as has been suggested, cannot be determined at the present time. In terms of 1-α-hydroxylase effects, PTH stimulates this enzyme. PHF, when injected into normotensive rats, resulted in an increase in circulating $1,25(OH)_2D$ levels after 2 h.[78] Whether this was due to direct effects on 1-α-hydroxylase or to other indirect actions could not be determined from the experimental design. PTH has been reported to increase intracellular calcium in red blood cells.[28] PHF, in a recent study, also led to an increase in intracellular calcium in red blood cells as measured by nuclear magnetic resonance spectroscopy.[79] Other actions of PTH, such as effects on bone, have not yet been studied in relation to PHF. To summarize, therefore, PTH and PHF generally have opposite actions at an organ level and opposite mechanisms of action at a cellular level in the vasculature. Some effects in other tissues, however, appear to be similar for the two substances. It is hoped that further study will more fully elucidate the mechanisms of action of these two parathyroid substances and thereby aid in the understanding of their physiology at the cellular and organ levels.

D. Physiological Role and Pathophysiological Effects of PHF and PTH

The traditionally assigned and still major actions of PTH are to maintain bone structure and function and to maintain serum calcium levels. Pathophysiologically, increases in PTH lead to osteopenia and hypercalcemia. Hypercalcemia, in turn, leads to adverse effects such as renal stones, abdominal pain, and mental confusion. These roles and effects of PTH will not be discussed any further in this chapter. Rather, the focus will be on the vascular effects of PTH.

As mentioned previously, PTH causes vasorelaxation and decreases blood pressure. The question arises, therefore, as to whether this is a physiological action of PTH or merely an interesting pharmacological phenomenon. The answer to this question is probably the latter. Although one can never rely entirely on circulating levels of a hormone to predict its physiological effects and sites of action because of potential paracrine effects, circulating levels of PTH are less than the minimum concentration necessary for vascular actions. While circulating levels of intact PTH range from approximately 10 to 65 pg/ml, minimal effective concentrations for a hypotensive effect *in vivo* begin at approximately 25 ng/ml, and for a vasorelaxant effect *in vitro* at approximately 300 ng/ml. Immunocytochemical study of the vasculature and perivascular areas shows no evidence for local production of PTH, thus a paracrine role is probably ruled out. Pathophysiologically, PTH may exert hypotensive effects. In some patients with primary hyperparathyroidism, parathyroidectomy leads to a postoperative increase in blood pressure.[38,39,41-44] In such cases, it is possible that the elevated levels of PTH are exerting a hypotensive effect and that normalization of these levels by parathyroidectomy leads to an increase in blood pressure. In cases where no blood pressure change is observed, PTH levels may not have been high enough to have caused a decrease in blood pressure. In cases where blood pressure falls postparathyroidectomy, this may be due to the removal of a parathyroid gland secreting PHF. Why then does PTH have the pharmacological effect of decreasing blood pressure? Again, as discussed earlier, PTH-rP is much more potent in causing vasorelaxation than PTH.[31-33] Although circulating levels of PTH-rP are normally undetectable, immunocytochemical evidence suggests that PTH-rP may be locally produced and secreted (i.e., have paracrine effects).[80] Thus, the natural ligand for the "PTH" receptor on vascular smooth muscle may be PTH-rP. Because of their structural similarity, PTH, at high concentrations, may interact with this receptor, causing the observed vasodilation. This leads to the question as to what the role of PTH-rP in the vasculature is. This, however, is not a subject for this chapter.

The next question to be addressed is whether PHF has a physiological role. At the present time, PHF has not been detected in the plasma of normotensive animals, nor has a "normal" range for PHF in humans been established. Although PHF is detected in some normotensive individuals, many of these subjects manifest changes in cation metabolism characteristic of the low-renin hypertensive state, such as an increased urinary calcium excretion.[81] Currently the PHF bioassay is too insensitive to determine whether PHF does circulate at low levels under normal circumstances. Thus, at the present time, one can only speculate as to whether PHF has a physiological role. In experimental animals, PHF production can be induced by treatment with DOCA[82] and possibly by a low-calcium diet.[83] This indicates that the genetic information necessary for the synthesis and secretion of PHF is present in normal animals. To date, no attempts have been made to induce PHF production in normal humans.

One possible role for PHF might be in regulating baseline vascular tone. As mentioned above, PHF does not cause vasoconstriction itself but potentiates the actions of other vasoconstrictors. PHF may therefore play a role in maintaining vascular tone under circumstances when blood pressure is reduced. For example, in shock, parathyroid hormone levels are elevated, yet serum calcium and ionized calcium are often reduced.[84] These features are reminiscent of low-renin hypertension where PHF plays a role. In a similar manner, if PHF regulates baseline vascular tone, it may be functioning as a regulator of intracellular calcium levels. If PTH regulates extracellular calcium levels, might it not be expected that an intracellular calcium-regulating hormone exists? These suggestions are purely speculative, and any physiological role for PHF will need to await the development of a more sensitive PHF assay.

In terms of pathophysiology, PHF seems to be linked to low-renin essential hypertension. Indeed, the effects of PHF are all seen in this condition: increased PTH levels in the face of apparently decreased PTH activity, decreased ionized calcium (possibly due to PHF-promoted intracellular calcium entry), increased sensitivity to pressor agents, decreased urinary sodium excretion, and enhanced responsiveness to calcium channel blockade, suggesting an increase in the open state of calcium channels. In a survey of unselected human subjects, PHF level did correlate with renin profile and salt sensitivity.[70] Similarly, the PHF level in the plasma from such patients correlated with their intracellular calcium levels in red blood cells,[79] PHF having been shown to be able to increase intracellular calcium levels in red blood cells *in vitro*.[79] In rats, PHF was found to be present in low-renin hypertension models but absent in high-renin hypertensive models.[82] In addition, maneuvers that decrease PHF secretion *in vitro* also lower PHF level and blood pressure *in vivo*. Specifically, an increase in calcium intake decreases PHF levels in SHRs in parallel with a reduction in their blood pressure.[69] In human hypertension, the effect of calcium supplementation has been more confusing. Although a low calcium intake is epidemiologically associated with a higher incidence of hypertension,[85-87] interventional studies have given inconsistent results. In some cases calcium supplementation has been reported to decrease blood pressure,[88-90] but in other cases it has been reported to have no effect.[91-93] A solution to this inconsistent situation, however, has been provided by Lyle et al., who reported that those hypertensive patients who respond favorably to calcium supplementation are characterized by increased levels of PTH.[94] This situation is, of course, one of the characteristics of low-renin hypertension. Thus, calcium supplementation may be of use in PHF-positive patients and not useful in other hypertensive patients.

E. Structural Comparison of PTH and PHF

Active PTH is an 84–amino acid peptide. It is synthesized as preproPTH but enzymatically clipped prior to secretion. In the circulation, PTH is degraded into two fragments: a 34–amino acid N-terminal fragment and a 50–amino acid C-terminal fragment. Traditionally, the activity of the molecule has been described as residing in the N-terminal region. Recently, however, some bone-related activity has been reported to reside in the C-terminal portion as well.[95] Nevertheless, all the vascular actions of the molecule reside in the N-terminal portion, the C-terminal fragment being inert to the vasculature. Within the N-terminal portion of the molecule, the first two amino acids, as well as amino acids 24 to 28, are important for the vascular activity; 3-34 PTH has no vascular activity.

The structure of PHF has still not been fully elucidated. Without question, the structure is exceedingly complex and novel. Currently, on the basis of much circumstantial evidence, a proposed core structure for PHF has been suggested. This structure was deduced after 4 years of work. Evidence for the structure of PHF is as follows.

After many difficulties, PHF was first purified to a single peak on high-performance liquid chromatography (HPLC) in 1991.[96] The availability of pure PHF then allowed certain structural studies to be carried out. One of the first studies carried out on PHF, even before the pure substance was isolated, was the determination of heat sensitivity. PHF was shown to be insensitive to boiling for 10 min. From this information, it was concluded that PHF was neither a large peptide nor a complex heat-sensitive molecule. Dialysis and ultrafiltration of PHF confirmed the relatively small size of PHF, as PHF-like activity was recovered between 1000 and 5000 mol wt by these studies. The next set of studies involved enzyme treatment of PHF.

First, trypsin sensitivity was assessed and PHF was shown to be trypsin sensitive. This suggested that PHF might be a small peptide, although, in retrospect, it was important to remember that trysin can cleave ester linkages as well as peptide bonds. Other enzymes such as carboxypeptidases and chymotrysin also destroyed PHF activity, apparently confirming a peptidic nature of PHF. Despite such indications, however, PHF was found to be extremely hydrophobic — much more hydrophobic than would be expected for a peptide. Thus, the possibility of another structural component linked to a peptide was considered. Alternatively, a nonpeptide structure that would nonspecifically respond to peptidases was also considered.

Histological examination of the novel parathyroid cells gave a clue as to possible structural components. When the SHR parathyroid gland was stained with Sudan black, a lipid-specific stain, it was found that the novel cells, but not the normal cells, were stained by this procedure. This suggested a lipid component or structure for PHF. In unrelated studies, work was being carried out on the vascular actions of phospholipids and lysophospholipids. It had previously been found that lysophosphatidyl inositol had pressor actions that were prolonged and of somewhat delayed onset, though not as delayed as those of PHF.[76] In addition, it was known that phosphatidic acid had vascular actions as well, although these were of more immediate nature. It was thus hypothesized that PHF might have both a peptide and a phospholipid component. Such a structure would have been consistent with findings to that point. Accordingly, the relative partitioning of PHF was tested in hydrophilic, hydrophobic, and intermediate environments. These studies showed that PHF partitioned into the chloroform-methanol phase of a water: chloroform-methanol: ether extraction mixture. Thus, the findings were consistent with an amphipathic molecule. The next studies involved testing the sensitivity of PHF to a variety of lipases, including phospholipase A_2, phospholipase C, and phospholipase D. Results from this experiment showed that PHF activity was preserved with phospholipase A_2 treatment but was abolished by treatment with phospholipases C and D. It was concluded, therefore, that PHF may have a lysophospholipid component in its structure as well as a peptide component.

To summarize, PTH and PHF tend to have totally opposite physiological effects, although certain functional characteristics are similar. This would suggest a closely related structure, with both substances acting at the same receptor, one substance being an agonist and the other being antagonistic. It is therefore surprising to find that the structures of the two substances are apparently so different. Moreover, a peptide-lysophosholipid with physiological functions has not been previously described; thus, PHF may represent an entirely new class of molecule. It should be emphasized, however, that this structural information on PHF is preliminary and awaits more rigorous confirmation. Similarly, the synthetic pathway for PHF has not yet been investigated. This synthetic pathway for such a unique molecule will also no doubt prove to be of great interest. In addition, the way in which PHF initiates its signal will also prove to be interesting, as it is not known whether PHF binds to a cell surface receptor, whether it binds to a cytoplasmic site, or whether it incorporates into and acts at the cell membrane.

V. CONCLUSION

Both parathyroid hormone and parathyroid hypertensive factor are produced in and secreted from the parathyroid gland. Both substances also have vascular actions, PTH being hypotensive and PHF being hypertensive. A comparative summary of their respective actions is given in Table 2. At present, it seems that the vascular actions of PTH do not have a physiological role and may be manifest only in pathophysiological states. Whether the vascular effects of PHF represent its primary function or whether it has a yet undiscovered physiological role remains to be determined. One possible explanation for the presence of these two substances in the parathyroid gland, however, is that one (PTH) is a whole body calcium-regulating hormone,

TABLE 2   Comparison of PTH and PHF

Parameter	PTH	PHF
Glandular origin	Parathyroid	Parathyroid
Effect on blood pressure	Decrease	Increase
Cellular origin	Chief cells	Novel cells
Effect on other pressors	Inhibits	Potentiates
Effect on $^{45}Ca^{2+}$ uptake	Decreases	Increases
Effect on L-channels	Blocks	Increases opening
Effect on cAMP	Increases	Decreases
Effect of Ca^{2+} on secretion	Decreases	Decreases
Effect on $U_{Na}V$	Increases	Decreases
Structure	Peptide	Peptide + phospholipid ?
Occurrence	All humans/mammals	Low-renin hypertension

whereas the other (PHF) is a cellular calcium regulator. Thus, integrated control of total body calcium regulation may be centered in one gland. This hypothesis is quite speculative and needs to be studied further. In addition, further studies are necessary on the structure, synthesis, mechanism of action, and physiological role of PHF. Similarly, the functional interrelationship between PTH and PHF needs to be addressed. One can therefore look forward to developments in these areas over the years. Such findings will more fully define the role of the parathyroid gland in cardiovascular function.

REFERENCES

1. Collip, J. B. and Clark, E. P., Further studies on the parathyroid hormone, *J. Biol. Chem.*, 66, 132, 1925.
2. McCann, W. S., Diuretic action of parathyroid extract-Collip in certain edematous patients, *J. Am. Med. Assoc.*, 90, 249, 1928.
3. Handler, P., Cohn, D. V., and De Maria, W. J. A., Effect of parathyroid extract on renal excretion of phosphate, *Am. J. Physiol.*, 165, 434, 1951.
4. Crass, M. F., III and Pang, P. K. T., Parathyroid hormone: a coronary artery vasodilator, *Science*, 207, 1087, 1980.
5. Pang, P. K. T., Tenner, T. E., Jr., Yee, J. A., Yang, M., and Janssen, H. F., Hypotensive action of parathyroid hormone preparations on rats and dogs, *Proc. Natl. Acad. Sci. U.S.A.*, 77, 675, 1980.
6. Pang, P. K. T., Yang, M., Oguro, C., Phillips, J. G., and Yee, J. A., Hypotensive actions of parathyroid hormone preparations in vertebrates, *Gen. Comp. Endocrinol.*, 41, 135, 1980.
7. Pang, P. K. T., Yang, M. C. M., Keutmann, H. T., and Kenny, A. D., Structure-activity relationship of parathyroid hormone: separation of the hypotensive and the hypercalcemic properties, *Endocrinology*, 112, 284, 1983.
8. Suzuki, Y., Lederis, K., Huang, M., Le Blanc, F. E., and Forstad, O. P., Relaxation of bovine, porcine and human brain arteries by parathyroid hormone, *Life Sci.*, 33, 2497, 1983.
9. Ellison, D. and McCarron, D. A., Structure pre-requisites for the hypotensive action of parathyroid hormone, *Am. J. Physiol.*, 246, F551, 1984.
10. Nickols, G. A. and Cline, W. H., Jr., Parathyroid hormone-induced changes in cyclic nucleotide levels during relaxation of the rabbit aorta, *Life Sci.*, 40, 2351, 1987.
11. Berthelot, A. and Gairard, A., Action of parathormone on arterial pressure and on contraction of isolated aorta in the rat, *Experientia*, 31, 457, 1975.
12. Schleiffer, R., Berthelot, A., and Gairard, A., Action of parathyroid extract on arterial blood pressure and on contraction and ^{45}Ca exchange in isolated aorta of the rat, *Eur. J. Pharmacol.*, 58, 163, 1979.
13. Rambausek, M., Ritz, E., Rascher, W., Kreusser, W., Mann, J. F. E., Kreye, V. A. W., and Mehls, O., Vascular effects of parathyroid hormone (PTH), *Adv. Exp. Med. Biol.*, 151, 619, 1982.

14. Pang, P. K. T., Yang, M. C. M., Shew, R., and Tenner, T. E., Jr., The vasorelaxant action of parathyroid hormone fragments on isolated rat tail artery, *Blood Vessels*, 22, 57, 1985.
15. Nickols, G. A., Metz, M. A., and Cline, W. H., Jr., Endothelium-independent linkage of parathyroid hormone receptors of rat vascular tissue with increased adenosine 3',5'-monophosphate and relaxation of vascular smooth muscle, *Endocrinology*, 119, 349, 1986.
16. Wang, H. H., Drugge, E. D., Yen, Y. C., Blumenthal, M. R., and Pang, P. K. T., Effects of synthetic parathyroid hormone on hemodynamics and regional blood flows, *Eur. J. Pharmacol.*, 97, 298, 1984.
17. Hashimoto, K., Nakagawa, Y., Shibuya, T., Satoh, H., Ushijima, T., and Imai, S., Effects of parathyroid hormone and related polypeptides on the heart and coronary circulation of dogs, *J. Cardiovasc. Pharmacol.*, 3, 668, 1981.
18. Katoh, Y., Klein, K. L., Kaplan, R. A., Sanborn, W. G., and Kurokawa, K., Parathyroid hormone has a positive inotropic action in the rat, *Endocrinology*, 109, 2252, 1981.
19. Bogin, E., Massry, S. G., and Harary, I., Effect of parathyroid hormone on rat heart cells, *J. Clin. Invest.*, 67, 1215, 1981.
20. Pang, P. K. T., Zhang, R. H., and Yang, M. C. M., Hypotensive action of parathyroid hormone in chicken, *J. Exp. Zool.*, 232, 691, 1984.
21. Pang, P. K. T., Yang, M. C. M., and Sham, J. S. K., Parathyroid hormone and calcium entry blockade in a vascular tissue, *Life Sci.*, 42, 1395, 1988.
22. Wang, R., Karpinski, E., and Pang, P. K. T., Parathyroid hormone selectively inhibits L-type calcium channels in single vascular smooth muscle cells of the rat, *J. Physiol.*, 441, 325, 1991.
23. Wang, R., Karpinski, E., and Pang, P. K. T., Two types of voltage-dependent calcium channel currents and their modulation by parathyroid hormone in neonatal rat ventricular cells, *J. Cardiovasc. Pharmacol.*, 17, 990, 1991.
24. Nickols, G. A., Increased cAMP in cultured vascular smooth muscle cells and relaxation of aortic strips by parathyroid hormone, *Eur. J. Pharmacol.*, 116, 137, 1985.
25. Nickols, G. A. and Cline, W. H., Jr., Parathyroid hormone-induced changes in cyclic nucleotide levels during relaxation of the rabbit aorta, *Life Sci.*, 40, 2351, 1987.
26. Pang, P. K. T., Yang, M. C. M., Tenner, T. E., Jr., Kenny, A. D., and Cooper, C. W., Cyclic AMP and the vascular action of parathyroid hormone, *Can. J. Physiol. Pharmacol.*, 64, 1543, 1987.
27. Wang, R., Wu, L. Y., Karpinski, E., and Pang, P. K. T., The effects of parathyroid hormone on L-type voltage-dependent calcium channel currents in vascular smooth muscle cells and ventricular myocytes are mediated by a cyclic AMP-dependent mechanism, *FEBS Lett.*, 282, 331, 1991.
28. Bogin, E., Massry, S. G., Levi, J., et al., Effect of parathyroid hormone on osmotic fragility of human erythrocytes, *J. Clin. Invest.*, 69, 1017, 1982.
29. Bogin, E., Massry, S. G., and Harary, I., Effect of parathyroid hormone on rat heart cells, *J. Clin. Invest.*, 67, 1215, 1981.
30. Chausmer, A. B., Sharmar, B. S., and Wallach, S., The effect of parathyroid hormone in hepatic cell transport of calcium, *Endocrinology*, 90, 663, 1972.
31. Winquist, R. J., Baskin, E. P., and Vlasuk, G. P., Synthetic tumor derived human hypercalcemic factor exhibits PTH-like vasorelaxation in renal arteries, *Biochem. Biophys. Res. Commun.*, 149, 227, 1987.
32. Nickols, G. A., Nana, A. D., Nickols, M. A., Di Pette, D. J., and Asimakis, G. K., Hypotension and cardiac stimulation due to the parathyroid hormone-related protein, humoral hypercalcemia of malignancy factor, *Endocrinology*, 125, 834, 1989.
33. Shan, J., Pang, P. K. T., Lin, H.-C., and Yang, M. C. M., Cardiovascular effects of human parathyroid hormone and parathyroid hormone-related peptide, *J. Cardiovasc. Pharmacol.*, 23(Suppl. 2), S38, 1994.
34. Schleiffer, R., Berthelot, A., Pernot, F., and Gairard, A., Parathyroids, thyroid and development of hypertension in SHR, *Jpn. Circ. J.*, 45, 1272, 1981.
35. McCarron, D. A., Yung, N. H., Ugoretz, B. A., and Brutzik, S., Disturbances in calcium metabolism in the spontaneously hypertensive rat, *Hypertension*, 3 (Suppl I), I161, 1981.
36. Stern, N., Lee, D. B. N., Silis, V., Beck, F. W. J., Deftos, L., Manolagas, S. C., and Sowers, J. R., Effects of high calcium intake on blood pressure and calcium metabolism in young SHR, *Hypertension*, 6, 639, 1984.

37. Resnick, L. M., Müller, F. B., and Laragh, J. H., Calcium regulating hormones in essential hypertension, *Ann. Intern. Med.*, 105, 649, 1986.
38. Hellstrom, J., Birke, G., and Edvall, C. A., Hypertension in hyperparathyroidism, *Br. J. Urol.*, 30, 13, 1958.
39. Madhaven, T., Frame, B., and Block, M. A., Influence of surgical correction of primary hyperparathyroidism on associated hypertension, *Arch. Surg.*, 100, 212, 1970.
40. Lueg, M. C., Hypertension and primary hyperparathyroidism: a five-year case review, *South. Med. J.*, 75, 1371, 1982.
41. Jones, D. B., Lucas, P. A., Jones, J. H., Lloyd, H. J., Wilkins, W. E., Lloyd, H. J., and Walker, D. A., Changes in blood pressure and renal function after parathyroidectomy in primary hyperparathyroidism, *Postgrad. Med. J.*, 59, 350, 1983.
42. Ringe, J. D., Reversible hypertension in primary hyperparathyroidism: pre- and postoperative blood pressure in 75 cases, *Klin. Wochenschr.*, 62, 465, 1984.
43. Rapado, A., Arterial hypertension and primary hyperparathyroidism, *Am. J. Nephrol.*, 6 (Suppl. 1), 49, 1986.
44. Niederle, B., Roka, R., Woloszczyk, W., Klaushofer, K., Kovarik, J., and Schernthaner, G., Successful parathyroidectomy in primary hyperparathyroidism: a clinical follow-up study of 212 consecutive patients, *Surgery*, 102, 903, 1987.
45. Hulter, H. N., Melby, J. C., Peterson, J. C., and Cooke, C. R., Chronic continuous PTH infusion results in hypertension in normal subjects, *J. Clin. Hypertens.*, 2, 360, 1986.
46. Kishimoto, H., Tsumura, K., Fujioka, S., Uchimoto, S., and Morii H., Chronic parathyroid hormone administration reverses the antihypertensive effect of calcium loading in young spontaneously hypertensive rats, *Am. J. Hypertens.*, 6, 234, 1993.
47. Berthelot, A., Pernot, F., Schleiffer, R., and Gairard, A., Correlations between parameters of parathyroid activity and blood pressure during the onset of DOCA + saline hypertension in the rat, *Contrib. Nephrol.*, 41, 146, 1984.
48. Grobbee, D. E., Hackeng, W. H. L., Birkenhager, J. C., and Hofman, A., Intact parathyroid hormone (1-84) in primary hypertension, *Clin. Exp. Hypertens.*, 8, 299, 1986.
49. Lewanczuk, R. Z. and Pang, P. K. T., Vascular and calcemic effects of spontaneously hypertensive rat plasma in normotensive rats, *Am. J. Hypertens.*, 3, 189S, 1990.
50. Lewanczuk, R. Z., Wang, J., Zhang, Z. R., and Pang, P. K. T., Effects of spontaneously hypertensive rat plasma on blood pressure and tail artery calcium uptake in normotensive rats, *Am. J. Hypertens.*, 2, 25, 1989.
51. Dahl, L. K., Knutsen, K. D., and Iwai, J., Humoral transmission of hypertension: evidence from parabiosis, *Circ. Res.*, 24/25 (Suppl. 1), 21, 1969.
52. Knudsen, K. D., Iwai, J., Heine, M., Leitl, G., and Dahl, L. K., Genetic influence on the development of renoprival hypertension in parabiotic rats, *J. Exp. Med.*, 130, 1353, 1969.
53. Dahl, L. K., Heine, M., and Thompson, K., Genetic influence of homografts on blood pressure of rats from different strains, *Proc. Soc. Exp. Biol. Med.*, 140, 852, 1972.
54. Zidek, W., Heckmann, U., Losse, H., and Vetter, H., Effects on blood pressure of cross circulation between spontaneously hypertensive and normotensive rats, *Clin. Exp. Hypertens.*, A8, 347, 1986.
55. Iwai, J., Knudsen, K. D., Dahl, L. K., and Tassinari, L., Effect of adrenalectomy on blood pressure in salt-fed, hypertension-prone rats: failure of hypertension to develop in the absence of evidence of adrenal cortical tissue, *J. Exp. Med.*, 129, 663, 1969.
56. Olsen, F., Transfer of arterial hypertension by splenic cells from DOCA-salt hypertensive and renal hypertensive rats to normotensive recipients, *Acta Pathol. Microbiol. Scand.*, 88, 1, 1980.
57. Pang, P. K. T. and Lewanczuk, R. Z., Parathyroid origin of a new circulating hypertensive factor in spontaneously hypertensive rats, *Am. J. Hypertens.*, 2, 898, 1989.
58. Benishin, C. G., Labedz, T., Guo, D. D., Lewanczuk, R. Z., and Pang, P. K. T., Identification and purification of parathyroid hypertensive factor (PHF) from organ culture of parathyroid glands from spontaneously hypertensive rats, *Am. J. Hypertens.*, 6, 134, 1993.
59. Benishin, C. G., Tang, L., Lewanczuk, R. Z., and Pang, P. K. T., Production of polyclonal antisera to parathyroid hypertensive factor from spontaneously hypertensive rats, *J. Hypertens.*, 11, 245, 1993.

60. Nerke, J., Lucas, P. A., Szabo, A., Cournot-Witmer, G., Mall, G., Bouillon, R., Drüeke, T., Mann, J., and Ritz, E., Hyperparathyroidism and abnormal calcitriol metabolism in the spontaneously hypertensive rats, *Hypertension*, 13, 233, 1989.

61. Kaneko, T., Ohtani, R., Lewanczuk, R. Z., and Pang, P. K. T., A novel cell type in the parathyroid glands of spontaneously hypertensive rats, *Am. J. Hypertens.*, 2, 549, 1989.

62. Lewanczuk, R. Z. and Pang, P. K. T., Expression of parathyroid hypertensive factor in primary hyperparathyroid patients, *Blood Pressure*, 2, 22, 1993.

63. Sherwood, L. M., Mayer, G. P., Ramberg, C. J., Kronfeld, D. S., Aurbach, G. D., and Potts, J. J., Regulation of parathyroid hormone secretion: proportional control of calcium, lack of effect of phosphate, *Endocrinology*, 93, 1043, 1968.

64. Care, A. D., Sherwood, L. M., Potts, J. J., and Aurbach, G. D., Perfusion of the isolated parathyroid gland of the goat and sheep, *Nature*, 209, 55, 1966.

65. Brown, E. M., Hurwitz, S., and Aurbach, G. D., Preparation of viable isolated bovine parathyroid cells, *Endocrinology*, 99, 1582, 1976.

66. Morrissey, J. J. and Cohn, D. V., The effects of calcium and magnesium on the secretion of parathormone and parathyroid secretory protein by isolated porcine parathyroid cells, *Endocrinology*, 193, 2081, 1978.

67. Adami, S., Nuirhead, N., and Manning, R. M., Control of secretion by parathyroid hormone in secondary hyperparathyroidism, *Clin. Endocrinol.*, 16, 463, 1982.

68. Fasciotto, B. H., Gorr, S.-U., Bourdeau, A. M., and Cohn, D. V., Autocrine regulation of parathyroid secretion: inhibition of secretion by chromogranin-A (secretory protein-I) and potentiation of secretion by chromogranin-A and pancreostatin antibodies, *Endocrinology*, 127, 1329, 1990.

69. Lewanczuk, R. Z., Chen, A., and Pang, P. K. T., The effect of dietary calcium on blood pressure in spontaneously hypertensive rats may be mediated by a circulating hypertensive factor, *Am. J. Hypertens.*, 3, 349, 1990.

70. Resnick, L. M., Lewanczuk, R. Z., Laragh, J. H., and Pang, P. K. T., Parathyroid hypertensive factor (PHF) in human essential hypertension: relation to plasma renin activity and dietary salt sensitivity, *J. Hypertens.*, 11, 235, 1993.

71. Lewanczuk, R. Z. and Pang, P. K. T., The occurrence of parathyroid hypertension factor (PHF) in Dahl rats, *Am. J. Hypertens.*, 6, 758, 1993.

72. Zemel, M. B., Gualdoni, S.M., and Walsh, M., Effects of sodium and calcium metabolism and blood pressure regulation in hypertensive black adults, *J. Hypertens.*, 4 (Suppl. 5), S364, 1986.

73. Zemel, M. B., Bedford, B. A., Standley, P. R., and Sowers, J. R., Saline infusion causes rapid increase in parathyroid hormone and intracellular calcium levels, *Am. J. Hypertens.*, 2, 185, 1989.

74. Habener, J. F., Rosenblatt, M., and Potts, J. T., Jr., Parathyroid hormone: biochemical aspects of biosynthesis, secretion, action and metabolism, *Physiol. Rev.*, 64, 985, 1984.

75. Mok, L. L. S., Nickols, G. A., Thompson, J. C., and Cooper, C. W., Parathyroid hormone as a smooth muscle relaxant, *Endocr. Rev.*, 10, 420, 1989.

76. Shan, J., Benishin, C. G., Lewanczuk, R. Z., and Pang, P. K. T., The mechanism of the vascular action of parathyroid hypertensive factor, *J. Cardiovasc. Pharmacol.*, 23(Suppl. 2), S1, 1994.

77. Lewanczuk, R. Z. and Pang, P. K. T., *In vivo* potentiation of vasopressors by spontaneously hypertensive rat plasma: correlation with blood pressure and calcium uptake, *Clin. Exp. Hypertens.*, A11, 1471, 1989.

78. Lewanczuk, R. Z. and Pang, P. K. T., Specific renal effects of parathyroid hypertensive factor, *Am. J. Hypertens.*, 6, 46A, 1993.

79. Barbagallo, M., Gupta, R. K., Lewanczuk, R. Z., Pang, P. K. T., and Resnick, L. M., Serum-mediated intracellular calcium changes in normotensive and hypertensive red blood cells: role of parathyroid hypertensive factor (PHF), *J. Cardiovasc. Pharmacol.*, 23(Suppl. 2), S14, 1994.

80. Hongo, T., Kupfer, J., Enomoto, H., Sharifi, B., and Giannella, N. D., Abundant expression of parathyroid hormone-related protein in primary aortic smooth muscle cells accompanies serum-induced proliferation, *J. Clin. Invest.*, 88, 1841, 1991.

81. Resnick, L. M., Lewanczuk, R. Z., Laragh, J. H., and Pang, P. K. T., Plasma hypertensive factor in essential hypertension, *J. Hypertens.*, 8 (Suppl. 3), S101, 1990.

82. Lewanczuk, R. Z. and Pang, P. K. T., Parathyroid hypertensive factor (PHF) is present in DOCA-salt, but not two-kidney, one-clip hypertension, *Am. J. Hypertens.*, 4, 802, 1991.
83. Tchurina, S. K., Rijov, D. B., Klueva, N. Z., and Eschanova, G. T., Dietary Ca deficiency as a cause of PHF activity in WKY rats, *Ricerca Scient. Educaz. Perm.*, (Suppl. 95), 744, 1993.
84. Zaloga, G. P., Calcium homeostasis in the critically ill patients, *Magnesium*, 8, 190, 1989.
85. Ackley, S., Barrett-Conor, E., and Suarez, L., Dairy products, calcium and blood pressure, *Am. J. Clin. Nutr.*, 38, 457, 1983.
86. Garcia-Palmieri, M. R., Costas, M., Cruz-Vidal, P. D., Sorlie, P. D., Tillotson, J., and Havlik, R. J., Milk consumption, calcium intake and decreased hypertension in Puerto Rico, *Hypertension*, 6, 322, 1984.
87. McCarron, D. A., Morris, C. D., Henry, H. J., and Stanton, J. L., Blood pressure and nutrient intake in the United States, *Science*, 224, 1392, 1984.
88. Belizan, J. M., Villar, J., Pineda, O., Gonzalez, A. E., Sainz, E., Garrera, G., and Sibrian, R., Reduction of blood pressure with calcium supplementation in young adults, *JAMA*, 248, 1161, 1983.
89. McCarron, D. A. and Morris, C. D., Blood pressure response to oral calcium supplementation in mild to moderate hypertension, *Ann. Intern. Med.*, 103, 825, 1985.
90. Grobbee, D. E. and Hofman, A., Effect of calcium supplementation on diastolic blood pressure in young people with mild hypertension, *Lancet*, 8509, 703, 1986.
91. Cappuccio, F. P., Nirmula, M. D., Singer, D. R. F., Singer, D. R. J., Smith, S. J., Shore, A. C., and MacGregor, G. A., Does oral calcium supplementation lower high blood pressure? A double blind study, *J. Hypertens.*, 5, 67, 1987.
92. Siani, A., Strazzullo, P., Guglielmi, S., Pacioni, D., Giacco, A., Iacone, R., and Mancini, M., Controlled trial of low calcium versus high calcium intake in mild hypertension, *J. Hypertens.*, 6, 253, 1988.
93. Zoccali, C., Mallamaci, F., Delfino, D., Ciccarelli, M., Parlongo, S., Iellamo, D., Moscato, D., and Maggiore, Q., Double blind randomized crossover trial of calcium supplementation in essential hypertension, *J. Hypertens.*, 6, 451, 1988.
94. Lyle, R. M., Melby, C. L., and Hyner, G. C., Metabolic differences between subjects whose blood pressure did or did not respond to oral calcium supplementation, *Am. J. Clin. Nutr.*, 47, 1030, 1988.
95. Murray, T. M., Rao, L. G., Muzaffar, S. A., and Ly, H., Human parathyroid carboxy-terminal peptide (53-84) stimulates alkaline phosphatase activity in dexamethasone-treated rat osteosarcoma cells *in vitro*, *Endocrinology*, 124, 1097, 1989.
96. Benishin, C. G., Lewanczuk, R. Z., and Pang, P. K. T., Purification of parathyroid hypertensive factor from plasma of spontaneously hypertensive rats, *Proc. Natl. Acad. Sci. U.S.A.*, 88, 6372, 1991.

6

Local Expression and Action of Parathyroid Hormone-Related Protein in the Cardiovascular System

Mark A. Thiede and G. Allen Nickols

CONTENTS

I. ACTIONS OF PARATHYROID HORMONE ON THE CARDIOVASCULAR SYSTEM

A discussion of the actions of parathyroid hormone-related protein (PTHrP) in the mammalian cardiovascular system should consider the roots of this line of research. The concept of PTHrP as an autocrine or paracrine modulator of blood pressure and cardiac function is based on the observations of the actions of parathyroid hormone (PTH) on this organ system. A detailed review of these effects of PTH is presented by Crass in Chapter 2. However, concepts fundamental to the consideration of the importance of PTHrP as a modifier of heart and blood vessel activity are generally discussed here. Because the amino terminal bioactivity of both PTH and PTHrP are attributed to interaction with the same receptor class(es) in target organs, similarities between the physiological effects of the two are discussed throughout this chapter.

Parathyroid hormone and PTH/PTHrP receptors appear to be well conserved across species and class lines. Parathyroid hormone has been shown to relax vascular smooth muscle in a number of mammalian, avian, and amphibian species.[1-4] Responsiveness also appears to be universal to smooth muscles. Besides vascular smooth muscle, PTH relaxes smooth muscle from the uterus,[5,6] trachea,[7] and gastrointestinal tract.[8-10] In most cases smooth muscle relaxation responses to PTH have been linked to increases in smooth muscle cell adenosine 3':5'-cyclic phosphate (cAMP) concentrations[11-14] as a potential intracellular mechanism of action.

The observation that PTH produced hypotensive effects in animals was made several decades ago. While Collip and Clark[15] reported a reduction in systemic blood pressure in dogs after the administration of bovine parathyroid extract, Charbon[16,17] established that this activity was not due to a contaminant in the extract. They observed vasodilatory effects of synthetic bovine PTH-(1-34) [bPTH-(1-34)] were not blocked by pharmacological antagonists of common vasoactive agents. Thus, PTH appeared to have direct activity on the vasculature, which was attributed to the amino terminal portion of the molecule. Also, it was likely that these actions were specific and not due to indirect stimulation of receptors for vasodilators such as catecholamine, histamine, or serotonin.

Data indicate that blood vessels from one anatomical area or organ appear to be more sensitive to PTH than vessels from other regions. For instance, coronary arteries in dog and rat dilate in response to picomolar doses of the hormone.[18-21] Mesenteric vasculature,[4,22-24] cerebral arteries,[14,25,26] tail artery,[27] and renal arteries[28-30] are relaxed or dilated with EC_{50} in the low nanomolar range. However, for some vessels, including the aorta,[12,31,32] relaxation requires relatively high concentrations of PTH. Vessel sensitivity may be related to the density of PTH/PTHrP receptors on the specific vessel and the efficiency of "coupling" of receptors to intracellular second messengers. Also, the physiological function of the vessel in regulating regional flow (i.e., resistance vessels are more sensitive than capacitance vessels) may play a role in the sensitivity of vessels to vasoactive agents, including PTH.

Besides the hypotensive activity of PTH, positive chronotropic and inotropic activity has been observed. *In vivo*, PTH has been shown to increase heart rate in a dose-dependent fashion independent of cardiovascular reflexes.[18,21,33,34] Parathyroid hormone also increased myocardial contractile force in the conscious, unrestrained rat.[21] Isolated heart preparations and myocardial strips displayed an enhanced rate of contraction as well as an increased force of contraction.[35-38] Isolated rat heart cells in culture increased their beating frequency in response to PTH via a cAMP-dependent mechanism.[39] Therefore, in addition to its direct vasodilatory effects, PTH also is a stimulant of cardiac function.

The actions of PTH in the cardiovascular system are similar to those of β-adrenergic agonists and have been compared to the effects of isoproterenol.[40] Thus, acute administration of PTH produces reduced blood pressure and tachycardia. While these actions of PTH are reproducible and substantial, a number of inconsistencies prevented the acceptance of the hypothesis of PTH as a physiological mediator or modulator of cardiovascular function. First, even with the sensitivity of the heart and vasculature to PTH in the same low nanomolar range as that demonstrated for more traditional target tissues such as bone and kidney,[41-43] it is difficult to postulate a feedback system whereby the parathyroid gland may respond to the cardiovascular system, and thus control secretion of the hormone in order to regulate cardiovascular activity. Also, circulating levels of PTH are generally in the picomolar range, below that which are required to activate vascular and cardiac PTH receptors.

However, with the discovery of PTHrP[44-46] and the determination that PTHrP can interact with the same receptors as PTH in specific tissues, a more reasonable hypothesis could be proposed. As an autocrine and/or paracrine factor, locally produced and released PTHrP would interact with local receptors, responding to local factors and producing tissue-specific effects. Thus, while PTH administration will produce significant alterations in systemic cardiovascular hemodynamics, probably the most physiologically relevant actions are those produced by autocrine or paracrine activity of PTHrP serving to modulate regional vascular hemodynamics and cardiac function.

II. BRIEF HISTORY OF PARATHYROID HORMONE-RELATED PROTEIN

A. Origin of Parathyroid Hormone-Related Protein — Production by Tumors Associated with Hypercalcemia of Malignancy

For nearly five decades following Fuller Albright's intuitive postulation that tumors associated with the clinical syndrome of humoral hypercalcemia of malignancy (HHM) secrete a PTH-like activity,[47] scientists pursued the tumor-borne hypercalcemic factor responsible for HHM. In the late 1980s this hypercalcemic factor was finally isolated from the conditioned media of cultures of human lung, breast, renal, and squamous carcinomas, in part as a result of the striking similarities between the biological activities of the N-terminal fragment of PTH and the tumor product.[44-46] N-terminal peptide sequences derived from the purified tumor product revealed for the first time that tumors associated with HHM produce a protein that shares sequence identity with PTH. Because the protein shares both N-terminal sequence homology and biological activity with PTH, it was called parathyroid hormone-related protein, or PTHrP, a name which has endured since 1987. The subsequent cloning of human

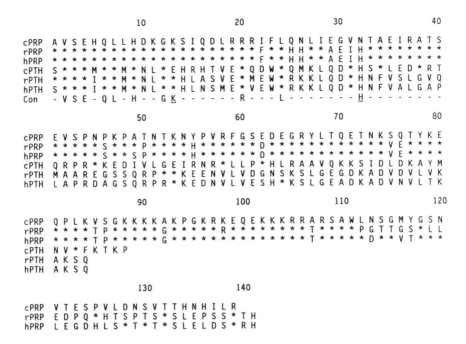

FIGURE 1   Comparison of the amino acid sequences of PTHrP and PTH from chicken, rat, and human. The top line (cPRP) represents the 139 amino acid sequence of chicken PTHrP that was deduced from a cDNA isolated from a 10-d chicken embryo library.[58] This sequence is compared to the corresponding sequences of the rat (rPRP)[54,55] and human (hPRP) PTHrP-(1-141)[48-50] and the chicken, rat, and human PTH.[48] Only the 139 and 141 amino acid hPTHrP sequences are presented. Residues which show identity with the chicken PTHrP are designated (*). A consensus (Con) sequence for those residues between 1 and 40 that are shared by chicken, rat, and human PTHrP and PTH is presented on the last line at the top.

cDNA[48-50] and genomic DNA[51-53] revealed the complete primary structures of the PTHrP molecules and eventually led to the isolation of PTHrP cDNA and genomic DNA from species such as the rat,[54-56] mouse,[57] and chicken.[58-60] As seen in Figure 1, a comparison of both the length and amino acid sequences of PTHrPs from these species demonstrates a remarkably strong phylogenetic conservation of the PTHrP structure, which in turn emphasizes the potential biological importance of this molecule. Amino acid sequences of PTHrP have now been used to generate a number of useful antibodies for immunohistochemical analysis of PTHrP, and the results of RNA blot hybridization and immunohistochemical studies have now demonstrated that human,[48-50,61-65] rat,[54,55] and canine[61,66] tumors associated with HHM produce PTHrP. In addition, the results of numerous clinical studies have shown a good correlation between the synthesis and secretion of PTHrP by tumors and the formation of well-defined hypercalcemia.[67-70] Kukreja et al.[71] further defined this correlation by showing that the infusion of anti-PTHrP antiserum reduced the hypercalcemia in nude mice implanted with human PTHrP-producing tumor cells. In other studies using this passive immunity approach researchers have failed to alter calcium levels in lactating[72] and neonatal mice,[73] suggesting that normally low circulating levels of PTHrP do not function in modulating calcium homeostasis.

B. Structural and Functional Similarities of Parathyroid Hormone and Parathyroid Hormone-Related Protein

Lending to their similar biological activities, the N-termini of PTHrP and PTH share 8 of the first 13 residues (Figure 1). *In vivo*, synthetic N-terminal fragments of both PTH and PTHrP are essentially equipotent in their calciotropic properties, including the stimulation of osteo-clastic bone resorption,[74,75] renal synthesis of 25-(OH) vitamin D_{1a}-hydroxylase,[76] and renal calcium reabsorption.[74,77,78] To date, N-terminal peptides of both PTH and PTHrP have been shown to stimulate the same intracellular second messenger systems[79-85] via their interaction with a membrane-associated receptor present in traditional (bone and kidney)[86-91] and nontraditional (e.g., vascular, gastric)[8,41,92] PTH target tissues. The broad tissue distribu-tion of both PTHrP and PTH/PTHrP receptor messenger RNA (mRNA)[93-96] in the rat strongly suggests that together they represent an important autocrine/paracrine activity. Although it is possible that PTHrP also may interact with a membrane receptor that is unique to the one that has been cloned,[90,91] there is no direct evidence to support the existence of such a molecule at this time.

C. Parathyroid Hormone-Related Protein as a Multifunctional Precursor Protein

As seen in Figure 1, beyond residue 32, the sequences of PTH and PTHrP completely diverge, with PTHrP molecules being nearly twice as long as PTH. In comparison to the human PTHrP, residues 1 to 110 of the avian and rodent molecules have been remarkably well conserved, with only 2 or 17 amino acid substitutions being seen between the human and rodent or avian molecules, respectively. In likeness to the preproopiomelanocortin (POMC) gene product which can be proteolytically processed into several bioactive species,[97] PTHrP-(1-110) con-tains multiple potential sites for proteolytic processing of the molecule. Such a structure suggests that PTHrP may contain a number of cryptic bioactive peptides, the bioactivities of which may require proteolytic release. In support of this possibility, Soifer et al.[98] have recently presented evidence to support the specific intracellular proteolysis of PTHrP into at least two molecular species: the N-terminal 1-36 amino acid and a 7-kDa C-terminal fragment, with residue 38 at its N-terminus. The two proteolytic fragments appear to be packaged into different intracellular secretory granules. The 7-kDa fragment of PTHrP may have physiologi-cal relevance to calcium translocation because it contains residues 67 to 86, a peptide sequence shown to stimulate placental calcium transfer in sheep.[99-102] Proteolysis between residues 106 and 107 also may be important for the release of an additional biological activity, as Fenton et al.[103,104] showed that both PTHrP-(107-111) and PTHrP-(107-139) can inhibit osteoclastic resorptive activity *in vitro*. Thus, evidence is mounting to indicate that the scope of biological actions of PTHrP will extend well beyond the calciotropic actions that it shares with PTH. Though it is quite possible that specific proteolytic fragments of PTHrP serve important biological functions, direct evidence for the physiological production and action of these fragments *in vivo* remains to be shown.

D. Organization, Expression, and Regulation of the Parathyroid Hormone-Related Protein Gene

In contrast to the simple structure of the gene encoding human PTH (hPTH),[105] the hPTHrP gene is a complex transcriptional unit containing multiple promoter elements[51-53,106,107] and alternatively spliced 3′ untranslated exons.[48-50,108] Comparison of the human, rat, mouse, and avian PTHrP genes shows a remarkable conservation of both the organization and structure of exon-intron boundaries.[109] Transcription of hPTHrP is initiated from up to three indepen-dent promoter elements including a GC (guanidine and cytosine)-rich promoter element[107] that is similar to those found in the 5′ regulatory region of genes encoding housekeeping func-tions.[110,111] The basal levels of PTHrP mRNA that are seen in many unstimulated cells and tissues may reflect a "housekeeping" level of PTHrP gene transcriptional activity. Multiple AU (adenine and uracil)-rich motifs found within the 3′ untranslated sequence of all known PTHrP mRNAs may be important for regulating PTHrP mRNA stability because these sequences, which are also present in mRNAs encoding a number of cytokines and protooncogenes, have been shown to decrease the half-life of normally stable mRNA.[112] One additional interesting feature of the human PTHrP mRNAs is that they encode molecules of either 139,[50] 141,[48,49] or 173[108] amino acids as a result of alternative RNA splicing of the 3' exons. Although the chicken PTHrP gene can produce mRNAs encoding 139 or 141 amino acid PTHrP molecules,[58-60] analysis of genomic sequences together with RNA blot hybridization data indicate that the rat and mouse PTHrP gene produces a single transcript encoding only the 141 amino acid form.[56,57] The alternative use of promoter elements and splicing of exons may be important in regulating the expression of the human PTHrP gene in a developmental or tissue-specific manner; however, currently the biological significance of these pathways remains unknown.

To better understand the role of PTHrP in normal physiology, a considerable effort has been put toward establishing the spatial organization of PTHrP expression in cells and tissues of developmental and adult origin. Unlike PTH, which is essentially a product of the parathyroid gland, PTHrP is produced by numerous cells and tissues.[113] During development, both PTHrP mRNA and PTHrP immunoreactivity are widely distributed in fetal tissues.[59,113-118] In the adult PTHrP is expressed in many tissues, including the skin, skeletal muscle, lung, kidney, esophagus, stomach, intestine, spleen, lymphocytes, long bones, urinary bladder, ovary, uterus, amnion, cervix, mammary tissue, prostate, testes, and central and peripheral nervous tissues.[49,54,55,57,59,60,93,94,96,99,113,119-135] Both PTHrP mRNA and immunoreactivity have been found in both abnormal as well as normal glandular tissues such as the adrenals,[93,119] parathyroid/thyroids,[129,136-138] pituitary,[128,129,136] and pancreas.[139] The expression of PTHrP by epithelial cells,[114,118,140-142] smooth muscle cells,[118,119,126,143] keratinocytes,[120-123,144,145] and secretory cells[136,139,142] suggests diverse functions for this protein. As discussed in greater detail later in the chapter, PTHrP mRNA and PTHrP immunoreactivity is also present throughout tissues of the cardiovascular system such as the atria, ventricle, aorta, and peripheral blood vessels. In view of the production of PTHrP by isolated peripheral blood vessels[115,119,120,126] and nerves,[128] a substantial amount of PTHrP mRNA that is detected by RNA blot analysis of whole tissue RNA may originate from associated neurovascular tissues.

Early data showing that PTHrP is produced by fetal parathyroids and lactating mammary tissue suggested a possible endocrine function for PTHrP. The results of several recent studies support this view;[146-148] however, increasing evidence indicates that PTHrP most likely serves an autocrine/paracrine function. This view has gained support from the results of recent RNA blot hybridization studies which show that PTH/PTHrP receptor and PTHrP share a similar tissue distribution.[94-96] To better understand the biological importance of PTHrP, Karaplis et al.[149] have developed a mouse strain in which the PTHrP gene has been genetically "knocked-out". In preliminary studies they found homozygous PTHrP *null* offspring died during the perinatal period and exhibited multiple bone abnormalities involving both the axial and appendicular skeleton. At the time of this writing, the effect of this mutation on the development of other organ systems such as the cardiovascular system has not been reported.

Results of studies designed to understand the spatial and temporal regulation of PTHrP expression has generated a sizable list of important molecular and environmental factors that regulate the synthesis of this molecule in cells and tissues. To date, the expression and secretion of PTHrP has been shown to be regulated by numerous factors, including peptide hormones such as prolactin[150] and calcitonin;[151] steroids such as glucocorticoids,[143,152-154] vitamin D,[143,153] and estrogens;[155,156] phorbol esters;[157,158] serum;[143,158] growth factors such as epidermal growth factor (EGF)[144, 145,157] and transforming growth factor-α[144] and -β[159,160] (TGF-α and β); interleukins;[161] prostaglandins;[161] vasoconstrictor substances;[143, 162] the virus-encoded transcriptional factor *tax;*[163] and biomechanical stretch.[131,132,164]

In vitro and *in vivo*, the response of the PTHrP gene to certain stimuli generates a transient increase in both the transcription of the gene and accumulation of mRNA, a response indicative of an early response gene.[143,155,158,162,165] *In vivo*, removal of the stimulus (e.g., parturition in the gravid rat uterus) results in a rapid decrease in the levels of PTHrP mRNA within the uterus.[131] Stabilization of cellular levels of PTHrP mRNA by treatment with cycloheximide supports a role for *de novo* protein synthesis in the rapid turnover of PTHrP mRNA.[143,157,158,162,165] On the other hand, recent data[159,160] which shows that TGF-β increases both PTHrP gene transcription and mRNA half-life in cells adds another dimension to the posttranscriptional regulation of this gene. Secretion of N-terminal PTHrP appears to be coupled to increases in intracellular PTHrP mRNA in cultures treated with calcium,[145] calcitonin,[151] phorbol esters,[157] and EGF.[144,145,157] During lactation, levels of PTHrP secreted into the milk correlate well with the expression of PTHrP mRNA in the mammary gland.[166] Therefore, one can conclude that PTHrP is not only a widely distributed and utilized gene product, but that its synthesis is under diverse, yet tight regulation.

E. Potential Physiological Roles of Parathyroid Hormone-Related Protein

Although it has been only 7 years since the structure of PTHrP was identified, great strides have been made to elucidate the potential physiological functions of this molecule. Evidence now supports a role for the N-terminal fragment of PTHrP in the proliferation/differentiation of keratinocytes.[144,145,167,168] Evidence to support a role for PTHrP in the proliferation and differentiation of cells other than keratinocytes was also reported.[169-171] In keratinocytes, PTHrP may serve to inhibit cell growth because blockade of endogenous PTHrP synthesis via the expression of antisense RNA for PTHrP effectively induced proliferation in these cells.[168]

Both the N-terminus[99,100,172] and the mid-molecular[101,102] portion of PTHrP may function in stimulating the transfer of calcium and magnesium by the ovine placenta. In addition, the molecule may possess reciprocal biological activities: the N-terminus can stimulate osteoclastic bone resorption,[75,173] while the C-terminus can inhibit[103,104] this activity.

It has become evident that perhaps one of the most important bioactivities of PTHrP is not related to calcium homeostasis, but instead to the function(s) of cardiovascular tissues and tissues containing nonvascular smooth muscle. N-terminal fragments of PTHrP have been shown to inhibit the contractile activity of smooth muscle in the gut,[8,174] uterus,[92,175,176] urinary bladder,[132] and cardiovascular tissues.[21,28,126] Previously described actions of PTH on the cardiovascular system (see Chapter 2) have largely defined the actions of PTHrP on cardiovascular tissues. However, unlike PTH, which is essentially a product of the adult parathyroid gland, PTHrP is produced within cardiovascular tissues and most likely represents a local mediator of previously described cardiovascular actions of PTH (see below).

III. LOCAL PRODUCTION AND ACTIONS OF PARATHYROID HORMONE-RELATED PROTEIN IN CARDIOVASCULAR TISSUES

A. Expression and Action of Parathyroid Hormone-Related Protein in Heart

As mentioned above, an appreciation for the physiological relevance for the actions of PTHrP on cardiovascular tissue has begun to emerge. Early immunohistochemistry studies on fetal tissues have localized PTHrP immunoreactivity to small blood vessels found in the lung.[115] Subsequent to these early studies, PTHrP immunoreactivity has been localized to blood vessels within tissues of both developmental and adult origin.[119,126] Soon after the cloning of the PTHrP cDNA, initial RNA blot studies failed to identify PTHrP mRNA in the heart.[54] However, subsequent application of sensitive reverse transcriptase-polymerase chain reaction (RT-PCR)[93] and RNase protection techniques[57] showed that low levels of PTHrP mRNA are present in this tissue. Using a current protocol for RNA blot hybridization (Figure 2), PTHrP mRNA is readily identified in total RNA prepared from both male and female rat atria and

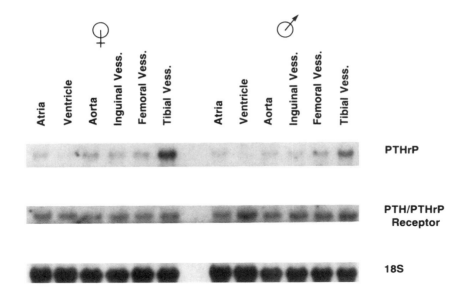

FIGURE 2 Coexpression of PTHrP and PTH/PTHrP receptor mRNA in the heart, aorta and peripheral blood vessels. Total RNA prepared from pools of either female or male atria (20 µg/lane), ventricle (20 µg/lane), aorta (10 µg/lane), inguinal mammary gland nutrient blood vessels (10 µg/lane), superficial femoral blood vessels (10 µg/lane), or tibial nutrient blood vessels (10 µg/lane) was sequentially hybridized to a radiolabeled rat PTHrP cDNA,[54] a rat PTH/PTHrP receptor cDNA,[91] and an 18S ribosomal RNA-specific DNA.[177] The 1.4-kb PTHrP mRNA, 2.5-kb rat PTH/PTHrP receptor mRNA, and 1.8-kb 18S RNA are shown.

ventricle. Based on total RNA, atria produce relatively more PTHrP message than ventricle; however, the functional significance of such findings is not known. In the human fetal heart, PTHrP was immunolocalized in both the cardiac muscle and smooth muscle of the coronary blood vessels.[130] While absent in valve tissue, immunoreactive PTHrP is present in the bundle of His and in isolated nerve cells. Expression of the 2.5-kb mRNA encoding the PTH/PTHrP receptor (Figure 2) in both atria and ventricle demonstrate the potential of this tissue to synthesize both PTHrP and its receptor, suggesting that chronotropic and inotropic actions of PTHrP may be mediated via an autocrine/paracrine mechanism.

Chronotropic and inotropic actions of PTHrP are similar to those demonstrated for PTH in isolated rat atrial preparations,[178,179] papillary muscle,[37,38] heart cells in culture,[39,180] ventricular strips,[181] and heart tissues from a number of lower vertebrates.[35,36] As shown in Figure 3, rat atria in muscle bath preparations were utilized to examine the effects of PTHrP-(1-34) on beating frequency and contractile force. Parathyroid hormone-related protein increased both

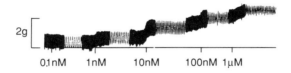

FIGURE 3 Positive inotropic and chronotropic effects of PTHrP in rat atria. Continuous atrial strips of both left and right rat atria were prepared from male Sprague-Dawley rats. Strips were equilibrated in Krebs bicarbonate buffer bubbled with 95% O_2/5% CO_2 for 1 h under 1-g resting tension. Contractions were detected using a strain gauge connected to a physiograph and strip chart recorder. As shown, chart speeds were increased and reduced to allow detection of beating frequency (chronotropic) as well as contractile (inotropic) activity. hPTHrP-(1-34) was added to the muscle bath chamber at the doses and times indicated.

the rate of contraction and the force of contraction in a dose-dependent manner. The EC_{50} was in the low nanomolar range, and the positive chronotropic effect occurred over the same PTHrP concentration range as the positive inotropic effect. In an isolated perfused rat heart preparation Nickols et al.[21] observed that PTHrP produced rapid and dose-related increases in heart rate and contractility. Interestingly, human PTHrP-(1-34) was significantly more potent and efficacious than rat PTH-(1-34) [rPTH-(1-34)] for stimulating heart rate in these studies. Also, rPTH-(1-34) produced a small increase in contractility compared to that induced by hPTHrP-(1-34). This increase may be attributed to an increased stability of PTHrP in this preparation, but may also indicate that the cardiac receptor mediating this chronotropic and inotropic activity has greater affinity for PTHrP as the local endogenous autocrine/paracrine ligand. Certainly others have reported variable results with PTH in enhancing cardiac function.[178] The effects of PTHrP on dromotropic activity (conduction velocity) have not been assessed as yet. However, based upon the evidence cited above indicating localization of PTHrP and receptor in cardiac nervous tissue, and the similarities of the cardiovascular effects of PTHrP and β-adrenergic agonists, one may postulate a positive dromotropic effect for PTHrP in the mammalian myocardium.

B. Expression and Action of Parathyroid Hormone-Related Protein in Large Blood Vessels

PTHrP likely functions locally in regulating the activity of the large conduit blood vessels, including the abdominal aorta (Figure 2) and inferior vena cava,[93] because PTHrP mRNA has been identified in total RNA prepared from these tissues. In the aorta, PTHrP immunoreactivity is localized to the tunica media and adventitial layers.[182] In support of a local function for PTHrP in the aorta, both PTHrP and PTH/PTHrP receptor mRNA are easily detected in total RNA prepared from this tissue (Figure 2). In addition to these RNA blot data, Orloff et al.[183] demonstrated the presence of specific binding sites for PTH and PTHrP on membranes derived from the renal artery. Relaxation of rat aorta,[21,255] rabbit aorta,[184] and rat renal vasculature[185,186] to PTHrP-(1-34) has been reported. As discussed in more detail below, the production of both PTHrP and its receptor in primary cultures of rat aorta smooth muscle cells further supports a local mode of action for PTHrP in aorta smooth muscle contractility.[143]

C. Expression and Action of Parathyroid Hormone-Related Protein in Peripheral Blood Supply

PTH or PTHrP-(1-34) administered systemically to laboratory animals are essentially equipotent in their ability to alter regional and systemic hemodynamics. In peripheral tissues, PTHrP increases blood flow by opening vascular beds via interactions with local membrane receptors.[41] To investigate whether PTHrP is produced in peripheral vascular tissues, pools of three individual vascular tissues that branch from the rat iliac artery and vein were used to produce total RNA for blot analysis.[95] Included in this analysis were RNAs prepared from (1) the inguinal mammary gland artery and vein, the main blood supply for the inguinal mammary gland, (2) the superficial femoral artery and vein, which runs subcutaneously along the exterior medial aspect of the thigh musculature, and (3) what we the authors refer to as the tibial blood vessels (a.k.a., popliteal), the major blood supply of the lower limb, which courses through the gluteal musculature and branches in several directions, including into the posterior of the proximal tibia via a series of foramen.

As seen in Figure 2, PTHrP mRNA is easily detected in samples of total RNA prepared from all peripheral vascular tissues branching from the iliac vessels. Relative to other peripheral vasculature, tibial vessel preparations are found to contain the greatest quantities of PTHrP mRNA. It is also worth noting that PTHrP mRNA is also abundant in the tibial nutrient blood vessels obtained from rabbits and *Cynomolgus macaques*.[187] Though the physiological

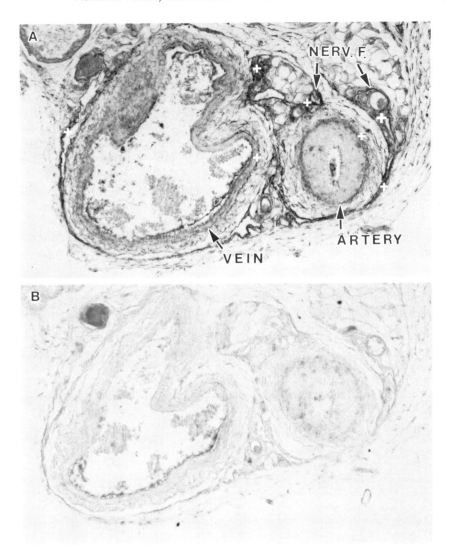

FIGURE 4   Immunolocalization of PTHrP in the nutrient vasculature of the rat inguinal mammary gland. Sequential cross-sections of paraffin-embedded samples of nutrient vasculature of the rat inguinal mammary gland were incubated with an (A) affinity-purified anti-PTHrP-(34-53) antibody or (B) the same antibody which had been preincubated with a 40 × (μg/μg) excess of PTHrP-(34-53). Following incubation with an anti-rabbit immunoglobulin G antibody conjugated to horseradish peroxidase, the slides were developed using diaminobenzadine. Specific PTHrP immunoreactivity is seen as brown staining, which is present on slide A, yet absent on slide B. Specific staining of PTHrP is seen in the artery and vein, with dense staining also localizing to the nerve fascicle (NERV. F.).

significance of these findings is unclear, one cannot help but consider a local role for PTHrP in regulating hemodynamics of the lower limb in light of the demonstrated action of PTH on blood flow to bone[188] and its actions in the perfused rat hind limb.[1] As seen in Figure 4, immunohistochemical analysis of a representative cross-section of the inguinal blood vessels show that PTHrP is localized to the outer layer of the tunica media of the inguinal artery as well as in the thin smooth muscle layer of the vein.[124] Dense PTHrP immunoreactivity of the thin fibrous membrane that encapsulates the major as well as some minor blood vessels of this tissue suggests that the protein may originate from local nervous tissue. A similar pattern of immunostaining of PTHrP is seen in cross-section analysis of superficial femoral and tibial blood vessels. The potential importance of the expression of PTHrP by a peripheral nervous tissue as well as the nutrient vasculature of the inguinal mammary gland during lactation is discussed below.

Parathyroid hormone-related protein has been shown to stimulate the placental transfer of calcium in sheep,[99-102,172] and because of its potential importance in eggshell calcification, the expression of PTHrP by the oviduct shell gland of the egg-laying hen was investigated. In those studies, the expression of PTHrP in the oviduct shell gland was found to be regulated during the egg-laying cycle,[126] and elevated levels of PTHrP in the shell gland were associated with shell gland activity. In the oviduct shell gland (uterus) of the egg-laying hen, PTHrP mRNA is enriched in the serosa (Figure 5), a thin outer membrane that is enriched in blood vessels and nerves. Furthermore, large blood vessels isolated from the shell gland serosa are highly enriched in PTHrP mRNA, indicating that these structures represent a major site of PTHrP synthesis in the oviduct shell gland. Immunohistochemical analysis of the shell gland demonstrated that PTHrP immunoreactivity is also highly enriched in the serosal membrane as well as in the tunica media and adventitia (Figure 5) of nutrient arterioles on the surface of the tissue.

As described above, a number of different blood vessels from a large variety of species respond to PTH with a dose-dependent reduction in contractile tone. The N-terminal fragment of chicken PTHrP apparently shares this quality. As seen in Figure 6, chicken PTHrP-(1-34)NH$_2$ relaxed chicken shell gland blood vessels in a concentration-dependent fashion. Specificity of the response was demonstrated by blockade of the relaxation to PTHrP by preincubation of the peptide with anti-PTHrP antiserum. These findings indicate that PTHrP is a local product of the peripheral vasculature of the chicken and support a role for PTHrP in eggshell calcification via the ability of PTHrP to increase shell gland blood flow, an important parameter of calcium transfer by the shell gland.[189,190]

In addition to aorta and shell gland vessels, dog coronary artery,[184] rat renal vasculature,[185] rabbit renal artery,[28] and rat tail artery[184] appear to respond to PTHrP. These responses generally are similar to those reported for PTH.[1,12,27,31,185,191,193] As shown in Figure 7, PTHrP-(1-34) relaxed ring preparations from rat superior mesenteric artery dose-dependently with an EC$_{50}$ of approximately 4 nM, similar to that seen for PTH in the isolated rat mesenteric vasculature preparation.[22] The EC$_{50}$ for vascular relaxation by PTH or PTHrP appears to be at least 1 log order lower in smaller blood vessels as compared to aortic preparations. The coronary vasculature of rats, dogs, and pigs is several logs more sensitive to PTH and PTHrP than corresponding large vessels.[18,19,21,193] As suggested earlier, regional differences in the density of PTH/PTHrP receptors and functional differences of the vessels in controlling blood pressure may contribute to these differences in sensitivity.

In the rat superior mesenteric artery rings, mid-region [PTHrP-(38-64) and PTHrP-(67-86)] and C-terminal [PTHrP-(107-138)] fragments of PTHrP were without effect, indicating that the amino terminal portion of the molecule mediates the vascular smooth muscle relaxation effect. In *in vitro* vascular relaxation experiments, the 3-34 and 7-34 analogues of PTH and PTHrP act as antagonists of the relaxation responses to PTHrP, albeit at 50- to 100-fold higher concentrations than agonist PTHrP.[194]

D. Production of Parathyroid Hormone-Related Protein in Peripheral Nervous Tissue

Additional evidence in support of the synthesis of PTHrP in peripheral nervous tissue comes from RNA blot hybridization and immunohistochemical studies of the sciatic nerve.[128] As seen in Figure 8A, PTHrP mRNA is easily detected in total RNA prepared from pools of rat sciatic nerve and also can be seen in RNA prepared from rabbit and primate sciatic nerve. Levels of

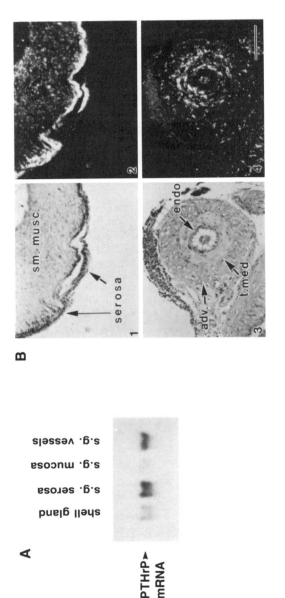

FIGURE 5   (A) Localization of PTHrP mRNA in the chicken oviduct shell gland. Total RNA (10 µg/lane) prepared from whole shell gland (s.g.), shell gland serosa, mucosa, and blood vessels (vessels) was hybridized to a radiolabeled chicken PTHrP cDNA.[58] The position of the 1.5-kb chicken PTHrP mRNA is shown with an arrow. (B) Immunohistochemical localization of PTHrP to the shell gland serosa and the tunica media of a shell gland arteriole. Bright field (1 and 3) micrographs of hematoxylin-stained tissue sections (×200) representing a cross-sectional sample of the shell gland (1) and an arteriole present within the serosa (3). Dark field micrographs (2 and 4) are of the corresponding section after sequential incubation with affinity-purified anti-PTHrP-(1-34) antibodies and anti-rabbit immunoglobulin G-conjugated to colloidal gold. Micrograph 2, abundant immunoreactive PTHrP, is localized to the thin serosa covering the shell gland. Some faint staining is also seen within cells of the underlying smooth muscle (sm. musc.) layer. Micrograph 4 is a dark field micrograph of this section incubated with the affinity-purified anti-PTHrP antibodies. Note the intense immunostaining of the tunica media (t. med.). PTHrP immunoreactivity is also localized to the adventitia (adv.) Bar = 100 µm. (From Thiede, M. A. et al., *Endocrinology*, 129, 1958, 1991, © The Endocrine Society. With permission.)

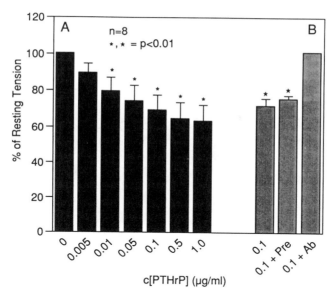

FIGURE 6   Relaxation of isolated shell gland blood vessels by synthetic chicken PTHrP-(1-34)NH$_2$. (A) Chicken PTHrP-(1-34)NH$_2$ induces concentration-dependent relaxation in isolated chicken shell gland vasculature. Large blood vessels were dissected from the serosa of occupied shell gland, placed in an isolated tissue bath, and a 1-g force was applied. After the tissue was equilibrated, increasing amounts of synthetic chicken PTHrP-(1-34)NH$_2$ were added to the bath, and the change in tension was recorded. (B) Antibody neutralization of chicken PTHrP-(1-34)NH$_2$-induced relaxation on isolated shell gland vasculature. Aliquots of chicken PTHrP-(1-34)NH$_2$ were incubated alone (25 μg/ml) at 37°C for 30 min or in the presence of antiPTHrP antiserum (Ab) or preimmune serum (Pre). The mixtures were then added to the bath (1:250 dilution), and the effect on resting tension was measured. (From Thiede, M. A. et al., *Endocrinology*, 129, 1958, 1991, © The Endocrine Society. With permission.)

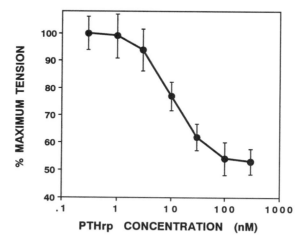

FIGURE 7   Dose-response relationship of PTHrP-induced relaxation of rat superior mesenteric artery. Ring segments (3-mm length) were prepared from male Sprague-Dawley rats and were allowed to equilibrate under 1-g tension in Krebs bicarbonate buffer in muscle bath chambers bubbled with 95% O/5% CO$_2$. Rings were rubbed to remove endothelium (confirmed by lack of relaxtion responses to acetylcholine). Tone was induced in the ring segments by the addition of 0.1 μM norepinephrine. Relaxation responses to the indicated doses of hPTHrP-(1-34) were recorded on a physiograph.

A.

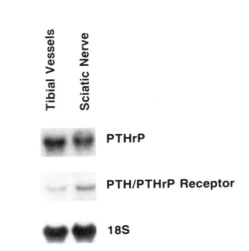

FIGURE 8   (A) Expression of PTHrP mRNA in the tibial nutrient blood vessels and sciatic nerve of the rat. Total RNA (10 μg/lane) prepared from pooled samples of rat tibial nutrient blood vessels or sciatic nerve was hybridized sequentially to a radiolabeled rPTHrP cDNA,[54] rat PTH/PTHrP receptor cDNA,[91] and an 18S ribosomal RNA cDNA.[177] Autoradiographic signals representing hybridization to the 1.4-kb PTHrP cDNA, 2.5-kb rat PTH/PTHrP mRNA, and 1.8-kb 18S RNA are shown. (B) Immunolocalization of PTHrP to rat sciatic nerve. Paraffin-embedded cross-sections of the rat sciatic nerve were incubated with affinity-purified anti-PTHrP-(34-53) antibodies alone (1) or following preincubation with a 40 × (mol/mol) excess of PTHrP-(34-53) (2). Following incubation with an anti-rabbit immunoglobulin G antibody conjugated to horseradish peroxidase, the sections were developed using diaminobenzidine. Specific PTHrP immunoreactivity is seen as brown staining, which is present on slide 1, yet absent on slide 2. Abundant PTHrP immunoreactivity is localized to the perineurium (Perin.) and local blood vessels (BV).

PTHrP mRNA in the sciatic nerve are quite abundant and comparable to those seen in an equal amount of total RNA from tibial vessel tissue. Immunohistochemical studies of PTHrP in sciatic nerve show dense staining of PTHrP in the perineurium and the smooth muscle layer of associated arterioles. PTHrP is likely to serve a local function in the sciatic nerve because mRNA for the PTH/PTHrP receptor (Figure 8A) is coexpressed in this tissue. Potential functions for PTHrP in the peripheral nerve may include the regulation of intracellular calcium for axonal transport of neurotransmitters, analgesia, and local vascular tone. The results of *in situ* hybridization analyses of both PTHrP and PTH/PTHrP receptor mRNA in the sciatic nerve and peripheral vascular tissues will be critical for elucidating the exact spatial organization of the cells which express genes for PTHrP and the PTH/PTHrP receptor in order to better understand the function(s) of PTHrP in this tissue.

Together these findings further emphasize the potential importance of the local production and action of PTHrP at all levels within the cardiovascular system. The ability of these tissues to regulate the activity of PTHrP may be in part dependent on the local synthesis of the PTH/PTHrP receptors.

IV. RECEPTORS AND SIGNALING PATHWAYS

A. Vascular Mechanism of Action

The mechanism of action of PTH or PTHrP on the cardiovascular system appears to resemble that of β-adrenergic agonists in many respects. Considering the actions of PTHrP on the vasculature, the vascular smooth muscle relaxation is a direct interaction with specific PTH/

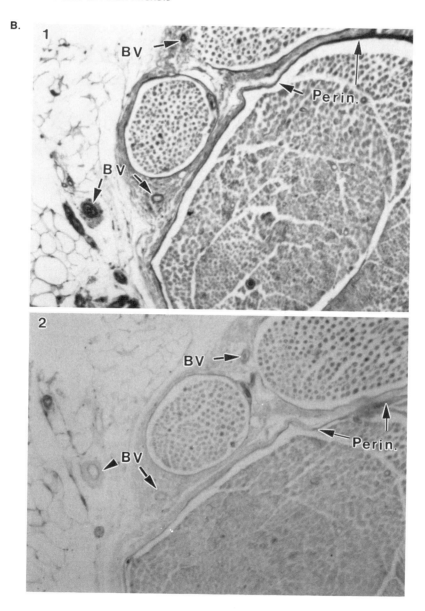

FIGURE 8 (continued)

PTHrP receptors.[41,183] As shown in Figure 9, radioligand binding studies indicate similar affinity of rabbit vascular smooth muscle for hPTHrP-(1-34) and rPTH-(1-34). The K_D for PTHrP was 1.8 nM and 0.4 nM for PTH. These values were very similar to those measured for PTHrP and PTH in renal tissue.[41] Computer analysis of binding parameters, including Hill coefficients of 1, predict one population of receptor sites. Orloff et al.[183] have performed elegant studies indicating that covalent labeling of bovine renal artery membranes with iodinated PTHrP yields a single receptor binding form of 85 kDa, which is similar to the size of the renal and bone PTH/PTHrP receptors.[79,87] Hongo et al.[143] have identified PTH/PTHrP receptors in rat aortic vascular smooth muscle cells using radioligand binding studies. Additionally, a 2.5-kb PTH/PTHrP receptor mRNA transcript was identified in smooth muscle

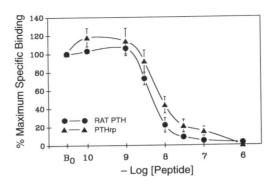

FIGURE 9   Competition for binding sites in rabbit renal microvessels. Competition curves for both rPTH-(1-34) and hPTHrP-(1-34) vs. ^{125}I-PTHrP-(1-34) binding to the vascular smooth muscle of rabbit renal microvessels are shown. The indicated doses of peptides were used to compete with the iodinated tracer. B_0 represents no added competitor. One hundred percent maximum specific binding = 2649 ± 371 cpm (PTHrP) and 2084 ± 234 cpm (PTH). Means ± SEMs are shown. (From Nickols, G.A. et al., *Endocrinology*, 126, 721, 1990, © The Endocrine Society. With permission.)

cells[143] using recently cloned rat cDNA from renal and bone tissue.[90,91] Ureña et al.[256] have recently described a wide tissue distribution of the PTH/PTHrP receptor mRNA in the rat using Northern blot analysis. They observed transcripts for the receptor in aorta, heart, spleen, and a large number of noncardiovascular tissues. Such a wide distribution suggests a physiological role for PTHrP and possibly PTH other than calcium homeostasis.

In the vascular cells PTH/PTHrP receptors are linked to cAMP production. To date, these studies suggest that PTHrP interacts with one receptor type in vascular tissue. In other target tissues radioligand binding studies indicate a two-site model for PTHrP binding.[43,195,196] Pharmacological and molecular biological studies of renal and bone PTH/PTHrP receptors indicate that receptors from these tissues are very similar, if not identical.[90,91,197] This is also likely to be the case in vascular smooth muscle as suggested by the studies of Hongo et al.[143] Perhaps differences in the density of PTH/PTHrP receptors from one target tissue to another or local factors impart varying affinities which may be interpreted as separate subtypes.

PTH and PTHrP activate adenylate cyclase and increase intracellular cAMP in the traditional target tissues (kidney and bone), and these peptides also appear to act similarly in the vasculature. A number of studies have shown that the interaction of PTH and PTHrP with specific receptors on vascular tissue stimulate adenylate cyclase and elicit cAMP responses.[11-14,25,30,185,198,255] The adenylate cyclase response to PTH has been found in the tunica media of rabbit aorta, associated with the vascular smooth muscle layer.[22] Additionally, cultured aortic vascular smooth muscle cells generate cAMP after PTH treatment.[12] Relaxation responses to PTH are potentiated in the presence of forskolin and cyclic nucleotide phosphodiesterase inhibitors.[12,13,22] Crass and Scarpace[255] recently presented evidence that PTHrP-(1-34) increases cAMP in the smooth muscle cells from rat aorta over the same dosage range as the peptide relaxed the perfused rat aorta. In contrast, PTH and PTHrP do not appear to alter cyclic guanosine monophosphate (cGMP) levels in vascular tissue.[13]

On the other hand, there have been reports of no detectable adenylate cyclase response or cAMP response to PTH or PTHrP from vascular tissue that relaxed to the peptides.[28,199] These may represent unique systems or vessels or possibly down regulation of target tissue responses to PTHrP. However, Martin et al.[200] presented evidence that in systems in which there was no measurable cAMP response to PTH or PTHrP analogues, protein kinase A (PKA) activity was found to be elevated and could account for cyclic nucleotide-mediated agonist activity. In fact, their data indicated that some amino truncated analogues of PTHrP thought to be antagonists

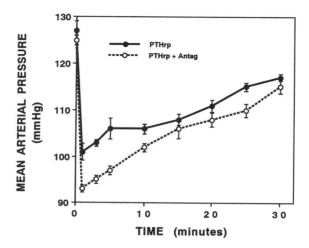

FIGURE 10   Hypotensive response of conscious, unrestrained rat to PTHrP. Male Sprague-Dawley rats were anesthetized, the carotid arteries were cannulated for measurement of systemic blood pressure, and the jugular veins were cannulated for administration of compounds. Catheters were burrowed subcutaneously and exited at the back of the neck. The animals were allowed to awaken and equilibrate for 2 h prior to the start of the experiment. hPTHrP-(1-34) (3 μg/kg) was administered as a bolus dose with (open circles) or without (closed circles) 150 μg/kg of the putative PTH/PTHrP receptor antagonist, [D-Trp^{12},Tyr^{34}]-bPTH-(7-34)NH$_2$. The antagonist was administered by I.V. bolus 2 min prior to administration of the agonist, PTHrP. Blood pressure was monitored using pressure transducers and a physiograph.

in vitro actually increased PKA activity. This could explain the often-reported agonist activity of some of these compounds in *in vivo* systems (see Figure 10). Activation of PKA is a necessary intermediary in the mechanism of action of PTHrP in different systems. For example, PKA activity appears to mediate the regulation of collagen synthesis[201] as well as the inhibition of cell proliferation and homologous desensitization in UMR-106 cells.[202] Thus, even if no increase in adenylate cyclase activity or intracellular cAMP levels is detected in a tissue known to respond to PTHrP physiologically, the examination of PKA activity in the presence and absence of PTHrP would be justified. While renal and bone PTH/PTHrP receptors are linked to both the adenylate cyclase and phospholipase C pathways for cellular signaling,[203-206] as yet there are no reports of PTH or PTHrP induced direct alterations in protein kinase C (PKC) activity or increases in inositol phosphates in smooth muscle systems.

While vasorelaxation associated with cyclic nucleotides is linked to a reduction in smooth muscle cell cytosolic calcium concentrations and ionic membrane fluxes,[207,208] in renal and osteoblastic cells PTH and PTHrP produced increases in cytosolic calcium as measured by fluorescent dyes.[82,83,209] However, in single smooth muscle cells from rat tail artery, bPTH-(1-34) relaxed KCl contractions.[210] The effect of PTH was antagonized by nifedipine, indicating that PTH exerted its cellular relaxant action via a calcium channel-related mechanism. Pang and co-workers[211,212] have demonstrated using patch clamp studies that bPTH-(1-34) decreased L-type voltage-dependent calcium channel currents in vascular smooth muscle cells. This effect of PTH was antagonized by the L-channel agonist, Bay K-8644, and mimicked by dibutyryl cAMP (dbcAMP). Moreover, the cAMP antagonist, Rp-cAMP, abolished the effect of PTH on L-channels. In other studies, Schleiffer et al.[192] observed a reduction in lanthanum-resistant ^{45}Ca influx and an increase in efflux in rat aortic tissue. Thus, in vascular smooth muscle the PTH/PTHrP receptor appears to be linked to a cAMP-mediated blockade of L-type calcium channels, yielding a reduction in intracellular calcium channels and relaxation.

B. Nitric Oxide and Prostaglandins

While the studies discussed above point to a direct effect of PTHrP and PTH on the vascular smooth muscle cell, it is possible that the interaction of PTHrP with its receptor may also liberate nitric oxide or vasodilatory prostaglandins such as prostacyclin to produce vasodilation and hypotension. However, removal of the intimal endothelial cell layer (the primary source of constitutive nitric oxide) from vascular tissue does not affect the ability of the tissue to relax to PTH or PTHrP.[21,22,27,31,213] In aortas in which the endothelium was damaged or removed by saponin treatment relaxation to PTH was not different from control, untreated aortas.[31] Additionally, rats treated *in vivo* with the constitutive nitric oxide synthase inhibitor, N^G-methyl-L-arginine, still produce dose-related hypotensive responses to PTHrP identical to control, untreated animals.[184]

Prostaglandins do not appear to mediate smooth muscle relaxation to PTH because indomethacin treatment of rat aortas[31] or rabbit aortic strips[213] does not alter relaxation responses to PTH. Therefore, the vasoactive effects of PTHrP and PTH are probably direct in nature, as suggested by receptor localization studies, and not linked to nitric oxide release or prostaglandin formation.

C. Myocardial Cell Interactions

As discussed in the chapter by Karpinski, PTH/PTHrP receptors in cardiac tissue are linked to calcium channels. Unlike the vascular smooth muscle cell in which PTH decreased the peak amplitude of the L-type calcium channel by up to 40%,[212] in cardiac cells PTH has an entirely opposite effect. Pang's group[211] showed that bPTH-(1-34) increased L-channel current in neonatal rat ventricular myocytes. This action was additive to that of dbcAMP[211] and was similar to that of Bay K-8644.[210] Nifedipine inhibited PTH effects on L-channels.[214,215] Rampe et al.[215] observed that PTH increased Ca^{2+} influx probably by increasing the probability of channel opening. They further demonstrated that PTH increased cAMP levels in rat ventricular myocytes,[215] an observation similar to that of Bogin et al.[39] We are not aware of reports of PTHrP stimulation of cAMP in heart tissue.

Taken together, these results are consistent with the currently held hypothesis that positive chronotropic and inotropic activity may be produced by increased cAMP activity in cardiac cells.[216] Elevated cAMP produces an increase in the influx of extracellular calcium, an increase in sarcoplasmic reticulum uptake of calcium, and an altered sensitivity of the contractile proteins to calcium. Such changes in calcium metabolism cause an increase in cardiac contractility and an increase in the rate of contraction and relaxation.[216] Thus, by enhancing calcium entry into the myocardial cell, PTHrP and PTH may stimulate cardiac function *in vivo* in a manner analogous to that of the β-adrenergic agonists.[40]

V. ACTIONS OF PARATHYROID HORMONE-RELATED PROTEIN *IN VIVO*

A. Hemodynamic Actions of Parathyroid Hormone-Related Protein

Parathyroid hormone-related protein produces marked, dose-dependent alterations in cardiovascular hemodynamics. As shown in Figure 10, PTHrP-(1-34) caused a rapid fall in mean arterial blood pressure, which was sustained for 30 min or more, depending upon the dose of PTHrP. The hypotensive effect of PTHrP has been demonstrated in several species, including rat, dog, and rabbit.[21,28,183,217-219] Administration of PTHrP-(1-34) to the conscious, unrestrained rat caused a reduction in total peripheral resistance and blood pressure concurrent with an increase in heart rate and cardiac output, all in a concentration-dependent manner.[218]

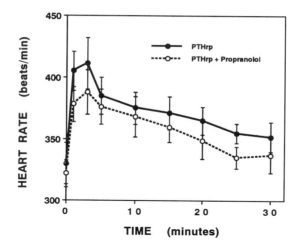

FIGURE 11 *In vivo* positive chronotropic response to PTHrP. Heart rate responses were monitored in conscious, unrestrained male rats. The animals were prepared as described in the legend to Figure 10 and hPTHrP-(1-34) (3 µg/kg) was administered as a bolus injection (closed circles). Propranolol (2 mg/kg) was administered with PTHrP (open circles) or isoproterenol (data not shown) as a positive control. Heart rate was detected from the blood pressure signal via a Gould tachygraph.

Like PTH,[33] PTHrP caused a greater fall in diastolic pressure than systolic blood pressure, indicating that the hypotension produced by PTHrP was likely a result of regional vasodilation. Indeed, radioactive microsphere studies have indicated that a number of vascular beds respond to PTHrP with a reduction in organ vascular resistance and an increase in blood flow through that organ system.[218,219] Hind limb muscle, forelimb muscle, sections of the gastrointestinal tract, brain, kidney, skin, and both the atria and ventricles of the heart respond with dose-related decreases in organ resistance.

In addition to increasing blood flow in the atria and ventricles of the heart, PTHrP also elevates heart rate and cardiac output.[218] The protein appears to produce direct inotropic and chronotropic actions on the heart and as shown in Figure 11, propranolol does not block the increase in beating frequency produced by PTHrP in the intact rat. Identical observations have been made with the PTH-(1-34) fragment.[1,18,33] Similar to its effect on blood pressure, stimulation of heart rate by PTHrP is dose-related and substantial; PTH and PTHrP can produce increases in heart rate of up to 150 beats per minute (bpm) in the rat. Parathyroid hormone-related protein also caused a dose-related increase in contractile force of up to 40%, as measured by the increase in dP/dt in the rat *in vivo*. Furthermore, cardiac output was enhanced by 30 ml/min in the intact rat by PTHrP.[218] β-adrenergic antagonists have no effect on PTHrP-induced hypotension and only slightly reduce the positive chronotropic responses to PTHrP (Figure 11), indicating that baroreceptor-mediated reflex mechanisms cannot account for the tachycardia following PTHrP treatment. Thus, PTHrP appears to have direct actions on the cardiac muscle to promote increased heart rate, similar to the actions observed *in vitro*.

The effects of PTHrP on blood vessels and the heart appear to be mediated by interaction with PTH/PTHrP receptors on the vascular smooth muscle and myocardial cells, as described above. However, the putative specific receptor antagonist [D-Trp^{12},Tyr^{34}]-bPTH-(7-34)NH$_2$ was found to have weak agonist activity in the cardiovascular system of the intact rat, potentiating the hypotensive actions of PTHrP-(1-34) (Figure 10). This agonist activity of 3-34 and 7-34 fragments of PTH and PTHrP is not peculiar to cardiovascular tissues because similar data have been obtained in other PTH- and PTHrP-responsive systems.[196,220]

TABLE 1   Cardiovascular profile and bone mineral density of Leydig tumor-bearing rats

	Day 0	Control Day 20	Leydig Day 20	Leydig + CT Day 20
MAP (mmHg)	122 ± 6	130 ± 6	96 ± 8	94 ± 7
HR (bpm)	357 ± 20	372 ± 24	462 ± 28	447 ± 23
Spine BMD (mg/cm^2)	153 ± 3.2	157 ± 2.4	140 ± 1.1	154 ± 1.3
Femur BMD (mg/cm^2)	136 ± 1.2	145 ± 3.1	129 ± 1.2	137 ± 1.6
Serum Ca (mg/dl)	10.2 ± 0.6	10.4 ± 0.7	18.7 ± 2.1	10.9 ± 0.8

Note: Male Fischer 344 rats were implanted with Leydig tumor cells on day 0 as described.[223,224] On day 20, mean arterial pressure (MAP) in millimeters of mercury and heart rate (HR) in beats per minute were monitored as described.[217,218] Serum calcium was measured by atomic absorption spectrometry. Bone mineral density (BMD) was measured by a Hologic QDR 1000 dual energy X-ray absorptiometer. Calcitonin (CT) was administered using an Alzet osmotic minipump delivering a dose of 26 U/kg/d of synthetic salmon calcitonin. Control rats were sham operated and received no tumor implantation.

B. Humoral Hypercalcemia of Malignancy

While we know of no reports of the effects of acute PTHrP administration on the cardiovascular system in humans, HHM may yield insights into the effects of PTHrP in humans. The HHM syndrome is characterized by high circulating PTHrP concentrations released by squamous cell tumors.[221,222] Mundy[221] has reported two patients diagnosed with HHM with striking features in their cardiovascular profiles. One patient had a serum calcium of 16 mg% and a blood pressure of 80/40. Another patient displayed a serum calcium of 15 mg/dl with resting blood pressure of 90/60 and heart rate of 120 bpm. While controlled studies of the actions of PTHrP on the cardiovascular system of humans are necessary, it appears that based on the limited data in HHM patients PTHrP may have vasodilatory and cardiac stimulatory actions in humans similar to those observed in other species.

C. Leydig Tumor-Bearing Rats

The Fischer 344 rat bearing a transplantable Leydig cell tumor has been shown to be a model of humoral hypercalcemia of malignancy.[223,224] These animals display increases in both circulating PTHrP and serum calcium levels within 10 d after tumor implantation and, as shown in Table 1, these rats are severely hypercalcemic 20 d after tumor implantation (serum calcium of 18.7 vs. normocalcemic controls). Upon examination of the bone mineral content and density of the spines and femurs of these animals by dual energy X-ray absorptiometry, the tumor-bearing rats displayed substantial bone losses as compared to the control group (day 20). Tumor-bearing rats displayed a greater net loss in bone mineral density in the L2-L6 spinal vertebrae as compared to the femur due to the greater proportion of trabecular to cortical bone in the vertebral segments. Interestingly, these animals also displayed hypotension and tachycardia, alterations in cardiovascular indices that may reflect the high circulating PTHrP levels produced by the Leydig tumor.

When bone resorption was inhibited in tumor-bearing rats by continuous administration with calcitonin (26 U/kg/d via osmotic minipump), hypercalcemia was prevented (Table 1). Additionally, the loss of bone mineral density associated with this HHM model was greatly reduced or blocked in both the spinal and femoral regions. However, mean arterial blood pressure was still reduced and heart rate was elevated in the Leydig cell tumor rats, even in the presence of calcitonin. Thus, while calcitonin served as a physiological antagonist of bone resorption induced by PTHrP, calcitonin had no detectable effect on the cardiovascular actions of PTHrP.

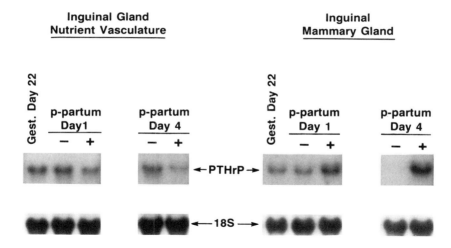

FIGURE 12 Reciprocal relationship of the expression of PTHrP mRNA in the mammary gland and its nutrient vasculature during lactation. Pairs of inguinal mammary gland nutrient vasculature and pieces of inguinal mammary gland were pooled from either pregnant or postpartum (p-partum) rats. Tissue samples were taken from dams on gestation (Gest.) day 22, just following parturition (day 1) without (–) or with (+) suckling for 3 h and postpartum day 4 after litters were removed for 8 h (–) or were removed for 4 h then replaced for 4 h (+). Total RNA from inguinal mammary gland nutrient vasculature (10 μg/lane) and inguinal mammary gland (20 μg/lane) were sequentially hybridized to a rPTHrP cDNA[54] and then an 18S ribosomal RNA-specific DNA[177] in order to monitor loading of RNA.

VI. REGULATED EXPRESSION OF PARATHYROID HORMONE-RELATED PROTEIN IN VASCULAR TISSUES AND CELLS

A. Altered Expression in the Rat Mammary Gland Nutrient Blood Vessels

As discussed above, the ability of PTHrP to modulate regional blood flow may result from the local production and action of PTHrP. Theoretically, if PTHrP is to play a role in regulating local blood flow, it would be necessary to increase local production of PTHrP, the responsiveness (i.e., receptor number) of the peripheral vascular beds to the protein, or both. At the same time, the nutrient vasculature would need to experience an increase in pressure in order to attain a net increase in blood flow. To support a local role for PTHrP in this process, one would predict that increased tissue blood flow would be correlated with an increase in the expression/action of PTHrP in the tissue and a concomitant decrease in PTHrP expression/action in the nutrient vasculature. An excellent model system with which to examine this relationship is the rat inguinal mammary gland and its nutrient vasculature during pregnancy and lactation.

Lactation is associated with increases in both cardiac output[225] and increased blood flow[226-228] to the mammary glands and other organs. During pregnancy in the rat, elevations in PTHrP mRNA levels in the mammary gland appear just prior to parturition (Figure 12). Following parturition, mammary gland expression of PTHrP mRNA is tightly linked to lactation[54] in response to suckling-induced elevations in serum prolactin.[150] Large quantities of PTHrP are secreted into the milk, suggesting a potential yet undetermined function for the protein in neonatal development. To date, experimental evidence in support of an endocrine function for PTHrP during lactation has been mixed. Early immunological-based analyses of PTHrP in plasma failed to detect suckling-associated elevations in lactating women and animals.[229,230] In support of an endocrine function for PTHrP during lactation, a 1992 study indicates that circulating levels of PTHrP are elevated during lactation.[147] Such elevations may be responsible for the suckling-associated phosphaturia in lactating rats.[146] If PTHrP synthesized by the lactating breasts is released into the circulation, it may also act on the heart to increase cardiac output.[225] Although not yet reported, it is also quite plausible that increased expression of PTHrP by the heart could possibly alter cardiac function during lactation.

On the other hand, the main biological target of PTHrP produced by the breasts may be the mammary gland itself. Immunohistochemical and *in situ* hybridization analyses of breast tissue[142] indicate that PTHrP is synthesized by epithelial cells throughout the gland. To support a role for PTHrP in epithelial cell function and perhaps milk production, Barlet[231] has found PTHrP to stimulate calcium secretion by the mammary gland of the goat. Parathyroid hormone-related protein may also modulate myoepithelial cell tone and milk ejection because immunoreactive PTHrP has been localized to myoepithelial cells in human breast[232] and can antagonize the actions of oxytocin on cultures of myoepithelial cells.[233]

As discussed above, PTHrP is produced in the nutrient vasculature of the inguinal mammary gland (Figure 2) and thus may regulate the activity of this tissue. The nutrient blood vessels of the inguinal mammary gland are amenable to studies of gene regulation because: (1) they produced PTHrP mRNA (Figure 2) and immunoreactive PTHrP (Figure 5), (2) their size (~2 cm in length) makes them easy to isolate, (3) they represent the major blood supply of the tissue, and (4) only four pairs of vessels are needed to produce adequate amounts of RNA for blot hybridization studies. Preparation of RNA from mammary glands from the same animals allows for the direct comparison of the effects of lactation on the expression of PTHrP mRNA in the inguinal gland and its blood supply. As shown in Figure 12, PTHrP mRNA is produced in both the inguinal gland and nutrient vasculature just prior to parturition (gestation day 22). If the pups are removed as they are born, and the dam not suckled for 3 h, PTHrP mRNA levels in the breast and vasculature remain unchanged relative to samples obtained just prior to parturition. However, if dams are suckled *ad libitum* in the first 3 h post partum, PTHrP mRNA levels in the breast increase while those in the nutrient vasculature decline. This reciprocal relationship in the expression of PTHrP mRNA by the mammary gland and its nutrient vasculature is consistently seen in the first week of the postpartum period (Figure 12).

In view of the action of PTHrP on regional blood flow and its synthesis in response to biomechanical stretch,[131,132,164] these data can be interpreted in the following manner: parturition without suckling (day −1) does not alter the expression of PTHrP in the naïve gland and its nutrient vasculature. On the other hand, the initiation of suckling results in a rapid increase in levels of PTHrP expressed by the mammary gland. By virtue of its vasodilatory action, this would lead to a decreased vascular resistance within the breast. The concomitant decrease in PTHrP expression that is seen in the nutrient vasculature may arise from lowered stress on the walls of the nutrient blood vessels resulting from decreased vascular resistance within the breast. Alternatively, glucocorticoids which are released during suckling may directly decrease the expression of PTHrP by the nutrient vasculature because these steroids have been shown to suppress the transcription of the PTHrP gene in cultured cells,[152-154] including rat aorta smooth muscle cells.[143] A decrease in local production of PTHrP would theoretically increase vascular resistance, and in concert with the increase in PTHrP within the breast would result in the enhancement of blood flow to the mammary gland.

An inverse relationship in the expression of PTHrP in these tissues is also seen following the removal of the suckling stimulus. However, this treatment, which rapidly reduces blood flow to the tissue,[226,227] causes a rapid reduction in the levels of PTHrP mRNA in the mammary gland and a time-dependent increase in PTHrP mRNA in the nutrient vasculature (Figure 12). Thus, this model predicts that increased vascular resistance within the breast can potentially increase fluid load in the nutrient vasculature, resulting in the accumulation of PTHrP mRNA in this tissue. In support of this view, PTHrP mRNA levels within the nutrient vasculature of the inguinal mammary gland indeed increase in the absence of suckling.[234] An additional explanation for this finding is that local or systemically derived vasoconstrictor substances

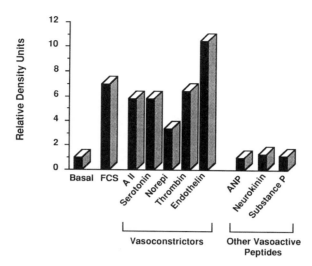

FIGURE 13 Vasoactive substances alter the accumulation of PTHrP mRNA in cultures of aorta smooth muscle cells. The expression of PTHrP mRNA by smooth muscle cells is increased by the addition of 2% fetal calf serum (FCS). Several vasoconstrictor substances, including angiotensin II (A II), serotonin, norepinephrine (Norepi), thrombin, and endothelin, increase the level of PTHrP mRNA in smooth muscle cells. Other vasoactive substances, including atrial natriuretic peptide (ANP), α-neurokinin, and substance P, failed to increase PTHrP mRNA. All measurements were made on cultures taken 4 h after addition of serum or vasoactive agent. Relative density units represent a semiquantitative comparison of the autoradiographic signals (i.e., specific hybridization to PTHrP mRNA) from blot analyses of total RNA from treated vs. control (Basal) cultures.

such as endothelin, which have been shown to increase PTHrP expression in cultures of rat aorta smooth muscle cells[143] (Figure 13), may act to increase PTHrP expression in the nutrient vasculature of the unsuckled breast.

The lactating mammary gland is an excellent tissue model with which to study the expression and actions of PTHrP on peripheral vascular tissues. In the breast, PTHrP may represent a tightly regulated multifunctional substance that in part may modulate blood flow to the gland. Barlet and colleagues,[235] using an ultrasonic flow probe, recently found the infusion of PTHrP-(1-34) into the mammary artery of the sheep to stimulate a rapid, dose-dependent increase in mammary blood flow. The reciprocal regulation of PTHrP expression in the nutrient vasculature of the breast suggests the possible dual action of PTHrP in modulating hemodynamics of the lactating mammary gland.

B. Expression of Parathyroid Hormone-Related Protein by Cultured Aorta Smooth Muscle Cells

It is now clear that PTHrP is widely distributed in cardiovascular tissues and immunoreactive PTHrP is localized in part to the media of isolated vascular tissues. To further support the view that PTHrP is produced by vascular smooth muscle cells, recent studies have examined the expression of PTHrP in primary cultures of rat aorta smooth muscle cells. Hongo et al.[143] were the first to demonstrate that serum stimulates a rapid, yet transient increase in the accumulation of PTHrP mRNA by smooth muscle cells. This transitory regulation of PTHrP mRNA, a common feature of the expression of PTHrP mRNA both *in vitro*[144,145,157,158] and *in vivo*,[54,128,131,134,146,150,155] results from a combination of transcriptional and posttranscriptional controls.[162] A concomitant increase in secretion of PTHrP by smooth muscle cells in response to serum suggests that a serum component(s) regulates the synthesis and release of PTHrP by smooth muscle cells. Smooth muscle cells also harbor receptors for PTHrP as assessed by their ability to bind ^{125}I PTHrP-(1-36)NH$_2$ and produce cAMP in response to exogenous PTHrP-(1-34) and PTHrP-(1-141).[143] Thus, smooth muscle cells are a very useful *in vitro* system with which to study both the expression and action of PTHrP in the vasculature.

Growth factors such as EGF and TGF-α stimulate the synthesis of PTHrP by tumor cells[157] as well as cultures of normal human epidermal keratinocytes (NHEK).[144,145] In their initial studies, Hongo et al.[143] demonstrated that insulin-like growth factor-1 and platelet-derived growth factor failed to increase PTHrP gene expression in smooth muscle cells, suggesting that these growth factors may not be involved in the action of serum on the expression of PTHrP by these cells. Whether other growth factors such as EGF or TGF-α, which stimulate PTHrP expression in other cells,[144,145,157] can stimulate PTHrP in smooth muscle cells has not been reported. Though several studies have shown that PTHrP can regulate the proliferative activity of cultured NHEK,[144,168] addition of PTHrP-(1-141) to smooth muscle cells in the absence or presence of serum did not alter the proliferation of these cells, suggesting that PTHrP may not regulate mitogenesis of vascular smooth muscle.

Glucocorticoids, which down regulate the expression of the PTHrP gene in other cell systems,[151-154] also block the serum-stimulated increase in PTHrP expression in smooth muscle cells. *In vivo* the decrease of PTHrP mRNA that is seen in the nutrient vasculature of the lactating inguinal mammary gland (Figure 12) may result from the direct repression of PTHrP gene transcription by steroids.[152-154] With less potency than glucocorticoids, 1,25-(OH)$_2$ vitamin D$_3$ partially inhibits the serum-stimulated increase in PTHrP mRNA. Such an observation may offer insight toward understanding the mechanisms underlying the effects of vitamin D on the contractile activity of vascular smooth muscle, a topic discussed in Chapter 7. Repression of PTHrP mRNA expression is likely mediated via the direct interaction of the ligand/ receptor complex with nucleotide recognition sites present within the 5′ regulatory sequences of the PTHrP gene.[154]

C. Regulation by Vasoactive Substances

In addition to the potential importance of growth factors and steroids in the expression of PTHrP by smooth muscle cells, a role for vasoactive substances in the expression of PTHrP in vascular smooth muscle cells is beginning to emerge (Figure 13). Studies to date have shown that vasodilators such as substance P, α-neurokinin, and atrial natriuretic peptide do not alter the levels of PTHrP mRNA in smooth muscle cells.[162] However, the expression of PTHrP mRNA in smooth muscle cells is sharply up-regulated by a number of known vasoconstrictors including endothelin, thrombin, norepinephrine, bradykinin, serotonin, and angiotensin II.[143,162] In recent work, Pirola et al.[162] demonstrated that angiotensin II stimulates a rapid and transient increase in the levels of PTHrP mRNA in smooth muscle cells. The effect of angiotensin II on PTHrP expression in smooth muscle cells is mediated in part by prostanoids and PKC through an increase in both the rate of PTHrP gene transcription and the half-life of the PTHrP mRNA. The addition of inhibitors of the renin-angiotensin systems (e.g., saralasin, captopril) to serum-treated smooth muscle cells reduced the normal serum-induced increase of PTHrP mRNA levels in smooth muscle cells, suggesting that angiotensin II plays a major role in the serum-associated up-regulation of PTHrP by smooth muscle cells. As mentioned above, addition of PTHrP does not alter the proliferation of smooth muscle cells however, when added with angiotensin II, PTHrP-(1-141) caused a decrease in [^{3}H]-thymidine incorporation relative to cultures treated with angiotensin alone. Thus, as in cultures of NHEK, PTHrP may influence smooth muscle cell proliferation under certain conditions.

Finally, angiotensin II may modulate the responsiveness of the cultures to PTHrP, because addition of the vasoconstrictor to smooth muscle cells decreases the levels of mRNA encoding the PTH/PTHrP receptor.[236] Whether this results from the direct action of angiotensin II on PTH/PTHrP receptor gene expression or on the potential of locally produced PTHrP to down-regulate the expression of its receptor needs to be determined. Understanding the mechanisms by which vasoconstrictors such as angiotensin II regulate the expression and action of PTHrP in cultured vascular smooth muscle cells will likely lead to important insights toward elucidating the biological regulation of vascular contractility *in vivo*.

VII. EXPRESSION AND ACTION OF PARATHYROID HORMONE-RELATED PROTEIN IN RESPONSE TO VOLUME LOAD

The cardiovascular system represents a series of elastic tissues that can expand or contract in response to changes in fluid load and increased blood volume resulting from normal physiology or pathology. One possible mechanism by which these tissues adapt to increases in blood volume is via the local production of substance(s) which will inhibit their contractile activity. In normal physiology — for example, during pregnancy — changes in blood volume are transient and thus the local production of such a substance would be short-lived. In pathology, such as volume-dependent hypertension or congestive heart failure, one would predict that the local production of this agent would exist as long as the stimulus was present. To contrast, loss of such a feedback loop may occur in the case of congestive heart failure and volume-dependent hypertension, with the chronic high blood volumes eventually leading to compensatory tissue hypertrophy.

Strong evidence exists to indicate that local synthesis of PTHrP in expandable tissues such as the rat uterus,[131,164] urinary bladder,[132] and stomach[237] is increased in response to the biomechanical stretch imposed by an increase in lumenal volume. Though direct evidence for stretch-related expression of PTHrP has been demonstrated in these three rat tissues, elevated levels of PTHrP are also found in the preterm human amnion[134] and chicken oviduct shell gland during the egg-laying cycle.[126] Stretching of the rat uterus during fetal growth is linked to local synthesis of high levels of PTHrP in the myometrium as demonstrated in natural and experimental unilateral pregnancy[131] (Figure 14), as well as in uteri which have been expanded by the insertion and inflation of a balloon catheter.[164] Parathyroid hormone-related protein produced by the uterus may function in the control of myometrial tone, as contractile activity of the uterus of estrogen-primed immature rats is inhibited by PTHrP-(1-34) *in vitro*[92,176] and *in vivo*.[175] Though the inhibitory action of PTHrP on smooth muscle contraction is dependent on the production of cAMP, Shew and Yee[238] showed that the inhibition of myometrial contraction by PTHrP may be dependent on the synthesis of nitric oxide, based upon the observation that PTHrP relaxation of the uterus *in vitro* is blocked by N^G-monomethyl arginine, a competitive inhibitor of nitric oxide synthase. In contrast to the estrogen-primed immature uterus, the pregnant rat uterus is refractory to this action of the peptide when the expression of PTHrP in the uterus is high. A plausible explanation for this lack of responsiveness to PTHrP on the part of the tissue is that specific PTHrP receptors are down-regulated in response to the high level of the protein. Parathyroid hormone-related protein desensitization has been observed in vascular,[217] renal,[217] and gastrointestinal tissue.[8,10]

The rat urinary bladder, a simple, expandable organ that repeatedly accumulates and dispenses urine, expresses PTHrP in response to filling in both a time- (Figure 14) and volume-dependent manner.[131] In tissue bath analysis, PTHrP-(1-34) inhibits the contractile activity of bladder smooth muscle; however, when the bladder expresses high levels of PTHrP, as seen after 4 h of filling, bladder smooth muscle becomes refractory to added peptide.[132] The molecular regulators of this response are unknown, but recent evidence supports a role for prostaglandins, which are released in response to tissue perturbation, in the upregulation of PTHrP expression in human cells.[161] The universal nature of the stretch responsiveness of the PTHrP gene is further supported in the results of studies which show that PTHrP mRNA accumulates in the rat stomach in both a time- and dose-dependent manner after acute filling of the stomach following duodenal ligature.[237] A role for PTHrP in gastric smooth muscle tone

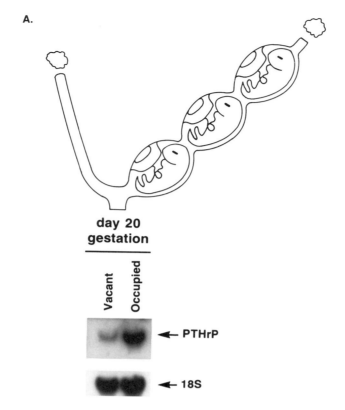

FIGURE 14   Stretch responsiveness of the PTHrP gene in expandable tissues. (A) High levels of PTHrP mRNA are associated with the gravid horn in the unilaterally pregnant rat uterus on gestation day 20. Total RNA (20 μg/lane) prepared from either the occupied or vacant horn was sequentially hybridized to a rPTHrP cDNA[54] and 18S ribosomal RNA-specific DNA.[177] (B) Time-dependent increase in PTHrP mRNA accumulation in the urinary bladder during filling. Urinary bladders were emptied (0 h) by removing urine by aspiration with a large-gauge needle and syringe and then allowed to fill for 2, 4, or 6 h. Total RNA (20 μg/lane) prepared from pools of bladders (*n* = 3) recovered at each time point was sequentially hybridized to a rPTHrP[54] and chicken β-actin cDNA.[54] The drawing above the autoradiographic panels depicts the relative increase in bladder size during this time course.

is supported by previous studies by Mok et al.,[8] in which they demonstrated the inhibitory action of PTHrP-(1-34) on the contractile activity of isolated gastric smooth muscle. Together these findings indicate that PTHrP is a locally synthesized smooth muscle relaxant produced in response to tissue stretch and that the levels of PTHrP produced by some tissues may in part dictate the contractile activity of the local smooth muscle. In this context, the local production and actions of PTHrP in heart and peripheral vasculature described above suggest that this calciotropic protein may function in the ability of the cardiovascular system to adapt to increases in fluid load. Collectively, one would then predict from these observations that the expression of PTHrP would be increased in the tissues of animal models of fluid excess such as in the DOCA-salt-induced hypertensive rat.

VIII. EXPRESSION AND ACTION OF PARATHYROID HORMONE-RELATED PROTEIN IN THE HYPERTENSIVE RAT

A long-recognized and as yet unexplained correlation exists between hyperparathyroidism and genetic hypertension (see Chapters 4 and 13). Parathyroid gland removal has been shown to

B. Time Of Bladder Filling (Hours)

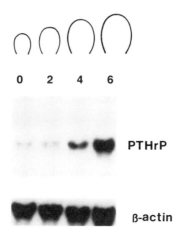

0   2   4   6

PTHrP

β-actin

FIGURE 14 (continued)

impair the development of hypertension in the spontaneously hypertensive rat (SHR)[239,240] and in the DOCA-salt hypertensive rat.[241,242] It appears that a factor of parathyroid gland origin other than PTH may be involved in the onset and development of hypertension in rats and humans (see Chapter 5). However, the acute administration of PTH-(1-34) or PTHrP-(1-34) to hypertensive rats still causes a fall in blood pressure due to systemic vasodilation.[217,239,243] Thus, exogenously added PTH or PTHrP are still potent in inducing cardiovascular changes in hypertensive animals. Both peptides reduced blood pressure and increased heart rate in conscious, unrestrained SHR and WKY rats in a concentration-dependent manner.[217] While the hypotensive response to both PTH and PTHrP was essentially identical when normalized for differences in resting blood pressure between the two groups, renal responses and cardiac responses were depressed in the hypertensive rats. Urinary cAMP, magnesium, calcium, and phosphorus responses to PTH were blunted in the SHR,[244] probably due to an apparent reduction in renal cortical PTH/PTHrP receptor density.[217] Insensitivity of the SHR renal excretory responses and heart rate responses to PTHrP suggest a state of tachyphylaxis to agonist produced by the high circulating PTH levels in the SHR.[217,245,246] The lack of tachyphylaxis of the hypotensive response to PTHrP in the SHR further underscores the potential for differences in the mechanism of action of PTHrP and in the PTH/PTHrP receptor population or coupling to second messengers in different tissues.

As proposed earlier, elevated systemic blood pressure may be expected to induce an increase in the expression of PTHrP locally in various cardiovascular tissues due to stretch of the muscle cells. Examination of PTHrP gene expression by Northern blot analysis indicates that this is indeed the case.[247] Compared to the levels of PTHrP mRNA in tissues from normotensive WKY rats, PTHrP mRNA was more abundant in heart and kidney from SHR. The enhanced expression in SHR appears to be tissue specific because no elevation in PTHrP expression was seen in brain tissue from the same animals. Essentially identical results were observed in the salt-sensitive Dahl hypertensive rat model. As shown in Figure 15, levels of PTHrP expression were slightly elevated in heart tissue from the salt-sensitive Dahl rat compared to hearts from the salt-resistant, normotensive rat. Interestingly, the expression of PTHrP mRNA in the heart of both the salt-sensitive and salt-resistant Dahl rats appeared

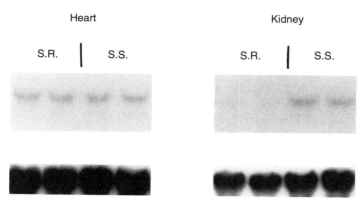

FIGURE 15   Increased expression of PTHrP in the salt-sensitive Dahl hypertensive rat. Salt-sensitive (SS) and salt-resistant (SR) Dahl rats were maintained on a high salt diet (Harlan Sprague-Dawley) *ad libitum* for 4 weeks. At that time, blood pressure measured by tail cuff plethysmography was 132 ± 2.2 mmHg in the SR rats and 213 ± 4.7 mmHg in the SS rats (*n* = 8). The animals were sacrificed and the indicated tissues were removed and immediately frozen for preparation of mRNA. Total RNA (20 μg/sample) prepared from heart and kidney was sequentially hybridized to a rPTHrP cDNA[54] and then to a chicken β-actin cDNA[126] in order to monitor the loading of RNA.

elevated compared to rats not supplemented with salt. In contrast, clear increases in PTHrP gene expression were detected in renal tissue from the salt-sensitive Dahl rats as compared to salt-resistant animals. Here again, brain tissue showed no elevations in PTHrP gene expression in either salt-sensitive or -resistant rats.

Mineralocorticoid-induced hypertension is clearly associated with marked increases in vascular fluid volume.[248] Thus, the DOCA-salt-treated rat model of hypertension was examined for alterations in PTHrP gene expression. As shown in Figure 16, atria, ventricle, and renal tissues showed distinct elevations of PTHrP mRNA expression by Northern blot analysis of at least threefold at 3 weeks as compared to pretreatment (week 0). As can be seen systemic blood pressure was also elevated at this time. Upon removal of the DOCA-salt treatment regimen, both blood pressure and PTHrP mRNA were reduced toward normal. Northern blots from the DOCA-salt rat tissues were also probed for atrial natriuretic polypeptide as a marker of fluid overload.[249] Atrial natriuretic peptide (ANP) mRNA, which was basally high in normotensive atria, did not appear increased as a result of DOCA-salt hypertension.[250] However, in ventricular tissue the expression of ANP mRNA increased in parallel with both the expression of PTHrP mRNA and the elevation in systemic blood pressure. It is possible that production of PTHrP and ANP by local or atrial sources in response to distension of vascular components due to fluid overload may produce compatible effects to relax the vasculature and enhance renal electrolyte excretion. Interestingly, PTH has been shown to modulate the release of ANP and to interact with ANP to regulate fluid homeostasis.[251] Thus, it is likely that PTHrP has similar properties, although this has not been demonstrated.

These data indicate that PTHrP gene expression appears to be increased in cardiovascular tissues from hypertensive rats, especially in models with a volume component. While this is consistent with the increase in local production of PTHrP in mammalian bladder and uterus upon stretch as discussed previously, up-regulation of PTHrP gene expression may also be under cytokine or neurotransmitter modulation. The SHR and Dahl hypertensive models both display a sympathetic neural contribution to the elevation in blood pressure marked by enhanced neuronal norepinephrine release.[252-254] Hongo et al.[143] have observed that vasoactive mediators such as norepinephrine and endothelin stimulate PTHrP expression in vascular smooth muscle cells. Therefore, increased levels of vasoconstrictor mediators and volume overload may both contribute to the increased PTHrP expression in hypertensive disease.

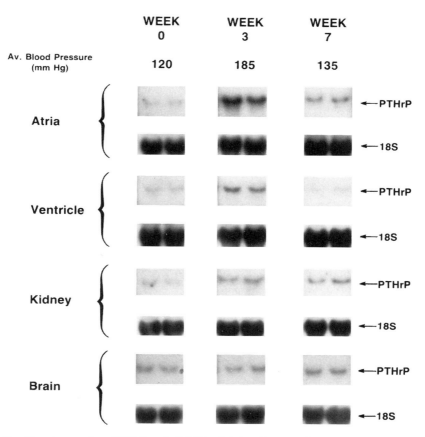

FIGURE 16 Altered expression of PTHrP in the DOCA-salt-induced hypertensive rat. Acute hypertension due to fluid overload was accomplished by the subcutaneous implantation of a time-released pellet (21-d duration) of deoxycorticosterone acetate and supplementation with 0.9% NaCl in the drinking water. Blood pressure was monitored by tail cuff and the mean blood pressure (mmHg) for each group of rats used to generate each sample is noted. Control rats (Week 0) were used to establish baseline expression of PTHrP mRNA in pools of atria ($n = 2$) as well as individual ventricle, kidney, and brain samples. Similar tissue samples were dissected from hypertensive rats (Week 3) and partially recovered rats (Week 7) for which the treatment was stopped after 3 weeks. Total RNA (20 μg/sample) was sequentially hybridized to a rPTHrP cDNA[54] and then to an 18S ribosomal RNA DNA[177] in order to monitor the loading of RNA.

PTHrP would act in a compensatory manner to reduce the elevated systemic blood pressure toward normal and obviate deleterious effects of chronic hypertension.

IX. CONCLUSIONS AND PERSPECTIVES

A major goal of this chapter was to integrate the experimental findings of two independent lines of investigation as a means of understanding a third: the biological role of the novel calciotropic protein, PTHrP, in cardiovascular function. In Chapter 2, Crass reviewed the extensive literature describing the potent actions of the calciotropic peptide endocrine hormone PTH on cardiovascular tissues. Here, we discussed the current understanding of the cardiovascular origins and actions of PTHrP, a protein that was identified as the hypercalcemic factor produced by tumors associated with the clinical syndrome of HHM by virtue of its functional similarities with PTH. In contrast to PTH, which is essentially a product of the adult parathyroid gland, PTHrP has a wide tissue distribution including sites throughout the cardiovascular system. Although PTHrP may potentially represent a calciotropic endocrine protein, coexpression of both PTHrP and PTH/PTHrP receptors in numerous tissues supports an autocrine/paracrine action for the protein. The complex regulation of PTHrP gene expression also argues against a classical endocrine feedback control of the PTHrP gene but instead favors a local means of regulating the synthesis and action of the protein. In support of a role for PTHrP in regulating cardiovascular function, recent studies have shown that synthetic N-terminal fragments of PTHrP and PTH are equipotent in modulating cardiovascular responsiveness. The demonstrated regulation of PTHrP expression by cardiovascular tissues and cultured vascular smooth muscle cells further emphasizes the potential importance of PTHrP in the local control of cardiovascular function. In view of its potent vasodilatory action, tumoral production of PTHrP may represent a selective advantage by which certain tumors increase local blood flow in the area of invasion.

In organizing this review, we hoped to present current developments that support the view that previously described actions of PTH on cardiovascular tissue most likely reflect the activities of locally produced PTHrP. Thus, while PTH may be the preferred agonist acting on bone and kidney to maintain serum calcium concentrations within narrow physiological limits, it appears that PTHrP may have little if any role in the normal regulation of serum calcium. On the other hand, locally produced PTHrP, interacting with local receptors, may have profound effects on local blood pressure and flow and on cardiac function. As pointed out by Nissenson and Strewler,[196] at normal circulating PTH levels (low picomolar range), $\leq 0.1\%$ of target cell PTH/PTHrP receptors ($K_D \approx 1$ nM) would be occupied. They suggest that this level of occupancy may be sufficient to regulate renal and skeletal responses because of the high density of receptors in these target tissues. However, in cardiovascular tissues with lower receptor densities, local production of PTHrP would produce biologically relevant effects. As we have described, the regulation of PTHrP gene expression, peptide production, and receptor density in pathology (volume-dependent hypertension) and during normal physiology (e.g., lactation, pregnancy) provide a system that is responsive to the local environment and in turn affects that environment.

We feel that the local production of PTHrP and its interaction with local PTH/PTHrP receptors in the heart, blood vessels, and other smooth muscles in general provide a unique mechanism of considerable efficacy which can modulate systemic and regional hemodynamics. In normal physiology (bladder filling, uterine distension in pregnancy) and in pathology (congestive heart failure, volume-dependent hypertension), PTHrP provides a mechanism whereby compensation for temporary or abnormal volume loads may be achieved. As we learn more of the basic science of the PTHrP system in the vasculature and heart, we will gain a greater appreciation of its role in cardiovascular function. Accordingly, a better understanding of the regulation of the expression of both PTHrP and PTH/PTHrP receptors in tissues of the cardiovascular system should also provide greater insights into the role of this protein in the control of local and systemic blood flow and cardiac function.

ACKNOWLEDGMENTS

We wish to thank J. A. Fagin and T. L. Clemens for their generous contribution of original data to this work, to J.-P. Barlet for sharing unpublished results, and to William A. Grasser and Donna Petersen for their help in preparing some of the original data presented in this chapter. We also wish to extend heartfelt thanks to Melissa and Maureen for their untiring support during the preparation of this review and to Ellen Christine for her incredible sense of good timing.

Portions of this work were supported by American Heart Association Grant-In-Aid #900885 to G. A. N.

REFERENCES

1. Pang, P. K. T., Tenner, T. E., Jr., Yee, J. A., Yang, M., and Janssen, H. F., Hypotensive action of parathyroid hormone preparations on rats and dogs, *Proc. Natl. Acad. Sci. U.S.A.*, 77, 675, 1980.
2. Sham, J. S. K., Chiu, K. W., and Pang, P. K. T., Hypotensive actions of snake parathyroid glands, *Gen. Comp. Endocrinol.*, 52, 365, 1983.
3. Pang, P. K. T., Yang, M. C. M., Oguro, C., Phillips, J. G., and Yee, J. A., Hypotensive actions of parathyroid hormone preparations in vertebrates, *Gen. Comp. Endocrinol.*, 41, 135, 1980.
4. Pang, P. K. T., Zhang, R. H., and Yang, M. C. M., Hypotensive action of parathyroid hormone in chicken, *J. Exp. Zool.*, 232, 691, 1984.
5. Shew, R. L. and Pang, P. K. T., Effects of bPTH fragments (1-34), (3-34) and (7-34) on uterine contraction, *Peptides*, 5, 485, 1984.
6. Shew, R. L., Kenny, A. D., and Pang, P. K. T., Uterine relaxing action of parathyroid hormone: effect of oxidation and methionine substitution (41818), *Proc. Soc. Exp. Biol. Med.*, 175, 444, 1984.
7. Yen, Y. C., Yang, M. C. M., Kenny, A. D., and Pang, P. K. T., Parathyroid hormone (PTH) fragments relax the guinea-pig trachea in vitro, *Can. J. Physiol. Pharmacol.*, 61, 1324, 1983.
8. Mok, L. L. S., Cooper, C. W., and Thompson, J. C., Parathyroid hormone and parathyroid hormone-related protein inhibit phasic contraction of pig duodenal smooth muscle, *Proc. Soc. Exp. Biol. Med.*, 191, 337, 1989.
9. Mok, L. L. S., Nickols, G. A., Thompson, J. C., and Cooper, C. W., Parathyroid hormone as a smooth muscle relaxant, *Endocr. Rev.*, 10, 420, 1989.
10. Cooper, C. W., Seitz, P. K., McPherson, M. B., Selvanayagam, P., and Rajaraman, S., Effects of parathyroid hormonal peptides on the gut, *Contrib. Nephrol.*, 91, 26, 1991.
11. Pang, P. K. T., Yang, M. C. M., Tenner, T.E., Jr.,Kenny, A. D., and Cooper, C. W., Cyclic AMP and the vascular action of parathyroid hormone, *Can. J. Physiol. Pharmacol.*, 64, 1543, 1986.
12. Nickols, G. A., Increased cyclic AMP in cultured vascular smooth muscle cells and relaxation of aortic strips by parathyroid hormone, *Eur. J. Pharmacol.*, 116, 137, 1985.
13. Nickols, G. A. and Cline, W. H., Jr., Parathyroid hormone-induced changes in cyclic nucleotide levels during relaxation of the rat aorta, *Life Sci.*, 40, 2351, 1987.
14. Huang, M. and Rorstad, O. P., Cerebral vascular adenylate cyclase: evidence for coupling to receptors for vasoactive intestinal peptide and parathyroid hormone, *J. Neurochem.*, 43, 849, 1984.
15. Collip, J. B. and Clark, E. P., Further studies on the physiological action of a parathyroid hormone, *J. Biol. Chem.*, 64, 133, 1925.
16. Charbon, G. A., A diuretic and hypotensive action of parathyroid extract, *Acta Physiol. Pharmacol. Neerld.*, 14, 52, 1966.
17. Charbon, G. A. and Hulstaert, P. F., Augmentation of arterial hepatic and renal flow by extracted and synthetic parathyroid hormone, *Endocrinology*, 95, 621, 1974.
18. Crass, M. F., III, Moore, P. L., Strickland, M. L., Pang, P. K. T., and Citak, M. S., Cardiovascular responses to parathyroid hormone, *Am. J. Physiol.*, 249, E187, 1985.
19. Crass, M. F., III, Jayaseelan, C. L., and Darter, T. C., Effects of parathyroid hormone on blood flow in different regional circulations, *Am. J. Physiol.*, 253, R634, 1987.
20. Crass, M. F., III and Pang, P. K. T., Parathyroid hormone: a coronary vasodilator, *Science*, 207, 1087, 1980.
21. Nickols, G. A., Nana, A. D., Nickols, M. A., DiPette, D. J., and Asimakis, G. K., Hypotension and cardiac stimulation due to the parathyroid hormone-related protein, humoral hypercalcemia of malignancy factor, *Endocrinology*, 125, 834, 1989.
22. Nickols, G. A., Metz, M. A., and Cline, W. H., Jr., Vasodilation of the rat mesenteric vasculature by parathyroid hormone, *J. Pharmacol. Exp. Ther.*, 236, 419, 1986.
23. Wang, H. H., Drugge, E. D., Yen, Y. C., Blumenthal, M. R., and Pang, P. K. T., Effects of synthetic parathyroid hormone on hemodynamics and regional blood flows, *Eur. J. Pharmacol.*, 97, 209, 1984.

24. Lepak, K., Lippton, H. L., Hyman, A. L., and Kadowitz, P. J., Parathyroid hormone: a potent vasodilator in the intestinal circulation, *Fed. Proc.,* 46, 949, 1987.

25. Huang, M., Hanley, D. A., and Rorstad, O. P., Parathyroid hormone stimulates adenylate cyclase in rat cerebral microvessels, *Life Sci.,* 32, 1009, 1983.

26. Suzuki, Y., Lederis, K., Huang, M., LeBlanc, F. E., and Rorstad, O. P., Relaxation of bovine, porcine, and human brain arteries by parathyroid hormone, *Life Sci.,* 33, 2497, 1983.

27. Pang, P. K. T., Yang, M. C. M., Shew, R., and Tenner, T. E., Jr., The vasorelaxant action of parathyroid hormone fragments on isolated rat tail artery, *Blood Vessels,* 22, 57, 1985.

28. Winquist, R. J., Baskin, E. P., and Vlasuk, G. P., Synthetic tumor-derived human hypercalcemic factor exhibits parathyroid hormone-like vasorelaxation in renal arteries, *Biochem. Biophys. Res. Commun.,* 149, 227, 1987.

29. Musso, M.-J., Barthelmebs, M., Imbs, J.-L., Plante, M., Bollack, C., and Helwig, J.-J., The vasodilator action of parathyroid hormone fragments on isolated perfused rat kidney, *Naunyn-Schmiedeberg's Arch. Pharmacol.,* 340, 246, 1989.

30. Helwig, J. J., Burgmeier, N., Gairard, A., Yang, M. C. M., and Pang, P. K. T., Renal adenylate cyclase stimulating action of normal and oxidized parathyroid hormone (1-34), in *Advances in Experimental Medicine and Biology, Phosphate and Mineral Homeostasis, Vol. 208,* Massry, S. G., Olmer, M., and Ritz, E., Eds., Plenum Press, New York, 1986, 351.

31. Crass, M. F., III, Hulsey, S. M., and Bulkley, T. J., Use of a new pulsatile perfused rat aorta preparation to study the characteristics of the vasodilator effect of parathyroid hormone, *J. Pharmacol. Exp. Ther.,* 245, 723, 1988.

32. Tenner, T. E., Jr., Yang, M. C. M., Chang, J. K., and Pang, P. K. T., The potency and efficacy of parathyroid hormone and other peptides as hypotensive agents, *Proc. West. Pharmacol. Soc.,* 23, 53, 1980.

33. Nickols, G. A. and Cline, W. H., Jr., Vasodilation of canine vascular beds by parathyroid hormone, *Pharmacologist,* 25, 724, 1983.

34. Crass, M. F., III, Moore, P. L., Strickland, M. L., and Citak, M. L., Cardiovascular responses to human PTH-(1-34) in the dog, *Proc. West. Pharmacol. Soc.,* 25, 269, 1982.

35. Furspan, P. B., Sham, J. S. K., Shew, R. L., Peng, G., and Pang, P. K. T., Cardiac actions of bovine parathyroid hormone fragment (1-34) in some lower vertebrates, *Gen. Comp. Endocrinol.,* 56, 246, 1984.

36. Sham, J. S. K., Kenny, A. D., and Pang, P. K. T., Cardiac actions and structural-activity relationship of parathyroid hormone on isolated frog atrium, *Gen. Comp. Endocrinol.,* 55, 373, 1984.

37. Kurokawa, K. and Katoh, Y., Effect of parathyroid hormone on the isolated papillary muscle of the rat heart, in *Advances in Experimental Medicine and Biology, Regulation of Phosphate and Mineral Metabolism,* Vol. 151, Massry, S. G., Letteri, J. M., and Ritz, E., Eds., Plenum Press, New York, 1982, 649.

38. Katoh, Y., Klein, K. L., Kaplan, R. A., Sanborn, W. G., and Kurokawa, K., Parathyroid hormone has a positive inotropic action in the rat, *Endocrinology,* 109, 2252, 1981.

39. Bogin, E., Massry, S. G., and Harary, I., Effect of parathyroid hormone on rat heart cells, *J. Clin. Invest.,* 67, 1215, 1981.

40. Pang, P. K. T., Yang, M. C. M., and Tenner, T. E., Jr., Beta-adrenergic-like actions of parathyroid hormone, *TIPS,* 7, 340, 1986.

41. Nickols, G. A., Nickols, M. A., and Helwig, J. J., Binding of parathyroid hormone and parathyroid hormone-related protein to vascular smooth muscle of rabbit renal microvessels, *Endocrinology,* 126, 721, 1990.

42. Nickols, G. A., Metz-Nickols, M. A., Pang, P. K. T., Roberts, M. S., and Cooper, C. W., Identification and characterization of parathyroid hormone receptors in rat renal cortical plasma membranes using radioligand binding, *J. Bone Min. Res.,* 4, 615, 1989.

43. Seitz, P. K., Nickols, G. A., Nickols, M. A., McPherson, M. B., and Cooper, C. W., Radioiodinated rat parathyroid hormone-(1-34) binds to its receptor on rat osteosarcoma cells in a manner consistent with two classes of binding sites, *J. Bone Min. Res.,* 5, 353, 1990.

44. Moseley, J. M., Kuboto, M., Diefenbach-Jagger, H., Wettenhall, R. E. H., Kemp, B. E., Suva, L. J., Rodda, C. P., Ebeling, P. R., Hudson, P. J., Zajac, J. D., and Martin, T. J., Parathyroid-related protein purified from human lung cancer cell line, *Proc. Natl. Acad. U.S.A.,* 84, 5048, 1987.

45. Stewart, A. F., Wu, T., Goumas, D., Burtis, W. J., and Broadus, A. E., N-terminal amino acid sequence of two novel tumor-derived adenylate cyclase-stimulating proteins: identification of parathyroid hormone-like and parathyroid-unlike domains, *Biochem. Biophys. Res. Comm.*, 146, 72, 1987.

46. Strewler, G. J., Stern, P. H., Jacobs, J. W., Eveloff, J., Klein, R. F., Leung, S. C., Rosenblatt, M., and Nissenson, R. A., Parathyroid hormone-like protein from human renal carcinoma cells. Structural and functional homology with parathyroid hormone, *J. Clin. Invest.*, 80, 1803, 1987.

47. Albright, F., Case records of the Massachusetts General Hospital. Case 27461, *N. Engl. J. Med.*, 225, 789, 1941.

48. Suva, L. J., Winslow, G. A., Wettenhall, R. E. H., Hammonds, R. G., Moseley, J. M., Diefenbach-Jagger, H., Rodda, C. P., Kemp, B. E., Rodriguez, H., Chen, E. Y., Hudson, P. J., Martin, T. J., and Wood, W. I., A parathyroid hormone-related protein implicated in malignant hypercalcemia: cloning and expression, *Science*, 237, 893, 1987.

49. Mangin, M., Webb, A. C., Dreyer, B. E., Posillico, J. T., Ikeda, K., Weir, E. C., Stewart, A. F., Bander, N. H., Milstone, L., Barton, D. E., Franke, U., and Broadus, A. E., Identification of a cDNA encoding a parathyroid hormone-like peptide from a human tumor associated with hypercalcemia of malignancy, *Proc. Natl. Acad. Sci. U.S.A.*, 85, 597, 1988.

50. Thiede, M. A., Strewler, G. J., Nissenson, R. A., Rosenblatt, M., and Rodan, G. A., Human renal carcinoma expresses two messages encoding a parathyroid hormonelike peptide: evidence for the alternative splicing of a single copy gene, *Proc. Natl. Acad. Sci. U.S.A.*, 85, 4605, 1988.

51. Mangin, M., Ikeda, K., Dreyer, B. E., and Broadus, A. E., Isolation and characterization of the human parathyroid hormone-like peptide gene, *Proc. Natl. Acad. Sci. U.S.A.*, 86, 2408, 1989.

52. Yasuda, T., Banville, D., Hendy, G. N., and Goltzman, D., Characterization of the human parathyroid hormone-like peptide gene, *J. Biol. Chem.*, 264, 7720, 1989.

53. Suva L. J., Mather, K. A., Gillespie, M. T., Webb, G. C., Ng, K. W., Winslow, G. A., Wood, W. I., Martin, T. J., and Hudson, P. J., Structure of the 5′ flanking region of the gene encoding human parathyroid hormone-related protein (PTHrP), *Gene*, 77, 95, 1989.

54. Thiede, M. A. and Rodan, G. A., Expression of a calcium-mobilizing parathyroid hormone-like peptide in lactating mammary tissue, *Science*, 242, 278, 1988.

55. Yasuda, T., Banville, D., Rabbani, S. A., Hendy, G. N., and Goltzman, D., Rat parathyroid hormone-like peptide: comparison with the human homologue and expression in malignant and normal tissue, *Mol. Endocrinol.*, 3, 518, 1989.

56. Karaplis, A. C., Yasuda, T., Hendy, G. N., Goltzman, D., and Banville, D., Gene-encoding parathyroid hormone-like peptide: nucleotide sequence of the rat gene and comparison with the human homolog, *Mol. Endocrinol.*, 4, 441, 1990.

57. Mangin, M., Ikeda, K., and Broadus, A. E., Structure of the mouse gene encoding parathyroid hormone-related peptide, *Gene*, 95, 195, 1990.

58. Thiede M. A. and Rutledge, S. J., Nucleotide sequence of a parathyroid hormone-related peptide by the 10 day chicken embryo, *Nucleic Acids Res.*, 18, 3062, 1990.

59. Schermer D. T., Chan, S. D. H., Bruce, R., Nissenson, R. A., Wood, W. I., and Strewler, G. J., Chicken parathyroid hormone-related protein and its expression during embryologic development, *J. Bone Min. Res.*, 6, 149, 1991.

60. Haddad, J. G., Jr., Rutledge, S. J., and Thiede, M. A., Structure and expression of the parathyroid hormone-related peptide gene in the chicken, *J. Bone Min. Res.*, 5(Suppl. 2), A732, 1990.

61. Ikeda, K., Mangin, M., Dreyer, B. E., Webb, A. C., Posillico, J. T., Stewart, A. F., Bander, N. H., Weir, E. C., Insogna, K. L., and Broadus, A. E., Identification of transcripts encoding a parathyroid hormone-like peptide in messenger RNAs from a variety of human and animal tumors associated with humoral hypercalcemia of malignancy, *J. Clin. Invest.*, 81, 2010, 1988.

62. Honda, S., Akiyama, Y., Maeda, Y., Koike, M., Alper, O., Kimura, S., and Abe, K., Parathyroid hormone-related protein in tumor tissues obtained from patients with humoral hypercalcemia of malignancy, *J. Natl. Cancer Inst.*, 82, 40, 1990.

63. Heath, D. A., Senior, P. V., Varley, J. M., and Beck, F., Parathyroid hormone-related protein in tumors associated with hypercalcemia, *Lancet*, 335, 66, 1990.

64. Danks, J. A., Ebeling, P. R., Hayman, J., Chou, S. T., Moseley, J. M., Dunlap, J., Kemp, B. E., and Martin, T. J., Parathyroid hormone-related protein: immunohistochemical localization in cancers and in normal skin, *J. Bone Min. Res.,* 4, 273, 1989.

65. Motokura, T., Fukumoto, S., Matsumoto, T., Takahashi, S., Fujita, A., Yamashita, T., Igarashi, T., and Ogata, E., Parathyroid hormone-related protein in adult T-cell leukemia-lymphoma, *Ann. Intern. Med.,* 111, 484, 1989.

66. Rosal, T. J., Capen, C. C., Danks, J. A., Suva, L. J., Steinmeyer, C. L., Hayman, J., Ebeling, P. R., and Martin, T. J., Identification of parathyroid hormone-related protein in canine apocrine adenocarcinoma of the anal sac, *Vet. Pathol.,* 27, 89, 1990.

67. Budayr, A. A., Nissenson, R. A., Klein, R. F., Pun, K. K., Clark, G. H., Diep, D., Arnaud, C. D., and Strewler, G. J., Increased serum levels of a parathyroid hormone-like protein in malignancy-associated hypercalcemia, *Ann. Intern. Med.,* 111, 807, 1989.

68. Burtis, W. J., Brady, T. G., Orloff, J. J., Ersbak, J. B., Warrell, R. P., Olson, T. L., Wu, T. L., Mitnick, M. E., Broadus, A. E., and Stewart, A. F., Immunochemical characterization of circulating parathyroid hormone related protein in patients with humoral hypercalcemia of cancer, *N. Engl. J. Med.,* 322, 2206, 1989.

69. Henderson, J. E., Shustik, C., Kremer, R., Rabbani, S. A., Hendy, G. N., and Goltzman, D., Circulating concentrations of parathyroid hormone-related peptide in malignancy and in hyperparathyroidism, *J. Bone Min. Res.,* 5, 105, 1990.

70. Kao, P. C., Klee, G. G., Taylor, R. L., and Heath, H., III, Parathyroid hormone-related peptide in plasmas of patients with hypercalcemia and malignant lesions, *Mayo Clin. Proc.,* 65, 1399, 1990.

71. Kukreja, S. C., Shevrin, D. H., Wimbiscus, S. A., Ebeling, P. R., Danks, J. A., Rodda, C. P., Wood, W. I., and Martin, T. J., Antibodies to parathyroid hormone-related protein lower serum calcium in athymic mouse models of malignancy-associated hypercalcemia due to human tumors, *J. Clin. Invest.,* 82, 1798, 1988.

72. Melton, M. E., D'Anza, J. J., Wimbiscus, S. A., Grill, V., Martin, T. J., and Kukreja, S. C., Parathyroid hormone-related protein and calcium homeostasis in lactating mice, *Am. J. Physiol.,* 259, E792, 1990.

73. Kukreja, S. C., D'Anza, J. J., Melton, M. E., Wimbiscus, S. A., Grill, V., and Martin, T. J., Lack of effects of neutralization of parathyroid hormone-related protein in calcium homeostasis in neonatal mice, *J. Bone Min. Res.,* 6, 1197, 1991.

74. Horiuchi, N., Caulfield, M. P., Fisher, J. E., Goldman, M. E., McKee, R. L., Levy, J. J., Nutt, R. F., Rodan, S. B., Schofield, T. L., Clemens, T. L., and Rosenblatt, M., Similarity of synthetic peptide from human tumor to parathyroid hormone in vivo and in vitro, *Science,* 238, 1566, 1987.

75. Thompson, D. D., Seedor, J. G., Fisher, J. E., Rosenblatt, M., and Rodan, G. A., Direct action of the parathyroid hormone-like human hypercalcemic factor on bone, *Proc. Natl. Acad. Sci. U.S.A.,* 85, 5673, 1988.

76. Walker, A. T., Stewart, A. F., Korn, E. A., Shiratori, T., Mitnick, M. A., and Carpenter, T. O., Effect of parathyroid hormone-like peptides on 1,25-hydroxyvitamin D-1 alpha-hydroxylase activity in rodents, *Am. J. Physiol.,* 256(Endocrinol. Metab. 19), E309, 1989.

77. Kemp, B. E., Moseley, J. M., Rodda, C. P., Ebeling, P. R., Wettenhall, R. E. H., Stapleton, D., Diefenbach-Jagger, H., Ure, F., Michelangeli, V. P., Simmons, H. A., Raisz, L. G., and Martin, T. J., Parathyroid hormone-related protein of malignancy: active synthetic fragments, *Science,* 238, 1568, 1987.

78. Zhou, H., Leaver, D. D., Moseley, J. M., Kemp, B., Ebeling, P. R., and Martin, T. J., Actions of parathyroid hormone-related protein on the kidney in vivo, *J. Endocrinol.,* 122, 229, 1989.

79. Nissenson, R. A., Diep, D., and Strewler, G. J., Synthetic peptides comprising the amino-terminal sequence of a parathyroid hormone-like protein from human malignancies. Binding to parathyroid hormone receptors and activation of adenylate cyclase in bone cells and kidney, *J. Biol. Chem.,* 263, 12866, 1988.

80. Fukayama, S., Bosma, T. J., Goad, D. L., Voelkel, E. F., and Tashjian, A. H., Jr., Human parathyroid hormone (PTH)-related protein and human PTH: comparative biological activities on human bone cells and bone resorption, *Endocrinology,* 123, 2841, 1988.

81. Rodan, S. B., Noda, M., Wesolowski, G., Rosenblatt, M., and Rodan, G. A., Comparison of postreceptor effects of 1-34 human parathyroid hormone (PTH) and PTH-related protein, *Endocrinology*, 124, 397, 1989.

82. Civitelli, R., Martin, T. J., Fausto, A., Gunsten, S. L., Hruska, K. A., and Avioli, L. V., Parathyroid hormone-related peptide transiently increases cytosolic calcium in osteoblast-like cells: comparison with parathyroid hormone, *Endocrinology*, 125, 1204, 1989.

83. Donahue, H. J., Fryer, M. J., and Heath, H., III, Structure-function relationships for full-length recombinant parathyroid hormone-related peptide and its amino-terminal fragments: effects on cytosolic calcium ion mobilization and adenylate cyclase activation in rat osteoblast-like cells, *Endocrinology*, 126, 1417, 1990.

84. Yamada, H., Tsutsumi, M., Fukase, M., Fujimori, A., Yamamoto, Y., Miyauchi, A., Fujii, Y., Noda, T., Fujii, N., and Fujita, T., Effects of human PTH-related peptide and human PTH on cyclic AMP production and cytosolic free calcium in an osteoblastic cell clone, *Bone Min.*, 6, 45, 1989.

85. Sugimoto, T., Kano, J., Fukase, M., and Fujita, T., Second messenger signaling in the regulation of cytosolic pH and DNA synthesis by parathyroid hormone (PTH) and PTH-related peptide in osteoblastic osteosarcoma cells: role of Na^+/H^+ exchange, *J. Cell. Physiol.*, 152, 28, 1992.

86. Shigeno, C., Yamamoto, I., Kitamura, N., Noda, T., Lee, K., Sone, T., Shiomi, K., Ohtaka, A., Fujii, N., Yajima, H., and Konishi, J., Interaction of human parathyroid hormone-related peptide with parathyroid hormone receptors in clonal rat osteosarcoma cells, *J. Biol. Chem.*, 263, 12866, 1988.

87. Juppner, H., Abou Samra, A. B., Uneno, S., Gu, W. X., Potts, J. T., and Segre, G. V., The parathyroid hormone-like peptide associated with humoral hypercalcemia of malignancy and parathyroid hormone bind to the same receptor on the plasma membrane of ROS 17/2.8 cells, *J. Biol. Chem.*, 263, 8557, 1988.

88. Orloff, J. J., Wu, T. L., Heath W. H., Brady, T. G., Brines, M. L., and Stewart, A. F., Characterization of canine renal receptors for the parathyroid hormone-like protein associated with hypercalcemia of malignancy, *J. Biol. Chem.*, 264, 6097, 1989.

89. Orloff, J. J., Goumas, D., Wu, T. L., and Stewart, A. F., Interspecies comparison of renal cortical receptors for parathyroid hormone and parathyroid hormone-related protein, *J. Bone Min. Res.*, 6, 279, 1991.

90. Juppner, H., Abou-Samra, A. B., Freeman, M., Kong, X. F., Schipani, E., Richards, J., Kolakowski, L. F., Jr., Hock, J., Potts, J. T., Jr., Kronenberg, H. M., and Segre, G. V., A G protein-linked receptor for parathyroid and parathyroid hormone-related peptide, *Science*, 254, 1024, 1991.

91. Abou-Samra, A. B., Jüppner, H., Force, T., Freeman, M. W., Kong, X. F., Schipani, E., Ureña, P., Richards, J., Bonventre, J. V., Potts, J. T., Jr., and Kronenberg, H. M., Expression cloning of a common receptor for parathyroid hormone and parathyroid hormone-related peptide from rat osteoblast-like cells: a single receptor stimulates intracellular accumulation of both cAMP and inositol trisphosphates and increases intracellular free calcium, *Proc. Natl. Acad. Sci. U.S.A.*, 89, 2732, 1992.

92. Shew, R. L., Yee, J. A., Kliewer, D. B., Keflemariam, Y. J., and McNeill, D. L., Parathyroid hormone-related protein inhibits stimulated uterine contraction in vitro, *J. Bone Min. Res.*, 6, 955, 1991.

93. Selvanayagam, P., Graves, K., Cooper, C., and Rajaraman, S., Expression of parathyroid hormone-related peptide gene in rat tissues, *Lab. Invest.*, 64, 713, 1991.

94. Ureña, P., Lee, K., Weaver, D., Kong, X. F., Brown, D., Bond, A. T., Abou-Samra, A. B., and Segre, G. V., PTH/PTHrP receptor mRNA expression as assessed by northern blot and in situ hybridization analysis, *J. Bone Min. Res.*, 7(Suppl. 1), A102, 1992.

95. Thiede, M. A., Petersen, D. D., Grasser, W. A., Jüppner, H., Abou-Samra, A. B., and Segre, G. V., Coexpresion of PTHrP and PTH/PTHrP receptor mRNA in vasculature supports a local mechanism of action in cardiovascular tissues, *J. Bone Min. Res.*, 7(Suppl. 1), A590, 1992.

96. Lee, K., Weaver, D. R., Bond, A. T., and Segre, G. V., Localization of PTHrP and PTH / PTHrP receptor mRNAs in the rat central nervous system by in situ hybridization, *J. Bone Min. Res.*, 7(Suppl. 1), A614, 199.

97. Mains, R. E. and Eipper, B. A., The tissue-specific processing of pro-ACTH/endorphin — recent advances and unsolved problems, *Trends Endocrinol. Metab.*, 1, 388, 1990.
98. Soifer, N. E., Dee, K. E., Insogna, K. L., Burtis, W. J., Matovik, L. M., Wu, T. L., Milstone, L. M., Broadus, A. E., Philbrick, W. M., and Stewart, A. F., Parathyroid hormone-related protein: evidence for secretion of a novel mid-region fragment by three different cell types, *J. Biol. Chem.*, 267, 18236, 1992.
99. Rodda, C. P., Kubota, M., Heath, J. A., Ebeling, P. R., Moseley, J. M., Care, A. D., Caple, I. W., and Martin, T. J., Evidence for a novel parathyroid hormone-related protein in fetal parathyroid glands and sheep placenta: comparisons with a similar protein implicated in humoral hypercalcemia of malignancy, *J. Endocrinol.*, 117, 261, 1988.
100. Abbas, S. K., Pickard, D. W., Rodda, C. P., Heath, J. A., Hammonds, R. G., Wood, W. I., Caple, I. W., Martin, T. J., and Care, A. D., Stimulation of ovine placental calcium transport by purified natural and recombinant parathyroid hormone-related protein (PTHrP) preparations, *J. Exp. Physiol.*, 74, 549, 1989.
101. Care A. D., Abbas, S. K., Pickard, D. W., Barri, M., Drinkhill, M., Findlay, J. B., White, I. R., and Caple, I. W., Stimulation of ovine placental transport of calcium and magnesium by mid-molecule fragments of human parathyroid hormone-related protein, *J. Exp. Physiol.*, 75, 605, 1990.
102. MacIsaac, R. J., Heath, J. A., Rodda, C. P., Moseley, J. M., Care, A. D., Martin, T. J., and Caple, I. W., Role of the fetal parathyroid glands and parathyroid hormone-related protein in the regulation of placental transport of calcium magnesium, and inorganic phosphate, *Reprod. Fertil. Dev.*, 3, 447, 1991.
103. Fenton, A. J., Kemp, B. E., Kent, G. N., Moseley, J. M., Zheng, M. H., Rowe, D. J., Britto, J. M., Martin, T. J., and Nicholson, G. C., A carboxyl-terminal peptide from the parathyroid hormone-related protein inhibits bone resorption by osteoclasts, *Endocrinology*, 129, 1762, 1991.
104. Fenton, A. J., Kemp, B. E., Hammonds, R. G., Mitchelhill, K., Moseley, J. M., Martin, T. J., and Nicholson, G. C., A potent inhibitor of osteoclastic bone resorption within a highly conserved pentapeptide region of parathyroid hormone-related protein; PTHrP (107-111), *Endocrinology*, 129, 3424, 1991.
105. Vasicek, T. J., McDevitt, B. E., Freeman, M. W., Fennick, B. J., Hendy, G. N., Potts, J. T., Jr., Rich, A., and Kronenberg, H. M., Nucleotide sequence of the human parathyroid hormone gene, *Proc. Natl. Acad. Sci. U.S.A.*, 80, 2127, 1983.
106. Mangin, M., Ikeda, K., Dreyer, B. E., and Broadus, A. E., Identification of an up-stream promoter of the human parathyroid hormone-related peptide gene, *Mol. Endocrinol.*, 4, 851, 1990.
107. Vasavada, R., Wysolmerski, J. J., Broadus, A. E., and Philbrick, W. M., Identification and characterization of a GC-rich promoter of the human parathyroid hormone related peptide gene, *Mol. Endocrinol.*, 7, 273, 1992.
108. Mangin, M., Ikeda, K., Dreyer, B. E., Milstone, L., and Broadus, A. E., Two distinct tumor-derived parathyroid hormone-like peptides result from alternative ribonucleic acid splicing, *Mol. Endocrinol.*, 2, 1049, 1988.
109. Hendy, G. N. and Goltzman, D., Molecular biology of parathyroid hormone-like peptide, in *Parathyroid Hormone-Related Protein: Normal Physiology and Its Role in Cancer*, Halloran, B.P. and Nissenson, R.A., Eds., CRC Press, Boca Raton, FL, 1992, 25.
110. Shtivelman, E., Lifshitz, B., Gale, R. P., Roe, B. A., and Canaanai, E., Alternative splicing of RNAs transcribed from the human *abl* gene and from the *bcr-abl* fused gene, *Cell*, 47, 277, 1986.
111. Chretien, S., Dubart, A., Beaupain, D., Raich, N., Grandchamp, B., Rosa, J., Goossens, M., and Romeo, P. H., Alternative transcription and splicing of the human porphobilinogen deaminase gene results either in tissue-specific or in housekeeping expression, *Proc. Natl. Acad. Sci. U.S.A.*, 85, 6, 1988.
112. Shaw, G. and Kamen, R., A conserved AU sequence from the 3'-untranslated region of GM-CSF mRNA mediates selective mRNA degradation, *Cell*, 46, 659, 1986.
113. Thiede, M. A., Expression and regulation of the parathyroid hormone-related protein gene in tumors and normal tissues, in *Parathyroid Hormone-Related Protein: Normal Physiology and Its Role in Cancer*, Halloran, B. P. and Nissenson, R. A., Eds., CRC Press, Boca Raton, FL, 1992, 57.

114. Moseley, J. M., Hayman, J. A., Danks, J. A., Alcorn, D., Grill, V., Southby, J., and Horton, M. A., Immunohistochemical detection of parathyroid hormone-related protein in fetal epithelia, *J. Clin. Endocrinol. Metab.*, 73, 478, 1991.

115. Moniz, C., Burton, P. B. J., Malik, A. N., Dixit, M., Banga, J. P., Nicolaides, K., Quieke, P., Knight, D. E., and McGregor, A. M., Parathyroid hormone-related peptide in normal human fetal development, *J. Mol. Endocrinol.*, 5, 259, 1990.

116. Senior, P. V., Heath, D. A., and Beck, F., Expression of parathyroid hormone-related protein mRNA in the rat before birth: demonstration by hybridization histochemistry, *J. Mol. Endocrinol.*, 6, 281, 1990.

117. Abbas, S. K., Pickard, D. W., Illingworth, D., Storer, J., Purdie, D. W., Moniz, C., Dixit, M., Caple, I. W., Ebeling, P. R., Rodda, C. P., Martin, T. J., and Care, A. D., Measurement of parathyroid hormone-related protein in extracts of fetal parathyroid glands and placental membranes, *J. Endocrinol.*, 124, 139, 1990.

118. Campos, R. V., Asa, S. L., and Drucker, D. J., Immunocytochemical localization of parathyroid hormone-like peptide in the rat fetus, *Cancer Res.*, 51, 6351, 1991.

119. Kramer, S., Reynolds, F. H., Castillo, M., Valenzuela, D. M., Thorikay, M., and Sorvillo, J. M., Immunological identification and distribution of parathyroid hormone-like protein polypeptides in normal and malignant tissues, *Endocrinology,* 128, 1927, 1991.

120. Merendino, J. J., Insogna, K. L., Milstone, L. M., Broadus, A. E., and Stewart, A. F., A parathyroid hormone-like protein from cultured human keratinocytes, *Science,* 231, 388, 1986.

121. Danks, J. A., Ebeling, P. R., Hayman, J., Chou, S. T., Moseley, J. M., Dunlap, J., Kemp, B. E., and Martin, T. J., Parathyroid hormone-related protein: immunohistochemical localization in cancers and in normal skin, *J. Bone Min. Res.*, 4, 273, 1989.

122. Hayman, J. A., Danks, J. A., Ebeling, P. R., Moseley, J. M., Kemp, B. E., and Martin, T. J., Expression of parathyroid hormone related protein in normal skin and in tumors of skin and skin appendages, *J. Pathol.*, 158, 293, 1989.

123. Atillasoy, E. J., Burtis, W. J., and Milstone, L. M., Immunohistochemical localization of parathyroid hormone-related protein (PTHrP) in normal human skin, *J. Invest. Dermatol.*, 96, 277, 1991.

124. Thiede, M. A., Grasser, W. A., and Petersen, D. N., Regulated expression of parathyroid hormone-related protein in mammary blood supply supports a role in mammary blood flow, *Bone Min.*, 17(Suppl. 1), A8, 1992.

125. Burton, P. B. J., Moniz, C., Quirke, P., Tzannatos, C., Pickles, A., Dixit, M., Triffit, J. T., Jüppner, H., Segre, G. V., and Knight, D. E., Parathyroid hormone-related peptide in the human fetal uro-genital tract, *Mol. Cell. Endocrinol.*, 69, R13, 1990.

126. Thiede, M. A., Harm, S. C., McKee, R. L., Grasser, W., Duong, L. T., and Leach, R. M., Expression of the parathyroid hormone-related protein gene in the avian oviduct: potential role as a local modulator of vascular smooth muscle tension and shell gland motility during the egg-laying cycle, *Endocrinology,* 129, 1958, 1991.

127. Weir, E. C., Brines, M. L., Ikeda, K., Burtis, W. J., Broadus, A. E., and Robbins, R. J., Parathyroid hormone-related peptide gene is expressed in the mammalian central nervous system, *Proc. Natl. Acad. Sci. U.S.A.*, 87, 108, 1990.

128. Grasser, W. A., Petersen, D. N., Smock, S. L., and Thiede, M. A., Estrogen regulation of PTHrP gene expression in the rat nervous system is tissue-specific, *J. Bone Min. Res.*, 7(Suppl. 1), A589, 1992.

129. Ikeda, K., Weir, E. C., Mangin, M., Dannies, P. S., Kinder, B., Deftos, L. J., Brown, E. M., and Broadus, A. E., Expression of messenger ribonucleic acids encoding a parathyroid hormone-like peptide in normal human and animal tissues with abnormal expression in parathyroid adenomas, *Mol. Endocrinol.*, 2, 1230, 1988.

130. Moniz, C., Bui, T., Burton, P., Moscoso, G., Malik, A., Al-Mahdawi, A., and Shallal, A., Parathyroid hormone-related peptide expression in normal human heart, *J. Bone Min. Res.,* 6(Suppl. 1), A597, 1991.

131. Thiede, M. A., Daifotis, A. G., Weir, E. C., Brines, M. L., Burtis, W. J., Ikeda, K., Dreyer, B. E., Garfield, R. E., and Broadus, A. E., Intrauterine occupancy controls expression of the parathyroid hormone-related peptide gene in preterm rat myometrium, *Proc. Natl. Acad. Sci. U.S.A.,* 87, 6969, 1990.

132. Yamamoto, M., Harm, S. C., Grasser, W. A., and Thiede, M., Parathyroid hormone-related protein in the rat urinary bladder: a smooth muscle relaxant produced locally in response to mechanical stretch, *Proc. Natl. Acad. Sci. U.S.A.*, 89, 5326, 1992.

133. Kitazawa, S., Kitazawa, R., Fukase, M., Fujimori, T., and Maeda, S., Immunohistochemical evaluation of parathyroid hormone-related protein (PTHrP) in the uterine cervix, *Int. J. Cancer*, 50, 731, 1991.

134. Ferguson, J. E., Gorman, J. V., Bruns, D. E., Weir, E. C., Burtis, W. J., Martin, T. J., and Bruns, M. E., Abundant expression of parathyroid hormone-related protein in human amnion and its association with labor, *Proc. Natl. Acad. Sci. U.S.A.*, 89, 8384, 1992.

135. Nijs-de Wolf, N., Pepersack, T., Corvilain, J., Karmali, R., and Bergmann, P., Adenylate cyclase stimulating activity immunologically similar to parathyroid hormone-related peptide can be extracted from rat long bones, *J. Bone Min. Res.*, 6, 921, 1991.

136. Asa, S. L., Henderson, J., Goltzman, D., and Drucker, D. J., Parathyroid hormone-like peptide in normal and neoplastic human endocrine tissues, *J. Clin. Endocrinol. Metab.*, 71, 1112, 1990.

137. MacIsaac, R. J., Caple, I. W., Danks, J. A., Diefenbach-Jagger, H., Grill, V., Moseley, J. M., Southby, J., and Martin, T. J., Ontogeny of parathyroid hormone-related protein in the ovine parathyroid gland, *Endocrinology*, 129, 757, 1991.

138. Conner, C. S., Drees, B. M., Thurston, A., Forte, L., Hermreck, A. S., and Hamilton, J. W., Bovine parathyroid tissue: a model to compare the biosynthesis and secretion of parathyroid hormone-related peptide, *Surgery*, 106, 1057, 1989.

139. Drucker, D. J., Asa, S. L., Henderson, J., and Goltzman, D., The parathyroid hormone-like peptide gene is expressed in the normal and neoplastic human endocrine pancreas, *Mol. Endocrinol.*, 3, 1589, 1989.

140. Docherty, H. M., Dixon-Lewis, M. J., Milton, P. G., Blight, A., and Heath, D. A., Parathyroid hormone-related proteins in cultured epithelial cells, *J. Endocrinol.*, 123, 487, 1989.

141. Ferrari, S. L., Rizzoli, R., and Bonjour, J. P., Parathyroid hormone-related protein production by primary cultures of mammary epithelial cells, *J. Cell Physiol.*, 150, 304, 1992.

142. Rakopoulos, M., Vargus, S. J., Gillespie, M. T., Ho, P. W. M., Diefenbach-Jagger, H., Leaver, D. D., Grill, V., Moseley, J. M., Danks, J. A., and Martin, T. J., Production of parathyroid hormone-related protein by the lactating mammary gland in pregnancy and lactation, *Am. J. Physiol.*, 263(Endocrinol. Metab.), E1077, 1992.

143. Hongo, T., Kupfer, J., Enomoto, H., Sharafi, B., Giiannella-Neto, D., Forrester, J. S., Singer, F. R., Goltzman, D., Hendy, G. N., Fagin, J. A., and Clemens, T. L., Abundant expression of parathyroid hormone-related protein in primary rat aortic smooth muscle cells accompanies serum-induced proliferation, *J. Clin. Invest.*, 88, 1841, 1991.

144. Ernst, M., Rodan, G. A., and Thiede, M. A., Rapid induction of parathyroid hormone-like peptide (PTH-LP) in keratinocytes: implication of PTH-LP in the proliferative response to epidermal growth factor, *J. Bone Min. Res.*, 4(Suppl. 1), A309, 1989.

145. Kremer, R., Henderson, J., Gulliver, W., Hendy, G. N., and Goltzman, D., Regulation of parathyroid hormone-like peptide in cultured normal human keratinocytes, *J. Clin. Invest.*, 87, 884, 1991.

146. Yamamoto, M., Duong, L. T., Fisher, J. E., Thiede, M. A., Caulfield, M. P., and Rosenblatt, M., Suckling-mediated increases in urinary phosphate and 3′,5′-cyclic adenosine monophophate excretion in lactating rats: possible systemic effects of parathyroid hormone-related protein, *Endocrinology*, 129, 2614, 1991.

147. Ratcliffe, M. A., Thompson, G. E., Care, A. D., and Peaker, M., Production of parathyroid hormone-related protein by the mammary gland of the goat, *J. Endocrinol.*, 133, 87, 1992.

148. Grill, V., Hillary, J., Ho, P. M. W., Law, F. M. K., MacIsaac, R. J., MacIsaac, I. A., Moseley, J. M., and Martin, T. J., Parathyroid hormone-related protein: a possible endocrine function in lactation, *Clin. Endocrinol.*, 37, 45, 1992.

149. Karaplis, A., Tybulewicz, V., Mulligan, R., and Kronenberg, H., Disruption of parathyroid hormone-related peptide gene leads to a multitude of skeletal abnormalities and perinatal mortality, *J. Bone Min. Res.*, Suppl. 1, A1, 1992.

150. Thiede, M. A., The mRNA encoding a parathyroid hormone-like peptide is produced in mammary tissue in response to elevations in serum prolactin, *Mol. Endocrinol.*, 3, 1443, 1989.

151. Deftos, L. J., Hogue-Angeletti, R., Chalberg, C., and Tu, S., PTHrP secretion is stimulated by CT and inhibited by CgA peptides, *Endocrinology,* 125, 563, 1989.

152. Lu, C., Ikeda, K., Deftos, L. J., Gazdar, A. F., Mangin, M., and Broadus, A. E., Glucocorticoid regulation of parathyroid hormone-related peptide gene transcription in a human neuroendocrine cell line, *Mol. Endocrinol.,* 3, 2034, 1989.

153. Ikeda, K., Lu, C., Weir, E. C., Mangin, M., and Broadus, A. E., Transcriptional regulation of the parathyroid hormone-related peptide by glucocorticoids and vitamin D in a C-cell line, *J. Biol. Chem.,* 264, 15743, 1989.

154. Gillespie, M. T., Glatz, J. A., Suva, L. J., Kiriyama, T., Moseley, J. M., and Martin, T. J., Transcriptional down-regulation of the human parathyroid hormone-related protein gene by dexamethasone, *J. Bone Min. Res.,* 5(Suppl. 2), A214, 1989.

155. Thiede, M. A., Harm, S. C., Hasson, D. M., and Gardner, R. M., In vivo regulation of parathyroid hormone-related peptide messenger ribonucleic acid in the rat uterus by 17 β-estradiol, *Endocrinology,* 128, 2317, 1991.

156. Thiede, M. A., Harm, S. C., and Gardner, R. M., In vivo regulation of the parathyroid hormone-related protein by estrogens and antiestrogens, *J. Bone Min. Res.,* 6(Suppl. 2), A599, 1991.

157. Rodan, S. B., Wesolowski, G., Ianacone, J., Thiede, M. A., and Rodan, G. A., Production of parathyroid hormone-like peptide in a human osteosarcoma cell line: stimulation by phorbol esters and epidermal growth factor, *J. Endocrinol.,* 122, 219, 1989.

158. Allinson, E. T. and Drucker, D. J., Parathyroid hormone-like peptide shares features with members of the early response gene family: rapid induction by serum, growth factors, and cycloheximide, *Cancer Res.,* 52, 3103, 1992.

159. Casey, M. L., Mibe, M., Erk, A., and MacDonald, P. C., Transforming growth factor-β1 stimulation of parathyroid hormone-related protein expression in human uterine cells in culture: mRNA levels and protein secretion, *J. Clin. Endocrinol. Metab.,* 74, 950, 1992.

160. Zakalik, D., Diep, D., Hooks, M. A., Nissenson, R. A., and Strewler, G. J., Transforming growth factor beta increases stability of parathyroid hormone related protein messenger RNA, *J. Bone Min. Res.,* 7(Suppl. 1), A104, 1992.

161. Ikeda, K., Okazaki, R., Inoue, D., and Matsumoto, T., Transcription of human PTH-related peptide gene is activated through a cAMP-dependent pathway by prostaglandin E1 in HTLV-1 infected cells, *J. Bone Min. Res.,* 7(Suppl. 1), A105, 1992.

162. Pirola, C. J., Wang, H., Kamyar, A., Wu, S., Enomoto, H., Sharifi, B., Forrester, J. S., Clemens, T. L., and Fagin, J. A., Angiotensin II regulates parathyroid hormone-related protein expression in cultured rat aortic smooth muscle cells through transcriptional and post-transcriptional mechanisms, *J. Biol. Chem.,* 268, 1987, 1993.

163. Watanabe, T., Yamaguchi, K., Takatsuki, K., Osame, M., and Yoshida, M., Constitutive expression of parathyroid hormone-related protein gene in human T cell leukemia virus type 1 (HTLV-1) carriers and adult T cell leukemia patients that can be *trans*-activated by HTLV-1 *tax* gene, *J. Exp. Med.,* 172, 759, 1990.

164. Daifotis, A. G., Weir, E. C., Dreyer, B. E., and Broadus, A. E., Stretch-induced parathyroid hormone-related peptide gene expression in the rat uterus, *J. Biol Chem.,* 267, 23455, 1992.

165. Ikeda, K., Lu, C., Weir, E.C., Mangin, M., and Broadus, A.E., Regulation of parathyroid hormone-related peptide gene expression by cycloheximide, *J. Biol. Chem.,* 265, 5398, 1990.

166. Yamamoto, M., Fisher, J. E., Thiede, M. A., Caulfield, M. P., Rosenblatt, M., and Duong, L. T., Concentration of parathyroid hormone-related protein in rat milk changes with the duration of lactation and interval from previous suckling, but not with milk calcium, *Endocrinology,* 130, 741, 1992.

167. Holick, M. F., Nussbaum, S., and Persons, K. S., PTH-like humoral hypercalcemia factor (HHF) of malignancy may be a epidermal differentiation factor: synthetic hHHF (1-34)NH$_2$ inhibits proliferation and induces terminal differentiation of cultured human keratinocytes, *J. Bone Min. Res.,* 3, A582, 1988.

168. Kaiser, S. M., Laneuville, P., Bernier, S. M., Shim, J. S., Kremer, R., and Goltzman, D., Enhanced growth of a human keratinocyte cell line induced by antisense RNA for parathyroid hormone-related peptide, *J. Biol. Chem.,* 267, 13623, 1992.

169. Burton, P. B. J., Moniz, C., and Knight, D. E., Parathyroid hormone-related peptide can function as an autocrine growth factor in human renal cell carcinoma, *Biochem. Biophys. Res. Comm.,* 167, 110, 1990.

170. Adachi, N., Yamaguchi, K., Miyake, Y., Honda, S., Nagasaki, K., Akiyama, Y., Adachi, I., and Abe, K., Parathyroid hormone-related protein is a possible autocrine growth inhibitor for lymphocytes, *Biochem. Biophys. Res. Commun.,* 166, 1088, 1990.

171. Chan, S. D. H., Strewler, G. J., King, K. L., and Nissenson, R. A., Expression of a parathyroid hormone-like protein and its receptor during differentiation of embryonal carcinoma cells, *Mol. Endocrinol.,* 4, 638, 1990.

172. Barlet, J.-P., Davicco, M. J., and Coxam, V., Synthetic parathyroid hormone-related peptide(1-34) fragment stimulates placental calcium transfer in ewes, *J. Endocrinol.,* 127, 33, 1990.

173. Evely, R. S., Bonomo, A., Schneider, H. G., Moseley, J. M., Gallaghe, J., and Martin, T. J., Structural requirements for the action of parathyroid hormone-related protein (PTHrP) on bone resorption by isolated osteoclast, *J. Bone Min. Res.,* 6, 85, 1991.

174. Cooper, C. W., Seitz, P. K., McPherson, M. B., Selvanayagam, P., and Rajaraman, S., Effects of parathyroid hormonal peptides on the gut, *Contrib. Nephrol.,* 91, 26, 1991.

175. Barri, M. E., Abbas, A. B., and Care, A. D., The effects in the rat of two fragments of parathyroid hormone-related protein on uterine contractions in situ, *Exp. Physiol.,* 77, 481, 1992.

176. Paspaliaris, V., Vargas, S. J., Gillespie, M. T., Williams, E. D., Danks, J. A., Moseley, J. M., Story, M. E., Pennefather, J. N., Leaver, D. D., and Martin, T. J., Oestrogen enhancement of the myometrial response to exogenous parathyroid hormone-related protein (PTHrP), and tissue localization of endogenous PTHrP and its mRNA in the virgin uterus, *J. Endocrinol.,* 134, 415, 1992.

177. Bowman, L. H., Rabin, B., and Schlessinger, D., Multiple ribosomal RNA cleavage pathways in mammalian cells, *Nucleic. Acids Res.,* 9, 4951, 1981.

178. Tenner, T. E., Jr., Ramanadham, S., Yang, M. C. M., and Pang, P. K. T., Chronotropic actions of bPTH(1-34) in the right atrium of the rat, *Can. J. Physiol. Pharmacol.,* 61, 1162, 1983.

179. Tenner, T. E. and Pang, P. K. T., Cardiac actions of parathyroid hormone, *Proc. West. Pharmacol. Soc.,* 25, 263, 1982.

180. Massry, S.G., Parathyroid hormone and the heart, in: *Advances in Experimental Medicine and Biology, Regulation of Phosphate and Mineral Metabolism,* Vol. 151, edited by Massry, S. G., Letteri, J. M., and Ritz, E., Eds., Plenum Press, New York, 1982, 607.

181. Sham, J. S. K., Wong, V. C. K., Chiu, K. W., and Pang, P. K. T., Comparative study of the cardiac actions of bovine parathyroid hormone (1-34), *Gen. Comp. Endocrinol.,* 61, 148, 1986.

182. Thiede, M. A., unpublished observation, 1992.

183. Orloff, J. J., Wu, T. L., and Stewart, A. F., Parathyroid hormone-like proteins: biochemical responses and receptor interactions, *Endocr. Rev.,* 10, 476, 1989.

184. Nickols, G. A., unpublished observation, 1992.

185. Musso, M.-J., Plante, M., Judes, C., Barthelmebs, M., and Helwig, J.-J., Renal vasodilatation and microvessel adenylate cyclase stimulation by synthetic parathyroid hormone-like protein fragments, *Eur. J. Pharmacol.,* 174, 139, 1989.

186. Trizna, W. and Edwards, R. M., Relaxation of renal arterioles by parathyroid hormone and parathyroid hormone-related protein, *Pharmacology,* 42, 91, 1991.

187. Thiede, M. A., unpublished observation, 1991.

188. Cochrane, E. and McCarthy, I. D., Rapid effects of parathyroid hormone (1-34) and prostaglandins E2 on bone blood flow and strontium clearance in the rat in vivo, *J. Endocrinol.,* 131, 359, 1991.

189. Moynihan, J. B. and Edwards, N.A., Blood flow in the reproductive tract of the domestic hen, *Comp. Biochem. Physiol.,* 51A, 745, 1975.

190. Wolfenson, D., Frei, Y., and Berman, A., Responses of the reproductive vascular system during the egg-formation cycle in unanaesthetised laying hens, *Br. Poult. Sci.,* 23, 425, 1982.

191. Nickols, G. A., Metz, M. A., and Cline, W. H., Jr., Endothelium-independent linkage of parathyroid hormone receptors of rat vascular tissue with increased adenosine 3',5'-monophosphate and relaxation of vascular smooth muscle, *Endocrinology,* 119, 349, 1986.

192. Schleiffer, R., Berthelot, A., and Gairard, A., Action of parathyroid extract on arterial blood pressure and on contraction and ⁴⁵Ca exchange in isolated aorta of the rat, *Eur. J. Pharmacol.*, 58, 163, 1979.

193. Crass, M. F., III and Brewer, K. S., Vasorelaxant effect of parathyroid hormone on isolated segments of porcine coronary artery, *Artery*, 15(2), 61, 1988.

194. Nickols, G. A., unpublished observation, 1991.

195. Henderson, J. E., Kremer, R., Rhim, J. S., and Goltzman, D., Identification and functional characterization of adenylate cyclase-linked receptors for parathyroid hormone-like peptides on immortalized human keratinocytes, *Endocrinology*, 130, 449, 1992.

196. Nissenson, R. A. and Strewler, G. J., Molecular mechanism of action of PTHrP, in *Parathyroid Hormone-Related Protein: Normal Physiology and Its Role in Cancer*, Halloran, B. P. and Nissenson, R. A., Eds., CRC Press, Boca Raton, FL, 1992, 145.

197. Orloff, J. J., Ribaudo, A. E., McKee, R. L., Rosenblatt, M., and Stewart, A. F., A pharmacological comparison of parathyroid hormone receptors in human bone and kidney, *Endocrinology*, 131, 1603, 1992.

198. Bergmann, C., Schoeffter, P., Stoclet, J. C., and Gairard, A., Effect of parathyroid hormone and antagonist on aortic cAMP levels, *Can. J. Physiol. Pharmacol.*, 65, 2349, 1987.

199. Stanton, R. C., Plant, S. B., and McCarron, D. A., cAMP response of vascular smooth muscle cells to bovine parathyroid hormone, *Am. J. Physiol.*, 10, E822, 1984.

200. Martin, K. J., McConkey, C. J., Jr. and Caulfield, M. P., The role of protein kinase-A activity in the evaluation of agonist/antagonist properties of analogs of parathyroid hormone-related protein in opossum kidney cells, *Endocrinology*, 131, 2161, 1992.

201. Kano, J., Sugimoto, T., Fukase, M., and Chihara, K., The direct involvement of cAMP-dependent protein kinase in the regulation of collagen synthesis by parathyroid hormone (PTH) and PTH-related peptide in osteoblast-like osteosarcoma cells (UMR-106), *Biochem. Biophys. Res. Commun.*, 184, 525, 1992.

202. Sugimoto, T., Kano, J., Fukase, M., and Fujita, T., The activation of cAMP-dependent protein kinase is directly linked to homologous desensitization by parathyroid hormone (PTH) and PTH-related peptide in osteoblastic osteosarcoma cells, *Horm. Metab. Res.*, 24, 347, 1992.

203. Civitelli, R., Reid, I. R., Westbrook, S., Avioli, L. V., and Hruska, K. A., PTH elevates inositol polyphosphates and diacylglycerol in a rat osteoblast-like cell line, *Am. J. Physiol.*, 255, E660, 1988.

204. Dunlay, R. and Hruska, K., PTH receptor coupling to phospholipase C is an alternate pathway of signal transduction in bone and kidney, *Am. J. Physiol.*, 258, F223, 1990.

205. Cole, J. A., Eber, S. L., Poelling, R. E., Thorne, P. K., and Forte, L. R., A dual mechanism for regulation of kidney phosphate transport by parathyroid hormone, *Am. J. Physiol.*, 253, E221, 1987.

206. Cole, J. A., Forte, L. R., Eber, S., Thorne, P. K., and Poelling, R. E., Regulation of sodium-dependent phosphate transport by parathyroid hormone in opossum kidney cells: adenosine 3'5'-monophosphate-dependent and -independent mechanisms, *Endocrinology*, 122, 2981, 1988.

207. Dominiczak, A. F. and Bohr, D. F., Mechanisms of vasorelaxation, *Cardiovasc. Drug Rev.*, 10, 243, 1992.

208. Jones, A. W., Bylund, D. B., and Forte, L. R., cAMP-dependent reduction in membrane fluxes during relaxation of arterial smooth muscle, *Am. J. Physiol.*, 246, H306, 1984.

209. Hruska, K. A., Goligorsky, M., Scoble, J., Tsutsumi, M., Westbrook, S., and Moskowitz, D., Effects of parathyroid hormone on cytosolic calcium in renal proximal tubular primary cultures, *Am. J. Physiol.*, 251, F188, 1986.

210. Wang, R., Wu, L., Karpinski, E., and Pang, P. K. T., The changes in contractile status of single vascular smooth muscle cells and ventricular cells induced by bPTH(1-34), *Life Sci.*, 52, 793, 1993.

211. Wang, R., Wu, L., Karpinski, E., and Pang, P. K. T., The effects of parathyroid hormone on L-type voltage-dependent calcium channel currents in vascular smooth muscle cells and ventricular myocytes are mediated by a cyclic AMP dependent mechanism, *FEBS Lett.*, 282, 331, 1991.

212. Wang, R., Karpinski, E., and Pang, P. K. T., Parathyroid hormone selectively inhibits L-type calcium channels in single vascular smooth muscle cells of the rat, *J. Physiol. (London)*, 441, 325, 1991.

213. Nickols, G. A., Actions of parathyroid hormone in the cardiovascular system, *Blood Vessels*, 24, 120, 1987.

214. Wang, R., Karpinski, E., and Pang, P. K. T., Two types of voltage-dependent calcium channel currents and their modulation by parathyroid hormone in neonatal rat ventricular cells, *J. Cardiovasc. Pharmacol.*, 17, 990, 1991.

215. Rampe, D., Lacerda, A. E., Dage, R. C., and Brown, A. M., Parathyroid hormone: an endogenous modulator of cardiac calcium channels, *Am. J. Physiol. Heart Circ. Physiol.*, 261, H1945, 1991.

216. Evans, D. B., Modulation of cAMP: mechanism for positive inotropic action, *J. Cardiovasc. Pharmacol.*, 8(Suppl. 9), S22, 1986.

217. DiPette, D. J., Christenson, W., Nickols, M. A., and Nickols, G. A., Cardiovascular responsiveness to parathyroid hormone (PTH) and PTH-related protein in genetic hypertension, *Endocrinology*, 130, 2045, 1992.

218. Roca-Cusachs, A., DiPette, D. J., and Nickols, G. A., Regional and systemic hemodynamic effects of parathyroid hormone-related protein: preservation of cardiac function and coronary and renal flow with reduced blood pressure, *J. Pharmacol. Exp. Ther.*, 256, 110, 1991.

219. Kishimoto, H., Tsumura, K., Fujioka, S., Uchimoto, S., Yamashita, N., Suzuki, R., Yoshimaru, K., Shimura, M., Sasakawa, O., and Morii, H., Effects of parathyroid hormone-related protein on systemic and regional hemodynamics in conscious rats. A comparison with human parathyroid hormone, *Contrib. Nephrol.*, 90, 72, 1991.

220. McKee, R. L., Caulfield, M. P., and Rosenblatt, M., Treatment of bone-derived ROS 17/2.8 cells with dexamethasone and pertussis toxin enables detection of partial agonist activity for parathyroid hormone antagonists, *Endocrinology*, 127, 76, 1990.

221. Mundy, G. R., The hypercalcemia of malignancy, *Kidney Int.*, 31, 142, 1987.

222. Soifer, N. E. and Stewart, A. F., *Parathyroid Hormone-Related Protein: Normal Physiology and Its Role in Cancer*, CRC Press, Boca Raton, FL, 1992, 93.

223. Sica, D. A., Martodam, R. R., Aronow, J., and Mundy, G. R., The hypercalcemic rat Leydig cell tumor-A model of the humoral hypercalcemia of malignancy, *Calcif. Tissue Int.*, 35, 287, 1983.

224. Insogna, K. L., Stewart, A. F., Vignery, A. M. C., Weir, E. C., Namnum, P. A., Baron, R. E., Kirkwood, J. M., Deftos, L. M., and Broadus, A. E., Biochemical and histomorphometric characterization of a rat model for humoral hypercalcemia of malignancy, *Endocrinology*, 114, 888, 1984.

225. Hanwell, A. and Linzell, J. L., Determination of cardiac output and mammary blood flow in the conscious lactating rat, *J. Physiol.*, 226, 24, 1972.

226. Cowie, A. T. and Folley, S. J., The measurement of lactational performance in the rat in studies of the endocrine control of lactation, *J. Endocrinol.*, 5, 9, 1947.

227. Hanwell, A. and Linzell, J. L., The time course of cardiovascular changes in lactation in the rat, *J. Physiol.*, 233, 93, 1973.

228. Reynolds, M., Increases in udder blood flow associated with initiation of lactation, *Fed. Proc.*, 24, 451, 1965.

229. Budayr, A. A., Halloran, B. P., King, J. C., Diep, D., Nissenson, R. A., and Strewler, G. J., High levels of a parathyroid hormone-like protein in milk, *Proc. Natl. Acad. Sci. U.S.A.*, 86, 7183, 1989.

230. Khosla, S., Johanson, K. L., Ory, S. J., O'Brien, P.C., and Kao, P. C., Parathyroid hormone-related peptide in lactation and in umbilical cord blood, *Mayo Clin. Proc.*, 65, 1408, 1990.

231. Barlet, J.-P., Champredon, C., Coxam, V., Davicco, M. J., and Tressol, J. C., Parathyroid hormone-related peptide might stimulate calcium secretion into milk of goats, *J. Endocrinol.*, 132, 353, 1992.

232. Khosla, S., van Heerden, J. A., Gharib, H., Jackson, I. T., Danks, J., Hayman, J. A., and Martin, T. J., Parathyroid hormone-related protein and hypercalcemia secondary to massive mammary hyperplasia, *N. Engl. J. Med.*, 322, 1157, 1989.

233. Cooper, K. M., Ives, K. L., Seitz, P. K., Ishizuka, J., Townsend, C. M., Jr., and Cooper, C. W., Parathyroid hormone-related peptide 1-34 blocks the oxytocin-induced increase in intracellular Ca^{++} in cultured human breast myoepithelial cells, *J. Bone Min. Res.*, 7(Suppl. 1), A566, 1992.

234. Thiede, M. A., unpublished observation, 1992.

235. Barlet, J. P. et al., unpublished observation, 1993.

236. Pirola, C. J., Wang, H. M., Wu, S., Okano, K., Jüppner, H., Abou-Samra, A. B., Segre, G. V., Forrester, J. S., Fagin, J. A., and Clemens, T. L., Regulated expression of parathyroid hormone-related protein and its receptor mRNA in rat aortic smooth muscle cells suggests an autocrine vasoactive role, *J. Bone Min. Res.,* 7(Suppl. 1), A206, 1992.

237. Thiede, M. A., unpublished observation, 1992.

238. Shew, R. L. and Yee, J. A., Inhibition of uterine contraction by parathyroid hormone related-peptide is dependent on nitric oxide, *J. Bone Min. Res.,* 7(Suppl. 1), A579, 1992.

239. Mann, J. F. E., Wiecek, A., Bommer, J., Ganten, U., and Ritz, E., Effects of parathyroidectomy on blood pressure in spontaneously hypertensive rats, *Nephron,* 45, 46, 1990.

240. Schleiffer, R., Pernot, F., and Gairard, A., Parathyroidectomy, cardiovascular reactivity and calcium distribution in aorta and heart of spontaneously hypertensive rats, *Clin. Sci.,* 71, 505, 1986.

241. Pernot, F., Berthelot, A., Schleiffer, R., and Gairard, A., Effect of parathyroidectomy on sodium metabolism in DOCA-NaCl treated and spontaneously hypertensive rats, *Arch. Int. Pharmacol. Ther.,* 264, 110, 1983.

242. Berthelot, A. and Gairard, A., Effect of parathyroidectomy on cardiovascular reactivity in rats with mineralocorticoid-induced hypertension, *Br. J. Pharm.,* 62, 199, 1978.

243. McCarron, D. A., Ellison, D. H., and Anderson, S., Vasodilation mediated by human PTH 1-34 in the spontaneously hypertensive rat, *Am. J. Physiol.,* 246, F96, 1984.

244. McCarron, D. A., Shneidman, R. J., and Lee, D. M., Ca2+ defects in experimental hypertension: SHR's renal response to chronic infusion of human PTH(1-34), *Kidney Int.,* 32(Suppl. 22), s249, 1987.

245. McCarron, D. A., Yung, N. N., Ugoretz, B. A., and Krutzik, S., Disturbances of calcium metabolism in the spontaneously hypertensive rat: attenuation of hypertension by calcium supplementation, *Hypertension,* 3(Suppl. I), I-162, 1981.

246. McCarron, D. A., Calcium, magnesium, and phosphorus balance in human and experimental hypertension, *Hypertension,* 4(Suppl. III), III-27, 1982.

247. Nickols, G. A., DiPette, D. J., Nickols, M. A., and Thiede, M. A., Altered PTHrP gene expression in hypertensive rats, *J. Bone Min. Res.,* 6(Suppl. 1), S230, 1991.

248. Schenk, J. and McNeill, J. H., The pathogenesis of DOCA-salt hypertension, *J. Pharmacol. Methods,* 27, 161, 1992.

249. Matsubara, H., Yamamoto, J., Hirata, Y., Mori, Y., Oikawa, S., and Inada, M., Changes of atrial natriuretic peptide and its messenger RNA with development and regression of cardiac hypertrophy in renovascular hypertensive rats, *Circ. Res.,* 66, 176, 1990.

250. Nickols, G. A. and Thiede, M. A., unpublished observation, 1992.

251. Geiger, H., Bahner, U., Meissner, M. et al., Parathyroid hormone modulates the release of atrial natriuretic peptide during acute volume expansion, *Lab. Invest.,* 12, 259, 1992.

252. Yamamoto, R. and Cline, W. H., Jr., Release of endogenous NE from the mesenteric vasculature of WKY and SHR in response to PNS, *J. Pharmacol. Exp. Ther.,* 241, 826, 1987.

253. Cline, W. H., Jr. and Yamamoto, R., Is presynaptic modulation of norepinephrine release altered in the mesenteric vasculature of adult spontaneously hypertensive rats?, *Blood Vessels,* 24, 100, 1986.

254. Mark, A. L., Sympathetic neural contribution to salt-induced hypertension in Dahl rats, *Hypertension,* 17, I-86, 1991.

255. Crass, M. F., III and Scarpace, P. J., Vasoactive properties of a parathyroid hormone-related protein in the rat aorta, *Peptides,* 14, 179, 1993.

256. Ureña, P., Kong, X.-F., Abou-Samra, A.-B., Jüppner, H., Kronenberg, H. M., Potts, J. T., Jr., and Segre, G. V., Parathyroid hormone (PTH)/PTH-related peptide receptor messenger ribonucleic acids are widely distributed in rat tissues, *Endocrinology,* 133, 617, 1993.

7

Vascular Actions of 1,25-Dihydroxyvitamin D$_3$

Richard D. Bukoski and Patsy A. Perry

CONTENTS

I. INTRODUCTION

Our understanding of the basic processes that regulate vascular smooth muscle growth and contraction has grown tremendously over the past decade and is important in terms of the impact of cardiovascular disease on our society. One aspect of vascular control that is still not widely appreciated, however, is modulation by long-term effectors such as the steroid hormone 1,25-dihydroxycholecalciferol-vitamin D$_3$ [1,25(OH)$_2$D$_3$]. Studies of the vascular actions of this seco-steroid were prompted by two separate lines of investigation. One was the general search for actions of 1,25(OH)$_2$D$_3$ on nonclassic target tissues, including skeletal[1] and cardiac muscle.[2] The other and perhaps more driving reason arose from the observations that systemic Ca^{2+} metabolism is disturbed in humans with the hypertension of primary hyperparathyroidism,[3-6] in a subgroup of humans with essential hypertension,[7,8] and in some experimental models of this disorder.[9,10] The present review summarizes what is currently known about the vascular actions of $1,25(OH)_2D_3$, including effects of both smooth muscle and endothelial elements. For in-depth reviews of the vascular actions of the other calciotropic hormones or factors including parathyroid hormone (PTH), parathyroid hormone related peptide (PTHrP), calcitonin gene-related peptide (CGRP), and parathyroid hypertensive factor (PHF), the reader is referred to other chapters of this volume as well as to recent reviews.[11,12]

II. PHYSIOLOGY OF VASCULAR SMOOTH MUSCLE

To facilitate our subsequent discussion of the vascular actions of $1,25(OH)_2D_3$ we will first present an overview of our current understanding of the mechanisms that are involved in the regulation of vascular smooth muscle contractility and its modulation by endothelium-derived factors.

A. Contractile Machinery

The major contractile proteins in the smooth muscle cell are actin and myosin. Actin is a 45-kDa protein that is expressed as three isoforms in intact vascular smooth muscle including the smooth muscle specific α-actin.[13] Native myosin is a hexamer consisting of two heavy chains, two 20-kDa regulatory light chains, and two 17-kDa essential light chains. Two distinct heavy chain subunits (200 kDa and 204 kDa) are expressed and result from differential processing of RNA arising from a single gene.[14] Each heavy chain is an asymmetric molecule with a filamentous tail and a globular head region that contains the hydrolytic ATPase site. The regulatory light chain can be phosphorylated and is a key regulator of the myosin ATPase activity. The two known regulatory light chain isoforms (RLC-A and RLC-B) are encoded by separate genes with high sequence homology in the translated region and significant differences in the 3′ untranslated region.[15,16] Although mRNA encoding both genes has been detected in multiple tissues, the RLC-A is expressed to a greater extent in vascular smooth muscle[17] and was believed until recently to be constitutively expressed. Intermediate filaments and thin filament-associated regulatory proteins are also present. For example, caldesmon is an actin-binding protein that inhibits actin-activated Mg-ATPase activity of phosphorylated myosin, and this inhibition is relieved by Ca^{2+}/calmodulin and phosphorylation.[18,19] Similar properties have been described for calponin, which is a 34-kDa actin-binding protein.[20,21]

B. Excitation-Contraction Coupling

Contractile agonists such as norepinephrine initiate contraction of vascular smooth muscle by binding to specific receptors on the cell membrane and inducing a rise in free intracellular Ca^{2+} via flux of the cation into the cell through voltage-dependent Ca^{2+} channels.[22] Two types of Ca^{2+} current are carried by voltage operated channels, the transient (T-type) current and the long-lasting (L-type) current that is blocked by dihydropyridine class of Ca^{2+} channel antagonists.[23] Through the family of GTP-binding proteins,[24] contractile agonists modulate a number of downstream effectors including adenylyl cyclase, Ca^{2+} and K^+ channels, and phospholipase C. The latter is particularly important in vascular smooth muscle since activation of phospholipase C results in the hydrolysis of phosphatidylinositol-4,5-bisphosphate, producing diacylglycerol and inositol-1,4,5-trisphosphate (IP_3).[25]

Diacylglycerol activates protein kinase C, which in turn modulates contractile force generation. For example, activation of protein kinase C by phorbol esters results in enhanced force generation in intact smooth muscle[26,27] and increases myofilament Ca^{2+} sensitivity in skinned fibers.[28,29] IP_3 releases Ca^{2+} from the sarcoplasmic reticulum, presumably by opening a caffeine-sensitive Ca^{2+} release channel.[30,31] Ca^{2+}, which is mobilized during agonist-induced activation, can be removed from the cytoplasm by active extrusion/sequestration processes[32] including a calmodulin-activated Ca^{2+}-ATPase located in the cell membrane[33] and a Ca-ATPase located in the sarcoplasmic reticulum, which can be inhibited by thapsigargin.[34] A Na^+-Ca^{2+} exchange carrier is also present in vascular smooth muscle, but its contribution to the regulation of free intracellular Ca^{2+} concentration is still debated.[35]

Ca^{2+} initiates contraction by forming a complex with calmodulin that activates myosin light chain kinase, which in turn phosphorylates the 20-kDa myosin regulatory light chain.[13] Phosphorylation of the regulatory myosin light chain is associated with an increase in myosin Mg-ATPase activity, which roughly correlates with steady state force generation.[36] Light chain phosphorylation is transient and falls to a low level while peak stress is maintained.[37] It has been proposed that dephosphorylation of attached cross bridges prevents their cycling and provides the mechanism for high stress maintenance (latch-bridge hypothesis).[38]

There has also been considerable work on the question of whether additional Ca^{2+}-dependent mechanisms contribute to steady-state force maintenance. Morgan[39] showed that force generated per unit of intracellular Ca^{2+} is greater during agonist-induced contraction than when a depolarizing stimulus is employed. This work has been confirmed and extended using permeabilized preparations that showed a role for G-proteins and suggested additional regulatory roles for protein kinase C and cyclic guanosine 3′,5′ monophosphate (cGMP).[40,41] Somlyo[42] and Kitazawa[43] proposed that a regulated phosphatase is responsible for enhanced Ca^{2+} sensitivity during agonist activation, and this is supported by work of Kubota[44] using a receptor-coupled saponin-permeabilized preparation of bovine trachea. Recently, Moreland[45] has provided evidence that a Ca^{2+}-dependent mechanism in addition to the regulatory myosin light chain (such as a thin-filament-associated protein) contributes to steady-state stress maintenance.

C. Modulation by the Endothelium

Extrinsic factors such as those generated by the endothelium also modulate vascular force generation.[46] It is now understood that the endothelium mediates relaxation of arterial muscle induced by numerous vasodilators including acetylcholine, thrombin, and adenosine diphosphate by the release of an endothelium-derived relaxing factor (EDRF).[47] Endothelium-derived factors also modulate the contractile response of isolated arteries to several agonists. Cocks[48] demonstrated that norepinephrine (NE), through an α_2 receptor, and serotonin (5-HT), through a non-5-HT_2 receptor, induce the release of vasodilator substances from the endothelium that depress force generation in the coronary artery. Similarly, Randall[49] and more recently our laboratory[50] have shown that arginine vasopressin (AVP) promotes the release of an endothelium-derived factor from mesenteric arteries of the rat that depresses contraction and facilitates relaxation.

It is generally agreed that a major form of EDRF is nitric oxide (NO)[51,52] or a related compound.[53] Nitric oxide has many of the properties of EDRF and is synthesized from L-arginine in endothelial and other cell types by NO synthetase.[54] Two forms of NO synthetase have been identified: a Ca^{2+}-dependent form found in the endothelial cell[55] and a non-Ca^{2+}-dependent form that can be induced in several cell types by cytokines, including interleukin-1 (IL-1) and α-tumor necrosis factor (αTNF).[56] One characteristic of the inducible NO synthetase is that it produces NO upon addition of L-arginine. Both NO synthetase pathways can be inhibited by structural analogs of L-arginine such as N^G-monomethyl L-arginine (L-NMMA),[57] and the inhibition can be overcome by L-arginine.[58,59]

In addition to NO, other relaxing factors are produced by the endothelium. One is the cyclooxygenase product prostacyclin (PGI$_2$), which is believed to relax vascular muscle by elevating cAMP. An endothelium-derived hyperpolarizing factor has also been proposed but has not yet been chemically identified.[60] Of interest is the observation that NO hyperpolarizes vascular tissue, suggesting that the hyperpolarizing factor may be NO in some tissues.[61]

The endothelium also produces several contracting factors (EDCFs).[62] One group is the family of endothelin peptides (ET-1, ET-2, and ET-3) derived from preproendothelin molecules, which yield proendothelins, which in turn are acted on by endothelin-converting enzyme to produce active endothelin. These constrictor peptides cause Ca^{2+}-dependent contraction of vascular smooth muscle by activating a specific receptor (ET$_A$) and producing IP$_3$.[62] Endothelin also stimulates an endothelial cell receptor (ET$_B$) and induces the release of EDRF and prostacyclin.[63] Nonendothelin contracting factors produced by the endothelium include thromboxane A$_2$ (TBX A$_2$), PGH$_2$, and superoxide anion. The latter is of interest because it is capable of reducing and inactivating NO and can thus depress NO-mediated relaxation.[64]

While many *in vitro* experiments indicate that EDRF (NO) modulates vascular smooth muscle function, an important question is whether EDRF modulates resistance to flow *in vitro*. Randall[65] found that resistance to blood flow occurs in blood-perfused mesenteric and hindlimb preparations of the spontaneously hypertensive rat (SHR) after destruction of the endothelium. Gardiner[66] showed that L-NMMA infused into the normotensive rat increases blood pressure. Recently, Chu[59] showed that blockade of NO production with L-NMMA increases mean arterial pressure in Dahl salt-sensitive and salt-resistant rats as well as the SHR, and that the effect is reversed by L-arginine. These results indicate that the EDRF (NO) pathway can modulate vascular resistance in both blood perfused preparations and the intact animal.

III. PHYSIOLOGY OF 1,25(OH)$_2$D$_3$

From the above discussion it is obvious that regulation of contractile force generation is very complex and there are multiple sites at which an effector such as 1,25(OH)$_2$D$_3$ can potentially act. Before we discuss the known mechanisms of action of 1,25(OH)$_2$D$_3$ on vascular smooth muscle, however, it will be necessary to consider how it affects classic target tissues.

It is recognized that serum ionized Ca^{2+} is tightly regulated by endocrine mechanisms (Figure 1). A fall in serum ionized Ca^{2+} induces the release of parathyroid hormone (PTH) from the parathyroid gland. In the renal proximal tubule PTH activates 1-hydroxylase resulting in the conversion of 25-OHD$_3$ to 1,25(OH)$_2$D$_3$. 1,25(OH)$_2$D$_3$ is then transported by a serum-binding protein to target tissues including intestinal and renal epithelia, where it induces transcription of genes encoding the 9-kDa and 28-kDa calcium-binding proteins (calbindin$_{9k}$[67] and calbindin$_{28k}$[68]). The increased calbindin levels, by mechanisms that are incompletely understood, stimulate Ca^{2+} absorption in the gut and Ca^{2+} reabsorption by the kidney to restore serum Ca^{2+}.

While numerous metabolites of vitamin D$_3$, including 25-OH and 24,25(OH)$_2$, are present in the circulation, it is recognized that the 1,25(OH)$_2$ metabolite is the biologically active form.[69] Furthermore, it is understood that 1,25(OH)$_2$D$_3$ acts on target tissues via the gene transcription mechanism that has been delineated for other steroid hormones.[70] Upon entry into the cell, 1,25(OH)$_2$D$_3$ binds to a specific receptor, which in turn binds to specific sites located in the promoter regions of responsive genes, called vitamin D response elements (DRE). The interaction of the 1,25(OH)$_2$D$_3$–receptor complex with the DRE results in an increase in gene transcription and subsequent protein synthesis.

In addition to the calbindins, 1,25(OH)$_2$D$_3$ also stimulates or suppresses the synthesis of a large variety of other proteins including osteocalcin,[71] and the proto-oncogene product c-*myc*,[72] which contributes to the growth-promoting and differentiating actions of the

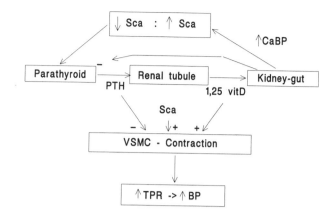

FIGURE 1 Our view of the potential role of $1,25(OH)_2D_3$ in blood pressure regulation. The top illustrates a classic PTH-vitD axis: a decrease in serum Ca (S_{Ca}) causes secretion of PTH, which stimulates renal production of $1,25(OH)_2D_3$. $1,25(OH)_2D_3$, through a gene transcription mechanism, then enhances expression of the calbindins (CaBP) in intestinal and renal epithelia, which enhance Ca^{2+} transport and restore serum Ca^{2+}. $1,25(OH)_2D_3$ can also affect other target organs including vascular smooth muscle (VSMC), where it acts through a gene transcription mechanism to enhance force generating capacity. This could result in enhanced peripheral resistance that would contribute to blood pressure regulation. Thus, during periods of relative Ca^{2+} deficit, $1,25(OH)_2D_3$ can help maintain blood pressure. In conditions where $1,25(OH)_2D_3$ and Ca^{2+} metabolism are disturbed (i.e., low-renin human hypertension), $1,25(OH)_2D_3$ could contribute to a chronic increase in peripheral resistance. Other mechanisms by which $1,25(OH)_2D_3$ could act are by inducing a state of hypercalcemia and by suppressing the secretion of PTH.

hormone.[73] Furthermore, $1,25(OH)_2D_3$ has been shown to alter cell Ca^{2+} metabolism in both intestinal and striated muscle via rapid nongenomic actions. For example, Nemere[74] showed that administration of $1,25(OH)_2D_3$ to chick intestine results in a rapid increase in ^{45}Ca uptake into the gut. This action is termed *transcaltachia* and requires a nifedipine-sensitive Ca^{2+} channel and functional protein kinase C pathway.[70,74] Similarly, de Boland[1] showed that $1,25(OH)_2D_3$ rapidly increases ^{45}Ca entry into skeletal muscle myoblasts, and the action is associated with cAMP- and protein kinase C-dependent translocation of calmodulin to the cell membrane.

Because of the potential therapeutic importance of the actions of $1,25(OH)_2D_3$, considerable effort has been made toward the development of structural analogues that exhibit antiproliferative properties without the side effect of hypercalcemia. One such compound (22-oxacalcitriol) has been shown to exert multiple $1,25(OH)_2D_3$-specific actions, including modulation of growth and differentiation without raising serum Ca^{2+}.[75,76]

IV. VASCULAR ACTIONS OF $1,25(OH)_2D_3$

A. Ca^{2+} Metabolism

In 1986, two groups working independently[77,78] described specific receptors with a high affinity for $1,25(OH)_2D_3$ in cultured vascular smooth muscle cells, indicating that this tissue is a target for the steroid. Shortly thereafter, we assessed the effect of $1,25(OH)_2D_3$ on ^{45}Ca uptake by primary cultures of aortic myocytes of spontaneously hypertensive (SHR) and normotensive Wistar-Kyoto (WKY) rats.[79] We found that after a 7-d exposure to 1 ng/ml $1,25(OH)_2D_3$, there was a significant increase in basal ^{45}Ca uptake. Inoue and Kawashima[80] confirmed these data and showed that in A7r5 cells, the stimulation of ^{45}Ca uptake by $1,25(OH)_2D_3$ is specific and depends on protein synthesis. Kawashima[81] later reported that treatment of A7r5 cells with $1,25(OH)_2D_3$ for a 12-h period results in an increase in Ca^{2+}-activated ATPase activity and that the increase can be inhibited by cycloheximide. While this is an interesting observation, no explanation of how an increase in Ca^{2+}-ATPase activity can be linked to enhanced Ca^{2+} uptake by the muscle cell has been offered.

More recently we demonstrated that $1,25(OH)_2D_3$ stimulates ^{45}Ca uptake by subcultured mesenteric artery myocytes of the SHR and WKY.[82] This action occurs over a physiologic concentration range and requires the synthesis of an intracellular protein. While the protein that is involved has not been identified, we have very recently discovered that vascular smooth muscle expresses a 34-kDa protein that is immunoreactive with a monoclonal antibody raised against the vitamin D dependent calbindin$_{28k}$.[83] We have tentatively named this protein immunoreactive D band 34k (irdb-34k). Control experiments have been performed to rule out the possibility that irdb-34k is calponin, which is a 34-kDa thin-filament-associated calcium-binding protein. Two lines of evidence indicate that the protein is distinct from calponin. Using two-dimensional gel electrophoresis, we have established that irdb-34k has a pK_i of 7.5, whereas the pK_i of native calponin is 8.5. The second line of evidence is the fact that the calbindin antibody that we have employed does not recognize calponin purified from either dog stomach or chicken gizzard. Additional work is in progress to further identify and characterize this protein.

In addition to genomic actions, we also have assessed potential rapid, nongenomic effects of $1,25(OH)_2D_3$. In very early experiments we examined the effect of $1,25(OH)_2D_3$ on intracellular Ca^{2+} of isolated mesenteric resistance arteries using fura-2 and found that acute administration of $1,25(OH)_2D_3$ does not increase basal levels of intracellular Ca^{2+}. The results did suggest, however, that $1,25(OH)_2D_3$ increases norepinephrine-induced Ca^{2+} mobilization in this preparation.[84] In abstract form, Shan and co-workers[85] recently reported that $1,25(OH)_2D_3$ increases intracellular Ca^{2+} in cultured vascular smooth muscle cells by opening L-type Ca^{2+} channels and that this effect is antagonized by $24,25(OH)_2D_3$. However, since no information regarding the concentrations of hormone that were used was provided, it is difficult to assess the physiologic relevance of these actions.

B. Contractility

Probably the largest effort put forth to date has been in the assessment of the ability of $1,25(OH)_2D_3$ to enhance contraction and/or increase peripheral resistance. The first report along these lines was our study that showed that short-term infusion of $1,25(OH)_2D_3$ potentiates the *in vivo* pressor response of normotensive rats to norepinephrine.[86] This work has recently been confirmed by Rocas-Cusachs et al.,[87] who used a radioactive microsphere technique and showed that renal vascular resistance was elevated 24 h after a single injection of $1,25(OH)_2D_3$. More recently, Shimosawa et al.[88] showed that more long-term administration of 1,25-vitamin D_3 or its noncalcemic analogue, 22-OCT, via osmotic minipumps increases the pressor response of rats to both norepinephrine and angiotensin II independently of changes in serum Ca^{2+}. Taken together, these results strongly indicate that $1,25(OH)_2D_3$ increases peripheral resistance, presumably by enhancing vascular reactivity.

Shortly after we performed the *in vivo* experiment described above,[86] we tested the hypothesis that acute administration of $1,25(OH)_2D_3$ alters force development by isolated vascular preparations. Mesenteric resistance arteries were isolated from SHR and WKY and studied using a wire myograph. Pretreatment of the vessel segments with 1 ng/ml $1,25(OH)_2D_3$ for 10 to 60 min was without effect on basal tone or the magnitude of active stress generation in response to norepinephrine and serotonin. There was, however, a significant increase in sensitivity of vessels of the SHR to both agonists.[89]

At this time we turned to more chronic regimens. In the first experiment, we injected 12-week-old SHRs and WKYs with 50 ng $1,25(OH)_2D_3$ on each of three consecutive mornings.[90]

On the fourth day serum was prepared and mesenteric resistance arteries were isolated and studied in the myograph. There was no effect of $1,25(OH)_2D_3$ injection on blood pressure or body weight. There was, however, a 5% increase in total and serum ionized Ca^{2+}, and total phosphate and $1,25(OH)_2D_3$ levels were increased 50% in SHRs and 75% in WKYs. Active stress generation in response to norepinephrine and serotonin was increased by 30% in $1,25(OH)_2D_3$-injected vs. vehicle-injected control animals. The fact that the heightened stress response was observed for two different agonists indicated that the action of $1,25(OH)_2D_3$ was a postreceptor event, and the fact that the effect was seen in isolated vessels indicated that we were not studying an acute response to a circulating factor.

We next addressed the question of whether the inotropic action of $1,25(OH)_2D_3$ occurs with a time course that is consistent with a genomic action.[91] SHRs were injected with 200 ng/kg $1,25(OH)_2D_3$, and serum and mesenteric resistance arteries were isolated 6 and 24 h after a single injection and 24 h after injections for 3 and 7 consecutive days. There was no effect of this level of $1,25(OH)_2D_3$ administration on serum ionized calcium over the 7-d period. Furthermore, an increase in serum $1,25(OH)_2D_3$ was observed only 6 h after the first injection. Thus, in this series, we achieved transient increases in serum $1,25(OH)_2D_3$ that were cleared by the animal each 24 h and resulted in no change in serum Ca^{2+}. When resistance arteries were studied, no change in tension or stress was detected 6 or 24 h after the first injection. However, after 3 and 7 d of injection, there was a 12% decrease in media thickness and a 12% increase in the tension response to norepinephrine and vasopressin, which resulted in an approximate 20% increase in active stress. These findings indicate that changes in vascular contractility and wall structure occurred with a time course consistent with a genomic mechanism of action.

Because the initial injection series resulted in a slight (5%) but significant increase in serum ionized and total Ca^{2+}, we could not be certain that the 30% increase in active stress generation that was observed was the result of a direct action of $1,25(OH)_2D_3$. We therefore adapted the organ culture system described by DeMey et al.[92] to assess the direct actions of $1,25(OH)_2D_3$.[93] Resistance arteries were isolated from Wistar-Kyoto rats and either studied immediately or placed in a standard medium that we use to maintain cultured smooth muscle cells in a quiescent state (DMEM/Hams F-12 (1:1) supplemented with insulin, transferrin and antibiotics) and incubated in a cell culture incubator at 37°C for 48 h. The vessels received 300 pg/ml $1,25(OH)_2D_3$ or vehicle. Vehicle-treated vessels incubated over the 48-h period underwent a 50 to 60% loss of their maximal stress response to norepinephrine, and this decrease was prevented by $1,25(OH)_2D_3$ such that there was only a 15% loss of force generation. The results of this study were therefore consistent with the hypothesis that 1,25-vitamin D exerts an inotropic action on vascular smooth muscle. Whether the action observed in the organ culture model is the result of the same mechanism that is operant *in vivo* remains to be established.

One potential mechanism by which $1,25-(OH)_2D_3$ might enhance contractile force generation is by increasing the synthesis of contractile proteins. Since the regulatory myosin light chain is a member of the superfamily of calcium-binding proteins that includes the vitamin D-dependent calbindins,[94] we tested the hypothesis that $1,25(OH)_2D_3$ modulates regulatory myosin light chain gene expression. In an early set of experiments, WKYs were given daily i.p. injections of $1,25(OH)_2D_3$ (20 ng/100 g) or vehicle for a 3-d period. On the fourth day, total RNA was extracted from thoracic aortas for Northern analysis using a 1.4 kb cDNA probe encoding the regulatory myosin light chain gene[15] and an 18S rDNA probe. Compared with control, $1,25(OH)_2D_3$ caused a 2.5-fold induction in regulatory myosin light chain message expression relative to 18S. To better define the time course, RNA was also prepared from aorta 6 h after a single injection of $1,25(OH)_2D_3$ and probed as described above. The results were quantitatively identical to those obtained after the 72-h treatment with $1,25(OH)_2D_3$. We have also assessed the effect of $1,25(OH)_2D_3$ on quiescent cultured cells of mesenteric artery myocytes derived from WKYs and SHRs and found that $1,25(OH)_2D_3$ induces a time-dependent increase in the expression of regulatory myosin light chain mRNA relative to 18S in both strains. These results have led to our hypothesis that 1,25-vitamin D enhances force generation by inducing myosin light chain gene expression.

In addition to this effect on the myosin light chain, there is a recent report that $1,25(OH)_2D_3$ stimulates the production of prostacyclin by cultured aortic smooth muscle cells and that the increase in prostacyclin is associated with an increase in mRNA encoding the cyclooxygenase enzyme. A similar action was described in aortic rings isolated from rats that were fed 22-oxacalcitriol or $1,25(OH)_2D_3$ in combination with mid-chain triglycerides.[95] Since prostacyclin is a vasodilator and inhibitor of growth, the described actions on prostacyclin are consistent with depressor and antiproliferative actions and are directionally inconsistent with the effects that we and others have described. Additional work needs to be carried out to address this discrepancy.

C. Growth

The effects of $1,25(OH)_2D_3$ on the growth of cultured vascular smooth muscle cells has been examined by several laboratories. In 1988, Koh et al[96] reported that aortic smooth muscle cells in culture have specific receptors for $1,25(OH)_2D_3$. Furthermore, they showed that the hormone caused a twofold increase in cell number over a 7-d period when added in the presence of 10% fetal calf serum. When this report appeared, we were completing a similar study in which we showed that 1 ng/ml $1,25(OH)_2D_3$ enhances proliferation of cultured mesenteric artery smooth muscle cells.[89] We subsequently found that the growth-promoting effects of $1,25(OH)_2D_3$ occur over a physiologic concentration range and have an absolute requirement for a competence factor (i.e., serum), since low levels of fetal calf serum are required for the growth effect to be detected.[11] In contrast with these reports, MacCarthy and colleagues have reported that $1,25(OH)_2D_3$ inhibits the growth of cultured vascular smooth muscle cells over a physiologic concentration range.[97] A recent report by Mitsuhashi et al.[72] may provide insight into these apparently discrepant actions of $1,25(OH)_2D_3$ on smooth muscle cell growth. These investigators demonstrated that $1,25(OH)_2D_3$ given to vascular smooth muscle cells made quiescent for a 3-d period causes a large increase in DNA synthesis and cell number. Moreover, this proliferative action is synergistic when assessed in combination with thrombin. However, when $1,25(OH)_2D_3$ is added to nonquiescent cells, it reduces the mitogenic response to thrombin and blunts thrombin-induced increases in c-*myc* RNA. Our current view is that $1,25(OH)_2D_3$ acts as a promoter of growth in cells that have undergone an event such as injury or enzymatic dispersion from the vessel wall and stimulates their migration or proliferation but acts as a differentiatagogue for quiescent cells in the intact vessel wall.

In addition to effects on cell number, there are reports that $1,25(OH)_2D_3$ modulates expression of structural proteins by vascular smooth muscle cells. Koh et al.[98] showed that 24-h exposure of rat aortic smooth muscle cells to $1,25(OH)_2D_3$ increases DNA synthesis and depresses glycosaminoglycan synthesis. The authors noted that glycosaminoglycans (i.e., heparin sulfate-1) inhibit platelet aggregation and smooth muscle cell growth and suggested that these effects of $1,25(OH)_2D_3$ are consistent with an atherogenic role for the steroid. Hinek and colleagues[99] assessed the effect of $1,25(OH)_2D_3$ on tropoelastin production by several cell lines including smooth muscle cells derived from intralobar pulmonary arteries. The primary action of $1,25(OH)_2D_3$ was to depress tropoelastin synthesis per unit of DNA. These authors conclude that $1,25(OH)_2D_3$ may be an important physiologic regulator of elastin expression.

D. Endothelial Actions

Given the importance of the endothelium as a modulator or vascular reactivity, it is wise to consider the potential role of $1,25(OH)_2D_3$ as a modulator of endothelial function. Merke and colleagues[100] showed that bovine aortic endothelial cells have receptors specific for $1,25(OH)_2D_3$ and are capable of hydroxylating $25-OHD_3$ at the 1-α position. Thus the machinery exists within the vessel wall for both an autocrine loop at the level of the endothelial cell and a paracrine loop in which $1,25(OH)_2D_3$ produced by the endothelial cell can modulate contraction and growth of the vascular myocyte.

As noted above, we used an organ culture model to assess the effect of 48-h incubation of resistance arteries with $1,25(OH)_2D_3$ on force generation.[93] The results showed that $1,25(OH)_2D_3$ prevents the loss in force generation and that this effect is independent of the endothelium. An additional and unexpected finding was that $1,25(OH)_2D_3$ prevented the decay in endothelium-dependent relaxation that resulted from the incubation process. Whether this action is the result of a suppression of an endothelium-derived contracting factor, suppression of the inducible and constitutively active nitric oxide synthase, or protection of the constitutively expressed form of nitric oxide synthase is not known. The results do, however, implicate a role for the steroid in the regulation of endothelial cell function.

V. PHYSIOLOGIC AND PATHOPHYSIOLOGIC CONSIDERATIONS

A. Role in Blood Pressure Regulation

An important question to be addressed is whether $1,25(OH)_2D_3$ contributes to the abnormal blood pressure regulation of hypertension. The majority of the animal work done in this area has been conducted using the SHR, which has been shown to have disturbed Ca^{2+} metabolism.[101] For example, it has been shown that serum $1,25(OH)_2D_3$ is elevated in the young SHR and becomes depressed as the animal ages (12 to 14 weeks).[102] This decrease in serum concentration of the hormone appears to result from decreased renal production in the adolescent SHR.[103,104] Therefore, while it is possible that elevated $1,25(OH)_2D_3$ in the young SHR contributes to the development of high blood pressure, a role for the hormone in the maintenance of hypertension is unlikely unless tissue sensitivity to the hormone (i.e., receptor number or affinity) or its local paracrine production is elevated in the older SHR.

Human clinical studies provide a picture that is somewhat different from the SHR model. Brickman et al.[105] found higher serum $1,25(OH)_2D_3$ concentrations in hypertensive vs. normotensive humans, although there was no correlation with blood pressure. In addition, Morimoto[106] found elevated $1,25(OH)_2D_3$ in patients with senile hypertension, and Yamakawa[107] demonstrated an enhanced $1,25(OH)_2D_3$ response to salt loading in offspring of essential hypertensive humans. In contrast, Young et al.[108] found an inappropriate suppression of $1,25(OH)_2D_3$ relative to serum Ca^{2+} and PTH in men with essential hypertension. Also of interest, van Hooft et al.[109] have recently shown that offspring of hypertensive humans in the Dutch population have inappropriately low levels of $1,25(OH)_2D_3$.

Although it appears that serum levels of $1,25(OH)_2D_3$ are not always elevated in the general human population with essential hypertension, a positive correlation between $1,25(OH)_2D_3$ and blood pressure does emerge when subclassification according to renin status is made. Resnick and coworkers[8,110] showed that humans with low-renin hypertension have elevated serum $1,25(OH)_2D_3$ levels. These observations have been recently confirmed.[111] Perhaps more importantly, it has been established that decreased Ca^{2+} intake or an enhanced Na^+ load causes a significant rise in serum levels of $1,25(OH)_2D_3$ in both the rat[9,10,112] and human.[113-115] These observations have led to the hypothesis that an elevation in serum $1,25(OH)_2D_3$ induced by decreased Ca^{2+} intake or increased salt load may contribute to some forms of hypertension. This is in part borne out by the report of Resnick et al.[116] that $1,25(OH)_2D_3$ administration increases blood pressure in humans, and the magnitude of the effect is relative to their initial renin status.

We have recently completed studies that assessed the blood pressure effect of relatively long-term daily i.p. injection of Wistar rats with 20 ng/100 g $1,25(OH)_2D_3$. Systolic blood

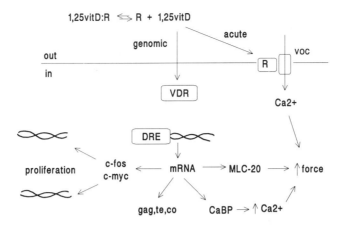

FIGURE 2   Model illustrating actions of 1,25(OH)₂D₃ on the vascular smooth muscle cell. 1,25(OH)₂D₃ could act via an acute action at a putative membrane receptor to increase intracellular Ca²⁺, perhaps at an L-type Ca²⁺ channel (voc), which could increase force generation. In the genomic mode, the hormone binds to the vitamin D receptor (VDR) and forms a complex that binds to the DRE of target genes and initiates mRNA synthesis. Genes that could contribute to an increase in force generation are the myosin regulatory light chain (MLC-20) and a putative calcium-binding protein (CaBP) such as irdb-34k, which could increase Ca²⁺ within the cell or serve in a regulatory capacity. Other genes that may be modulated by 1,25(OH)₂D₃ include glycosaminoglycans (*gag*), tropoelastin (*te*), cyclooxygenase (*co*), and the protooncogenes c-*myc* and c-*fos*. The latter may contribute to the proliferative and differentiating activity that has been defined in cultured vascular smooth muscle cells.

pressure was significantly elevated above baseline after 7 d and remained elevated for the 28 d of the study.[91] We did not assess serum cation levels from these rats and therefore have no information about whether there was a hypercalcemia induced over the extended period. We do know, however, that injection of similar levels of 1,25(OH)₂D₃ is without effect on serum ionized Ca²⁺ over a 5-d period.

More recently, we assessed the effect of 9 weeks of daily i.p. injection of 1,25(OH)₂D₃ (20, 30, and 40 ng/100 g) beginning at 6 weeks of age on the blood pressure of male SHRs (unpublished data). The results showed that there was little effect of the injection over the initial 3 to 4 weeks of the study. At 5 and 6 weeks, however, there was a rise in blood pressure in the groups receiving 20 and 40 ng 1,25(OH)₂D₃. Thereafter, blood pressure continued to rise in all groups and was associated with a decline in the rate of weight gain in the rats receiving the highest levels of 1,25(OH)₂D₃. The net result was an increase in the ratio of blood pressure to body weight without a significant effect on absolute blood pressure. Serum ionized Ca²⁺ was also elevated in all of the 1,25(OH)₂D₃ groups. Contractile force generation of mesenteric resistance arteries was significantly elevated in the rats that received 30 ng 1,25(OH)₂D₃, an effect that appeared to be independent of the level of hypercalcemia that was achieved. We concluded from this study that unlike the normotensive animal, chronic injection of 1,25(OH)₂D₃ significantly enhances active stress generation by resistance arteries but has little effect on blood pressure of the growing SHR. We propose that the underlying disease process in the SHR overwhelms any pressor action of 1,25(OH)₂D₃ in the SHR.

VI. SUMMARY AND FUTURE DIRECTIONS

This chapter presents an overview of the current state of knowledge of the vascular actions of 1,25(OH)₂D₃ and discusses the potential role of this hormone in the development or maintenance of high blood pressure in experimental models of hypertension and in the hypertensive human. Current data indicate that $1,25(OH)_2D_3$ can enhance pressor reactivity in intact animals, can induce long-term changes in force generation, and can induce a sustained rise in blood pressure in the normotensive animal. Figure 1 illustrates our model for how a disturbance of systemic Ca^{2+} metabolism might result in changes in blood pressure. Insight into the underlying cellular mechanisms of the vascular actions has also become available and is summarized in Figure 2. For example, it has been demonstrated that the hormone modulates vascular cell Ca^{2+} metabolism, increases expression of the myosin regulatory light chain gene, and modulates vascular prostacyclin synthesis. Finally, $1,25(OH)_2D_3$ has been shown to modulate the growth and synthesis of structural proteins, which indicates that the hormone may play a role in vascular development or as a modulator of the smooth muscle response to injury or the increased transmural pressure of hypertension.

ACKNOWLEDGMENTS

The authors would like to thank Wilma Frye for her expert secretarial assistance. Original work described in this review was supported by NIH grant HL41816.

REFERENCES

1. de Boland, A. R. and Boland, R., Suppression of 1,25-dihydroxy-vitamin D_3-dependent calcium transport by protein synthesis inhibitors and changes in phospholipids in skeletal muscle, *Biochim. Biophys. Acta*, 845, 237–241, 1985.
2. Walters, M. R., Ilenchuk, T., and Claycomb, W. C., 1,25-dihydroxyvitamin D_3 stimulates $^{45}Ca^{2+}$ uptake by cultured adult rat ventricular cardiac muscle cells, *J. Biol. Chem.*, 262, 2536–2541, 1987.
3. Mallette, L. E., Bilezikian, J. P., Heath, D. A., and Aurbach, G. D., Primary hyperparathyroidism: clinical and biochemical features, *Medicine*, 53, 127–138, 1974.
4. Massry, S. G., Iseki, K., and Campese, V. M., Serum calcium, parathyroid hormone and blood pressure, *Am. J. Nephrol.*, 6, 19–28, 1986.
5. Berthelot, A. and Gairard, A., Parathyroid hormone and deoxycorticosterone acetate induced hypertension in the rat, *Clin. Sci.*, 58, 365–370, 1980.
6. Gairard, A., Berthelot, A., Schleiffer, R., and Pernot, F., Parathyroidectomy significantly decreases hypertension in spontaneously hypertensive and deoxycorticosterone plus saline treated rats, *Can. J. Physiol. Pharmacol.*, 60, 208–212, 1982.
7. McCarron, D. A., Pingree, P. A., Rubin, R. J., Gaucher, S. M, Molitch, M., and Krutzik, S., Enhanced parathyroid function in essential hypertension: response to a urinary calcium leak, *Hypertension*, 2, 162–168, 1980.
8. Resnick, L. M., Laragh, J. H., Sealey, J. E., and Alderman, M. H., Divalent cations in essential hypertension. Relations between serum ionized calcium, magnesium, and plasma renin activity, *N. Engl. J. Med.*, 309, 888–891, 1983.
9. DiPette, D. J., Greilich, P. E., Kerr, N. E., Graham, G. A., and Holland, O. B., Systemic and regional hemodynamic effects of dietary calcium supplementation in mineralocorticoid hypertension, *Hypertension*, 13, 77–82, 1989.
10. Kotchen, T. A., Ott, C., and Whitescarver, S. A., Calcium and calcium regulating hormones in the "prehypertensive" Dahl salt sensitive rat (calcium and salt sensitive hypertension), *Am. J. Hypertens.*, 2, 747–753, 1989.
11. Bukoski, R. D. and Kremer, D., Vascular actions of the calciotropic hormones, *Am. J. Clin. Nutr.*, 54, 220S–226S, 1991.
12. McCarron, D. A., Calcium metabolism and hypertension, *Kidney Int.*, 35, 717–736, 1989.
13. Stull, J. T., Gallagher, P. J., Herring, P., and Kamm, K. E., Vascular smooth muscle contractile elements, *Hypertension*, 17, 723–732, 1991.

14. Babjib, P. and Periasamy, M., Myosin heavy chain isoform diversity in smooth muscle is produced by differential RNA processing, *J. Mol. Biol.,* 210, 673–679, 1988.

15. Taubman, M. B., Grant, J. W., and Nadal–Ginard, B., Cloning and characterization of mammalian myosin regulatory light chain (RLC) cDNA: the RLC gene is expressed in smooth, sarcomeric, and nonmuscle tissues, *J. Cell. Biol.,* 104, 1505–1513, 1987.

16. Kumar, C. C., Mohan, S. R., Zavodny, P. J., Narula, S. K., and Leibowitz, P. J., Characterization and differential expression of human vascular smooth muscle myosin light chain 2 isoform in nonmuscle cells, *Biochemistry,* 28, 4027–4035, 1989.

17. Grant, J. W., Taubman, M. B., Church, S. L., Johnson, R. L., and Nadal-Ginard, B. Mammalian nonsarcomeric myosin regulatory light chains are encoded by two differentially regulated and linked genes, *J. Cell. Biol.,* 111, 1127–1135, 1990.

18. Ngai, P. K. and Walsh, M. P., Inhibition of smooth muscle actin-activated myosin Mg^{2+}-ATPase activity by caldesmon, *J. Biol. Chem.,* 259, 13656–13659, 1984.

19. Sobue, K., Kanda, K., Tanaka, T., and Ueki, N., A common actin-linked regulatory protein in the smooth muscle and non-muscle contractile system. *J. Cell. Biochem.,* 37, 317–325, 1988.

20. Takahashi, K., Hiwada, K., and Kokubu, T., Vascular smooth muscle calponin: a novel troponin T-like protein, *Hypertension,* 11, 620–626, 1988.

21. Winder, S. J. and Walsh, M. P., Smooth muscle calponin: inhibition of MgATPase and regulation by phosphorylation. *J. Biol. Chem.,* 265, 10148–10155, 1990.

22. van Breemen, C., Leijten, P., Yamamoto, H., Aaronson, P., and Cauvin, C., Calcium activation of vascular smooth muscle, *Hypertension,* 8 (Suppl II), II-89–II-95, 1986.

23. Lory, P., Varadi, G., and Schwartz, A., Molecular insights into regulation of L-type Ca channel function, *NIPS,* 6, 277–281, 1991.

24. Harden, T. K., G-protein-regulated phospholipase C. Identification of component proteins, *Adv. Second Messenger Phosphoprotein Res.,* 26, 11–34, 1992.

25. Berridge, M. J. and Irvine, R. F., Inositol triphosphate, a novel second messenger in cellular signal transduction, *Nature,* 312, 315–321, 1984.

26. Rasmussen, H., Takuwa, Y., and Park, S., Protein kinase C in the regulation of vascular smooth muscle contraction, *FASEB J.,* 1, 177–185, 1987.

27. Danthuluri, N. R. and Deth, R. C., Phorbol ester-induced contraction of arterial smooth muscle and inhibition of α-adrenergic response, *Biochem. Biophys. Res. Commun.,* 125, 1103–1109, 1984.

28. Drenth, J. P. H., Nishimura, J., Nouailhetas, V. L. A., and van Breemen, C. Receptor-mediated C-kinase activation contributes to alpha-adrenergic tone in rat mesenteric resistance artery, *J. Hypertens.,* 7, S41–S45, 1989.

29. Brozovich, F. V., Walsh, M. P., and Morgan, K. G., Regulation of force in skinned, single cells of ferret aortic smooth muscle, *Pflugers Arch.,* 416, 742–749, 1990.

30. Somlyo, A. V., Bond, M., Somlyo, A. P., and Scarpa, A., Inositol triphosphate-induced calcium release and contraction in vascular smooth muscle, *Proc. Natl. Acad. Sci. U.S.A.,* 82, 5231–5235, 1985.

31. Saida, K., Twort, C., and van Breemen, C., The specific GTP requirement for inositol 1,4,5-triphosphate-induced Ca^{2+} release from skinned vascular smooth muscle, *J. Cardiovasc. Pharmacol.,* 12 (Suppl. 5), S47–S50, 1988.

32. Eggermont, J. A., Vrolix, M., Wuytack, F., Raeymaekers, L., and Casteels, R., The (Ca^{2+}-Mg^{2+})-ATPases of the plasma membrane and of the endoplasmic reticulum in smooth muscle cells and their regulation, *J. Cardiovasc. Pharmacol.,* 12, S51–S55, 1988.

33. De Jaegere, S., Wuytack, F., Eggermont, J. A., Verboonen, H., and Casteels, R., Molecular cloning and sequencing of the plasma-membrane Ca^{2+} pump of pig smooth muscle, *Biochem. J.,* 271, 655–660, 1990.

34. Wuytack, F., Kanmura, Y., Eggermont, J. A., Raeymaekers, L., Verbist, J., Hartweg, D., Gietzen, K., and Casteels, R., Smooth muscle expresses a cardiac/slow muscle isoform of the Ca^{2+}-transport ATPase in its endoplasmic reticulum, *Biochem. J.,* 257, 117–123, 1989.

35. Mulvany, M. J., Aalkjaer, C., and Jensen, P. E. Sodium-calcium exchange in vascular smooth muscle, *Ann. N.Y. Acad. Sci.,* 639, 498–504, 1991.

36. Rembold, C. M. and Murphy, R. A., Myoplasmic calcium, myosin phosphorylation, and regulation of the crossbridge cycle in swine arterial smooth muscle, *Circ. Res.,* 58, 803–815, 1986.

37. Dillon, P. F., Aksoy, M. O., Driska, S. P., and Murphy, R. A., Myosin phosphorylation and the cross-bridge cycle in smooth muscle, *Science*, 24, 495–497, 1981.

38. Hai, C. M. and Murphy, R. A., Ca^{2+}, cross-bridge phosphorylation, and contraction, *Annu. Rev. Physiol.*, 51, 285–298, 1989.

39. Morgan, J. P. and Morgan, K. G., Stimulus-specific patterns of intracellular calcium levels in smooth muscle of ferret portal vein, *J. Physiol.*, 351, 155–167, 1984.

40. Nishimura, J., Kolber, M., and van Breemen, C., Norepinephrine and GTP-gamma-S increase myofilament Ca^{2+} sensitivity in alpha-toxin permeabilized arterial smooth muscle, *Biochem. Biophys. Res. Commun.*, 157, 677–683, 1988.

41. Kitazawa, T. and Somlyo, A.P., Desensitization and muscarinic re-sensitization of force and myosin light chain phosphorylation to cytoplasmic Ca^{2+} in smooth muscle, *Biochem. Biophys. Res. Commun.*, 172(3), 1291–1297, 1990.

42. Somlyo, A. P., Kitazawa, T., Himpens, B., Matthijs, G., Horiuti, K., Kobayashi, S., Goldman, Y. E., and Somlyo, A. V., Modulation of Ca^{2+}-sensitivity and of the time course of contraction in smooth muscle: a major role of protein phosphatases? *Adv. Protein Phosphatases*, 5, 181–195, 1989.

43. Kitazawa, T., Gaylinn, B. D., Denney, G. H., and Somlyo, A. P., G-protein-mediated Ca^{2+} sensitization of smooth muscle contraction through myosin light chain phosphorylation, *J. Biol. Chem.*, 266, 1708–1715, 1991.

44. Kubota, Y., Nomura, M., Kamm, K. E., Mumby, M. C., and Stull, J. T., GTPαS-dependent regulation of smooth muscle contractile elements, *Am. J. Physiol.*, 262, C405–C410, 1992.

45. Moreland, S., Nishimura, J., van Breemen, C., Ahn, H. Y., and Moreland, R. S., Transient myosin phosphorylation at constant Ca^{2+} during agonist activation of permeabilized arteries, *Am. J. Physiol.*, 263, C540–C544, 1992.

46. Furchgott, R. F. and Zawadzky, J. V., The obligatory role of endothelial cells in the relaxation of arteries induced by acetylcholine, *Nature*, 288, 373–376, 1980.

47. Furchgott, R.F. and Vanhoutte, P.M. Endothelium-derived relaxing and contracting factors, *FASEB J.*, 3, 2007–2018, 1989.

48. Cocks, T. M. and Angus, J. A., Endothelium-dependent relaxation of coronary arteries by noradrenaline and serotonin, *Nature*, 305, 627–630, 1983.

49. Randall, M. D., Kay, A. P., and Hiley, C. R., Endothelium-dependent modulation of the pressor activity of arginine vasopressin in the isolated superior mesenteric arterial bed of the rat, *Br. J. Pharmacol.*, 95, 646–652, 1988.

50. Li, J. and Bukoski, R. D., Altered endothelium-dependent relaxation of resistance arteries of hypertensive and normotensive rats is a function of the contractile agonist, *Circ. Res.*, 72, 290–296, 1993.

51. Palmer, R. M. J., Ferrige, A. G., and Moncada, S., Nitric oxide release accounts for the biological activity of endothelium-derived relaxing factor, *Nature*, 327, 524–526, 1987.

52. Ignarro, L. J., Buga, G. M., Wood, K. S., Byrns, R. E., and Chaudhuri, G., Endothelium-derived relaxing factor produced and released from artery and vein is nitric oxide, *Proc. Natl. Acad. Sci. U.S.A.*, 84, 9265–9269, 1987.

53. Meyers, P. R., Minor, R. L., Guerra, R., Bates, J. N., and Harrison, D. G., Vasorelaxant properties of the endothelium-derived relaxing factor more closely resemble S-nitrosocysteine than nitric oxide, *Nature*, 345, 161–163, 1990.

54. Palmer, R. M. J., Ashton, D. S., and Moncada, S., Vascular endothelial cells synthesize nitric oxide from L-arginine, *Nature*, 333, 664–666, 1988.

55. Bredt, D. S. and Snyder, S. N., Isolation of nitric oxide synthetase, a calmodulin-requiring enzyme, *Proc. Natl. Acad. Sci. U.S.A.*, 87, 682–685, 1990.

56. Busse, R. and Mulsch, A., Induction of nitric oxide synthase by cytokines in vascular smooth muscle cells, *FEBS Lett.*, 275, 87–90, 1990.

57. Rees, D. D., Palmer, R. M. J., Hodson, H. F., and Moncada, S., A specific inhibitor of nitric oxide formation from L-arginine attenuates endothelium-dependent relaxation, *Br. J. Pharmacol.*, 96, 418–424, 1989.

58. Schini, V. B. and Vanhoutte, P. M., L-arginine evokes both endothelium-dependent and independent relaxations in L-arginine-depleted aortas of the rat, *Circ. Res.*, 68, 209–216, 1990.

59. Chen, P. Y. and Sanders, P. W. L-arginine abrogates salt-sensitive hypertension in Dahl/Rapp rats, *J. Clin. Invest.*, 88, 1559–1567, 1991.

60. Feletou, M. and Vanhoutte, P. M. Endothelium-dependent hyperpolarization of canine coronary smooth muscle, *Br. J. Pharmacol.*, 93, 515–524, 1988.

61. Tare, M., Parkington, H. C., Coleman, H. A., Neild, T. O., and Dusting, G. J., Hyperpolarization and relaxation of arterial smooth muscle caused by nitric oxide derived from the endothelium, *Nature*, 346, 69–71, 1990.

62. Luscher, T. F., Boulanger, C. M., Dohi, Y., and Yang, Z., Endothelium-derived contracting factors, *Hypertension*, 19, 117–130, 1992.

63. Fukuda, N., Izumi, Y., Soma, M., Watanabe, Y., Watanabe, M., Hatano, M., Sakuma, I., and Yasuda, H., L-N^G-monomethyl arginine inhibits the vasodilating effects of low dose of endothelin-3 on rat mesenteric arteries, *Biochem. Biophys. Res. Commun.*, 167, 739–745, 1990.

64. Rubanyi, G. M. and Vanhoutte, P. M., Superoxide anions and hyperoxia inactivate endothelium-derived relaxing factor, *Am. J. Physiol.*, 250, H822–H827, 1986.

65. Randall, M. D., Thomas, G. R., and Hiley, C. R., Effect of destruction of the vascular endothelium upon pressure/flow relations and endothelium-dependent vasodilatation in resistance beds of spontaneously hypertensive rats, *Clin. Sci.*, 80, 463–469, 1991.

66. Gardiner, S. M., Compton, A. M., Bennett, T., Palmer, R. M. J., and Moncada, S., Control of regional blood flow by endothelium-derived nitric oxide. *Hypertension*, 15, 486–492, 1990.

67. Thomassett, M., Parkes, C. O., and Cuisinier-Gleizes, P., Rat calcium-binding proteins: distribution, development, and vitamin D dependence, *Am. J. Physiol.*, 243, E483–E488, 1982.

68. Christakos, S., Gabrielides, C., and Rhoten, W. B., Vitamin D-dependent calcium binding proteins: chemistry, distribution, functional considerations, and molecular biology, *Endocr. Rev.*, 10, 3–26, 1989.

69. Tanaka, Y., DeLuca, H. F., and Holick, M. F., Mechanism of action on 1,25-dihydroxy-cholecalciferol on intestinal calcium transport, *Proc. Natl. Acad. Sci. U.S.A.*, 68, 1286, 1971.

70. Norman, A. W., Nemere, I., Zhou, L. X., Bishop, J. E., Lowe, K. E., Maiyar, A. C., Collins, E. D., Taoka, T., Sergeev, I., and Farach-Carson, M. C. 1,25(OH)$_2$-vitamin D$_3$, a steroid hormone that produces biologic effects via both genomic and nongenomic pathways, *J. Steroid Biochem. Mol. Biol.*, 41, 231–240, 1992.

71. DeMay, M. B., Gerardi, J. M., DeLuca, H. F., and Kronenberg, H. M., DNA sequences in the rat osteocalcin gene that bind the 1,25-dihydroxyvitamin D$_3$ receptor and confer responsiveness to 1,25-dihydroxyvitamin D$_3$, *Proc. Natl. Acad. Sci. U.S.A.*, 87, 369–373, 1990.

72. Mitsuhashi, T., Morris, R. C., and Ives, H. E., 1,25-dihydroxyvitamin D$_3$ modulates growth of vascular smooth muscle cells, *J. Clin. Invest.*, 87, 1889–1895, 1991.

73. Minghetti, P. P. and Norman, A. W., 1,25 (OH)$_2$-vitamin D$_3$ receptors: gene regulation and genetic circuitry, *FASEB J.*, 2, 3043–3053, 1988.

74. Nemere, I., Yoshimoto, Y., and Norman, A. W., Calcium transport in perfused duodena from normal chicks: enhancement within fourteen minutes of exposure to 1,25-dihydroxyvitamin D$_3$, *Endocrinology*, 115, 1476–1483, 1984.

75. Fubibayashi, S., Suzuki, S., Okano, K., Naitoh, T., Katabami, T., and Someya, K., The weak calcemic vitamin D$_3$ analogue 22-oxacalcitriol suppresses the production of tumor necrosis factor-α by peripheral mononuclear cells, *Immunol. Lett.*, 30, 307–312, 1991.

76. Finch, J. L., Brown, A. J., Mori, T., Nishii, Y., and Slatopolsky, E., Suppression of PTH and decreased action on bone are partially responsible for the low calcemic activity of 22-oxacalcitriol relative to 1,25-(OH)$_2$D$_3$, *J. Bone Miner. Metab.*, 7, 835–839, 1992.

77. Kawashima, H., Receptor for 1,25 dihydroxyvitamin D in a vascular cell line derived from rat aorta, *Biochem. Biophys. Res. Comm.*, 146, 1–6, 1987.

78. Merke, J., Hofmann, D., Goldschmidt, H., and Ritz, E., Demonstration of 1,25 (OH)$_2$ vitamin D$_3$ receptors and actions in vascular smooth muscle in vitro, *Calcif. Tissue Int.*, 41, 112–114, 1987.

79. Bukoski, R. D., Xue, H., and McCarron, D. A., Effect of 1,25(OH)$_2$ vitamin D$_3$ and ionized Ca^{2+} on ^{45}Ca uptake by primary cultures of aortic myocytes of spontaneously hypertensive and Wistar-Kyoto normotensive rats, *Biochem. Biophys. Res. Commun.*, 146, 1330–1335, 1987.

80. Inoue, T. and Kawashima, H., 1,25-dihydroxyvitamin D$_3$ stimulates ^{45}Ca-uptake by cultured vascular smooth muscle cells derived from rat aorta, *Biochem. Biophys. Res. Comm.*, 152, 1388–1394, 1988.

81. Kawashima, H., 1,25-dihydroxyvitamin D$_3$ stimulates Ca-ATPase in a vascular smooth muscle cell line, *Biochem. Biophys. Res. Commun.*, 150, 1138–1143, 1988.

82. Xue, H., McCarron, D. A., and Bukoski, R. D., 1,25(OH)$_2$ vitamin D$_3$ and ^{45}Ca uptake by vascular myocytes of hypertensive and normotensive rats, *Life Sci.*, 49, 651–659, 1991.

83. Bukoski, R. D. and Bo, J., Expression of a 34 kDa protein in vascular smooth muscle that is immunoreactive with the 28 kDa calcium binding protein (abstract), *FASEB J.*, 7, A533, 1993.

84. Bukoski, R. D., Xue, H., DeWan, P., and McCarron, D. A., Calciotropic hormones and vascular calcium metabolism in experimental hypertension, in *Resistance Arteries,* Halpern, W., Pegram, B. L., Brayden, J. E., Mackey, K., McLaughlin, M. K., and Osol, G., Eds., Perinatology Press, Ithaca, NY, 1988, 320–328.

85. Shan, J., Li, B., Wu, X., Karpinski, E., Lewanczuk, R., and Pang, P. K. T., Effects of 24,25 (OH)$_2$ vitamin D$_3$ intracellular calcium regulation in rat vascular smooth muscle, *FASEB J.*, 6, A1734, 1992.

86. Bukoski, R. D., DeWan, P., Hatton, D. C., and McCarron, D. A., 1,25(OH)$_2$ vitamin D$_3$ differentially modulates vascular metabolism in hypertensive (SHR) and normotensive rats (WKY), *Hypertension,* 12, 361, 1988.

87. Roca-Cusachs, A., DiPette, D. J., Carson, J., Graham, G. A., and Holland, O. B., Systemic and regional hemodynamic effects of 1,25 vitamin D$_3$ administration, *J. Hypertens.*, 10, 939–947, 1992.

88. Shimosawa, T., Ando, K., and Fujita, T., Enhancement of vasoconstrictor responses by a noncalcemic analogue of vitamin D$_3$, *Hypertension,* 21, 253–258, 1993.

89. Bukoski, R. D., DeWan, P., and McCarron, D. A., 1,25 (OH)$_2$ vitamin D$_3$ modifies growth and contractile function of vascular smooth muscle of spontaneously hypertensive rats, *Am. J. Hypertens.,* 2, 533–556, 1989.

90. Bukoski, R. D., Wagman, D. W., and Wang, D., Injection of 1,25 vitamin D enhances resistance artery contractile properties, *Hypertension,* 16, 523–531, 1990.

91. Bukoski, R. D. and Xue, H., On the vascular inotropic action of calcitriol, *Am. J. Hypertens.,* 6, 388, 1993.

92. DeMey, J. G. R., Uitendaal, M. P., Boonen, H. C. M., Vrijdag, M. J. J. F., Daemen, M. J. A. P., and Struyker-Boudier, H. A. J., Acute and long-term effects of tissue culture on contractile reactivity in renal arteries of the rat, *Circ. Res.*, 65,1125–1135, 1989.

93. Xue, H., McCarron, D. A., and Bukoski, R. D., 1,25 (OH)$_2$ vitamin D$_3$ attenuates the loss of resistance artery contractile function associated with incubation in culture media, *Biochem. Biophys. Res. Commun.*, 174, 11–17, 1991.

94. Messer, N. G. and Kendrick-Jones, J., Molecular cloning and sequencing of the chicken smooth muscle myosin regulatory light chain, *FEBS Lett.*, 234, 49–52, 1988.

95. Inoue, M., Wakasugi, M., Wakao, R., Gan, N., Tawata, M., Nishii, Y., and Onaya, T., A synthetic analogue of vitamin D$_3$, 22-oxa-1,25-dihydroxy-vitamin D$_3$, stimulates the production of prostacyclin by vascular tissues, *Life Sci.*, 51, 1105–1112, 1992.

96. Koh, E., Morimoto, S., Fukuo, K., Itoh, K., Hironaka, T., Shiraishi, T., Onishi, T., and Kumahara, Y., 1,25-dihydroxyvitamin D$_3$ binds specifically to rat vascular smooth muscle cells and stimulates their proliferation in vitro, *Life Sci.*, 42, 215–223, 1988.

97. MacCarthy, E. P., Yamashita, W., Hsu, A., and Ooi, B. S., Modulating effect of 1,25-dihydroxyvitamin D$_3$ (1,25D$_3$) on rat vascular smooth muscle cell (VSMC) growth, *Hypertension,* 13, 954–959, 1988.

98. Koh, E., Morimoto, S., Nabata, T., Takamoto, S., Kitano, S., and Ogihara, T., Effects of 1,25-dihydroxyvitamin D$_3$ on the synthesis of DNA and glycosaminoglycans by rat aortic muscle cells in vitro, *Life Sci.*, 46, 1545–1551, 1990.

99. Hinek, A., Botney, M. D., Mecham, R. P., and Parks, W. C., Inhibition of tropoelastin expression by 1,25-dihydroxyvitamin D$_3$, *Connect. Tissue Res.*, 26, 155–166, 1991.

100. Merke, J., Milde, P., Lewicka, S., Hugel, U., Klaus, G., Mangelsdorf, D. J., Haussler, M. R., Rauterberg, E. W., and Ritz, E., Identification and regulation of 1,25-dihydroxyvitamin D₃ receptor activity and biosynthesis of 1,25-dihydroxyvitamin D₃. Studies in cultured bovine aortic endothelial cells and human dermal capillaries, *J. Clin. Invest.*, 83, 1903–1915, 1989.

101. McCarron, D. A., Yung, N. N., Ugoretz, B. A., and Krutzig, S., Disturbances of calcium metabolism in the spontaneously hypertensive rat, *Hypertension*, 4, III-27–III-33, 1981.

102. Bourgouin, P., Lucas, P., Roullet, C., Pointillart, A., Thomasset, M., Brami, M., Conte, L., Lacour, B., Garabedian, M., McCarron, D. A., and Drueke, T., Developmental changes of Ca²⁺, PO₄, and calcitriol metabolism in spontaneously hypertensive rats, *Am. J. Physiol.*, 259, F104–F110, 1990.

103. Patel, S., Simpson, R. U., and Hsu, C. H., Calcitriol synthesis is decreased in spontaneously hypertensive rats, *Kidney Int.*, 345, 224–228, 1988.

104. Kawashima, H., Altered vitamin D metabolism in the kidney of the spontaneously hypertensive rat, *Biochem. J.*, 237, 893–897, 1986.

105. Brickman, A., Nyby, M. D., von Hungen, K., Eggena, P., and Tuck, M. L., Calciotropic hormones, platelet calcium, and blood pressure in essential hypertension, *Hypertension*, 16, 515–522, 1990.

106. Morimoto, S., Imaoka, M., Kitano, S., Imanaka, S., Fukuo, K., Miyashita, Y., Koh, E., and Ogihara, T., Exaggerated natri-calci-uiresis and increased circulating levels of parathyroid hormone and 1,25-dihydroxyvitamin D in patients with senile hypertension, *Contrib. Nephrol.*, 90, 94–98, 1991.

107. Yamakawa, H., Suzuki, H., Nakamura, M., Ohno, Y., and Saruta, T., Disturbed calcium metabolism in offspring of hypertensive patients, *Hypertension*, 19, 528–534, 1992.

108. Young, E. W., McCarron, D. A., and Morris, C. D., Calcium regulating hormones in essential hypertension. Importance of gender, *Am. J. Hypertens.*, 3, 161S–166S, 1990.

109. van Hooft, I. M. S., Grobbee, D. E., Frolich, M., Pols, H. A. P., and Hofman, A., Alterations in calcium metabolism in young people at risk for primary hypertension. The Dutch hypertension and offspring study, *Hypertension*, 21, 267–272, 1993.

110. Resnick, L. M., Muller, F. B., and Laragh, J. H., Calcium regulating hormones in essential hypertension. Relation to plasma renin activity and sodium metabolism, *Ann. Intern. Med.*, 105, 649–654, 1986.

111. Gomez, M. A. V., Cano, R. P., Olivan, J., Garcia, J. M., Garcia, R. M. M., and Peralta, M. G., Absorcion intestinal de calcio y vitamin D en la hipertension arterial esencial, *An. Med. Interna (Madrid)*, 7, 58–62, 1990.

112. Roullet, C. M., Roullet, J. B., Duchambon, P., Thomasset, M., Lacour, B., McCarron, D. A., and Drueke, T., Abnormal intestinal regulation of calbindin-D9K and calmodulin by dietary calcium in genetic hypertension, *Am. J. Physiol.*, 261, F474–F480, 1991.

113. Resnick, L. M., DiFabio, B., Marion, R., James, G. D., and Laragh, J. H., Dietary calcium modifies the pressor effects of dietary salt intake in essential hypertension, *J. Hypertens.*, 4, S679–S681, 1986.

114. Hughes, G. S., Oexmann, M. J., Margolius, H. S., Epstein, S., and Bell, N. H., Normal vitamin D and mineral metabolism in essential hypertension, *Am. J. Med. Sci.*, 296, 252–259, 1988.

115. Burgess, E. D., Hawkins, G. R., and Watanabe, M. Interaction of 1,25-dihydroxyvitamin D and plasma renin activity in high renin essential hypertension, *Am. J. Hypertens.*, 3, 903–905, 1990.

116. Resnick, L. M. and Laragh, J. H., Does 1,25 dihydroxyvitamin D (1,25D) cause low renin hypertension? (abstract) *Hypertension*, 6, 792, 1984.

8

1,25-Dihydroxyvitamin D₃ and Cardiac Muscle Structure and Function

Timothy D. O'Connell and Robert U. Simpson

CONTENTS

I. INTRODUCTION

During the last 20 years, studies in a number of laboratories have provided evidence to suggest that the endocrine system plays an important role in regulating cardiovascular function. These studies have shown that both insulin and thyroid hormone exert significant effects on elements involved in regulating the cardiovascular system. For instance, in experimental animals hyperthyroidism is associated with significant increases in cardiac output, heart rate, left ventricular systolic pressure, and left ventricular contractility.[1] Hyperthyroidism also has been shown to cause ventricular hypertrophy in several animal species.[2–4] In addition, changes in circulating levels of thyroid hormone can alter myosin isozyme distribution,[5–7] which in turn will alter the contractile function of the heart.[8] Diabetes mellitus was shown to produce changes in cardiac contractility.[9–12] It has been suggested that this is primarily caused by changes in the myocardial microcirculation leading to focal areas of anoxia and necrosis. Cellular metabolism, specifically glucose uptake, is reduced by diabetes.[13] In addition, circulating levels of free fatty acids, triglycerides, and cholesterol are increased in diabetic rats which is correlated with decreased contractility in isolated perfused hearts from these animals.[14,15] Finally, diabetes is associated with changes in subcellular metabolism regulating calcium homeostasis, such as calcium transport into the sarcoplasmic reticulum and mitochondria,[16–18] and changes in contractile function by altering myosin isozyme distribution.[19,20]

Vitamin D$_3$ regulates the cardiovascular system. These effects include an enhancement of myocardial contractile function, altered vascular muscle contractility, myocardial hypertrophy, and alterations in collagen content. This chapter focuses on summarizing the current knowledge regarding vitamin D$_3$ regulation of cardiac muscle function and structure. In addition, it provides insight into some of the cellular and subcellular processes that may account for the observed changes in heart function caused by altered circulating levels of vitamin D$_3$.

II. VITAMIN D$_3$ AND THE CARDIOVASCULAR SYSTEM

The importance of vitamin D$_3$ in regulating calcium and phosphate metabolism has been known for more than half a century.[21,22] Elegant studies from several laboratories have established that vitamin D$_3$ acting through its metabolite, 1,25-dihydroxyvitamin D$_3$ [1,25(OH)$_2$D$_3$], maintains circulating calcium and phosphate levels via concerted effects on several organ systems, including the intestine, bone, and kidney.[23–25] In the intestine, 1,25(OH)$_2$D$_3$ stimulates the inward movement of calcium and phosphate from the gut, through the intestine wall, and into the blood, and also induces intestinal hyperplasia.[24,26] These actions are mediated in part by a vitamin D$_3$-dependent calcium-binding protein, whose synthesis is induced by 1,25(OH)$_2$D$_3$.[27] In bone, this hormone is known to regulate cell maturation and cell function, leading to increased resorption of calcium and phosphate.[28] Recent studies have provided evidence that vitamin D$_3$, acting through 1,25(OH)$_2$D$_3$, may play a direct role in regulating metabolism in other organs and cells. Specific receptors for 1,25(OH)$_2$D$_3$ have been identified in over 20 organs, including skin,[29] pancreas,[30] and muscle.[31,32] More significantly, several investigators have demonstrated direct functional roles for 1,25(OH)$_2$D$_3$ in these tissues.[33–36]

In 1983, Simpson identified a specific receptor for 1,25(OH)$_2$D$_3$ in rat heart,[31] and later in cultured G-8 skeletal and H9c2 cardiac myoblast cells,[32] thus suggesting that cardiac muscle represents a target tissue for vitamin D$_3$. Walters et al.[37] also characterized a receptor for 1,25(OH)$_2$D$_3$ in a low-salt chromatin preparation from normal rat hearts. In addition, Thomasett and co-workers[38] have shown that myocardial tissue contains a vitamin D$_3$-dependent calcium-binding protein. Taken together, these observations suggest that 1,25(OH)$_2$D$_3$ may play a role in regulating calcium homeostasis in cardiac muscle.

Several studies have suggested that vitamin D$_3$ may play an important role in pathological conditions involving the heart, either through a direct action on cardiac muscle or indirectly through an effect on the level of other hormones or electrolytes. Administration of either 25-hydroxyvitamin D$_3$ (25-OHD$_3$) or 1α-hydroxyvitamin D$_3$ has been shown to improve left ventricular function in patients with cardiomyopathy subsequent to endstage renal disease.[39,40] Whether such improvement is due to restoration of a 1,25(OH)$_2$D$_3$-dependent metabolic process in cardiac muscle is not known. Scragg et al.[41] showed that a correlation exists between reduced blood levels of 25-OHD$_3$ and myocardial infarction. The possibility also exists that altered levels of vitamin D$_3$ may play a role in the changes in cardiac function which can accompany diabetes,[42] lengthy bedrest or immobilization,[43,44] and weightlessness.[44] In addition, a decrease in circulating levels of both 1,25(OH)$_2$D$_3$ and calcium occurs with increasing age.[45] This may be significant because a correlation has been demonstrated between elevated blood pressure and hypocalcemia in patient and animal models of hypertension.[40,46,47] Taken together, these studies suggest that the regulation of circulating levels of vitamin D$_3$ may have a strong impact on cardiovascular function with substantial clinical relevance.

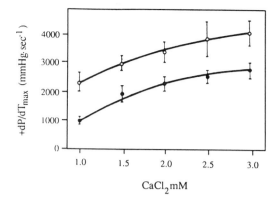

FIGURE 1 Changes in the development of left ventricular pressure (+dP/dt) in response to extracellular calcium in isolated, Langendorff-perfused hearts from rats maintained for 9 weeks on a vitamin D_3-deficient diet containing 0.4% calcium, 0.4% phosphate (open circles), or on a vitamin D_3-sufficient diet containing 0.4% calcium, 0.4% phosphate (closed circles). Each point represents the mean ± SEM of five to seven hearts. A statistically significant difference ($p < 0.05$) was observed between the two groups at each point. (From Weishaar, R. E. and Simpson, R. U., *Endocrine Review,* 10, 351, 1989, © The Endocrine Society. With permission.)

A. Effects of Vitamin D_3 on Cardiovascular Contractility

Although concentrations of $1,25(OH)_2D_3$ as high as $10^{-6} M$ do not exert an acute effect on the contractility of isolated cardiac muscle,[75] rats maintained on a vitamin D_3-deficient diet containing 0.4% calcium and 0.4% phosphate for 9 weeks exhibited a profound alteration in cardiac muscle contractile function.[48] As shown in Figure 1, large and statistically significant increases in ventricular pressure development (+dP/dt) are observed in perfused hearts from vitamin D_3-deficient rats compared to hearts from vitamin D_3-sufficient rats in response to increasing concentrations of extracellular calcium. In addition, enhanced cardiac contractile activity is observed in response to several other positive inotropic stimuli, including interventions that increase intracellular adenosine 3':5'-cyclic adenosine monophosphate (cAMP), such as dobutamine and isobutylmethylxanthine, and interventions that do not alter intracellular cAMP, such as ouabain. Whereas the maximum response to all these inotropic interventions was increased in hearts from vitamin D_3-deficient rats, it is interesting to note the sensitivity to these agents was not altered. EC_{50} values (the concentrations required to increase contractility by 50% of the maximum response) for the four inotropic stimuli studied was not significantly different when hearts from vitamin D_3-sufficient and vitamin D_3-deficient rats were compared.[75]

While lengthy periods of vitamin D_3 deficiency in rats were associated with profound changes in cardiac muscle function, it could not be stated for certain whether these changes were a direct response to vitamin D_3 deficiency or to hypocalcemia induced by vitamin D_3 depletion. To examine the relationship among vitamin D_3 deficiency, hypocalcemia, and changes in contractile function, a diet was developed that maintained serum calcium and phosphate at normal levels in vitamin D_3-deficient rats.[49] As Figure 2 illustrates, a vitamin D_3-deficient diet containing 2.5% calcium and 1.5% phosphate maintains both serum calcium and serum phosphate at normal levels. The latter diet was used to prevent or reverse hypocalcemia in vitamin D_3-deficient rats. Figure 3A shows that the profound increase in +dP/dt observed in hearts from rats maintained on the 0.4% calcium, 0.4% phosphate, vitamin D_3-deficient diet could not be prevented by maintaining vitamin D_3-deficient rats on the 2.5% calcium, 1.5% phosphate

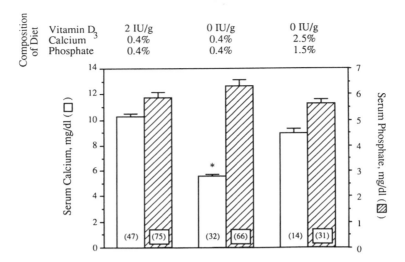

FIGURE 2   Levels of serum electrolytes after chronic administration of diets varying in calcium and phosphate
composition to vitamin D_3-sufficient and vitamin D_3-deficient rats. Each bar represents the mean ±
SEM of the number of samples in parentheses. * = p <0.05, compared to the value obtained for the
vitamin D_3-sufficient rats. (From Weishaar, R. E. and Simpson, R. U., *Endocrine Review*, 10, 351,
1989, © The Endocrine Society. With permission.)

phosphate diet. Furthermore, reversing vitamin D_3 deficiency, hypocalcemia, or both did not
return contractile function to the level observed in rats maintained throughout the study on
the vitamin D_3-sufficient diet (Figure 3B). The results of these experiments suggest that
hypocalcemia is not responsible for the change in the contractile function of isolated,
perfused hearts that accompanies lengthy periods of vitamin D_3 deficiency. Although these
results imply a direct role for vitamin D_3 in regulating cardiac contractile function, the
possibility that other hormonal factors also may be involved was not totally excluded. As
shown in Table 1, vitamin D_3 deficiency was not associated with chronic changes in
circulating catecholamines, thyroid hormones, or insulin. However, vitamin D_3 deficiency
was associated with an elevated plasma level of parathyroid hormone (PTH). Several
investigators have suggested that chronic elevations in PTH may play a role in the depression of left ventricular contractile function which has been reported in patients with
advanced renal failure.[39,40,50] Therefore, the involvement of PTH with the changes in cardiac
contractile function seems unlikely, as vitamin D_3 deficiency enhanced rather than decreased cardiac contractile function.

The results of the latter experiments, combined with the observations previously described,
demonstrate that vitamin D_3 plays an important role in regulating cardiovascular function.
Indeed, the profound increase in cardiac contractile function that is observed in vitamin D_3-
deficient rats appears to represent a direct response to vitamin D_3 deficiency.

B.   Mechanisms of Vitamin D₃ Regulation of Cardiac Contractile Function

1.   Effects of Vitamin D₃ on Calcium Regulatory Processes

The involvement of vitamin D_3 in regulating the contractile function of the heart was evaluated
at the cellular level by examining the activity of key elements that regulate calcium homeostasis and contractile activity in the cardiac myocyte. Changes in the calcium slow channel,
as determined by measuring the binding characteristics of the selective calcium slow channel
blocker [³H]nitrendipine to isolated cardiac membranes, calcium uptake by the sarcoplasmic
reticulum, as determined by measuring the postrest contraction response in isolated cardiac

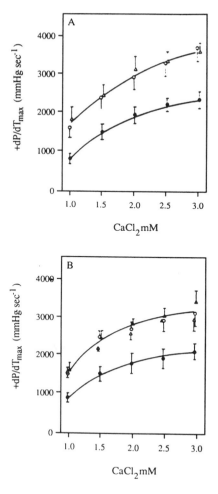

FIGURE 3   (A) Changes in the development of left ventricular pressure (+dP/dt) in response to changes in extracellular calcium in isolated, Langendorff-perfused hearts from rats maintained for 9 weeks on a vitamin D_3-deficient diet containing 0.4% calcium, 0.4% phosphate (open circles); a vitamin D_3-deficient diet containing 2.5% calcium, 1.5% phosphate (open triangles); and vitamin D_3-sufficient diet containing 0.4% calcium, 0.4% phosphate (closed circles). Each point represents the mean ± SEM of five to seven hearts. A statistically significant difference ($p < 0.05$) was observed between the two vitamin D_3-deficient groups and the vitamin D_3-sufficient group at each point. (B) Changes in development of left ventricular pressure (+dP/dt) in response to changes in extracellular calcium in isolated, Langendorff-perfused hearts isolated from rats maintained for 18 weeks on a vitamin D_3-sufficient diet (closed circles); rats maintained for 18 weeks on a vitamin D_3-deficient diet containing 0.4% calcium, 0.4% phosphate (open circles), and rats initially maintained for 9 weeks on a vitamin D_3-deficient diet containing 0.4% calcium, 0.4% phosphate, and subsequently maintained for an additional 9 weeks on either a vitamin D_3-deficient diet containing 2.5% calcium, 1.5% phosphate (open triangles) or a vitamin D_3-sufficient diet (closed triangles). Each point represents the mean ± SEM of four to seven hearts. A statistically significant difference ($p < 0.05$) was observed between the three groups originally maintained on the vitamin D_3-deficient diet and the vitamin D_3-sufficient group at each point. (From Weishaar, R. E. and Simpson, R. U., *American Journal of Physiology,* 253(Endocrinol. Metab. 16), E675, 1987, © The American Physiology Society. With permission.)

muscle, and cellular calcium uptake were examined in tissue preparations from control and vitamin D_3-deficient rats. Large decreases were observed in the number of [³H]nitrendipine binding sites on cardiac membranes. The postrest contraction response was also significantly less in heart muscle preparation from rats maintained for lengthy periods on the vitamin

TABLE 1   Levels of several hormones in plasma from vitamin D_3-sufficient and vitamin D_3-deficient rats maintained on diets containing varying amounts of calcium and phosphate

	Groups		
Hormone	Vitamin D_3-sufficient, normocalcemic rats	Vitamin D_3-deficient, hypocalcemic rats	Vitamin D_3-deficient, normocalcemic rats
$1,25(OH)_2D_3$ (pg/ml)	94.2 ± 2.4 (4)	<15[a] (4)	<15[a] (4)
$25(OH)D_3$[b] (ng/ml)	14.1	<0.1[a]	N.D.
Norepinephrine (pg/ml plasma)	384 ± 56 (5)	321 ± 59 (5)	312 ± 59 (4)
Epinephrine (pg/ml plasma)	107 ± 40 (5)	130 ± 41 (5)	104 ± 25 (6)
Dopamine (pg/ml plasma)	126 ± 10 (5)	104 ± 25 (6)	78 ± 5 (4)
T_4 (μg/100 ml plasma)	3.6 ± 0.4 (4)	4.2 ± 0.1 (4)	3.5 ± 0.2 (4)
T_3 (ng/ml plasma)	0.29 ± 0.01 (4)	0.34 ± 0.03 (4)	0.36 ± 0.02 (4)
Insulin (μU/ml plasma)	23 ± 1 (3)	28 ± 2 (4)	50 ± 18 (3)
Renin (ng AI/ml/h)	29 ± 7 (7)	33 ± 3[c] (3)	35 ± 6 (6)
PTH (pmol/l)	66 ± 17 (8)	99 ± 13[c] (3)	101 ± 23 (6)

Source: Weishaar, R. E. and Simpson, R. U., *American Journal of Physiology,* 258(Endocrinol. Metab. 21), E675, 1990, © The American Physiological Society. With permission.

Note: Data represent the mean ± SEM of the number of samples shown in parentheses. Each sample was drawn from a different rat. AI = angiotensin I.

[a] Below the level of detection (15 pg/ml for $1,25(OH)_2D_3$ and 0.1 ng/ml for $25(OH)D_3$.

[b] Value represents the level of $25(OH)D_3$ in pooled serum from five rats.

[c] p <0.05, compared to the vitamin D_3-sufficient group.

D_3-deficient, hypocalcemic diet. These changes are illustrated in Tables 2A and 2B, respectively. To determine whether these effects were directly related to vitamin D_3 deficiency or occurred secondary to the accompanying hypocalcemia, [³H]nitrendipine binding studies and postrest contraction responses also were evaluated in vitamin D_3-deficient rats maintained on the 2.5% calcium, 1.5% phosphate diet. In the latter group, the increase in [³H]nitrendipine binding sites previously observed in vitamin D_3-deficient, hypocalcemic rats was completely prevented (Table 2A). In addition, the reduction in the postrest contraction response observed in the vitamin D_3-deficient, hypocalcemic rats was completely blocked by preventing hypocalcemia (Table 2B). These observations suggest that the changes in [³H]nitrendipine binding capacity and postrest contraction response do not contribute to the changes in contractile function that accompany vitamin D_3 deficiency and are a result of hypocalcemia. Interestingly, small but reproducible increases in $^{45}Ca^{2+}$ uptake have been observed in cultured myocytes treated with 5 nM $1,25(OH)_2D_3$ for 24 h. This effect was not observed at an early time point (4 h), suggesting that the action may require *de novo* synthesis of proteins.[51] This observation was similar to data previously reported by Walters et al.[52]

TABLE 2A   Nitrendipine binding to cardiac membranes isolated from vitamin D_3-deficient and vitamin D_3-sufficient rats

Composition of diet			B_{max}	K_D
Vitamin D_3	Ca^{2+}	PO_4^-	(fmol/mg protein)	(nM)
2 IU/g	0.4%	0.4%	75 ± 7 (5)	0.30 ± 0.05 (5)
0 IU/g	0.4%	0.4%	176 ± 24[a] (5)	0.59 ± 0.04[a] (5)
0 IU/g	2.5%	1.5%	53 ± 6 (4)	0.55 ± 0.20[a] (4)

Source: Weishaar, R. E. and Simpson, R. U., *Endocrine Review,* 10, 351, 1989, © The Endocrine Society. With permission.

Note: Data represent the mean ± SEM of the number of samples in parentheses.

[a] p <0.05, compared to the vitamin D_3-sufficient group.

TABLE 2B   Postrest contraction response of left ventricular papillary muscles from vitamin D_3-deficient and vitamin D_3-sufficient rats

Composition of diet			Beats postrest (% of prerest force development after 2 min rest period)				
Vitamin D_3	Ca^{2+}	PO_4^-	1	3	5	7	9
2 IU/g	0.4%	0.4%	154 ± 11	134 ± 8	126 ± 6	119 ± 6	118 ± 6
0 IU/g	0.4%	0.4%	121 ± 4[a]	112 ± 3[a]	108 ± 3[a]	108 ± 2[a]	108 ± 2[a]
0 IU/g	2.5%	1.5%	155 ± 4	132 ± 5	124 ± 4	121 ± 4	118 ± 5

Source: Weishaar, R. E. and Simpson, R. U., *Endocrine Review,* 10, 351, 1989, © The Endocrine Society. With permission.

Note: Data represent the mean ± SEM of five to six papillary muscles from each group.

[a] p <0.05, compared to the vitamin D_3-sufficient group.

2. Effects of Vitamin D_3 on Myosin Isozyme Distribution

Another way in which cardiac contractile function can be regulated is by modulations of contractile proteins such as the myosin isozymes. It has been shown that increasing the amount of the V_1 myosin isozyme leads to increased myocardial contractility.[8] No shift in myosin isozyme distribution was observed for rats maintained for 9 weeks on the vitamin D_3-deficient, hypocalcemic diet. However, a shift toward myosin isozyme V_1 did occur for rats maintained for 9 weeks on the vitamin D_3-deficient diet containing 2.5% calcium, 1.5% phosphate.[53] These results are illustrated in Figures 4 and 5. Figure 4 depicts the electrophoretic separation and respective densitometric tracing of the three myosin isozymes from a rat maintained for 9 weeks on the vitamin D_3-sufficient diet with 0.4% calcium, 0.4% phosphate. Figure 5 shows representative densitometric tracings of the myosin isozymes for animals maintained for 9 weeks on the vitamin D_3-sufficient or vitamin D_3-deficient diet with 0.4% calcium, 0.4% phosphate and the vitamin D_3-deficient diet with 2.5% calcium, 1.5% phosphate. The findings of this study are summarized in Table 3, which shows V_3/V_1 and V_2/V_1 isozyme ratios for animals on the three diets. There was a significant (p <0.05) decrease in both the V_3/V_1 and V_2/V_1 ratios for animals on the vitamin D_3-deficient diet with 2.5% calcium, 1.5% phosphate, which suggests that vitamin D_3-deficiency induces a shift toward the V_1 myosin isozyme. A

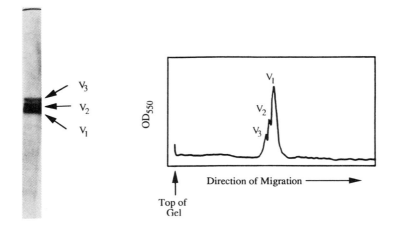

FIGURE 4 Distribution of myosin isozymes isolated from rats maintained on a 0.4% calcium, 0.4% phosphate vitamin D_3-sufficient diet for 9 weeks. A representative gel is shown on the left and the densitometric tracing of the gel is shown on the right. Peaks corresponding to the myosin isozymes are designated V_1, V_2, or V_3, respectively. (From O'Connell, T. D. and Simpson, R. U., *Endocrinology*, 134, 899, 1994, © The Endocrine Society. With permission.)

follow-up study was performed in which myosin isozyme distribution was measured in rats maintained for 9 weeks on a vitamin D_3-sufficient or -deficient diet with 2.5% calcium, 1.5% phosphate. The results are illustrated in Table 4, which shows that for animals raised on the vitamin D_3-deficient diet with 2.5% calcium, 1.5% phosphate there is a decrease in V_3/V_1 ratios, indicating a shift toward the V_1 myosin isozyme. These results corroborate the results of the first study mentioned above. These findings may partially explain the increased contractile function observed in vitamin D_3-deficient animals. However, it should be noted that in animals raised on the vitamin D_3-deficient, hypocalcemic diet, no shift in isozyme distribution occurred. These data would therefore suggest that while vitamin D_3 deficiency may regulate myosin isozyme expression, it is not the only factor leading to increased contractile function in vitamin D_3-deficient rats.

One possible explanation for rats raised on the vitamin D_3-deficient, hypocalcemic diet not expressing greater levels of the V_1 isozyme similar to animals raised on the vitamin D_3-deficient diet with 2.5% calcium, 1.5% phosphate is that these animals experienced a significant rise in blood pressure from weeks 2 through 6 of the 9-week diet regimen (Figure 6). Elevations in systolic blood pressure have been shown to increase V_3 myosin isozyme expression.[54–58] Therefore, it is likely that any increase in V_1 expression caused by vitamin D_3 deficiency in the hypocalcemic rat is offset by pressure overload-induced expression of the V_3 isozyme.

The results of the previous experiments suggest a direct action of vitamin D_3 on myosin isozyme expression. To examine if this was indeed the case, primary cultures of myocytes from 1-d-old rat hearts were used to test the effects of $1,25(OH)_2D_3$ on myosin isozyme expression. Figure 7 (lanes 1 to 5) shows the effects of increasing concentrations of $1,25(OH)_2D_3$ on myosin isozyme expression. From the gels in Figure 7 (lanes 1 to 4), it is apparent that $1,25(OH)_2D_3$ had no effect on myosin isozyme distribution but did significantly reduce total myosin levels.[53] This data is summarized in Table 5, which shows that the V_3/V_1 ratio is unaffected by $1,25(OH)_2D_3$, and total myosin levels are reduced relative to control. These experiments suggest that if $1,25(OH)_2D_3$ directly regulates myosin isozyme expression, it does so in a way not predicted by our studies using vitamin D_3-deficient rats. Those studies suggested that vitamin D_3 would increase V_3 expression or decrease V_1 expression. However,

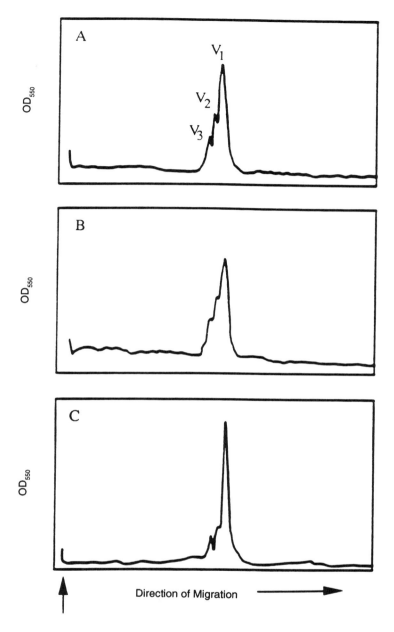

FIGURE 5 Distribution of myosin isozymes isolated from rats maintained for 9 weeks on (A) a vitamin D_3-sufficient diet containing 0.4% calcium, 0.4% phosphate; (B) a vitamin D_3-deficient diet containing 0.4% calcium, 0.4% phosphate; (C) a vitamin D_3-deficient diet containing 2.5% calcium, 1.5% phosphate. Peaks corresponding to the myosin isozymes are designated V_1, V_2, or V_3, respectively. (From O'Connell, T. D. and Simpson, R. U., *Endocrinology*, 134, 899, 1994, © The Endocrine Society. With permission.)

vitamin D_3 deficiency, by an unidentified mechanism, regulates myosin isozyme expression in the rat and may represent one of possibly several contributing factors leading to the increase in contractility observed in vitamin D_3-deficiency rats. This observation has important implications for the population of young and old that are vitamin D_3-deficient as a result of diet, environment, or disease.

TABLE 3   Relative distribution of myosin isozymes in rat ventricular muscle

Composition of diet			Distribution of myosin isozymes	
Vitamin D₃	Ca²⁺	PO₄⁻	V_3/V_1	V_2/V_1
2 IU/g	0.4%	0.4%	0.307 ± 0.045 (7)	0.428 ± 0.126 (7)
0 IU/g	0.4%	0.4%	0.284 ± 0.042 (7)	0.460 ± 0.116 (7)
0 IU/g	2.5%	1.5%	0.140 ± 0.018[a] (4)	0.231 ± 0.045[a] (4)

Source: O'Connell, T. D. and Simpson, R. U., *Endocrinology,* 134, 899, 1994, © The Endocrine Society. With permission.

Note: Data represent the mean ± SEM. The number of animal preparations is indicated in the parentheses. For each preparation at least four determinations of myosin isozyme ratios were made.

[a] $p < 0.05$, compared to vitamin D₃-sufficient groups.

TABLE 4   Relative distribution of myosin isozymes in rat ventricular muscle

Composition of diet			Distribution of myosin isozymes	
Vitamin D₃	Ca²⁺	PO₄⁻	V_3/V_1	V_2/V_1
2 IU/g	2.5%	1.5%	0.275 ± 0.036 (3)	0.607 ± 0.054 (3)
0 IU/g	2.5%	1.5%	0.121 ± 0.011[a] (3)	0.198 ± 0.015[a] (3)

Source: O'Connell, T. D. and Simpson, R. U., *Endocrinology,* 134, 899, 1994, © The Endocrine Society. With permission.

Note: Data represent the mean ± SEM. The number of animal preparations is indicated in parentheses. For each preparation at least four determinations of myosin isozyme ratios were made.

[a] $p < 0.0005$, compared to vitamin D₃-sufficient groups.

C.   Effects of Vitamin D₃ on Cardiovascular Morphology and Gene Expression

The potential effects of vitamin D₃ deficiency on the physical and morphological properties of the heart have been studied. As can be seen in Table 6, lengthy periods of vitamin D₃ deficiency were associated with a significant increase in heart weight to body weight ratio. This increase appears to represent a direct response to vitamin D₃ deficiency because it could not be averted by preventing hypocalcemia in vitamin D₃-deficient rats or reversed by restoring serum calcium to normal in vitamin D₃-deficient rats after an initial period of hypocalcemia. In addition, the increase in heart weight to body weight ratio was not accompanied by any evidence of myocardial edema or leakage of myocardial creatine phosphokinase. Interpretation of the changes in heart weight to body weight ratios were complicated by the fact that vitamin D₃-deficient rats gained slightly less weight than the vitamin D₃-replete rats. However, organ weight to body weight ratios for the kidneys, stomach, liver, and spleen were unchanged by vitamin D₃ deficiency,[75] suggesting that the increase in heart weight to body weight ratio was an organ-specific action of vitamin D₃ deficiency on the heart.

To obtain a clear understanding of the potential for physical changes to the heart during vitamin D₃ deficiency, thin sections of myocardial tissue were prepared from both vitamin D₃-

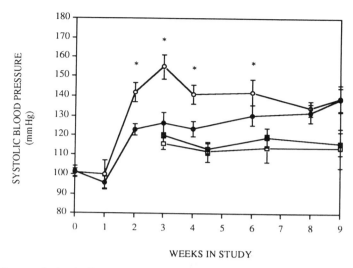

FIGURE 6 Influence of vitamin D_3 and dietary calcium on systolic blood pressure in rats. Blood pressure measurements for rats maintained for 9 weeks on a 0.4% calcium, 0.4% phosphate vitamin D_3-deficient (open circles) or vitamin D_3-sufficient diet (closed circles), or for 9 weeks on a 2.5% calcium, 1.5% phosphate vitamin D_3-deficient (open squares) or vitamin D_3-sufficient diet (closed squares). Data are representative of three separate time course experiments with triplicate measurements of each rat at the times indicated.

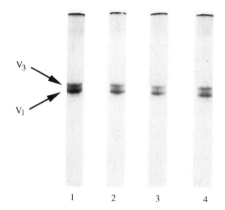

FIGURE 7 Distribution of myosin isozymes from primary cultures of rat ventricular myocytes treated for 72 h with (lane 1) 0.1% ethanol (all groups contained 0.1% ethanol); (lane 2) 1 nM 1,25(OH)$_2$D$_3$; (lane 3) 10 nM 1,25(OH)$_2$D$_3$; (lane 4) 100 nM 1,25(OH)$_2$D$_3$. Isozymes V_1 and V_3 are designated. (From O'Connell, T. D. and Simpson, R. U., *Endocrinology*, 134, 899, 1994, © The Endocrine Society. With permission.)

sufficient and vitamin D_3-deficient rats and examined microscopically (Figure 8). The results demonstrated that rather than increasing in size, total myofibrillar area was significantly reduced in the vitamin D_3-deficient rats (from $86.1 \pm 1.7\%$ to $74.0 \pm 4.1\%$, $p < 0.05$). This reduction was accompanied by a doubling in nonmyofibrillar material in hearts from the vitamin D_3-deficient rats (from $13.3 \pm 1.6\%$ to $25.5 \pm 4.0\%$, $p < 0.05$). In addition, both average myofibrillar area and average maximum fibril diameter were decreased (from 169.5 ± 24.1 mm^2 to 105.1 ± 9.3 mm^2, $p < 0.05$, and from 17.7 ± 1.5 mm to 13.3 ± 0.6 mm, $p < 0.05$, respectively) while the number of myofibrils per region scanned increased (from 58 ± 7 to 75 ± 6, $p < 0.05$). These results suggest that vitamin D_3 deficiency causes an increase in extracellular matrix material and myocyte hyperplasia.[59] The combination of these effects may account for the increase in heart weight to body weight ratio that accompanies vitamin D_3 deficiency.

TABLE 5   Relative distribution of myosin isozymes in primary cultures of ventricular myocytes from 1-d-old rats

$1,25(OH)_2D_3$ concentration (nM)[a]	Distribution of myosin isozymes, V_3/V_1	Total myosin (% of control)
0	0.622 ± 0.055 (3)	100
1	0.578 ± 0.064 (3)	56.63 ± 10.76[b]
10	0.582 ± 0.156 (3)	42.90 ± 4.87[b]
100	0.660 ± 0.043 (3)	64.53 ± 5.17[b]

Source: O'Connell, T. D. and Simpson, R. U., *Endocrinology,* 134, 899, 1994, © The Endocrine Society. With permission.

Note: Data represent the mean ± SEM. The number of determinations from individual cultures is in parentheses.

[a] Ethanol concentration 0.1% in all conditions.

[b] $p < 0.05$, compared to ETOH-treated group.

TABLE 6   Heart weight/body weight ratios for vitamin D₃-sufficient and vitamin D₃-deficient rats maintained on diets containing varying amounts of calcium and phosphate

Composition of diet			Duration of treatment (weeks)	Heart wt/body wt (×1000)
Vitamin D₃	Ca²⁺	PO₄⁻		
Prevention Study				
2 IU/g	0.4%	0.4%	9	3.06 ± 0.09 (14)
0 IU/g	0.4%	0.4%	9	3.50 ± 0.24[a] (10)
0 IU/g	2.5%	1.5%	9	3.71 ± 0.21[a] (6)
Reversibility Study				
2 IU/g	0.4%	0.4%	18	2.70 ± 0.059 (9)
0 IU/g	0.4%	0.4%	18	3.38 ± 0.10[a] (9)
0 IU/g	0.4%	0.4%	9	3.46 ± 0.09[a] (4)

Source: Weishaar, R. E. and Simpson, R. U., *American Journal of Physiology,* 253(Endocrinol. Metab. 16), E675, 1987, © The American Physiological Society. With permission.

Note: Data represent the mean ± SEM of the number of animals in parentheses.

[a] $p < 0.05$, compared to the vitamin D₃-sufficient group.

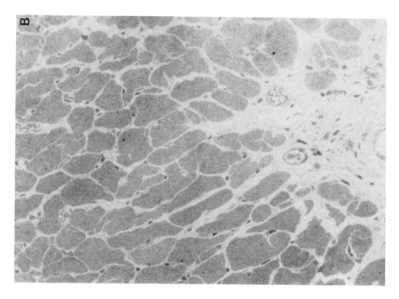

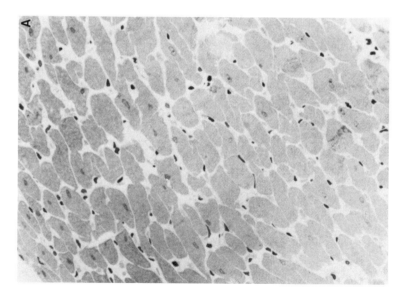

FIGURE 8 Representative examples of cross-sections of ventricular muscle prepared from rats maintained for 9 weeks on a vitamin D_3-sufficient (A) or -deficient (B) diet containing 0.4% calcium, 0.4% phosphate. The original magnification factor was 400× for both A and B. (From Weishaar, R. E. and Simpson, R. U., American Journal of Physiology, 258(Endocrinol. Metab. 21), E675, 1990, © The American Society of Physiology. With permission.)

TABLE 7   Collagen content of ventricular muscle of vitamin
D_3-sufficient and vitamin D_3-deficient rats
maintained on diets containing varying amounts of
calcium and phosphate

Composition of diet			Myocardial collagen
Vitamin D_3	Ca^{2+}	PO_4^-	(µg hydroxyproline/g wet wt)
2 IU/g	0.4%	0.4%	244.3 ± 13.5 (18)
0 IU/g	0.4%	0.4%	310.3 ± 12.4[a] (17)
0 IU/g	2.5%	1.5%	306.0 ± 41.3[a] (10)

Source: Weishaar, R. E., and Simpson, R. U., *American Journal of Physiology,* 258(Endocrinol. Metab. 21), E675, 1990, © The American Physiological Society. With permission.

Note: Data represent the mean ± SEM of the number of separate samples shown in parentheses.

[a] $p < 0.05$, compared to the vitamin D_3-sufficient group.

1.   Effects of Vitamin D_3 on Myocardial Collagen Levels

To characterize the nature of the increase in nonmyofibrillar material, myocardial collagen levels were measured in hearts from vitamin D_3-sufficient and vitamin D_3-deficient rats. As shown in Table 7, a significant increase in the levels of collagen was observed in myocardial tissue from rats maintained for 9 weeks on a vitamin D_3-deficient diet containing 0.4% calcium, 0.4% phosphate compared to rats maintained on a vitamin D_3-sufficient diet. This increase in myocardial collagen, like the previously described increases in heart weight to body weight ratio and cardiac contractile function, appeared to be a direct response to vitamin D_3 deficiency, because the increase could not be prevented by preventing hypocalcemia (Table 7). The relationship between the vitamin D_3-dependent increases in the heart weight to body weight ratio and myocardial collagen and the vitamin D_3-dependent changes in cardiac contractile function is unclear at the present time. This relationship is complicated by the fact that at least five genetically distinct subclasses of collagen have been characterized that can respond independently of each other.[60,61] Interestingly, Raisz and co-workers[62] have shown that in cultured bone cells from vitamin D_3-depleted rat fetuses, low concentrations of vitamin D_3 metabolites inhibit collagen synthesis. The rate of collagen synthesis is also enhanced in cartilage from vitamin D_3-deficient chicks.[63]

Investigations of the relationship between ventricular collagen content and the contractile properties of the heart have often reached contradictory conclusions.[64–66] This confusion may be due to several factors including differences in the animal models used, differences in the age of the animals studied (mature vs. immature), and differences in the experimental procedure used to determine mechanical properties. Bing and co-workers[67] examined the relationship among hypertrophy, myocardial collagen content, and the mechanical properties of the heart and demonstrated that both ventricular hypertrophy and increases in ventricular collagen appear to contribute to the alterations in cardiac contractile function.

2.   Effects of Vitamin D_3 on c-*myc* Expression in the Heart

To define the cause of the myocyte hyperplasia observed in vitamin D_3-deficient rats, the expression of the c-*myc* protooncogene was analyzed. $1,25(OH)_2D_3$ was shown to regulate the transcription of c-*myc* in HL-60 cells, tonsillar T lymphocytes, and U937 myelomonocytic

c-myc

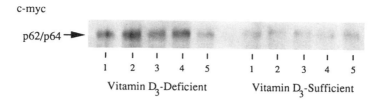

p62/p64 →

| 1   2   3   4   5   1   2   3   4   5 |
| Vitamin D₃-Deficient   Vitamin D₃-Sufficient |

FIGURE 9   Effect of vitamin D_3 depletion on c-*myc* protein levels in rat heart. Rats were maintained for 9 weeks either on a vitamin D_3-sufficient or a vitamin D_3-deficient diet containing 2.5% calcium, 1.5% phosphate. c-*myc* protein levels were determined by Western blot. The figure shows a representative Western blot depicting the c-*myc* 62/64 kDa doublet. Each lane represents protein samples from one rat.

c-myc

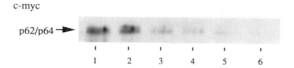

p62/p64 →

| 1   2   3   4   5   6 |

FIGURE 10   c-*myc* protein levels in primary cultures of rat ventricular myocytes treated for 72 h with: (lane 1) 0.1% ethanol (all groups contained 0.1% ethanol; (lane 2) 0.1 nM 1,25(OH)$_2$D$_3$; (lane 3) 1 nM 1,25(OH)$_2$D$_3$; (lane 4) 10 nM 1,25(OH)$_2$D$_3$; (lane 5) 100 nM 1,25(OH)$_2$D$_3$; and (lane 6) 600 nM 1,25(OH)$_2$D$_3$. The figure shows a representative Western blot depicting the c-*myc* 62/64 kDa doublet.

c-myc

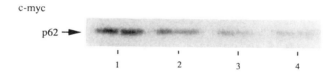

p62 →

| 1   2   3   4 |

FIGURE 11   c-*myc* protein levels in H9c2 cells treated for 72 h with: (lane 1) 0.1% ethanol (all groups contained 0.1% ethanol); (lane 2) 1 nM 1,25(OH)$_2$D$_3$; (lane 3) 10 nM 1,25(OH)$_2$D$_3$; (lane 4) 100 nM 1,25(OH)$_2$D$_3$. The figure shows a representative Western blot depicting the c-*myc* 62 kDa protein.

cells.[68–72] The down regulation of c-*myc* expression is also associated with cellular growth and differentiation in HL-60 cells.[68] In addition, Jackson et al.[73] used transgenic mice to demonstrate that overexpression of the c-*myc* gene in the heart causes myocyte hyperplasia. Therefore, we chose to examine c-*myc* protein levels in vitamin D_3-deficient rats. Figure 9 shows a Western blot for c-*myc* proteins isolated from animals maintained for 9 weeks on a vitamin D_3-sufficient or -deficient diet with 2.5% calcium, 1.5% phosphate. From this figure it is apparent that vitamin D_3 deficiency led to increased levels of c-*myc* and protein. The preceding observation suggests that vitamin D_3 deficiency directly regulates myocardial c-*myc* levels. To determine if the effect of vitamin D_3 deficiency to regulate c-*myc* was a direct effect of 1,25(OH)$_2$D$_3$ on myocytes and not other myocardial cell types, we measured c-*myc* protein levels in primary myocyte cultures from 1-d-old rat hearts treated with 1,25(OH)$_2$D$_3$. Figure 10 depicts a Western blot for the c-*myc* protein extracted from cultures treated with increasing concentrations of 1,25(OH)$_2$D$_3$. The results suggest that treatment with 1,25(OH)$_2$D$_3$ decreases c-*myc* protein levels in myocytes. Furthermore, to analyze myocyte proliferation in response to 1,25(OH)$_2$D$_3$, H9c2 cardiac myoblast cells were used. Figure 11 shows a Western blot for the c-*myc* protein from H9c2 cells treated with increasing concentrations of 1,25(OH)$_2$D$_3$. The decrease in c-*myc* protein levels caused by increasing 1,25(OH)$_2$D$_3$ concentration in the medium is consistent with the results seen with the primary cultured myocytes. In addition, cell growth and DNA synthesis were inhibited by 1,25(OH)$_2$D$_3$ treatment in the H9c2 cells (Figure 12). This suggests that 1,25(OH)$_2$D$_3$ regulates c-*myc* and cell growth in the H9c2 cells.

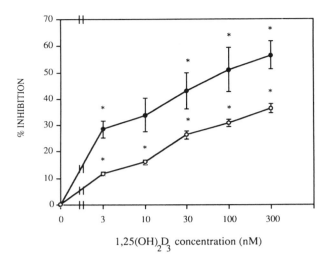

1,25(OH)₂D₃ concentration (nM)

FIGURE 12   Effects of $1,25(OH)_2D_3$ on DNA synthesis (closed circles) and cell proliferation (open circles) in the H9c2 cardiac myoblast cell line. H9c2 cells were treated for 72 h with the indicated concentrations of $1,25(OH)_2D_3$ (ethanol concentration 0.1% in all conditions). DNA synthesis was determined by [³H]thymidine incorporation, and cell growth was determined by cell number (EtOH concentration 0.1%). Data are expressed as % inhibition of control ethanol vehicle ± SEM. (*$p < 0.05$.)

The findings that c-*myc* protein levels are increased by vitamin D_3 deficiency and that $1,25(OH)_2D_3$ appears to regulate c-*myc* protein levels in cultured myocytes may explain the myocyte hyperplasia observed in the vitamin D_3-deficient rat heart.[59]

The results of the preceding studies demonstrate that lengthy periods of vitamin D_3 deficiency are associated with profound changes in the physical and morphological characteristics of the myocardium. As with the previously described increase in cardiac contractile function, increases in heart weight to body weight ratio, and increases in myocardial collagen levels that accompany vitamin D_3 deficiency, myocyte hyperplasia appears to represent a direct response to vitamin D_3 rather than a response to hypocalcemia. In addition, myocyte hyperplasia is correlated with increased c-*myc* levels in the heart, which has been suggested to cause myocyte hyperplasia.[73] These findings are corroborated by the studies in both primary cultures of ventricular myocytes and H9c2 cells, which show that $1,25(OH)_2D_3$ regulates c-*myc* protein levels. However, the precise role that changes in the physical and morphological properties of the myocardium which accompany vitamin D_3 deficiency have in the observed changes in myocardial contractile function (also observed in vitamin D_3-deficient rats) remains to be established.

III. CONCLUSION

Conventional approaches to characterizing the events that modulate myocardial function have tended to focus on factors such as the sympathetic and parasympathetic nervous systems, which via local release of various neurotransmitters can influence the inotropic and chronotropic activities of the heart. Other approaches have emphasized the role that pathological events such as hypoxia and ischemia play in altering myocardial contractility. Although these various factors all play a critical role in regulating contractile function, particularly on a beat-to-beat basis, investigations in a number of laboratories over the last decade have provided clear evidence to indicate that the endocrine system also plays an important role in modulating the performance of the heart. Studies by Morkin, Sonnenblick, Nadal-Ginard, Dhalla, and others have demonstrated that both thyroid hormone and insulin exert a major influence on the pumping capacity of the heart via alterations in the activity of key cellular processes involved in regulating calcium homeostasis and contractile activity in the cardiac cell.[2,14,54,74]

The hormone $1,25(OH)_2D_3$, the active metabolite of vitamin D_3, was shown to play an important role in regulating the function and physical characteristics of the heart. Weishaar and Simpson[49] demonstrated that vitamin D_3 deficiency causes an increase in myocardial contractility, and that this is the direct result of vitamin D_3 deficiency and not due to hypocalcemia that accompanies vitamin D_3 deficiency. It was also shown that the increase in contractility in the vitamin D_3-deficient rat heart was, at least in part, due to a shift in myosin isozyme distribution, which did not appear to be caused by hypocalcemia. However, from *in vitro* studies of primary cultures of ventricular myocytes treated with $1,25(OH)_2D_3$, it appears likely that this effect was not mediated directly by $1,25(OH)_2D_3$.[53] In addition to the changes in contractility that were observed, vitamin D_3 deficiency produces significant alterations in myocardial morphology. Vitamin D_3 deficiency causes an increase in heart to body weight ratio, which is not the result of hypocalcemia, suggesting that vitamin D_3 deficiency causes myocardial hypertrophy. Examinations of cross-sections of ventricular muscle, however, revealed that rather than a cellular hypertrophy, the increase in heart size was caused by a combination of increased collagen content and myocyte hyperplasia. Further studies revealed that myocardial levels of c-*myc* protein were increased in the hearts of these animals, which may be responsible for the myocyte hyperplasia. Studies in primary cultures of ventricular myocytes and H9c2 cardiac myoblast cells suggest that $1,25(OH)_2D_3$ directly regulates c-*myc* protein levels.[59] Although it appears clear that vitamin D_3 does regulate myocardial morphology, it remains to be determined if a direct link exists between changes induced by vitamin D_3 deficiency on the physical and morphological characteristics of the ventricular wall and alterations in contractility.

None of the three endocrine hormones mentioned — thyroid hormone, insulin or vitamin D_3 — exerts an acute effect on cardiac morphology or contractile function; rather, lengthy periods of hyper- or hypothyroidism, diabetes, or vitamin D_3 deficiency are required to produce measurable changes in cardiac structure and function. This suggests that the role that these endogenous substances play may be an adaptive one and may represent a mechanism for modifying the heart to adjust to altered hemodynamic loads caused by chronic changes in cardiovascular function induced by such states as hypertension, diabetes, and aging.

The possibility also exists that different endocrine hormones act synergistically to influence the heart, or that hormones can exert both direct and indirect effects on cardiovascular metabolism. Such possibilities could explain the observation that both insulin and thyroid hormone have been shown to alter the distribution of myosin enzymes. In addition, the observation that PTH levels can increase in response to vitamin D_3 deficiency suggests that the effects of vitamin D_3 deficiency on cardiovascular function may be influenced by PTH.

The existence of humoral factors capable of rapidly altering the contractile performance of the heart, such as catecholamines, as well as factors such as thyroid hormone, insulin, and $1,25(OH)_2D_3$ that alter gene expression and thus remodel the morphology of the heart, suggests the availability of both "short-term" and "long-term" planning for the heart. Such a dual system for regulating contractile function would enable the heart to alter its output in response to both acute and chronic environmental changes and still maintain steady perfusion of all peripheral organs and cells. The existence of both short- and long-term regulatory systems also suggests that future therapy for cardiovascular disorders such as heart failure and hypertension may be more properly directed toward those hormones that are responsible for the long-term regulation of heart function. Such an approach, by remodeling the diseased heart rather than simply providing acute relief of symptoms, may provide the means for actually reversing myocardial dysfunction, or at least retarding its progression.

REFERENCES

1. Goldman, S., Olajas, M., and Freidman, H., Left ventricular performance in conscious thyrotoxic calves, *Am. J. Physiol.*, 242, H113, 1981.
2. Morkin, E. and Flink, I. L., Biochemical and physiological effects of thyroid hormones on cardiac performance, *Prog. Cardiovasc. Dis.*, 25, 435, 1983.
3. Goodkind, M. J., Damback, G. E., and Thyrum, P. T., Effect of thyroxine on ventricular myocardial contractility and ATPase activity in guinea pigs, *Am. J. Physiol.*, 226, 66, 1974.
4. Korecky, B. and Beznak, M., Effect of thyroxine on growth and function in cardiac muscle, in *Cardiac Hypertrophy*, Alpert, N. R., Ed., Academic Press, New York, 1971, 55.
5. Hoh, J. Y., McGrath, P. A., and Hale, P. T., Electrophoretic analysis of rat cardiac myosin: effects of hypophysectomy and thyroxine replacement, *J. Mol. Cell. Cardiol.*, 10, 1053, 1977.
6. Chizzonite, R. A. and Zak, R., Regulation of myosin isoenzyme composition in fetal and neonatal rat ventricle by endogenous thyroid hormone, *J. Biol. Chem.*, 259, 12628, 1984.
7. Lompre, A. M., Nadal-Ginard, B., and Mahdavi, V., Expression of the cardiac ventricular α- and β-myosin heavy chain genes is developmentally and hormonally regulated, *J. Biol. Chem.*, 259, 6437, 1984.
8. Schwartz, K., Lecarpentier, Y., Martin, J. L., Lompre, A. M., Mercadier, J. J., and Swynghedauw, B., Myosin isoenzymatic distribution correlates with the speed of myocardial contraction, *J. Mol. Cell. Cardiol.*, 13, 1071, 1981.
9. Regan, T. J., Lyons, M. M., Ahmed, S. S., Levinson, G. E., Oldewurtle, H. A., Ahmed, M. R., and Haider, B., Evidence for cardiomyopathy in familial diabetes mellitus, *J. Clin. Invest.*, 60, 885, 1977.
10. Shah, S., Cardiomyopathy in diabetes mellitus, *Angiology*, 31, 502, 1980.
11. Shapiro, L. M., Leatherdale, B. A., Cayne, M. E., Fletcher, R. F., and Mackinnon, J., Prospective study of heart disease in untreated maturity onset diabetes, *Br. Heart J.*, 44, 342, 1980.
12. D'Elia, J. A., Weinrauch, L. A., Healy, R. W., Libertino, R. W., Bradley, R. F., and Leland, O. S., Myocardial dysfunction without coronary artery disease in diabetic renal failure, *Am. J. Cardiol.*, 43, 193, 1979.
13. Morgan, H. E., Cadenos, E., Regen, D. M., and Park, C. R., Regulation of glucose uptake in muscle. II. Rate limiting steps and effects of insulin and anoxia in heart muscle from diabetic rats, *J. Biol. Chem.*, 236, 262, 1961.
14. Dhalla, N. S., Pierce, G. N., Innes, I. R., and Beamisk, R. E., Pathogenesis of cardiac dysfunction in diabetes mellitus, *Can. J. Cardiol.*, 1, 263, 1985.
15. Rodrigues, B., Goyal, R. K., and McNeill, J. H., Effects of hydralizine on streptozotocin-induced diabetic rats: prevention of hyperlipidemia and improvement of cardiac function, *J. Pharmacol. Exp. Ther.*, 237, 292, 1976.
16. Penpargkal, S., Fein, F., Sonnenblick, E. H., and Scheuer, J., Depressed cardiac sarcoplasmic reticular function in diabetic rats, *J. Mol. Cell. Cardiol.*, 13, 303, 1981.
17. Ganguly, P. K., Pierce, G. N., Dhalla, K. S., and Dhalla, N. S., Defective sarcoplasmic reticular calcium transport in diabetic cardiomyopathy, *Am. J. Physiol.*, 244, E528, 1983.
18. Pierce, G. N. and Dhalla, N. S., Mitochondrial abnormalities in diabetic cardiomyopathy, *Can. J. Cardiol.*, 1, 48, 1985.
19. Malhorta, A., Penpargkul, S., Fein, F. S., Sonnenblick, E. H., and Scheuer, J., The effect of streptozocin-induced diabetes on cardiac contractile proteins, *Circ. Res.*, 49, 1243, 1981.
20. Pollack, P. S., Malhorta, A., Fein, F. S., and Scheuer, J., Effects of diabetes on cardiac contractile proteins in rabbits and reversal with insulin, *Am. J. Physiol.*, 251, H448, 1986.
21. Orr, W. J., Holt, L. E., Wilkins, L., and Boone, F. H., Calcium and phosphate metabolism in rickets, with special reference to ultraviolet ray therapy, *Am. J. Dis. Child.*, 26, 362, 1923.
22. Nicolaysen, R., Peg-Larsen, N., and Mahn, O. J., Physiology of calcium metabolism, *Physiol. Rev.*, 32, 424, 1952.
23. Wasserman, R. H. and Taylor, A. N., Vitamin D$_3$ inhibition of radiocalcium binding by chick intestinal homogenates, *Nature*, 198, 30, 1963.
24. DeLuca, H. F. and Schndes, H. L., Vitamin D$_3$. Recent advances, *Annu. Rev. Biochem.*, 52, 411, 1983.

25. Norman, A. W., Hormonal actions of vitamin D₃, *Curr. Top. Cell. Regul.*, 24, 35, 1984.

26. Rasmussen, H., Matsumoto, T., Fontaine, O., and Goodman, D. B. P., Role of changes in membrane lipid structure in the action of 1,25-dihydroxyvitamin D₃, *Fed. Proc.*, 41, 72, 1982.

27. Wasserman, R. H. and Fullner, C. S., Calcium transport proteins, calcium absorption and vitamin D, *Annu. Rev. Physiol.*, 45, 375, 1983.

28. Stern, P. H., Vitamin D and bone, *Kidney Int.*, 38(Suppl. 29), S17, 1990.

29. Simpson, R. U. and DeLuca, H. F., Characterization of receptor-like protein for 1,25-dihydroxyvitamin D₃ in rat skin, *Proc. Natl. Acad. Sci. U.S.A.*, 77, 5822, 1980.

30. Christakos, S. and Norman, A. W., Studies on the mode of action of calciferol. XXIV. Biochemical characterization of 1,25-dihydroxyvitamin D₃ receptors in chick pancreas and kidney cytosol, *Endocrinology*, 108, 140, 1981.

31. Simpson, R. U., Evidence for a specific 1,25-dihydroxyvitamin D₃ receptor in rat heart, *Circulation*, 68(Abstr.), 239, 1983.

32. Simpson, R. U., Thomas, G. A., and Arnold, A. J., Identification of 1,25-dihydroxyvitamin D₃ receptors and activities in muscle, *J. Biol. Chem.*, 260, 8882, 1985.

33. Hosoi, J., Abe, E., Suda, T., and Kuroki, T., Regulation of melanin synthesis of B₁₆ mouse melanoma cells by 1-alpha, 25-dihydroxyvitamin D₃ and retinoic acid, *Cancer Res.*, 45, 1474, 1985.

34. Norman, A. W., Roth, J., and Orci, L., The vitamin D endocrine system, *Endocr. Rev.*, 3, 331, 1982.

35. Schot, G. D. and Willis, M. R., Muscle weakness and osteomalacia, *Lancet*, 1, 626, 1976.

36. Rodman, J. S. and Baker, J., Changes in the kinetics of muscle contraction in vitamin D-depleted rats, *Kidney Int.*, 13, 109, 1978.

37. Walters, M. R., Wicker, D. C., and Riggle, P. C., 1,25-Dihydroxyvitamin D₃ receptors identified in the rat heart, *J. Mol. Cell. Cardiol.*, 18, 67, 1986.

38. Thomasett, M., Parkes, C. D., and Cuiseier-Eleizes, P., Rat calcium-binding proteins; distribution, development, and vitamin D-dependence, *Am. J. Physiol.*, 243, E483, 1982.

39. Coratelli, P., Petratulo, F., Biongiorno, E., Giannattasio, M., Antonelli, G., and Amerio, A., Improvement of left ventricular function during treatment of hemodialysis patients with 25-OHD₃, *Contrib. Nephrol.*, 41, 433, 1984.

40. McGonigle, R. J. S., Fowler, M. B., Timimis, A. B., Weston, M. J., and Parsons, V., Uremic cardiomyopathy: potential role of vitamin D and parathyroid hormone, *Nephrology*, 36, 94, 1984.

41. Scragg, R., Jackson, R., Holdaway, I. M., Lim, T., and Beaglehole, R., Myocardial infarction is inversely associated with plasma 25-hydroxyvitamin D₃ levels: a community-based study, *Int. J. Epidemiol.*, 19, 559, 1990.

42. Nixon, J. V., Murray, R. G., Bryant, C., Johnson, R. J., Mitchell, J. H., Holland, O. B., Gomez, S. C., Vergne, M. P., and Blomqvist, C. G., Early cardiovascular adaptation to simulated zero gravity, *J. Appl. Physiol.*, 46, 541, 1979.

43. Coratelli, P., Petrarulo, F., Giannattasio, M., Buongiorno, E., Passavanti, G., Antonelli, G., Capurso, A., Ferrannini, E., and Amerio, A., Clinical and metabolic effects of long-term treatment with 25(OH)D₃ in hemodialysis, *Contrib. Nephrol.*, 49, 20, 1985.

44. Leach, C. S., Altchular, S. I., and Cintron-Trivino, N. M., Circulating 1,25-(OH)₂D₃ decreased following prolonged weightlessness, *Med. Sci. Sports Exercise*, 15, 432, 1983.

45. Fugisawa, Y., Kaichi, K., and Matsuda, H., Role of change in vitamin D metabolism with age in calcium and phosphorus metabolism in normal human subjects, *Clin. Endocrinol. Metab.*, 59, 719, 1984.

46. McCarron, D. A., Yung, N. N., Ugoretz, I. A., and Krutzik, S., Disturbances of calcium metabolism in the spontaneously hypertensive rat, *Hypertension*, 3, I162, 1981.

47. McCarron, D. A., Lucas, P. A., Schneidman, B., and Lacour, B., Blood pressure development of the spontaneously hypertensive rat after concurrent manipulations of dietary Ca+ and Na+, *J. Clin. Invest.*, 76, 1147, 1985.

48. Weishaar, R. E. and Simpson, R. U., Vitamin D₃ and cardiovascular function in rats, *J. Clin. Invest.*, 79, 1706, 1987.

49. Weishaar, R. E. and Simpson, R. U., Involvement of vitamin D₃ with cardiovascular function. II. Direct and indirect effects, *Am. J. Physiol.*, 253, E675, 1987.

50. Massry, S. G., Parathyroid hormone and uremic myocardiopathy, *Contrib. Nephrol.*, 41, 231, 1984.

51. Simpson, R. U. and Weishaar, R. E., Involvement of 1,25-dihydroxyvitamin D₃ in regulating myocardial calcium metabolism: physiological and pathological actions, *Cell Calcium*, 9, 285, 1988.

52. Walters, M. R., Ilenchuk, T. T., and Claycomb, W. C., 1,25-Dihydroxyvitamin D₃ stimulates $^{45}Ca^{2+}$ uptake by cultured adult rat ventricular cardiac muscle cells, *J. Biol. Chem.*, 262, 2536, 1987.

53. O'Connell, T. D., Weishaar, R. E., and Simpson, R. U., Regulation of myosin isozyme expression by vitamin D₃ deficiency and 1,25 dihydroxy-vitamin D₃ in the rat heart, *Endocrinology*, 134, 899, 1994.

54. Izumo, S., Lompre, A. M., Matsuoka, R., Koren, G., Schwartz, K., Nadal-Ginard, B., and Mahdavi, V., Myosin heavy chain messenger RNA and protein isoform transitions during cardiac hypertrophy. Interaction between hemodynamic and thyroid hormone-induced signals, *J. Clin. Invest.*, 79, 970, 1987.

55. Mahdavi, V., Izumo, S., and Nadal-Ginard, B., Developmental and hormonal regulation of sarcomeric myosin heavy chain gene family, *Circ. Res.*, 60, 804, 1987.

56. Mahdavi, V., Matsuoka, R., and Nadal-Ginard, B., Molecular characterization and expression of the cardiac α- and β-myosin heavy chain gene, in *Cardiac Morphogenesis*, Ferrans, V. J., Rosenquist, G., and Weinstein, C., Eds., Elsevier, Amsterdam, 1985, 2.

57. Matsuoka, R., Nadal-Ginard, B., and Mahdavi, V., α- and β-Myosin heavy chain gene expression in response to systolic overload hypertrophy (abstract), *Circulation*, 70(Suppl. II), 196, 1984.

58. Imamura, S. I., Matsuoka, R., Hiratsuka, E., Kimura, M., Nakanishi, T., Nishikawa, T., Furutani, Y., and Takao, A., Adaptational changes of MHC gene expression and isozyme transition in cardiac overloading, *Am. J. Physiol.*, 260, H73, 1991.

59. O'Connell, T. D. and Simpson, R. U., The effects of vitamin D₃ on myocardial cell growth and c-*myc* expression, manuscript in preparation, 1994.

60. Bornstein, P. and Sage, H., Structurally distinct collagen types, *Am. Rev. Biochem.*, 49, 957, 1980.

61. Medugorac, I. and Jacob, R., Characterization of left ventricular collagen in the rat, *Cardiovasc. Res.*, 17, 15, 1983.

62. Raisz, L. G., Maina, D. M., Gworek, S. G., Dietrich, J. W., and Canalis, E. M., Hormonal control of bone collagen synthesis in vitro: inhibitory effect of 1-hydroxylated vitamin D₃ metabolites, *Endocrinology*, 102, 731, 1978.

63. Canas, F., Brand, J. S., Neuman, W. F., and Terepka, A. R., Some effects of vitamin D₃ on collagen synthesis in rachitic chicks cortical bone, *Am. J. Physiol.*, 216, 1092, 1969.

64. Weisfeldt, M. L., Lowen, W. A., and Shock, N. W., Resting and active mechanical properties of trabeculae corneal from aged rats, *Am. J. Physiol.*, 220, 1921, 1971.

65. Lee, J. C. and Downing, S. E., Left ventricular distensibility in new born piglets, adult swine, young kittens, and adult cats, *Am. J. Physiol.*, 226, 1484, 1974.

66. Cappelli, V., Forni, R., Poggesi, C., Reggiani, C., and Riccardi, L., Age dependent variations of diastolic stiffness and collagen content in rat ventricular myocardium, *Arch. Int. Physiol. Biochem.*, 92, 93, 1984.

67. Bing, O. H. L., Fanburg, B. L., Brooks, W. W., and Matsushita, S., The effect of the lathyrogen β-amino propionitrelo (BAPN) on the mechanical properties of experimentally hypertrophied rat cardiac muscle, *Circ. Res.*, 43, 632, 1978.

68. Miyaura, C., Abe, T., Kuribayeshi, T., Tanaka, H., Konno, K., Nishii, Y., and Suda, T., 1,25 Dihydroxyvitamin D₃ induces differentiation of human myeloid cells, *Biochem. Biophys. Res. Commun.*, 102, 937, 1981.

69. Reitsma, P. H., Rothberg, P. G., Astrin, S. M., Trial, J., Bar, S. Z., Hall, A., Teitelbaum, S. L., and Kahn, A. J., Regulation of myc gene expression in HL-60 leukemia cells by a vitamin D metabolite, *Nature*, 306, 492, 1983.

70. Simpson, R. U., Hsu, T., Begley, D. A., Mitchell, B. S., and Alizadeh, B. N., Transcriptional regulation of the c-myc protooncogene by 1,25-dihydroxyvitamin D_3 in HL-60 promyelocytic leukemic cells, *J. Biol. Chem.*, 262, 4104, 1987.

71. Karmali, R., Bhalla, A. K., Farrow, S. M., Williams, M. M., Lal, S., Lydyard, P. M., and O'Riordan, J. L., Early regulation of c-myc mRNA by 1,25-dihydroxyvitamin D_3 in human myelomonocytic U937 cells, *J. Mol. Endocrinol.*, 3, 43, 1989.

72. Karmali, R., Hewison, M., Rayment, N., Farrow, S. M., Brennan, A., Katz, D. R., and O'Riordan, J. L., $1,25(OH)_2D_3$ regulates c-myc mRNA levels in tonsillar T lymphocytes, *Immunology*, 74, 589, 1991.

73. Jackson, T., Allard, M. F., Sreenan, C. M., Doss, L. K., Bishop, S. P., and Swain, J. L., The c-myc proto-oncogene regulates cardiac development in transgenic mice, *Mol. Cell. Biol.*, 10, 3709, 1990.

74. Fein, F. S., Strobeck, L. E., Malhorta, A., Scheuer, J., and Sonnonblick, E. H., Reversibility of diabetic cardiomyopathy with insulin in rats, *Circ. Res.*, 49, 1251, 1981.

75. O'Connell, T. D. and Simpson, R. U., unpublished observation.

9

Sunlight, Vitamin D, and Cardiovascular Disease

Robert Scragg

CONTENTS

0-8493-8661-6/95/$0.00+$.50

I. INTRODUCTION

Recent laboratory investigations have shown that a number of calcium-regulating hormones, including vitamin D, affect cardiovascular function. (These investigations are reviewed in other chapters of this book.) However, while in-depth biochemical and physiological investigations can provide detailed and specific information on the mechanisms by which calcium-regulating hormones affect cardiovascular function, they do not allow us to see the wider picture of how these hormones may affect the risk of cardiovascular disease. This information can come only from epidemiological studies that measure both calciotropic hormones and cardiovascular disease status in large groups of people. These studies suggest that changes in body levels of calcium-regulating hormones, particularly vitamin D, may contribute to the variations in cardiovascular event rates which are known to occur with season, latitude, and altitude, possibly through some unknown mechanism that is influenced by changes in exposure to sunshine among populations.

This chapter aims to:

1. Review the epidemiology of cardiovascular disease in relation to season, latitude, and altitude;
2. Show that ultraviolet (UV) radiation exposure is inversely related, at the population level, to the occurrence of cardiovascular disease;
3. Put forward a hypothesis that increased sunlight exposure, by changing body levels of calciotropic hormones, in particular levels of vitamin D, may lower the risk of cardiovascular disease;
4. Briefly discuss the possible implications of this hypothesis as it may affect future research on vitamin D and cardiovascular function and public health policies relating to sunshine exposure.

II. GEOGRAPHICAL EPIDEMIOLOGY OF CARDIOVASCULAR DISEASE

Epidemiological studies from around the world show that mortality and morbidity from cardiovascular disease vary with latitude, season, and altitude. Changes in sociocultural factors, such as diet and lifestyle, are unlikely to be primarily responsible for these variations because most examples come from comparisons within individual countries. Rather, the results from these studies (described below) suggest that climatic factors, such as temperature, sunlight, or both, are more likely to be involved and therefore to have a role in the etiology of these diseases.

A. Latitude

Countries nearer the Equator, which are mainly developing nations, have lower cardiovascular mortality rates than those farther away.[1] A major part of this difference is due to international differences in lifestyle between developing and developed nations. However, climatic factors related to latitude also may be involved because a number of studies within countries have shown that latitude is positively associated with cardiovascular mortality.

In country boroughs of England and Wales, mortality rates from cardiovascular disease and all causes of death during 1948 to 1954 and 1958 to 1964 in men and women were significantly associated with latitude after adjusting for air pollution, rainfall, water calcium, and social factors.[2] This study also found that sunshine and temperature were each inversely associated with mortality from all causes, and therefore probably with mortality from cardiovascular disease as it is the major cause of death. A British cohort study begun in 1978, after 6.5 years of follow-up, found that coronary heart disease rates (fatal and nonfatal) were twice as high in Scottish participants as in those living in southern England, and that place of

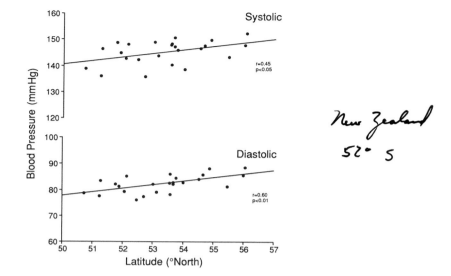

FIGURE 1   Relation between latitude and mean blood pressure level for men interviewed in 24 towns of the British Regional Heart Study. (Blood pressure data from Reference 5. Latitude data from *Gazetter of Great Britain,* 2nd ed., Macmillan, London, 1990.)

residence was a more important determinant of disease risk than place of birth.[3] For the 24 towns in this study, variations in cardiovascular mortality were related to blood pressure, cigarette smoking, and heavy alcohol consumption, but not with serum total and high density lipoprotein (HDL) cholesterol.[4] Moreover, a strong north-south gradient in blood pressure prevalence was found which was three times higher in Scotland and northern England than in the south.[5] The authors concluded that heavy alcohol drinking explained part of the variation in blood pressure prevalence. However, latitude also may be responsible because a plot of the mean blood pressure for each town with latitude shows a statistically significant positive correlation (Figure 1).

North-south gradients in cardiovascular disease also occur in a number of other European countries.[6] In the former West Germany, cardiovascular death rates show a general trend for rates to be higher in the north. Coronary heart disease mortality in Finland increases from southwest to northeast. Heart disease mortality rates in France are higher in the north than in the south, although the nonfatal incidence rates do not vary. Northern Italy has higher heart disease mortality rates than the south. In contrast, the direction of the gradient is reversed in Belgium, probably due to dietary differences between the ethnically distinct, butter-eating, French-speaking population in the south and the margarine-consuming Dutch speakers of the north.

There is also evidence for a north-south gradient in the Southern Hemisphere. The age-standardized mortality rate from coronary heart disease in New Zealand is about 5% higher on the South Island than the North Island, although the incidence for stroke is no different.[7]

In contrast, cardiovascular mortality in the U.S. is related to longitude, not latitude.[8] However, the role of latitude in U.S. mortality rates is complicated by altitude, which increases from south to north,[8] and is inversely associated with cardiovascular mortality (see below).

In summary, north-south gradients in cardiovascular mortality (rates are higher the farther from the Equator) have been described within several countries. The authors of these studies have tended to focus on the explanatory role of blood lipids and lifestyle factors. Rarely have they considered a possible role for climatic factors, such as temperature and sunshine. This is surprising given the substantial work carried out on the large seasonal variations in cardiovascular

TABLE 1   Proportion of winter deaths from major causes of
death for England and Wales, 1976 to 1983[9]

Cause of death	Male (%)	Female (%)
Coronary heart diseae	33.9	23.2
Stroke	11.1	16.2
Other circulatory disease	9.2	16.5
Respiratory disease	34.2	32.5
Injuries and violence	1.7	2.7
All other causes	9.9	8.9
Avg. no. of excess deaths each year	18,354	20,272

mortality (described below), which are most likely due to climatic factors and could involve a mechanism similar to that causing the variations in mortality related to latitude.

B.   Seasonal Variation

1.   Cardiovascular Mortality and Morbidity

Total mortality among developed countries typically follows a sinusoidal pattern each year, with a zenith in winter and a nadir in summer. The amplitude of the seasonal change varies from country to country. For example, an index of winter excess mortality from all causes of death, defined as the percentage excess of deaths in the four winter months of highest mortality (usually December to March in the Northern Hemisphere) compared with the average of deaths in the preceding and following 4-monthly periods, was found to range from 7 to 10% in North America, northern Europe, and Scandinavia and up to 20 to 25% in southern Europe, the U.K., Israel, and Australasia.[9]

Cardiovascular diseases are responsible for the major part of the winter increase in mortality. In England and Wales during the period 1976 to 1983, cardiovascular diseases (coronary heart disease, stroke, other circulatory diseases) accounted for more than one half (55%) of the winter excess in mortality, and respiratory disease for one third (33%) (Table 1).

The weakness of using the above index of winter excess mortality, which is based on total mortality, is that it does not provide information on seasonal mortality variations for specific diseases. Moreover, it is possible that countries with a low winter excess mortality index have an increased summer mortality from certain diseases (e.g., infectious) that is masking a pronounced winter increase in mortality from other diseases (e.g., cardiovascular).

Studies of specific diseases have shown that the seasonal variations in cardiovascular diseases are greater than the variations in total mortality described above. For example, an early Scottish report found that coronary heart disease mortality in the general population was about 30% higher in January than in August through September, and that the seasonal variation was age related, being greatest (about 40%) in people aged over 65 years.[10] Similar results were found in a recent study of the population living in northeast Scotland, where the peak mortality from coronary heart disease, stroke, and other circulatory disorders was about 30% higher in February than in the summer.[11] In the U.S. mortality from coronary heart disease, stroke, and, to a lesser extent, diabetes was higher in winter than in summer.[12] The population living in the Canadian province of Ontario experienced about a 25% higher coronary heart disease mortality in January as compared to August during the years 1958 to 1962.[13] In New Zealand a higher mortality occurs from coronary heart disease (by about 33% men and 40% women) and from stroke (by about 33% men and 50% women) in the middle of winter (July) compared with late summer–early autumn (January to March).[7] In contrast, a Swedish study found no evidence of a seasonal variation in mortality from myocardial infarction.[14]

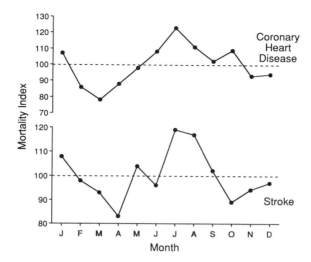

FIGURE 2 Seasonal variation in coronary heart disease and stroke mortality for the Northern and Far North Statistical Divisions of Queensland, men and women combined, 1968 to 1975. Average mortality index for year = 100. (Data from Australian Bureau of Statistics, Canberra.)

The seasonal mortality variations for cardiovascular disease are not confined to populations living in temperate climates. For example, winter increases in mortality during 1968 to 1975 in the subtropical Australian state of Queensland were found for coronary heart disease, stroke, diseases of the arteries, hypertensive diseases, other forms of heart disease, and respiratory diseases.[15] Similar seasonal patterns were found in the two northern coastal statistical divisions of Queensland (Figure 2). The main urban areas in these divisions are the cities of Cairns and Townsville, which have a warm tropical weather pattern at latitudes 17° and 19°S, respectively. In Kuwait at latitude 30°N the seasonal variation in cardiovascular mortality is very similar to that in northeast Scotland at 57°N.[11]

Despite the convincing results showing a seasonal variation in mortality from cardiovascular disease, the evidence for a similar seasonal variation in morbidity is less clear. An early British study described a doubling in the incidence of myocardial infarction in winter compared with summer,[16] while a Finnish study observed increased hospital admission rates on cold (i.e., winter) days of the year.[17] In Scotland from 1962 to 1966, nonfatal hospital admissions for coronary heart disease were 16% higher in winter.[10] However, a recent report on seasonality in northern Scotland during 1974 to 1988 found that hospital admissions for coronary heart disease did not increase in winter, although they did for stroke (by 12%).[18] Studies in Sweden and India have also failed to find any significant variation in myocardial infarction incidence by month.[14,19,20] The inconsistent findings for mortality and morbidity may be explained partly by evidence indicating a rise in the case-fatality rate for myocardial infarction from about 23% in summer to 27% in winter.[10] The same report also found that the seasonal variation in the case-fatality rate was greatest in people over 65 years.

With regard to cancer, while a summer increase occurs in the incidence of certain cancers such as malignant melanoma and breast cancer, mortality from cancer has been found consistently not to vary by season but to remain constant throughout the year.[15,18,21] This has important biological implications, because if winter weather acted to increase mortality among people already debilitated and weak from preexisting disease, one would expect to see a similar rise in cancer mortality during winter as seen for cardiovascular disease. Rather, the winter rise in mortality for cardiovascular disease only suggests some pathological mechanism specific to that system.

2. Cardiovascular Risk Factors

Evidence was found that two of the three major cardiovascular risk factors — blood pressure and serum total cholesterol, but not cigarette smoking — also vary by season. Large-scale epidemiological studies in a number of countries have generally found a winter increase in blood pressure. The British Medical Research Council's treatment trial for mild hypertension observed an increase in pressure of 6 mmHg systolic and 3 mmHg diastolic in winter as compared to summer among the placebo group aged 55 to 64 years.[22] The Tromso Heart Study reported a blood pressure increase of 10 mmHg systolic and 8 mmHg diastolic in February as compared to August.[23] A U.S. study found that blood pressure increased in winter.[24]

With regard to serum cholesterol, a 1981 review concluded that the evidence for a seasonal variation was not compelling;[25] however, results from subsequent larger epidemiological studies, better designed and analyzed, suggest that cholesterol levels are higher in winter. For instance, a cross-sectional study in Jerusalem found that cholesterol was about 8% higher in winter as compared to summer,[26] while serial blood measurements of the placebo group in the Lipid Research Clinics Coronary Primary Prevention Trial showed a nearly 3% winter increase in total cholesterol as compared to summer.[27] In the latter study, winter increases in weight and dietary saturated fat intake explained less than one third of the seasonal variations in plasma cholesterol levels.

Results from studies of seasonal variations in diet and exercise, both probable risk factors of cardiovascular disease, are limited and inconsistent. In agreement with the diet results from the Lipid Research Clinics Coronary Primary Prevention Trial mentioned above, a Dutch study of young adult women found a higher intake of fat in winter (39.4% of total dietary energy) as compared to summer (37.2%), although no seasonal change in total energy intake was observed.[28] However, a U.S. nationwide food consumption survey reported little variation in nutrient intake from season to season.[29] With regard to exercise, physical fitness was observed to be 9% higher in summer than in autumn in a cross-sectional survey of middle-aged Norwegian men,[30] while the Dutch study of young women found that they spent 17 min more each day walking and participating in sports in summer and spring as compared to winter and autumn.[28] The authors of the Dutch report concluded that the differences in time spent by the women in the various activity categories during the seasons were too small to have a noteworthy effect on energy intake and body weight, although the latter was 0.4 kg higher in winter than in summer.

Overall, the evidence suggests that winter increases in blood pressure and serum cholesterol and lifestyle factors such as diet and physical activity which affect them explain only part of the winter increase in cardiovascular mortality. (Apparently, no studies of seasonal variations in cigarette smoking exist.) Moreover, alterations in these risk factors are unlikely to be responsible for the seasonal variations in cardiovascular disease mortality. Aside from possible short-term changes in blood pressure increasing the risk of cerebral hemorrhage, changes in lipid metabolism and blood pressure are thought to take many years to manifest their effects as symptomatic disease. This finding is not consistent with the monthly changes in mortality that occur with coronary heart disease and stroke.

3. Seasonality of Thrombosis

Seasonal variations in cardiovascular mortality must involve other, more acute mechanism(s), such as winter increases in the risk of thrombosis, cardiac arrhythmias, or both. There is a growing body of evidence that thrombosis and risk factors for thrombosis increase in winter. Studies in the U.S. have reported winter increases in deep-vein thrombosis and pulmonary thrombosis[31] and in thromboembolic mortality.[32] The risk of postoperative deep-vein thrombosis was found to be higher in the winter months (May to October) in an Australian study,[33] while the postoperative mortality rate from pulmonary embolism was found to be higher during the winter (November to February) in England.[34] A similar increase in mortality from pulmonary embolism during January to April has been observed in Italy,[35] as has a winter increase in the incidence of peripheral arterial embolus in Edinburgh, Scotland.[36] Blood levels of the thrombotic risk factor, fibrinogen, are increased in winter by 23%,[37] an amount similar to the winter increase in cardiovascular mortality.

Evidence is limited for a winter increase in cardiac arrhythmias. Hospital admissions for atrial fibrillation in Helsinki were about 50% higher during both the first and the last 4 months of the year compared to the warmest 4 months, May to August.[38] However, while it is possible that an arrhythmic mechanism may partly explain the winter increase in coronary heart disease mortality, it seems unlikely to be a factor in the winter increase in stroke. In contrast, the thrombotic mechanism is a common factor in both coronary heart disease and stroke, and is the most likely mechanism to be involved with the winter increases in cardiovascular mortality.

4. Is Temperature Involved?

Cold winter temperatures have been proposed by many researchers as the most likely reason for the winter increase in mortality from coronary heart disease and stroke. An inverse association has been described between temperature and mortality from both diseases.[16,39,40] Cold weather is thought to increase the risk of developing cardiovascular disease either (1) by acting directly on the body to exert a cooling effect, which results in increased stress on the heart or a change in some other body parameter such as blood coagulability, or (2) by causing lifestyle changes such as diet and physical activity.[16]

Supporting evidence for temperature causing changes in body parameters comes from a study of healthy students in whom mild cooling in skin temperature, with only a slight fall in core temperature (0.4°C), produced significant increases in blood viscosity, blood pressure, and total plasma cholesterol.[41] A study of old and young adults showed that blood pressure increased when the ambient room temperature was decreased to 6°C, but little or no increase in blood pressure occurred at 12° and 15°C, respectively.[42]

With regard to seasonal changes in lifestyle, cardiovascular mortality is elevated for several days after snowfalls, particularly in men, which suggests that increased physical activity involved with clearing snow may in part increase the death rate.[40,43,44] In contrast, the limited evidence on seasonal changes in diet mentioned above suggests that this is small and unlikely to explain the large winter increases in cardiovascular mortality.

A number of findings that are inconsistent with the temperature hypothesis have emerged since it was first proposed. Studies that have controlled for the confounding effects of season have failed to find an association between temperature and mortality. A Canadian study, which examined the acute effect of temperature on mortality in the winter months only, found that an increase in the daily rate of sudden coronary death at the time of cold snaps occurred in men <65 years of age, but not in men or women >65 years, who are known to have the greatest seasonal variations in cardiovascular mortality.[44] A study of mortality during blizzards in eastern Massachusetts found no significant association between heart disease mortality and temperature during the weeks adjacent to the blizzard period.[43] A study of Greater London failed to show any association between cardiovascular mortality and temperature after the seasonal trends in each were removed.[45] The results of these studies suggest that the inverse association between temperature and cardiovascular mortality reported in earlier analyses may have been confounded by season.

International comparisons have found that the amplitudes in seasonal variation in temperature and cardiovascular mortality are not related. Anderson and Le Riche,[13] who compared Ontario to England and Wales, found that while the seasonal variations in temperature were greater in Ontario, the seasonal variations in coronary heart disease mortality were greater in

England and Wales. The higher seasonal variation in total mortality in southern Europe, where temperature swings are smaller, as compared to Scandinavia, is consistent with their finding.[9] Instead of cold temperatures, they suggested that the winter increase in respiratory infections may be responsible for the rise in coronary heart disease mortality.[13] Their hypothesis is supported by the increase in cardiovascular mortality during influenza epidemics[46–48] and the association of acute respiratory symptoms with the onset of acute myocardial infarction.[49]

Other studies have shown that the increased availability of household heating has not decreased the excess in cardiovascular mortality in winter. Elderly people in England with unrestricted home heating continued to experience a winter increase in total mortality similar to that in the general population,[50] while excess winter mortality from coronary heart disease and stroke did not fall during 1964 to 1984 as the percentage of households in Britain with central heating increased from 13 to 66%.[51] These results have been interpreted by their authors to suggest that outdoor excursions into cold weather, rather than cold houses, are the main cause for the winter excess in cardiovascular mortality. However, another possibility is that some seasonal factor related to temperature, rather than temperature itself, is responsible for the increase in mortality in winter.

C. Altitude

The strongest evidence against the temperature hypothesis comes from studies of altitude and cardiovascular disease. In the troposphere, the layer of the atmosphere closest to the earth's surface, temperature decreases by about 6.5°C/1000 m rise in altitude.[52] If the inverse association between temperature and cardiovascular mortality holds for all situations, then mortality should increase with altitude. However, this is not the case, as shown by studies in the U.S., that provide the best evidence because no other country has large populations living over such a wide range of altitudes together with a nationally standardized system for collecting mortality data.

Cardiovascular mortality from 1949 to 1951 among Caucasians was inversely correlated with altitude ($r = -0.45$) in the 163 metropolitan areas of the U.S.[53] Ten years later altitude was also found to be inversely associated with coronary heart disease mortality for Caucasian populations living in the largest U.S. cities.[54,55] Mortality from coronary heart disease was found to be reduced in men, but not women, residing at high altitudes in New Mexico,[56] although this association is partly due to the confounding factor of Hispanic ethnicity.[57]

The most systematic and extensive analysis of cardiovascular mortality and altitude involves mortality rates in 1968 to 1971 from coronary heart disease and stroke for Caucasians living in over 3000 counties in the contiguous U.S.[8] These rates were found to be inversely associated with both longitude and altitude. Of these, longitude was more strongly associated with mortality when both variables were included in multivariate analyses. Because of this finding, the authors concluded that variables related to longitude may offer the most fruitful approach to explaining differences in county cardiovascular mortality rates. However, juxtaposing data from Figure 7 of their report, which shows the relation between longitude and mortality, together with an altitude profile across the U.S. at the 40th parallel shows that they mirror each other. Their report also shows that the nadir in mortality, at a longitude between 110° and 100° W, coincides with the peak altitudes of the Rocky Mountains (Figure 3). This comparison suggests that longitude in the U.S. is only indirectly related to cardiovascular mortality through its relation with altitude.

Other populations living at the very high altitudes of the Himalayas of Tibet[58] and India[59] and the Andes of South America have been found to have low rates of coronary heart disease.[60] Clearly, a non-Western lifestyle is a major determinant of the low heart disease rates in these populations, but it is significant that those communities that claim longevity — Ecuador, Kashmir, and Soviet Georgia — are all situated at high altitudes.[61]

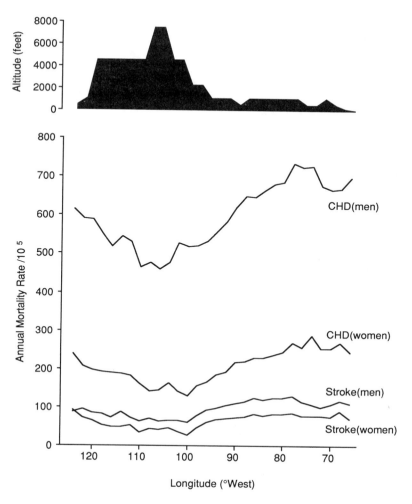

FIGURE 3 An altitude profile across the U.S. at latitude 40°N is the mirror image of the pattern for mortality from coronary heart disease (CHD) and stroke by longitude, with the peak in altitude and the nadir in mortality occurring between longitudes 110° and 100°W. (Mortality data redrawn from Reference 8. Altitude data (at latitude 44°N for longitudes <76°W) are the medians for the ranges given in *The Times Atlas of the World,* 6th ed., London, 1980.)

Previous explanations for the low rates of cardiovascular disease at high altitude have focused on the possible role of hypoxia at high altitude in inducing changes in the myocardium, such as increased vascularization, which in some way protects against cardiovascular disease.[54–56] However, while hypoxic-induced myocardial changes may explain the inverse relationship of altitude with coronary heart disease, it is unlikely the changes would explain its relationship with stroke.

The best evidence of a mechanism to explain the low rates of cardiovascular disease at high altitude is available for blood pressure. Many of these studies have been carried out in the Andes Mountains of South America. In a natural experiment, blood pressure in 100 Caucasian men born at sea level decreased by 13 mmHg systolic and 6 mmHg diastolic after residing at high altitudes (>12,000 ft) for more than 2 years.[62] A cross-sectional study of five Peruvian communities, two located at sea level and three above 13,000 ft, found hypertension prevalences more than tenfold higher in the sea level communities.[63] The same paper also described unpublished data which showed that blood pressure levels of native highlanders increased after prolonged residence at sea level. Part of these blood pressure differences may have been due to differences between sea level and highland living in other lifestyle factors such as physical activity and diet, although the five communities in the Ruiz and Penaloza paper had similar socioeconomic levels. The Aymara, living on the Chilean altiplano, were found to have lower blood pressures and lower body weights than those at sea level, although an inverse relation between blood pressure and altitude in women was still found after controlling for body mass index and age.[64]

In the former U.S.S.R., a cross-sectional study of ethnically homogeneous men in Kirghizia found a twofold higher prevalence of hypertension in those residing at 800 to 900 m above sea level as compared to those at 2800 to 3600 m.[65] Other studies from northern India, all without internal comparison groups, are conflicting, with some reporting blood pressure levels at high altitude that are lower than[66,67] and others similar[68,69] to those of sea level communities.

Only limited information is available regarding the association of altitude with other major cardiovascular risk factors. A cross-sectional study of populations living at altitudes between 3000 and 5500 m in the Indian Himalayas found that altitude was positively associated with HDL cholesterol, but unrelated to total cholesterol for which the mean values were similar to those for other communities living at sea level.[59] Tibetan highlanders also have lower serum total cholesterol, but similar HDL cholesterol, levels than those in healthy Japanese, although these differences also could be due to lifestyle factors.[58] Physiological studies of changes in cardiovascular function associated with short-term changes in altitude are unlikely to provide an understanding of how living for long periods at high altitude decreases cardiovascular mortality.[70,71]

In summary, epidemiological studies have mostly found that altitude is inversely associated with cardiovascular mortality and hypertension, although some have found no association. More importantly, *no* studies have reported a positive association between altitude and cardiovascular disease. Invoking Occam's razor, the latter finding should have been the norm if the inverse association between temperature and cardiovascular mortality, proposed to explain the winter excess in mortality, also applied to altitude because temperature decreases as altitude increases.

III. ULTRAVIOLET RADIATION

Given the above criticisms of the temperature hypothesis, it seems unlikely that cold temperatures cause the winter excess in cardiovascular mortality. Rather, other factors related to temperature are likely to be involved. One of these factors may be UV radiation from the sun, which is the major source of vitamin D in humans. Like temperature, UV radiation follows a sinusoidal pattern throughout the seasons, being strongest in summer and weakest in winter.[72–74] It is possible that previous associations found between temperature and cardiovascular mortality exist only because temperature and UV radiation are highly correlated (e.g., $r = 0.94$ in Queensland).[15]

A. Factors Affecting Ultraviolet Radiation

The solar UV spectrum can be divided into three wavelength bands: UVA, at 320 to 400 nm, is only slightly absorbed by ozone; UVB, at 280 to 320 nm, is highly dependent on ozone content; and UVC, at <280 nm, is totally absorbed by ozone.[75] The UV radiation at ground level is a combination of solar radiation, which travels directly in a straight line from the sun; sky radiation, which is scattered by minute particles in the atmosphere and hence is traveling in many directions; and reflected radiation from the ground.[76] Several factors affect the intensity of UV radiation at ground level, including:

1. The intensity of the sun's radiation, which varies with solar cycles;
2. The distance between the earth and the sun, which varies because of the earth's elliptical orbit;
3. The thickness of the atmosphere through which solar UV travels — ground level UV is higher with shorter path lengths through the atmosphere, such as at high ground altitude and at high sun elevations which are related to season, latitude, and time of day;
4. The amount of ozone in the atmosphere;
5. Atmospheric turbidity, which is the concentration of aerosols such as pollutants;
6. Cloud cover;
7. The albedo, i.e., the proportion of UV radiation that is reflected from the ground.[73]

These factors lead to the following observations about the intensity of UV radiation that are relevant to the epidemiology of cardiovascular disease (described above). (1) Because the elevation of the sun is high in summer and low in winter, UV radiation varies with the seasons, being strongest in summer and weakest in winter.[72,74] (2) UV radiation increases with altitude by about 15%/1000 m.[75] (3) Because the elevation of the sun decreases with latitude, so does UV radiation, which is strongest at the Equator and weakest at the Poles.[74] Combining these observations with the cardiovascular epidemiological data leads to the conclusion that UV radiation is inversely associated with cardiovascular mortality and possibly with the prevalence of hypertension.

B. Ultraviolet Radiation and Vitamin D

How might solar UV radiation decrease the risk of cardiovascular disease? Uncontrolled trials carried out on humans earlier in this century suggested that UV may lower serum cholesterol[77,78] and blood pressure.[79] A nonblinded study of college freshman in Illinois found that UV radiation given over 10 weeks increased both cardiovascular (assessed by pulse measurements) and motor fitness as compared to the control group.[80] The quality of these early studies, usually without controls and not double blind, casts doubt on the validity of their findings.

Ultraviolet radiation of skin has been shown to lower its cholesterol concentration,[81] although the biological significance of this effect is unclear because epidemiological studies have generally failed to find any association between blood levels of vitamin D and serum cholesterol. In addition, evidence from a controlled trial of young French adults showed that UV increases insulin secretion.[82] Some relevance may be attached to this finding as diabetes is an established risk factor for cardiovascular disease.[83] However, the possibility with the greatest supporting evidence is that UVB radiation acts on the skin to increase the synthesis of vitamin D, and that an increased body level of vitamin D by itself or through changes in some other related calciotropic hormone decreases cardiovascular risk.[84]

Ultraviolet radiation is the major source of vitamin D in humans.[85,86] This produces vitamin D_3 (cholecalciferol), as opposed to vitamin D_2 (ergocalciferol). The latter is exclusively of dietary origin, although vitamin D_3 is also ingested orally because in some countries, including the U.S., it is added as a supplement to foods such as milk.

Ultraviolet B radiation in the waveband of 290 to 315 nm acts on the stratum spinosum and stratum basale layers of skin to convert 7-dehydrocholesterol to previtamin D_3;[87] the peak of the action spectrum occurs at 295 nm.[88] The greatest variations in UV radiation with season and latitude occur in this waveband of peak vitamin D synthesis.[72,74] Previtamin D_3 is then converted to vitamin D_3 in skin at a rate that is temperature dependent[89] before travelling bound to protein via the blood to the liver where it is converted into 25-hydroxyvitamin D_3 (25-OHD$_3$) the main metabolite. Blood levels of this hormone are considered to be a measure of total body vitamin D_3 status because they are 1000 times higher than those of the most active metabolite, 1,25-dihydroxyvitamin D_3 (1,25(OH)$_2$D$_3$), which is formed in the mitochondria of cells in the proximal tubules of the kidney from 25-OHD$_3$.[86] Although 25-OHD$_3$

is not usually considered to be biologically active, there is evidence that it has metabolic effects.[90] The much higher blood level of 25-OHD$_3$ than 1,25(OH)$_2$D$_3$ suggests that the magnitude of its effects on the body may be similar to those of 1,25(OH)$_2$D$_3$.

Blood levels of 25-OHD$_3$ in humans vary with climate in the same directions as does UV. Numerous studies have shown that seasonal variations follow a sinusoidal pattern, with serum levels in summer being approximately double those in winter.[91–97] A study of people living in five U.S. cities (Boston, Denver, Detroit, Palm Beach, and Seattle) found that blood levels of 25-OHD were inversely associated with latitude,[98] while residents of Denver, living 1 mile higher than those of Seattle, Detroit, and Boston, had higher blood levels of vitamin D, despite residing at a similar latitude.

There is limited available information on climatic variations in other calciotropic hormones related to season. In contrast to 25-OHD$_3$, blood levels of 1,25(OH)$_2$D generally do not show any seasonal variation,[94,97,99] although a Dutch study reported a summer increase.[93] Exposure to sunlight by elderly rest home residents[100] and to artificial UV by healthy volunteers[101] had no effect on blood levels of 1,25(OH)$_2$D; only in vitamin D-deficient subjects did levels of metabolite increase.[101] However, blood levels of parathyroid hormone (PTH) show a seasonal pattern that is approximately 6 months out of phase with 25-OHD, having a zenith in winter and its nadir in summer.[99,102,103] Because PTH stimulates the conversion of 25(OH)$_2$D to 1,25(OH)$_2$D, collectively these results suggest that reduced body levels of vitamin D in winter result in a secondary hyperparathyroidism, with increased secretion of PTH and maintenance of body levels of 1,25(OH)$_2$D despite reduced amounts of its precursor 25(OH)$_2$D.

It is tempting to speculate that the winter hyperparathyroidism may have metabolic consequences that are related to the winter increase in cardiovascular disease. First, winter increases in the activity of the parathyroid gland may increase the secretion of other compounds from it, such as parathyroid hypertensive factor (PHF),[104] leading to the winter increase in blood pressure (described earlier), although no evidence has appeared as to whether parathyroid hypertensive factor is inversely related to vitamin D. Alternatively, vitamin D may be directly involved in the winter increase in cardiovascular mortality and blood pressure through seasonal changes in the ratio of its metabolites and their effects on intracellular calcium. With regard to blood pressure, vascular smooth muscle tone can be increased by increasing either the concentration of, or sensitivity to, intracellular calcium.[105] Increased intracellular cytoplasmic concentrations have been found in platelets,[106–108] erythrocytes,[109] and lymphocytes[110] from patients with essential hypertension as compared to normotensive controls. However, 25-OHD and 1,25(OH)$_2$D may have opposite effects on intracellular calcium levels in cardiac and smooth muscle. Experiments with chick skeletal muscle have shown that 25-OHD increases the calcium content of the slow turnover pool (e.g., intracellular organelles such as mitochondria and sarcoplasmic reticulum), whereas 1,25(OH)$_2$D increases the size of the fast exchangeable calcium pool (equivalent to the cytoplasmic pool).[111,112] 1,25-Dihydroxyvitamin D is known to increase cytosolic calcium in other tissues.[113,114] Because blood levels of this vitamin D metabolite are generally stable throughout the year, increased levels of 25-OHD in summer would have to lower intracellular calcium for this mechanism to explain the summer drop in blood pressure. However, no studies have been conducted on the effect of 25-OHD on intracellular calcium.

IV. VITAMIN D AND CARDIOVASCULAR DISEASE

A. History

Several experimental studies carried out in the early 1970s produced results suggesting that increased intake of dietary vitamin D increased the risk of coronary heart disease. For example, in a nonblinded study without controls, 50,000 IU of oral vitamin D, given daily for

21 d, increased serum levels of cholesterol but not triglycerides.[115] In another study, rachitic children aged less than 2 years developed raised levels of serum cholesterol and blood pressure after daily doses of up to 12,000 IU were taken for 1 month.[116] However, the relevance of the results from these studies must be questioned because they lacked control groups and used pharmacological doses of vitamin D. For instance, in the study by Fleischman et al.[115] vitamin D intake in the first 21-d period was >14 times the total amount a person adhering to the U.S. recommended daily allowance (200 IU) would consume in 1 year. The only study to give physiological doses of vitamin D and to use a control group found that daily doses of 500 and 1000 IU over 6 weeks had no effect on serum cholesterol or triglyceride levels in healthy men.[117]

Observational epidemiological studies carried out at the same time also suggested that dietary vitamin D adversely affected cardiovascular disease risk. An ecological comparison of eight regions in England and Wales found strong positive correlations between regional vitamin D intake and mortality from coronary heart disease and stroke, but not hypertension.[118] This type of epidemiological study, by its very nature, can only generate hypotheses and not test them. Stronger evidence was provided by a subsequent Norwegian case control study in Tromso which found a doubling in the risk of myocardial infarction for those consuming >30 μg (1200 IU) of vitamin D per day.[119] Supporting evidence for possible adverse consequences from dietary vitamin D came in a cross-sectional study on the same population in whom men ingesting more than the mean daily intake of vitamin D (2.5 μg or 100 IU) had higher serum cholesterol levels than those eating less than the mean.[120] However, the large difference in the mean daily vitamin D intake between men in this study and male myocardial infarction controls in the earlier case control study (22.68 μg or 907 IU), both from the same population, raises questions about the validity of the dietary instruments used in these two studies. A further criticism of these studies is that we now know that the sun and not diet is the major source of vitamin D in humans,[86] and hence these studies were not measuring total vitamin D exposure.

B. 25-Hydroxyvitamin D$_3$ and Coronary Heart Disease

The advent of assays for blood levels of specific vitamin D metabolites allowed a more valid assessment of the role of vitamin D, particularly sun-induced vitamin D$_3$, in heart disease. The first epidemiological study to report on the blood vitamin D levels of myocardial infarction cases found that serum 25-OHD$_3$ concentrations were normal or low in cases as compared to controls.[121] However, the statistical power of this study was limited because of the very small number of cases ($n = 15$). A subsequent, larger case control study in Denmark observed significantly lower serum 25-OHD$_3$ levels in cases compared to controls from May to August.[122] A further report from Tromso, in opposition to the earlier findings by Linden[119,120] from the same population, found that new cases of myocardial infarction in the first 5 years of followup had significantly lower 25-OHD levels than matched controls after adjusting for concentration of vitamin-D binding protein.[123] Because this latter case control comparison was nested within a larger cohort study, and blood samples were collected from all subjects at baseline prior to some experiencing coronary events, the lower vitamin D levels in cases could not have been caused by the acute phase reaction of the myocardial infarction.

Prior to carrying out a large case control study, researchers in Auckland, New Zealand, investigated whether the acute phase reaction from myocardial infarctions changed blood levels of 25-OHD$_3$. Levels were shown to remain unchanged for up to 12 h after the onset of myocardial infarction symptoms.[124] On the assumption that 25-OHD$_3$ levels in blood samples collected within this time were similar to those prior to the onset of symptoms, 179 new cases of myocardial infarction, presenting within 12 h of symptom onset, were individually matched with controls by age, sex, and time of year during a 2-year period.[125] Cases had significantly lower plasma levels of 25-OHD$_3$ compared to controls for the total year (32.0 vs. 35.0 nmol/l). The percentage difference in vitamin D blood levels between cases and controls (9%) is

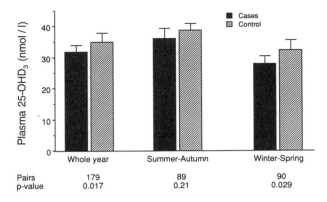

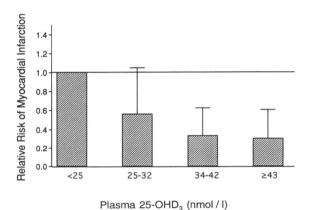

FIGURE 4   Mean (95% confidence interval) levels of plasma 25-OHD$_3$ in myocardial infarction cases and controls, matched for age, sex, and time of year.[125]

FIGURE 5   Relative risk (95% confidence interval) of myocardial infarction by plasma 25-OHD$_3$ quartile.[125]

similar to that reported for other major cardiovascular risk factors such as blood pressure and serum cholesterol.[126,127] Categorizing matched pairs by season showed that mean case control differences were greatest during the winter-spring period as compared to summer-autumn (4.5 vs. 2.5 nmol/l; Figure 4), although the decrease in the relative risk of myocardial infarction associated with raised vitamin D$_3$ levels was seen in all seasons of the year. When subjects were categorized into quartiles by plasma level of 25-OHD$_3$, the relative risk decreased progressively from the first (lowest) quartile to the second and third; however, little difference was found between the third and fourth (highest) quartile, suggesting that a threshold in the association may exist between myocardial infarction risk and plasma level of 25-OHD$_3$ (Figure 5).

Thus, the results of the larger epidemiological studies, both cohort and case control, which have assessed individual vitamin D status by using blood measurements, all show that cases have lower blood levels of vitamin D than controls.[122,123,125] Clearly, more studies are required to confirm these findings.

C. Vitamin D and Cardiovascular Risk Factors

If an inverse relation exists among sunlight, vitamin D, and coronary heart disease, does it involve any of the established cardiovascular risk factors? Again, only limited information is available, but the evidence favors a role for vitamin D acting through a possible association with blood pressure.

1. Blood Pressure

This evidence is described more fully in other chapters of this book, and only evidence from human studies is presented here. With regard to dietary vitamin D, an inverse association between systolic blood pressure and oral vitamin D intake has been observed in North American women,[128] while supplementation with a vitamin D analogue (1α-calcidol) has been shown to lower blood pressure in Swedes with intermittent hypercalcemia, possibly caused by primary hyperparathyroidism,[129] and with impaired glucose tolerance.[130] In contrast, a trial of white normotensive men in Oregon found no effect on blood pressure after calcium (1000 mg/d) and vitamin D_3 (1000 IU/d) supplementation over 3 years.[131]

Information on the association between blood levels of 25-OHD and blood pressure is inconsistent. A case control study in Poland observed significantly lower 25-OHD levels in cases, which the authors attributed to a possible depressive effect of antihypertensive drugs.[132] An Auckland cross-sectional study of 295 middle-aged men reported a weak inverse association between blood pressure and 25-OHD ($r = -0.15$).[133] However, other studies found either no association[131,134] or a positive association.[135,136] This contrasts with the results for blood levels of $1,25(OH)_2D$ which, aside from the Oregon study[131] have been found to be elevated in hypertension.[134–138]

Opposite blood pressure findings for vitamin D supplementation and $1,25(OH)_2D$ blood levels may be explained by the possibility that increased levels of the dihydroxy metabolite represent a homeostatic response to either vitamin D or calcium deficiency, or to other factors contributing to increased blood pressure. The latter possibility is supported by studies showing that increased dietary sodium leads to increases in $1,25(OH)_2D$ and blood pressure.[139,140]

2. Blood Lipids

In contrast to the extensive work on the relation between vitamin D and blood pressure, very limited research has been conducted on its relation with serum cholesterol in healthy populations. Epidemiological studies in Sweden,[122] Norway,[123] Belgium,[141] and New Zealand[133] found no association between blood levels of 25-(OH)D and serum total cholesterol. High density lipoprotein cholesterol was found to be associated with 25-OHD in one study[141] but not in another.[133] Treatment with 1α-calcidol had no effect on serum total and HDL cholesterol or on serum triglycerides.[142] Thus, in contrast to trials in the early 1970s, which gave pharmacological doses of vitamin D (above), the results of recent studies suggest that body levels of vitamin D in the general population are unrelated to serum lipids.

3. Physical Activity

There is increasing evidence that regular physical activity during leisure time protects against coronary heart disease.[143] While a number of biological mechanisms have been proposed, results from the cross-sectional study of middle-aged men in Auckland suggests that activity-related changes in vitamin D metabolism also may be involved.[133] Men who did leisure time aerobic activities at least weekly over the 3 months prior to interview had significantly higher plasma levels of 25-OHD$_3$ as compared to inactive men, and the increase in active men was greatest during the winter (July to September) (Figure 6). The raised 25-OHD$_3$ levels among physically active men did not appear to be due to increased sun exposure while exercising outdoors because plasma vitamin D remained elevated after controlling for weekly hours of sunshine exposure.

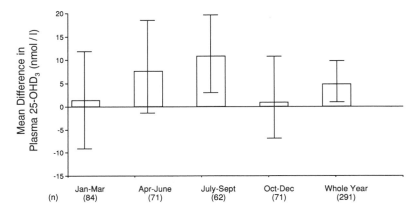

FIGURE 6   Mean increase (95% confidence interval) in plasma 25-OHD$_3$ level in men doing leisure time aerobic activities compared to those who were inactive (= 0), by time of year.[133]

This study confirms an earlier report of higher serum levels of both 25-OHD and 1,25(OH)$_2$D in healthy young adult males who did weightlifting exercises as compared to nonexercising controls.[144] Although not stated, it is probable that the major part of the weightlifters' exercise program was indoors, out of the sun because of their use of weights and body exercise machines. If increased sun exposure with exercise is not involved, the results from these two studies could be explained by the effect of increased body heat from physical activity, resulting in the increased formation of vitamin D$_3$ from previtamin D$_3$ because this reaction is temperature dependent.[87]

4.   Skin Pigmentation

Epidemiological studies in developed countries have found that cardiovascular disease is more common in some populations having increased skin pigmentation than in those having white skin. Blacks in the U.S. have a higher mortality from coronary heart disease and stroke.[145–147] Mortality rates from coronary heart disease in Britain are higher among immigrant Asians than in the native-born population.[148,149] In New Zealand, coronary heart disease mortality rates are higher in Polynesian Maoris than New Zealanders of European descent.[150] As compared to Caucasians, the prevalence of hypertension is higher among U.S. blacks[151–153] and among Asians and Afro-Caribbeans in Britain.[154] A study of 4000 urban Puerto Rican men found higher blood pressure levels in those with dark skin as compared to those with light skin.[155]

Low body levels of vitamin D in blacks, Indian Asians, and New Zealand Maoris could be partly responsible for their increased risk of cardiovascular disease and hypertension. Increased skin pigment reduces the capacity of skin to synthesize vitamin D$_3$ after exposure to UV radiation.[156,157] Blacks, Indian Asians, and Polynesians living at temperate latitudes have been found to have lower levels of 25-OHD$_3$ than Caucasians,[157–159] along with an associated secondary hyperparathyroidism.[158]

5.   Age

Body levels of vitamin D, as measured by blood levels of 25-OHD, decrease with increasing age[160–162] as a result of a decreased capacity of aged skin to produce vitamin D$_3$.[163] This association may explain, in part, the increased occurrence of cardiovascular disease with old age,[1] and the increased seasonality from cardiovascular disease that occurs in older age groups.[9,15,18,21]

V. CONCLUSIONS

A. Summary

The geographical epidemiology of cardiovascular disease, in particular coronary heart disease and stroke mortality and hypertension prevalence, shows that these conditions are related to season (higher in winter), increase with latitude, and decrease with increasing altitude. Thus, some climatic factors influence the occurrence of these conditions. A review of the evidence suggests that UV radiation is the climatic factor most likely to explain the geographical variations in cardiovascular disease, and that it is inversely associated with the occurrence of cardiovascular disease. The following hypothesis may explain how UV radiation protects against these diseases.

Ultraviolet radiation is the major source of vitamin D in humans. Low body levels of vitamin D are more likely to occur in winter, with residence at sea level or high latitude, with physical inactivity, and with increased skin pigmentation and age. Low vitamin D levels may have a direct effect on body tissues which increases the risk of cardiovascular disease. Alternatively, a low vitamin D status may lead to altered levels of other calciotropic hormones in the population that increase the risk of cardiovascular disease, for example, an increased prevalence of secondary hyperparathyroidism. The latter may increase the secretion of other compounds from the parathyroid gland such as PHF. The seasonality evidence suggests that low levels of vitamin D are likely to involve a thrombotic rather than a lipid mechanism to increase coronary heart disease and stroke mortality. Given the important role of vitamin D in calcium metabolism, it and other calciotropic hormones may influence cardiovascular risk by a mechanism involving changes in intracellular calcium.[164]

B. Implications for Research and Public Health Policy

A considerable body for international research has identified hypertension, serum cholesterol, and smoking as the major risk factors for coronary heart disease. More than 50% of new patients with this disease do not have raised levels of these risk factors, however.[165] This implies that there must be other important, but currently unknown, risk factors for coronary heart disease. The situation is likely to be the same for stroke. Research on the role of vitamin D and other calciotropic hormones in cardiovascular disease may offer an opportunity for identifying new risk factors, which may lead to new insights into the pathophysiology of coronary heart disease and stroke, and result in new options for preventing these diseases.

To date, the focus of vitamin D research at the biochemical and physiological levels has been on the active metabolite $1,25(OH)_2D$. However, it is possible that body levels of this hormone represent a homeostatic response to vitamin D or calcium deficiency or other cardiovascular etiological factors such as increased intake of dietary salt in hypertension. Thus, its role in the etiology of cardiovascular disease may be less important than that of vitamin D and 25-OHD because blood levels of the latter correlate better with the geographical variations in cardiovascular mortality; e.g., $1,25(OH)_2D$ blood levels do not vary by season, while 25-OHD levels are lowest in winter when cardiovascular mortality is highest. An increased research emphasis on the effects of vitamin D and 25-OHD rather than $1,25(OH)_2D$ on cardiovascular function will be necessary if the etiological role of vitamin D exposure in cardiovascular disease is to be properly determined.

Finally, confirmation of a link among sunlight, vitamin D, and cardiovascular disease would have implications for public health policies regarding sun exposure. Great concern has arisen recently about depletion of the earth's ozone layer, and with the appearance of a hole in the ozone over Antarctica during the Southern Hemisphere spring.[166] Scientific reports about the effects of the hole on human health have generally emphasized the harmful consequences of increased UV exposure arising from depletion of the ozone layer. These consequences include increased risk of skin cancers such as malignant melanoma, cataracts, and immunosuppression.[167,168] However, these reports do not mention that sunlight, particularly in summer, is the major source of vitamin D in humans. At latitudes above 42° N exposure to sunshine during the winter months does not produce vitamin D in skin.[169] Thus, vitamin D is a bit like firewood — each summer we need to store enough to tide us over the following winter.

Besides coronary heart disease, reduced blood levels of 25-OHD have been found in colon cancer[170] and fractured neck of femur,[171,172] while the antirachitic effect of UV radiation has been known since the 1920s.[173] Ultraviolet radiation may also protect against breast cancer.[174] If future research confirms an additional, protective role for sunlight and vitamin D in cardiovascular disease, current public health policies, which advise people to avoid the sun in summer, would need to be revised, particularly for the elderly and those with increased skin pigmentation.

Ozone depletion may not be all doom and gloom. Vitamin D receptors occur in many mammalian tissues.[175] Who knows? Further research may eventually show that the effect of the sun, like beauty, is more than skin deep.

REFERENCES

1. World Health Organization, *World Health Statistics Annual, 1990,* WHO, Geneva, 1991.
2. Gardner, M. J., Crawford, M. D., and Morris, J. N., Patterns of mortality in middle and early old age in the county boroughs of England and Wales, *Br. J. Prev. Soc. Med.,* 23, 133, 1969.
3. Elford, J., Phillips, A. N., Thomson, A. G., and Shaper, A. G., Migration and geographic variations in ischaemic heart disease in Great Britain, *Lancet,* 1, 343, 1989.
4. Shaper, A. G., Pocock, S. J., Walker, M., Cohen, N. M., Wale, C. J., and Thompson, A. G., British Regional Heart Study: cardiovascular risk factors in middle-aged men in 24 towns, *Br. Med. J.,* 283, 179, 1981.
5. Shaper, A. G., Ashby, D., and Pocock, S. J., Blood pressure and hypertension in middle-aged British men, *J. Hypertens.,* 6, 367, 1988.
6. Smith, W. C. and Tunstall-Pedoe, H., European regional variation in cardiovascular mortality, *Br. Med. Bull.,* 40, 374, 1984.
7. Douglas, A. S., Russell, D., and Allan, T. M., Seasonal, regional and secular variations of cardiovascular and cerebrovascular mortality in New Zealand, *Aust. N.Z. J. Med.,* 20, 669, 1990.
8. Fabsitz, R. and Feinleib, M., Geographic patterns in county mortality rates from cardiovascular disease, *Am. J. Epidemiol.,* 111, 315, 1980.
9. Curwen, M., Excess winter mortality: a British phenomenon?, *Health Trends,* 22, 169, 1990/91.
10. Dunnigan, M. G., Harland, W. A., and Fyfe, T., Seasonal incidence and mortality of ischaemic heart-disease, *Lancet,* 2, 793, 1970.
11. Douglas, A. S., Al-Sayer, H., Rawles, J. M., and Allan, T. M., Seasonality of disease in Kuwait, *Lancet,* 337, 1393, 1991.
12. Rogot, E., Fabsitz, R., and Feinleib, M., Daily variation in USA mortality, *Am. J. Epidemiol.,* 103, 198, 1976.
13. Anderson, T. W. and Le Riche, W. H., Cold weather and myocardial infarction, *Lancet,* 1, 291, 1970.
14. Ahlbom, A., Seasonal variations in the incidence of acute myocardial infarction in Stockholm, *Scand. J. Soc. Med.,* 7, 127, 1979.
15. Scragg, R., Seasonal variation of mortality in Queensland, *Community Health Stud.,* 6, 120, 1982.
16. Rose, G., Cold weather and ischaemic heart disease, *Br. J. Prev. Soc. Med.,* 20, 97, 1966.
17. Sotaniemi, E., Vuopala, U., Huhti, E., and Takkunen, J., Effect of temperature on hospital admissions for myocardial infarction in a subarctic area, *Br. Med. J.,* 4, 150, 1970.
18. Douglas, A. S., Allan, T. M., and Rawles, J. M., Composition of seasonality of disease, *Scot. Med. J.,* 36, 76, 1991.

19. Ohlson, G.-G., Bodin, L., Bryngelsson, I.-L., Helsing, M., and Malmberg, L., Winter weather conditions and myocardial infarctions, *Scand. J. Soc. Med.,* 19, 20, 1991.

20. Thakur, C. P., Anand, M. P., and Shahi, M. P., Cold weather and myocardial infarction, *Int. J. Cardiol.,* 16, 19, 1987.

21. Bull, G. M. and Morton, J., Environment, temperature and death rates, *Age Ageing,* 7, 210, 1978.

22. Brennan, P. J., Greenberg, G., Miall, W. E., and Thompson, S. G., Seasonal variation in arterial blood pressure, *Br. Med. J.,* 285, 919, 1982.

23. Thelle, D. S., Forde, O. H., Try, K., and Lehmann, E. H., The Tromso Heart Study: methods and main results of the cross-sectional study, *Acta Med. Scand.,* 200, 107, 1976.

24. Khaw, K. T., Barrett-Connor, E., and Suarez, L., Seasonal and secular variation in blood pressure in man, *J. Cardiac Rehab.,* 4, 440, 1984.

25. Rippey, R. M., Overview: seasonal variations in cholesterol, *Prev. Med.,* 10, 655, 1981.

26. Harlap, S., Kark, J. D., Baras, M., Eisenberg, S., and Stein, Y., Seasonal changes in plasma lipid and lipoprotein levels in Jerusalem, *Isr. J. Med. Sci.,* 18, 1158, 1982.

27. Gordon, D. J., Trost, D. C., Hyde, J., Whaley, F. S., Hannan, P. J., Jacobs, D. R., and Ekelund, L.-G., Seasonal cholesterol cycles: the Lipid Research Clinics coronary primary prevention trial placebo group, *Circulation,* 76, 1224, 1987.

28. Van Staveren, W. A., Deurenberg, P., Burema, J., De Groot, L. C. P. G. M., and Hautvast, J. G. A. J., Seasonal variation in food intake, pattern of physical activity and change in body weights in a group of young adult Dutch women consuming self-selected diets, *Int. J. Obesity,* 10, 133, 1986.

29. Windham, C. T., Wyse, B. W., Hansen, R. G., and Hurst, R. L., Nutrient density of diets in the USDA nationwide food consumption survey, 1977–1978. I. Impact of socioeconomic status on dietary density, *J. Am. Diet. Assoc.,* 82, 28, 1983.

30. Erikssen, J. and Rodahl, K., Seasonal variation in work performance and heart rate response to exercise: a study of 1,835 middle-aged men, *Eur. J. Appl. Physiol.,* 42, 133, 1979.

31. Allen, A. W., Linton, R. R., and Donaldson, G. A., Venous thrombosis and pulmonary embolism: further experience with thrombectomy and femoral vein interruption, *JAMA,* 128, 397, 1945.

32. Feinleib, M., Venous thrombosis in relation to cigarette smoking, physical activity and seasonal activity, *Milbank Mem. Fund Q.,* 50(Suppl. 2), 123, 1973.

33. Lawrence, J. C., Xabregas, A., Gray, L., and Ham, J. M., Seasonal variation in the incidence of deep vein thrombosis, *Br. J. Surg.,* 64, 777, 1977.

34. Wroblewski, B. M., Siney, P. D., and White, R., Fatal pulmonary embolism after total hip arthroplasty: seasonal variation, *Clin. Orthop.,* 276, 222, 1992.

35. Colantonio, D., Casale, R., Natali, G., and Pisqualetti, P., Seasonal periodicity in fatal pulmonary thromboembolism, *Lancet,* 335, 56, 1990.

36. Clark, C. V., Seasonal variation in incidence of brachial and femoral emboli, *Br. Med. J.,* 287, 1109, 1983.

37. Stout, R. W. and Crawford, V., Seasonal variations in fibrinogen concentrations among elderly people, *Lancet,* 338, 9, 1991.

38. Kupari, M. and Koskinen, P., Seasonal variation in occurrence of acute atrial fibrillation and relation to air temperature and sale of alcohol, *Am. J. Cardiol.,* 66, 1519, 1990.

39. Bull, G. M. and Morton, J., Seasonal and short term relationship of temperature with deaths from myocardial and cerebral infarction, *Age Ageing,* 4, 19, 1975.

40. Rogot, E. and Padgett, S. J., Association of coronary and stroke mortality with temperature and snowfall in selected areas of the United States, *Am. J. Epidemiol.,* 103, 565, 1976.

41. Keatinge, W. R., Coleshaw, S. R. K., Cotter, F., Mattock, M., Murphy, M., and Chelliah, R., Increases in platelet and red cell counts, blood viscosity, and arterial pressure during mild surface cooling: factors in mortality from coronary and cerebral thrombosis in winter, *Br. Med. J.,* 289, 1405, 1984.

42. Collins, K. J., Easton, J. C., Belfield-Smith, H., Exton-Smith, A. N., and Pluck, R. A., Effects of age on body temperature and blood pressure in cold environments, *Clin. Sci.,* 69, 465, 1985.

43. Glass, R. J. and Zack, M. M., Increase in deaths from ischaemic heart disease after blizzard, *Lancet,* 1, 485, 1979.

44. Anderson, T. W. and Rochard, C., Cold snaps, snowfall and sudden death from ischemic heart disease, *Can. Med. Assoc. J.,* 121, 1580, 1979.
45. Baghurst, P. A., Cardiovascular deaths in winter, *Lancet,* 1, 982, 1979.
46. Collins, S. D., Excess mortality from causes other than influenza and pneumonia during influenza epidemics, *Publ. Health Rep. (Wash.),* 47, 2159, 1932.
47. Bainton, D., Jones, G. R., and Hole, R., Influenza and ischaemic heart disease — a possible trigger for acute myocardial infarction, *Int. J. Epidemiol.,* 7, 231, 1978.
48. Scragg, R., The effect of influenza epidemics on Australian mortality, *Med. J. Aust.,* 142, 98, 1985.
49. Spodick, D. H., Flessas, A. P., and Johnson, R. N., Association of acute respiratory symptoms with onset of acute myocardial infarction: prospective investigation of 150 consecutive patients and matched control patients, *Am. J. Cardiol.,* 53, 481, 1984.
50. Keatinge, W. R., Seasonal mortality among elderly people with unrestricted home heating, *Br. Med. J.,* 293, 732, 1986.
51. Keatinge, W. R., Coleshaw, S. R. K., and Holmes, J., Changes in seasonal mortalities with improvement in home heating in England and Wales from 1964 to 1984, *Int. J. Biometeorol.,* 33, 71, 1989.
52. Trapasso, L. M., Temperature distribution, in *The Encyclopedia of Climatology,* Oliver, J. E. and Fairbridge, R. W., Eds., Van Nostrand Reinhold, New York, 1987, 830.
53. Sauer, H. L., Epidemiology of cardiovascular mortality — geographic and ethnic, *Am. J. Publ. Health,* 52, 94, 1962.
54. Voors, A. W. and Johnson, W. D., Altitude and arteriosclerotic heart disease mortality in white residents of 99 of the 100 largest cities in the United States, *J. Chron. Dis.,* 32, 157, 1979.
55. Weinberg, C. R. and Brown, K. G., Altitude, radiation and mortality from cancer and heart disease, *Radiat. Res.,* 112, 381, 1987.
56. Mortimer, E. A., Monson, R. R., and MacMahon, B., Reduction in mortality from coronary heart disease in men residing at high altitude, *N. Engl. J. Med.,* 296, 581, 1977.
57. Buechley, R. W., Key, C. R., Morris, D. L., Morton, W. E., and Morgan, M. V., Altitude and ischemic heart disease in tricultural New Mexico: an example of confounding, *Am. J. Epidemiol.,* 109, 663, 1979.
58. Fujimoto, N., Matsubayashi, K., Miyahara, T., Murai, A., Matsuda, M., Shio, H., Suzuki, H., Kameyama, M., Saito, H., and Shuping, L., The risk factors for ischemic heart disease in Tibetan highlanders, *Jpn. Heart J.,* 30, 27, 1989.
59. Sharma, S., Clinical, biochemical, electrocardiographic and noninvasive hemodynamic assessment of cardiovascular status in natives at high to extreme altitudes (3000–5500 m) of the Himalayan region, *Indian Heart J.,* 42, 375, 1990.
60. Ruiz, L., Figueroa, M., Horna, C., and Penaloza, D., Prevalencia de la hipertension arterial y cardiopatia isquemica en las grandes alturas, *Arch. Inst. Cardiol.,* 39, 474, 1969.
61. Leaf, A., A scientist visits some of the world's oldest people: "every day is a gift when you are over 100", *Natl. Geogr.,* 143, 93, 1973.
62. Marticorena, E., Ruiz, L., Severino, J., Galvez, J., and Penaloza, D., Systemic blood pressure in white men born at sea level: changes after long residence at high altitudes, *Am. J. Cardiol.,* 23, 364, 1969.
63. Ruiz, L. and Penaloza, D., Altitude and hypertension, *Mayo Clin. Proc.,* 52, 442, 1977.
64. Makela, M., Barton, S. A., Schull, A. J., Weidman, W., and Rothhammer, F., The multinational Andean genetic and health program. IV. Altitude and the blood pressure of the Aymara, *J. Chron. Dis.,* 31, 587, 1978.
65. Mirrakhimov, M. M., Rafibekova, Zh. S., Dzhumagulova, T. S., Meimanaliev, T. S., Murataliev, T. M., and Shatemirova, K. K., Prevalence and clinical peculiarities of essential hypertension in a population living at high latitude, *Cor Vasa,* 27, 23, 1985.
66. Ghosh, B. N., Bansai, R. D., Ganguly, S. S., and Sen, A. K., Polynomial regression analysis of arterial blood pressure in different population groups at higher altitude (Simla hills), *Indian J. Publ. Health,* 29, 338, 1985.
67. Puri, D. S., Pal, L. S., Gupta, B. P., Swami, H. M., and Dasgupta, D. J., Distribution of blood pressure and hypertension in healthy subjects residing at high altitude in the Himalayas, *J. Assoc. Phys. India,* 34, 477, 1986.

68. Dasgupta, D. J., Prasher, B. S., Vaidya, N. K., Ahluwalia, S. K., Sharma, P. D., Puri, D. S., and Mehrotra, A. N., Blood pressure in a community at high altitude (3000 m) at Pooh (North India), *J. Epidemiol. Commun. Health,* 36, 251, 1982.

69. Dasgupta, D. J., Study of blood pressure of a high altitude community at Spiti (4000 m), *Indian Heart J.,* 38, 134, 1986.

70. Hirata, K., Ban, T., Jinnouchi, Y., and Kubo, S., Echocardiographic assessment of left ventricular function and wall motion at high altitude in normal subjects, *Am. J. Cardiol.,* 68, 1692, 1991.

71. Scognamiglio, R., Ponchia, A., Fasoli, G., and Miraglia, G., Changes in structure and function of the human left ventricle after acclimatization to high altitude, *Eur. J. Appl. Physiol.,* 62, 73, 1991.

72. Bener, P., Spectral intensity of natural ultraviolet radiation and its dependence on various parameters, in *The Biologic Effects of Ultraviolet Radiation,* Urbach, F., Ed., Pergamon Press, Oxford, 1969, 351.

73. McKenzie, R. L. and Elwood, J. M., Intensity of solar ultraviolet radiation and its implications for skin cancer, *N.Z. Med. J.,* 103, 152, 1990.

74. Johnson, F. S., Mo, T., and Green, A. E. S., Average latitudinal variation in ultraviolet radiation at the earth's surface, *Photochem. Photobiol.,* 23, 179, 1976.

75. Barton, I. J. and Paltridge, G. W., The Australian climatology of biologically effective ultraviolet radiation, *Aust. J. Dermatol.,* 20, 68, 1979.

76. Urbach, F., Geographic pathology of skin cancer, in *The Biologic Effects of Ultraviolet Radiation,* Urbach, F., Ed., Pergamon Press, Oxford, 1969, 635.

77. Altschul, R., Ultraviolet irradiation and cholesterol metabolism, *Arch. Phys. Med. Rehab.,* 36, 394, 1955.

78. Altschul, R., Lowering of serum cholesterol by ultraviolet radiation, *Geriatrics,* 10, 208, 1955.

79. Johnson, J. R., Pollock, B. E., Mayerson, H. S., and Laurens, H., The effect of carbon arc radiation on blood pressure and cardiac output, *Am. J. Physiol.,* 114, 594, 1936.

80. Allen, R. M. and Cureton, T. K., Effect of ultraviolet radiation on physical fitness, *Arch. Phys. Med.,* 26, 641, 1945.

81. Rauschkolb, E. W., Farrell, G., and Knox, J. M., Effects of ultraviolet light on skin cholesterol, *J. Invest. Dermatol.,* 49, 6332, 1967.

82. Colas, C., Garabedian, M., Fontbonne, A., Guilozzo, H., Slama, G., Desplanque, N., Dauchy, F., and Tchobroutsky, G., Insulin secretion and plasma 1,25-$(OH)_2$D after UV-B irradiation in healthy adults, *Horm. Metab. Res.,* 21, 154, 1989.

83. Jarrett, R. J., McCartney, P., and Keen, H., The Bedford Survey: ten year mortality rates in the newly diagnosed diabetics, borderline diabetics and normoglycaemic controls and risk indices for coronary heart disease in borderline diabetics, *Diabetologia,* 22, 79, 1982.

84. Scragg, R., Seasonality of cardiovascular disease mortality and the possible protective effect of ultra-violet radiation, *Int. J. Epidemiol.,* 10, 337, 1981.

85. Haddad, J. G. and Hahn, T. J., Natural and synthetic sources of circulating 25-hydroxyvitamin D in man, *Nature,* 224, 515, 1973.

86. Audran, M. and Kumar, R., The physiology and pathophysiology of vitamin D, *Mayo Clin. Proc.,* 60, 851, 1985.

87. Holick, M. F., McLaughlin, J. A., Clark, M. B., Holick, S. A., Potts, J. T., Anderson, R. R., Blank, I. H., Parrish, J. A., and Elias, P., Photosynthesis of previtamin D_3 in human skin and the physiologic consequences, *Science,* 210, 203, 1980.

88. Maclaughlin, J. A., Anderson, R. R., and Holick, M. F., Spectral character of sunlight modulates photosynthesis of previtamin D_3 and its photoisomers in human skin, *Science,* 216, 1001, 1982.

89. Holick, M. F., Photosynthesis of vitamin D in the skin: effect of environmental and life-style variables, *Fed. Proc.,* 46, 1876, 1987.

90. Bell, N. H., Epstein, S., Shary, J., Greene, V., Oexmann, M. J., and Shaw, S., Evidence of a probable role for the 25-hydroxyvitamin D in the regulation of human calcium metabolism, *J. Bone Min. Res.,* 3, 489, 1988.

91. Stryd, R. P., Gilbertson, T. J., and Brunden, M. N., A seasonal variation study of 25-hydroxyvitamin D_3 serum levels in normal humans, *J. Clin. Endocrinol. Metab.,* 48, 771, 1979.

92. Beadle, P. C., Burton, J. L., and Leach, J. F., Correlation of seasonal variation of 25-hydroxycalciferol with UV radiation dose, *Br. J. Dermatol.,* 102, 289, 1980.

93. Juttmann, J. R., Visser, T. J., Buurman, C., de Kam, E., and Birkenhager, J. C., Seasonal fluctuations in serum concentrations of vitamin D metabolites in normal subjects, *Br. Med. J.,* 282, 1349, 1981.

94. Chesney, R. W., Rosen, J. F., Hamstra, A. J., Smith, C., Mahaffey, K., and DeLuca, H. F., Absence of seasonal variation in serum concentrations of 1,25-dihydroxyvitamin D despite a rise in 25-hydroxyvitamin D in summer, *J. Clin. Endocrinol. Metab.,* 53, 139, 1981.

95. Devgun, M. S., Paterson, C. R., Johnson, B. E., and Cohen, C., Vitamin D nutrition in relation to season and occupation, *Am. J. Clin. Nutr.,* 34, 1501, 1981.

96. Elomaa, I., Karonen, S.-L., Kairento, A.-L., and Pelkonen, R., Seasonal variation of urinary calcium and oxalate excretion, serum $25(OH)D_3$ and albumin level in relation to renal stone formation, *Scand. J. Urol. Nephrol.,* 16, 155, 1982.

97. Tjellesen, L. and Christiansen, C., Vitamin D metabolites in normal subjects during one year: a longitudinal study, *Scand. J. Clin. Lab. Invest.,* 43, 85, 1983.

98. Neer, R. M., Environmental light: effects on vitamin D synthesis and calcium metabolism in humans, *Ann. N.Y. Acad. Sci.,* 453, 14, 1985.

99. Lips, P., Hackeng, M. J., Jongen, F. C., van Ginkel, F. C., and Netelenbos, J. C., Seasonal variation in serum concentrations of parathyroid hormone in elderly people, *J. Clin. Endocrinol. Metab.,* 57, 204, 1983.

100. Reid, I. R., Gallagher, D. J. A., and Bosworth, J., Prophylaxis against vitamin D deficiency in the elderly by regular sunlight exposure, *Age Ageing,* 15, 35, 1986.

101. Adams, J. S., Clemens, T. L., Parrish, J. A., and Holick, M. F., Vitamin-D synthesis and metabolism after ultraviolet irradiation of normal and vitamin-D-deficient subjects, *N. Engl. J. Med.,* 306, 722, 1982.

102. Nordin, B. E. C., *Calcium, Phosphate and Magnesium Metabolism: Clinical Physiology and Diagnostic Procedures,* Churchill Livingstone, Edinburgh, 1976, 417.

103. von Knorring, J., Slatis, P., Weber, T. H., and Helenius, T., Serum levels of 25-hydroxyvitamin D, 24,25-dihydroxyvitamin D and parathyroid hormone in patients with femoral neck fracture in southern Finland, *Clin. Endocrinol.,* 17, 189, 1982.

104. Bukowski, R. D. and Kremer, D., Calcium-regulating hormones in hypertension: vascular actions, *Am. J. Clin. Nutr.,* 54, 220S, 1991.

105. Morgan, K. G., Role of calcium ion in maintenance of vascular smooth muscle tone, *Am. J. Cardiol.,* 59, 24A, 1987.

106. Erne, P., Bolli, P., Burgisser, E., and Buhler, F. R., Correlation of platelet calcium with blood pressure, *N. Engl. J. Med.,* 310, 1084, 1984.

107. Hvarfner, A., Larsson, R., Morlin, C., Rastad, J., Wide, L., Akerstrom, G., and Ljunghall, S., Cytosolic free calcium in platelets: relationships to blood pressure and indices of systemic calcium metabolism, *J. Hypertens.,* 6, 71, 1988.

108. McVeigh, G. E., Copeland, S., McKellar, J., and Johnston, D., Effect of low versus conventional dose cyclopenthiazide on platelet intracellular calcium in mild essential hypertension, *J. Hypertens.,* 6, 337, 1988.

109. Zidek, W., Spieker, C., and Vetter, H., Ca^{++}/K^+ ratio and total intracellular calcium in essential and renal hypertension, *J. Hypertens.,* 4(Suppl. 6), S321, 1986.

110. Oshima, T., Matsuura, H., Kido, K., Matsumoto, K., Inoue, I., Otsuki, T., Shingu, T., and Kajiyama, G., Abnormalities in intralymphocytic sodium and free calcium in essential hypertension: relation to plasma renin activity, *J. Hypertens.,* 4(Suppl. 6), S334, 1986.

111. Giuliani, D. L. and Boland, R. L., Effects of vitamin D_3 metabolites on calcium fluxes in intact chicken skeletal muscle and myoblasts cultured in vitro, *Calcif. Tissue Int.,* 36, 200, 1984.

112. de Boland, A. R. and Boland, R., In vitro cellular muscle calcium metabolism: characterization of effects of 1,25-dihydroxy-vitamin D_3 and 25-hydroxy-vitamin D_3, *Z. Naturforsch.,* 40c, 102, 1985.

113. Baran, D. T. and Milne, M. L., 1,25 Dihydroxyvitamin D increases hepatocyte cytosolic calcium levels: a potential regulation of vitamin-D-25-hydroxylase, *J. Clin. Invest.,* 77, 1622, 1986.

114. Sugimoto, T., Ritter, C., Reid, I., Morrissey, J., and Slatopolsky, E., Effect of 1,25-dihydroxyvitamin D_3 on calcium in dispersed parathyroid cells, *Kidney Int.,* 33, 859, 1988.

115. Fleischman, A. I., Bierenbaum, M. L., Raichelson, R., Hayton, T., and Watson, P., Vitamin D and hypercholesterolemia in adult humans, in *Proc. 2nd. Int. Symp. Atherosclerosis,* Jones, R. J., Ed., Springer-Verlag, Berlin, 1970, 468.

116. Curcic, V. G. and Curcic, B., Effect of vitamin D on serum cholesterol and arterial blood pressure in infants, *Nutr. Metabol.,* 18, 57, 1975.

117. Carlson, L. A., Derblom, H., and Lanner, A., Effect of different doses of vitamin D on serum cholesterol and triglyceride levels in healthy men, *Atherosclerosis,* 12, 313, 1970.

118. Knox, E. G., Ischaemic-heart-disease mortality and dietary intake of calcium, *Lancet,* 1, 1465, 1973.

119. Linden, V., Vitamin D and myocardial infarction, *Br. Med. J.,* 3, 647, 1974.

120. Linden, V., Vitamin D and serum cholesterol, *Scand. J. Soc. Med.,* 3, 83, 1975.

121. Schmidt-Gayk, H., Goossen, J., Lendle, F., and Seidel, D., Serum 25-hydroxycalciferol in myocardial infarction, *Atherosclerosis,* 26, 55, 1977.

122. Lund, B., Badskjaer, J., Lund, B., and Soerensen, O. H., Vitamin D and ischaemic heart disease, *Horm. Metab. Res.,* 10, 553, 1978.

123. Vik, T., Try, K., Thelle, D. G., and Forde, O. H., Tromso heart study: vitamin D metabolism and myocardial infarction, *Br. Med. J.,* 2, 176, 1979.

124. Scragg, R., Jackson, R., Holdaway, I., Woollard, G., and Woollard, D., Changes in plasma vitamin levels in the first 48 hours after myocardial infarction, *Am. J. Cardiol.,* 64, 971, 1989.

125. Scragg, R., Jackson, R., Holdaway, I. M., Lim, T., and Beaglehole, R., Myocardial infarction is inversely associated with plasma 25-hydroxyvitamin D3 levels: a community-based study, *Int. J. Epidemiol.,* 19, 559, 1990.

126. Yano, K., Reed, D. M., and McGee, D. L., Ten-year incidence of coronary heart disease in the Honolulu heart program: relationship to biologic and lifestyle characteristics, *Am. J. Epidemiol.,* 119, 653, 1984.

127. Heliovaara, M., Karvonen, M. J., Punsar, S., and Haapakoski, J., Importance of coronary risk factors in the presence or absence of myocardial ischemia, *Am. J. Cardiol.,* 50, 1248, 1982.

128. Sowers, M. R., Wallace, R. B., and Lemke, J. H., The association of intakes of vitamin D and calcium with blood pressure among women, *Am. J. Clin. Nutr.,* 42, 135, 1985.

129. Lind, L., Wengle, B., and Ljunghall, S., Blood pressure is lowered by vitamin D (alphacalcidol) during long-term treatment of patients with intermittent hypercalcaemia: a double-blind, placebo-controlled study, *Acta Med. Scand.,* 222, 423, 1987.

130. Lind, L., Lithell, H., Skarfors, E., Wide, L., and Ljunghall, S., Reduction of blood pressure by treatment with alphacalcidol: a double-blind, placebo-controlled study in subjects with impaired glucose tolerance, *Acta Med. Scand.,* 223, 211, 1988.

131. Orwoll, E. S. and Oviatt, S., Relationship of mineral metabolism and long-term calcium and cholecalciferol supplementation to blood pressure in normotensive men, *Am. J. Clin. Nutr.,* 52, 717, 1990.

132. Kokot, F., Pietrek, J., Srokowska, S., Wartenberg, W., Kuska, J., Jedrychowska, M., Duda, G., Zielinska, K., Wartenberg, Z., and Kuzmiak, M., 25-Hydroxyvitamin D in patients with essential hypertension, *Clin. Nephrol.,* 16, 188, 1981.

133. Scragg, R., Holdaway, I., Jackson, R., and Lim, T., Plasma 25-hydroxyvitamin D3 and its relation to physical activity and other heart disease risk factors in the general population, *Ann. Epidemiol.,* 2, 697, 1992.

134. Morimoto, S., Imaoka, M., Kitano, S., Imanaka, S., Fukuo, K., Miyashita, Y., Koh, E., and Ogihara, T., Exaggerated natricalciuresis and increased circulating levels of parathyroid hormone and 1,25-dihydroxyvitamin D in patients with senile hypertension, *Contrib. Nephrol.,* 90, 94, 1991.

135. Kokot, F., Schmidt-Gayk, H., Wiecek, A., Mleczko, Z., and Bracel, B., Influence of ultraviolet irradiation on plasma vitamin D and calcitonin levels in humans, *Kidney Int.,* 36(Suppl. 27), S-143, 1989.

136. Brickman, A. S., Nygy, M. D., von Hungen, K., Eggena, P., and Tuck, M. L., Calcitropic hormones, platelet calcium, and blood pressure in essential hypertension, *Hypertension,* 16, 515, 1990.

137. Resnick, L. M., Muller, F. B., and Laragh, J. H., Calcium-regulating hormones in essential hypertension: relation to plasma renin activity and sodium metabolism, *Ann. Intern. Med.,* 105, 649, 1986.

138. Sowers, M. R., Wallace, R. B., Hollis, B. W., and Lemke, J. H., Relationship between 1,25-dihydroxyvitamin D and blood pressure in a geographically defined population, *Am. J. Clin. Nutr.,* 48, 1953, 1988.

139. Hughes, G. S., Oexmann, M. J., Margolius, H. S., Epstein, S., and Bell, N. H., Normal vitamin D and mineral metabolism in essential hypertension, *Am. J. Med. Sci.,* 296, 252, 1988.

140. Burgess, E. D., Hawkins, R. G., and Watanabe, M., Interaction of 1,25-dihydroxyvitamin D and plasma renin activity in high renin essential hypertension, *Am. J. Hypertens.,* 3, 903, 1990.

141. Auwerx, J., Bouillon, R., and Kesteloot, H., Relation between 25-hydroxyvitamin D_3, apolipoprotein A-1, and high density lipoprotein cholesterol, *Arterioscler. Thromb.,* 12, 671, 1992.

142. Ljunghall, S., Lind, L., Lithell, H., Skarfors, E., Selinus, I., Sorensen, O. H., and Wide, L., Treatment with one-alpha-hydroxycholecalciferol in middle-aged men with impaired glucose tolerance — a prospective randomized double-blind study, *Acta Med. Scand.,* 222, 361, 1987.

143. Powell, K. E., Thompson, P. D., Caspersen, C. T., and Kendrick, J. S., Physical activity and the incidence of coronary heart disease, *Am. Rev. Publ. Health,* 8, 253, 1987.

144. Bell, N. H., Godsen, R. N., Henry, D. R., Shary, J., and Epstein, S., The effects of muscle-building exercise on vitamin D and mineral metabolism, *J. Bone Miner. Res.,* 3, 369, 1988.

145. Leaverton, P. E., Feinleib, M., and Thom, T., Coronary heart disease mortality rates in United States blacks, 1968–1978: interstate variation, *Am. Heart J.,* 108, 732, 1984.

146. Johnson, J. L., Heineman, E. F., Heiss, G., Hames, C. G., and Tyroler, H. A., Cardiovascular disease risk factors and mortality among black women and white women aged 40–64 years in Evans County, Georgia, *Am. J. Cardiol.,* 123, 209, 1986.

147. Lee, M. H., Borhani, N. O., and Kuller, L. H., Validation of reported myocardial infarction mortality in blacks and whites: a report from the Community Cardiovascular Surveillance Program, *Ann. Epidemiol.,* 1, 1, 1990.

148. McKeigue, P. M. and Marmot, M. G., Mortality from coronary heart disease in Asian communities in London, *Br. Med. J.,* 297, 903, 1988.

149. Fox, K. M. and Shapiro, L. M., Heart disease in Asians in Britain: commoner than in Europeans, but why?, *Br. Med. J.,* 297, 311, 1988.

150. Tipene-Leach, D., Stewart, A., and Beaglehole, R., Coronary heart disease mortality in Auckland Maori and Europeans, *N.Z. Med. J.,* 104, 55, 1991.

151. Boyle, E., Biological patterns in hypertension by race, sex, body weight, and skin color, *JAMA,* 213, 1637, 1970.

152. Harburg, E., Gleibermann, L., Roeper, P., Schork, M. A., and Schull, W. J., Skin color, ethnicity, and blood pressure. I. Detroit blacks, *Am. J. Publ. Health,* 68, 1177, 1978.

153. Winkleby, M. A., Ragland, D. R., Syme, L., and Fisher, J. M., Heightened risk of hypertension among black males: the masking effect of covariables, *Am. J. Epidemiol.,* 128, 1075, 1988.

154. McKeigue, P. M., Shah, B., and Marmot, M. G., Relation of central obesity and insulin resistance with high diabetes prevalence and cardiovascular risk in South Asians, *Lancet,* 337, 382, 1991.

155. Costas, R., Garcia-Palmieri, M. R., Sorlie, P., and Hertzmark, E., Coronary heart disease risk factors in men with light and dark skin in Puerto Rico, *Am. J. Publ. Health,* 71, 614, 1981.

156. Clemens, T. L., Adams, J. S., Henderson, S. L., and Holick, M. F., Increased skin pigment reduces the capacity of skin to synthesise vitamin D_3, *Lancet,* 1, 74, 1982.

157. Matsuoka, L. Y., Wortsman, J., Haddad, J. G., Kolm, P., and Hollis, B. W., Racial pigmentation and the cutaneous synthesis of vitamin D, *Arch. Dermatol.,* 127, 536, 1991.

158. M'Buyamba-Kabangu, J. R., Fagard, R., Lijnen, P., Bouillon, R., Lissens, W., and Amery, A., Calcium, vitamin D-endocrine system, and parathyroid hormone in black and white males, *Calcif. Tissue Int.,* 41, 70, 1987.

159. Reid, I. R., Cullen, S., Schooler, B. A., Livingston, N. E., and Evans, M. C., Calcitropic hormone levels in Polynesians: evidence against their role in interracial differences in bone mass, *J. Clin. Endocrinol. Metab.,* 70, 1452, 1990.

160. Lund, B. and Sorensen, O. H., Measurement of 25-hydroxyvitamin D in serum and its relation to sunshine, age and vitamin D intake in the Danish population, *Scand. J. Clin. Lab. Invest.*, 39, 23, 1979.

161. Parfitt, A. M., Gallagher, J. C., Heaney, R. P., Johnston, C. C., Neer, R., and Whedon, G. D., Vitamin D and bone health in the elderly, *Am. J. Clin. Nutr.*, 36, 1014, 1982.

162. Editorial, Vitamin D supplementation in the elderly, *Lancet*, 1, 306, 1987.

163. MacLaughlin, J. and Holick, M. K., Aging decreases the capacity of human skin to produce vitamin D_3, *J. Clin. Invest.*, 76, 1536, 1985.

164. Phair, R. D., Cellular calcium and atherosclerosis: a brief review, *Cell. Calcium*, 9, 275, 1988.

165. Heller, R. F., Chin, S., Tunstall-Pedoe, H. D., and Rose, G., How well can we predict coronary heart disease? — Findings in the United Kingdom heart disease prevention project, *Br. Med. J.*, 288, 1409, 1984.

166. Lemonick, M. D., The ozone vanishes, *Time Int.*, 139(February 17), 38, 1992.

167. Editorial, Protecting man from UV exposure, *Lancet*, 337, 1258, 1991.

168. National Health and Medical Research Council, *Health Effects of Ozone Layer Depletion*, Australian Government Publishing Service, Canberra, 1989.

169. Webb, R., Kline, L., and Holick, M. F., Influence of season and latitude on the cutaneous synthesis of vitamin D_3: exposure to winter sunlight in Boston and Edmonton will not promote vitamin D_3 synthesis in human skin, *J. Clin. Endocrinol. Metab.*, 67, 373, 1988.

170. Garland, C. F., Comstock, G. W., Garland, F. C., Helsing, K. J., Shaw, E. K., and Gorham, E. D., Serum 25-hydroxyvitamin D and colon cancer: eight year prospective study, *Lancet*, 2, 1176, 1989.

171. Baker, M. R., McConnell, H., Peacock, M., and Nordin, B. E. C., Plasma 25-hydroxyvitamin D concentrations in patients with fractures of the femoral neck, *Br. Med. J.*, 1, 589, 1979.

172. Pun, K. K., Wong, F. H. W., Wang, C., Lau, P., Ho, P. W. M., Pun, W. K., Chow, S. P., Cheng, C. L., Leong, J. C. Y., and Young, R. T. T., Vitamin D status among patients with fractured neck of femur in Hong Kong, *Bone*, 11, 365, 1990.

173. Steenbock, H. and Black, A., Fat soluble vitamins. XVIII. The induction of growth-promoting and calcifying properties in a ration by exposure to ultraviolet light, *J. Biol. Chem.*, 61, 405, 1924.

174. Garland, F. C., Garland, C. F., Gorham, E. D., and Young, J. F., Geographic variation in breast cancer mortality in the United States: a hypothesis involving exposure to solar radiation, *Prev. Med.*, 19, 614, 1990.

175. Reichel, H., Koeffler, P., and Norman, A. W., The role of the vitamin D endocrine system in health and disease, *N. Engl. J. Med.*, 320, 980, 1989.

10

Cardiovascular Actions of Calcitonin Gene-Related Peptide

Donald J. DiPette and Sunil J. Wimalawansa

CONTENTS

ABSTRACT

Calcitonin gene-related peptide (CGRP) is a 37-amino acid neuropeptide produced from the alternate splicing of the calcitonin/CGRP gene. The peptide is distributed throughout the central (CNS) and peripheral nervous systems (PNS) and is located in areas known to be involved in cardiovascular function. Peripherally, CGRP is located in the heart, particularly in association with the sinoatrial and atrioventricular nodes. In addition, CGRP is found in nerve fibers that form a dense periadventitial network throughout the peripheral vascular system, including the central, coronary, and renal arteries. Calcitonin gene-related peptide has prominent cardiovascular effects including vasodilation and positive chronotropic and inotropic effects. Because of these effects, CGRP may play an important role in normal cardiovascular function. Furthermore, alterations in CGRP may be involved in the pathophysiology of a spectrum of cardiovascular disease states, including cerebrovascular disease, coronary artery disease, and hypertension. The development of CGRP analogues may be potential therapeutic modalities in the treatment of these and other cardiovascular disorders.

I. INTRODUCTION

Calcitonin gene-related peptide (rat-CGRPα, r-CGRPα) is a 37-amino acid neuropeptide, the existence of which was predicted in the rat.[1,2] The peptide results from alternate splicing of the primary RNA transcript of the calcitonin/CGRP gene.[2] This alternate splicing of the primary RNA transcript leads to the translation of CGRP and calcitonin peptides in a tissue-specific manner. In the CNS, α-calcitonin/CGRP gene splicing leads to the production of CGRP, whereas in the C-cells of the thyroid gland it results in the formation of calcitonin. Another very similar peptide in the rat (r-CGRPβ), differing in one amino acid from r-CGRPα, and in humans (h-CGRPβ), differing in three amino acids from h-CGRPα, was predicted from cDNA analysis in the rat and in humans.[3] The existence of h-CGRPβ was proven by its isolation and full characterization by amino acid sequencing and fast atom bombardment-mass spectrometry (FAB-MS).[4] Both α- and β-calcitonin/CGRP genes are located on chromosome 11.[5,6] Calcitonin gene-related peptide mRNA has also been localized and characterized in the heart[7] and CGRP is present in the circulation in humans and in animals.[8,9] The α and β strains of CGRP are both present in plasma, cerebrospinal fluid, and the spinal cord.[10] Throughout evolution,[11] CGRP and its receptors are well conserved.

II. DISTRIBUTION OF IMMUNOREACTIVE CALCITONIN GENE-RELATED PEPTIDE AND ITS RECEPTORS IN THE CARDIOVASCULAR SYSTEM

The distribution of CGRP and its receptors is consistent with the known cardiovascular actions of CGRP. In many organs CGRP immunoreactivity is seen in close relation to blood vessels, and it is abundant in the cardiovascular and the CNS and PNS.[12-16] In the heart, CGRP immunoreactivity is found in the pericardium and around and parallel to the coronary arteries. Fibers that are CGRP enriched also penetrate into the heart muscles, particularly the papillary muscles, sinoatrial, atrioventricular nodes, and the conducting system. In blood vessels, the varicose and smooth CGRP-containing nerve fibers pass through the junction of the adventitia and the media and then into the smooth muscle cellular layer. A dense perivascular neural network is also seen around the inferior vena cava, renal arteries, superior mesenteric artery, the carotid arteries, the cerebral arteries, and most other vascular beds. Indeed, fibers to the carotid arteries can be traced to the ipsilateral trigeminal ganglion.[17] Most, if not all, of these peripheral CGRP-containing nerve fibers are sensory afferents which have their cell bodies in the respective dorsal root ganglia and their central termini in laminae I/II of the dorsal horn of the spinal cord. Thus, these afferent neurons innervate the heart and peripheral blood vessels. These afferents synapse centrally with neurons in the intermediolateral cell column of the spinal cord, which can connect to sympathetic preganglionic neurons. This connection could influence the activity of the sympathetic nervous system and therefore cardiovascular function. In addition, evidence is accumulating for the efferent release of peptides, including CGRP, from these CGRP-containing primary afferent endings in the periphery. Thus, CGRP could influence cardiovascular control via both afferent and efferent neuronal activity. In addition to CGRP peptide, the existence of subclasses of CGRP receptors in a similar target organ distribution has been demonstrated using CGRP-(8-37) fragment.[18]

III. BIOLOGICAL ACTIVITY OF CALCITONIN GENE-RELATED PEPTIDE

This peptide is the most potent endogenous vasodilatory peptide thus far discovered and its receptors are widely distributed in the body.[14,19-23] This effect of CGRP is induced through the relaxation of vascular smooth muscle. Calcitonin gene-related peptide has a number of other biological actions in the cardiovascular system, including positive inotropic and chronotropic effects on the heart[13,24-27] and control of blood supply to various organs.[28,29] These actions are discussed individually.

A. Chronotropic and Inotropic Effects

It has been known for some time that capsaicin, an agent found in peppers, results in the release of neuropeptides from sensory afferent neurons. Such neuropeptides include, but are not limited to, CGRP and substance P. Acute capsaicin administration induces both positive inotropic and chronotropic effects.[26,30,31] Evidence is accumulating that CGRP, in these cardiovascular nonadrenergic noncholinergic neurons, mediates these cardiovascular effects of capsaicin. The *in vitro* administration of CGRP to rat, guinea pig, or human atrial or porcine ventricular tissue increases contractile rate and force.[27,32-34] Similarly, the *in vitro* administration of CGRP to the isolated perfused intact heart produces positive chronotropic and inotropic effects.[24] The *in vivo* systemic intravenous administration of CGRP to intact animals and humans produces both positive chronotropic and inotropic effects.[35-37] Thus, in multiple species, including humans, CGRP mimics the known cardiovascular effects of capsaicin. Furthermore, capsaicin administration results in tachyphylaxis to its positive chronotropic and inotropic effects. Following tachyphylaxis to capsaicin, CGRP administration continues to produce positive chronotropic and inotropic effects. On the other hand, following tachyphylaxis to CGRP, the positive chronotropic and inotropic effects of capsaicin administration are abolished. In addition, capsaicin administration to the intact perfused isolated heart has been shown to release CGRP. Therefore, it is likely that CGRP mediates the acute cardiovascular effects of capsaicin.

The positive inotropic effects of CGRP have been compared to other agents in similar animal models. In studies using the isolated, electrically driven human atrium, both CGRP and vasoactive intestinal peptide (VIP) have been shown to increase the force of contraction in a dose-dependent manner.[25] Interestingly, CGRP was approximately ten times more potent than the positive inotrope norepinephrine. In this preparation neither the α-adrenergic blocker, phentolamine, or the β-adrenergic blocker, metoprolol, antagonized the response to CGRP, indicating that the effects of CGRP are likely to be mediated by specific myocardial CGRP receptors. In addition, neither neurokinin A or substance P, which are co-stored with CGRP in some cardiac sensory neurons had any effect on contractility in this preparation. The mechanisms of the positive chronotropic and inotropic effects of CGRP appear to be attributed to the activation of adenylate cyclase, adenosine $3':5'$-cyclic phosphate leading to increased intracellular (cAMP) levels, to an increase in the slow inward calcium current,[27,33,34] or both. In these studies, the time course of the increase in cAMP secondary to CGRP administration correlated closely with the chronotropic and inotropic effects. Administration of CGRP had no effect on myocardial cyclic guanosine monophosphate (cGMP) levels, and preincubation with either atenolol, a β-adrenergic receptor blocker, or indomethacin did not alter the chronotropic, inotropic, or cAMP responses to CGRP. In addition to these myocardial cellular processes, CGRP has also been shown to increase potassium permeability in single atrial cell preparations.

B. Vasodilatory Effects

Many organ bath preparations have shown vasorelaxation in response to CGRP: rat aorta;[38] rat coronary vasculature;[24] rat mesenteric vasculature;[39] cat cerebral vessels;[40] cat, rabbit, and human pial vessels;[41] and human pulmonary, coronary, gastric, splenic, brachial, and transverse cervical arteries.[42] Guinea pig cheek pouch arterial dilatation[19] and splenic vascular relaxation[43] also have been reported following local *in vivo* administration of CGRP. In the rat coronary vasculature, CGRP is a more potent vasodilator with a more prolonged duration of action than adenosine.[44]

Calcitonin gene-related peptide is also a potent cutaneous vasodilator. Intradermal injection of CGRP in rabbits and in humans causes a marked increased in local skin blood flow.[19] Not surprisingly, a systemic injection of CGRP in humans causes a rise in skin temperature and skin flushing, a fall in blood pressure, and a reflex-mediated release of catecholamine-associated tachycardia.[45,46] These effects and the increase in plasma catecholamines persist for a long time after the CGRP infusions are stopped and the levels of circulatory CGRP return to the baseline. Similarly, following intradermal injection of CGRP, both the flare and the vasodilation persist for several hours. Therefore, the vasodilatory effects of CGRP are prolonged, persisting long after the local levels have returned to baseline.

Administration of CGRP either directly to the CNS or systemically (i.e., intravenously or intraarterially) produces prominent cardiovascular effects including those upon the vasculature. Intracerebroventricular administration of CGRP to conscious, unrestrained rats produces a dose-dependent increase in blood pressure and heart rate.[47] These cardiovascular effects are accompanied by a marked increase in plasma norepinephrine levels.[47] This suggests that the central administration of CGRP may increase sympathetic outflow, which in turn could mediate the observed increase in blood pressure and heart rate. In addition other studies have shown that baroreceptor deafferentation by sinoaortic denervation may accentuate the increase in blood pressure following the central administration of CGRP.

The regional hemodynamic effect of central administration of CGRP also has been studied in several rat strains. In addition to the increase in blood pressure and heart rate, central CGRP administration to conscious Sprague-Dawley normotensive rats decreases hindquarter vascular resistance, but has no effect on renal or mesenteric vascular resistances.[48] Pretreatment with peripheral propranolol or hexamethonium attenuates but does not completely abolish the increase in heart rate, indicating that the mechanism of the central effect of CGRP may indeed be mediated, in part, by activation of the sympathetic nervous system. In the Long-Evans normotensive rat, the central administration of CGRP also produces an increase in heart rate and a modest increase in blood pressure.[49] These systemic hemodynamic changes are accompanied by renal hemodynamic changes, but no change in hindquarter vascular resistance. Interestingly, the central administration of CGRP to Brattleboro rats, which are deficient in vasopressin, causes regional hemodynamic effects similar to those observed in the Long-Evans rat, suggesting that these observed vascular effects are not due to the central release of vasopressin into the systemic circulation. Differences in rat strains or doses of CGRP employed may explain the differing results obtained in these normotensive rat studies. Direct injection of CGRP into the central amygdaloid in the rat produces an increase in blood pressure and heart rate.

Immunocytochemical and radioimmunoassay (RIA) techniques have demonstrated that CGRP is densely localized within the central amygdaloid and direct electrical stimulation of the central amygdaloid produces similar cardiovascular effects.[50] These results suggest that the amygdaloid is a site where CGRP may play a central modulatory cardiovascular role. Although CGRP is located in multiple CNS sites, whether these sites are also involved in the central hemodynamic effects of CGRP remains to be determined.

Homology between human and salmon calcitonins, calcitonin gene-related peptides and amylin.

```
  h-CT   -  C G N L S T C M L G T Y T Q D F N K - - - - - F H T F P Q T A I G V G A P

  s-CT   -  C S N L S T C V L G K L S Q D L H K - - - - - L Q T Y P R T N T G S G T P

 Amylin  -  K C N T A T C A T Q R L A N F L V H S S N N F G A I L S S T N V G S N T Y

 β-hCGRP -  A C N T A T C V T H R L A G L L R R S G G M V K S N F V P T N V G S K A F

 α-hCGRP -  A C D T A T C V T H R L A G L L R R S G G V V K N N F V P T N V G S K A F
```

FIGURE 1 Primary amino acid sequence homology of CGRP calcitonin and amylin.

The systemic and regional hemodynamic effects of the peripheral administration of CGRP has also been determined.[21,22,51,52] The systemic administration of CGRP to the conscious unrestrained normotensive rat results in a dose-dependent decrease in mean blood pressure. The mechanism of this decrease in blood pressure is due to peripheral arterial vasodilation because total peripheral resistance decreases in a dose-dependent manner while cardiac output does not significantly change.[21,22] As previously mentioned, the peripheral administration of CGRP consistently results in a dose-dependent increase in heart rate. Calcitonin gene-related peptide appears to have significant and selective regional hemodynamic effects and has been shown to increase blood flow and/or decrease the vascular resistance in the coronary, common carotid, renal, mesenteric, and hindquarter vascular beds, particularly at lower doses. The administration of CGRP at higher doses, which results in a significant decrease in blood pressure, produces variable regional vascular hemodynamic effects which are probably due to the resultant increase in endogenous pressors such as norepinephrine and epinephrine as a compensatory response to the induced systemic blood pressure reduction.[22]

IV. CALCITONIN GENE-RELATED PEPTIDE AND ITS RECEPTORS: RELATIONSHIP TO AMYLIN, CALCITONIN, AND BIOLOGIC EFFECTS

The primary amino acid sequence homology of CGRP, calcitonin, and amylin is shown in Figure 1. Calcitonin gene-related peptide (with 19% amino acid homology with fish calcitonins) can displace specific calcitonin binding in the osteoclast and vice versa, but only at a 1000-fold molar excess.[9] Amylin is a 37-amino acid peptide with 46% amino acid homology with CGRP[53-55] and can compete with ^{125}I-CGRP for specific CGRP binding in brain, but at a 50 to 60-fold molar excess.[11,56] Furthermore, both amylin and CGRP are capable of stimulating adenyl cyclase in CGRP receptor-rich cells in a dose-dependent manner.[57] This receptor cross-reactivity has been confirmed *in vivo* by demonstrating of the vasodilatory properties of amylin.[58,59] Amylin also has potent effects on calcium metabolism in animals[60,61] and in humans. In renal membranes and LLC-PK1 renal cells, CGRP can stimulate adenyl cyclase activity and plasminogen activator production, perhaps through interaction with calcitonin receptors. Similarly, it is possible that the actions of CGRP and amylin on the inhibition of bone resorption may be exerted via activation of at least one class of calcitonin receptor in the osteoclast.[61] The other effects of amylin include interference with the actions of insulin in the peripheral tissues,[62-64] suppression of appetite,[65] production of hypocalcemia secondary to suppression of osteoclastic activity, and vasodilation.[59]

The wide distribution of CGRP and its receptors in the cardiovascular system,[66,67] and the immunoreactive CGRP (iCGRP) in the perivascular nerves,[2] taken together with the potent vasodilatory activity of CGRP,[19,20,37,46,68] suggest that CGRP may have a major role in the regulation of peripheral vascular tone and the control of blood flow in various organs.[57] Although CGRP is a potent vasodilator,[19,20,37,46,68] the physiological significance of its presence in the circulation and the age-related increase of iCGRP levels in plasma,[69,70] are yet unknown. The increased iCGRP in the circulation with age suggests a number of possibilities: increased synthesis of CGRP due to down regulation of its receptors, hypersecretion in response to increasing rigidity of arterioles, increased protein binding of CGRP or increased CGRP-binding protein in the circulation, and decrease of CGRP clearance from the circulation with age.

Furthermore, CGRP is widely distributed in the mesenteric vasculature,[39] the gastrointestinal tract,[14] and the thyroid gland.[12,14] Liberation of CGRP into the circulation has been demonstrated following a meal or pentagastrin stimulation test (a potent stimulator of C-cells).[71,72] The vasodilatory response seen following a heavy or spicy meal and following pentagastrin stimulation test (acute stimulation of C-cells of the thyroid gland) is due to acute liberation of CGRP.

V. AGE-RELATED CHANGES OF CALCITONIN GENE-RELATED PEPTIDE IN THE CARDIOVASCULAR SYSTEM

An age-related decline of iCGRP contents has been observed in right and left atria and in the lungs.[70] This may indicate that CGRP has a prominent role to play during maturity (e.g., acting as a growth factor) in the lungs and in controlling cardiovascular function, particularly in the young. In this respect, as previously mentioned, CGRP has been shown to increase the chronotropic and inotropic actions of the heart and to increase cell replication in the human umbilical endothelial cells.[73,74] An age-related decrease of iCGRP contents in the arteries and the simultaneous increase in the veins may have a negative cardiovascular hemodynamic effect. Interestingly, such a hemodynamic profile is seen in aging, in which cardiac output decreases and total peripheral resistance and blood pressure increases. It is tempting to suggest that a casual relationship exists between some of the age-related vascular disorders and the changes of the content of iCGRP in various cardiovascular tissues, particularly the arteries. For example, the decrease of iCGRP contents with age demonstrated in the cerebral arteries[70] may well be associated with vasomotor instability and the likelihood of cerebrovascular episodes in older people. Furthermore, a circadian rhythm of CGRP levels is found in the circulation, the level of which lowest in the early morning hours (between 3 and 5 a.m.).[71] Taken together, the low content of CGRP present in the arteries (carotid, cerebral, and presumably coronary) in the elderly and the tendency to have a relative deficiency of circulatory CGRP during the early hours of the morning may be partially responsible for the increased incidence of early morning cardiovascular episodes in these individuals.

VI. CARDIOVASCULAR PATHOPHYSIOLOGY: RELATIONSHIP TO CALCITONIN GENE-RELATED PEPTIDE

Calcitonin gene-related peptide is primarily a neuropeptide and it participates in the modulation of sensory neurotransmission. Because of its potent vasodilatory effects, one of the most important roles of CGRP in the periphery may be the control of blood flow to various organs.[19,20,29,57] Although there appears to be no sex differences in plasma CGRP levels,[8,75] as opposed to those found with calcitonin,[76] circulating CGRP levels seem to increase with age.[69] This increase contrasts with the decline in tissue CGRP content with increasing age as previously detailed. The pathophysiological significance of these age-related changes in CGRP, particularly in the circulation, remains to be determined.

Receptors are widely distributed in the CNS,[11,12,77,78] which indicates the possibility of a range of important actions of CGRP in the brain.[65,79,80] In addition, CGRP receptors are also widely distributed in the periphery. The intradermal injection of CGRP not only increases skin blood flow, but also plasma protein extravasation and edema formation in the skin.[81,82] In this regard, the cutaneous vasodilatory effects of CGRP may increase the survival of tissue flaps in reconstructive surgery.[83] Similar effects of CGRP are seen in the knee joint;[84] some of these effects can be eliminated by administration of CGRP-(8-37),[85] a CGRP receptor antagonist.

A number of pharmacological studies have demonstrated various beneficial effects following the injection or infusion of h-CGRP-(1-37) in humans. For example, prolonged infusion of CGRP into patients with congestive heart failure has been shown to have a sustained beneficial effect on the hemodynamic functions (increased cardiac output and decreased total peripheral resistance) without adverse effects. Furthermore, unlike other vasodilators, CGRP also increases renal blood flow and glomerular filtration.[86] In animal models, CGRP has been shown to be useful in peripheral nerve regeneration following injury.

One of the major biological effects of CGRP is the relaxation of smooth muscle in the cardiovascular system. However, as previously mentioned, in the rat intra-cerebroventricular administration of CGRP causes a prompt rise in plasma norepinephrine and an elevation in the mean arterial pressure, while the intravenous administration of CGRP causes a fall in mean arterial pressure.[47] Intracoronary infusion of CGRP as well as the systemic administration of CGRP, even in low doses, produces a marked increase in coronary blood flow.[21,22,24] A similar effect is observed with the systemic administration of other known vasodilators such as verapamil, isosorbide dinitrate, and VIP, but at higher concentrations.[39] The vasodilatory effect observed in response to CGRPα or -β[19,20] is comparable. Thus, CGRP could play a significant role in the pathophysiology as well as treatment of coronary artery disease. For instance, if the neuronal levels and subsequent release of CGRP from coronary artery-associated neurons is diminished (e.g., in atherosclerosis) while local vasoconstrictors are preserved or augmented, then conditions would be favorable for coronary spasm with or without thrombosis. On the other hand, the administration of CGRP or CGRP-like agonist analogues would be useful in the treatment of ischemia in coronary artery disease from either coronary spasm or the atherosclerotic process. In addition to its vasodilatory activity, CGRP exerts proliferative effects on the endothelium,[73,74] which may have a role in revascularization and repair following ischemic injury.[83]

The systemic administration of CGRP in animals and humans causes a fall in blood pressure.[45] Because CGRP has such potent effects on the peripheral vascular system, the abundance of immunoreactive CGRP in perivascular nerves and accompanying specific binding sites in vascular smooth muscle, it is logical to speculate that CGRP may play an important role in the modulation of peripheral vascular tone and hypertension. In this regard, the role of CGRP in systemic hypertension recently has come under intense investigation. Similar to coronary artery disease, CGRP could play a pathophysiologic and/or therapeutic role in hypertension. The spontaneously hypertensive rat (SHR) is a genetic animal model of hypertension thought to most closely represent the pathophysiology of human essential hypertension. The SHR is also known to possess abnormalities of calcium homeostasis such as decreased serum ionized calcium and increased serum parathyroid levels.[87] Thus, the SHR appears to have a relative calcium deficiency. Because CGRP is a product of the calcitonin/CGRP gene, which is intricately linked to calcium homeostasis, it is logical to propose that alterations of CGRP (e.g., as a relative reduction) could lead to an increase in blood pressure and play a role in hypertension, particularly in this animal model. Furthermore, the neuronal level of CGRP is directly modulated by changes in dietary calcium in that a low calcium diet, which decreases the serum ionized calcium level, decreases the neuronal content of CGRP, while a high calcium diet, which increases the serum ionized calcium level, increases the neuronal content of CGRP.[88] Interestingly and consistent with these findings, the SHR has been shown to have significantly decreased neuronal levels of both CGRP messenger RNA (mRNA) and CGRP immunoreactive peptide.[89,90]

Therefore, in this genetic model of experimental hypertension the reduced neuronal production and content of CGRP may contribute to the blood pressure elevation and play a primary role in hypertension. In addition, the administration of CGRP markedly lowers the blood pressure and produces selective regional vasodilatory effects in the SHR.[91,92] Unfortunately, the role of CGRP in the hypertensive process appears more complex. In contrast to the results found in the SHR, more recent studies have shown that in mineralocorticoid-salt-induced (DOC-salt) hypertension, an acquired sodium-dependent model of experimental hypertension, the neuronal levels of CGRP mRNA and immunoreactive CGRP peptide are increased.[93] Therefore, in this acquired model of hypertension an increase in CGRP may represent a secondary compensatory vasodilatory response to elevation of blood pressure. As would be anticipated, less is known regarding the role of CGRP in human essential hypertension. The data concerning circulating CGRP levels in essential hypertensive patients have been conflicting, and investigators report an increased,[94] an unchanged,[95] or a decreased[96] level. Such results may be due to the heterogenous nature of essential hypertension or to differences in RIA. Of course, because CGRP is a neuropeptide, the relationship of circulating levels of CGRP to local neuronal release and vascular activity is unknown. In addition to a potential role in the pathophysiology of hypertension and due to its potent peripheral vasodilatory properties, the administration of CGRP or CGRP-like analogues may have potential therapeutic implications in hypertension.

Being a potent vasodilator, CGRP is likely to have a potential use in vascular (e.g., coronary or cerebral) disease, especially during acute episodes. The major limitations to the therapeutic use of CGRP are the necessity of infusions and the cost of the product. However, when a CGRP mimetic of simple structure is available, it will open the door for further therapeutic applications. Receptor-based peptide and nonpeptide CGRP-mimetic "super-analogues" are likely to be developed using the information obtained from the CGRP binding site. These can then be used for the prevention and treatment of cardiovascular disorders in man.

So far, no disease processes have been attributed solely to either a deficiency or an excess of CGRP. Variable but increased circulating CGRP levels have been described in patients with C-cell hyperplasia and medullary thyroid carcinoma.[75,97] Although the plasma iCGRP level is a poor marker for diagnosis of medullary thyroid carcinoma,[75] measurement of receptor-active CGRP by radioreceptor assay[78,98,99] is a sensitive tool for the diagnosis of both medullary thyroid carcinoma and C-cell hyperplasia. It has been suggested that the increased plasma levels of CGRP are responsible for the hemodynamic derangement present in hepatic cirrhosis.[100] Increased iCGRP has also been demonstrated in plasma and splanchnic organs following experimental endotoxemia, suggesting that CGRP may play a role in this disorder.[101] The only other disorder reported so far where there is altered sensitivity of CGRP to its receptor is Raynaud's syndrome. On the other hand, Brain et al.[102] reported that Raynaud's sufferers do not exhibit a diminished response to CGRP in the cutaneous microvasculature. Administration of synthetic CGRP-(1-37) has been shown to minimize the ischemic damage to the brain following subarachnoid hemorrhage, and alterations in CGRP have been proposed to play a primary role in cerebral vasospasm in this clinical disorder.[103-105] As previously mentioned, it is likely that infusion of CGRP into coronary arteries may decrease or reverse the vasospasm, and hence ischemic damage to the heart, during acute myocardial infarction. Similarly, administration of CGRP systemically or into an affected cerebral artery may reverse the vasospasm associated with subarachnoid hemorrhage or certain strokes in evolution.

CGRP receptors have been isolated and purified, and monoclonal antibodies have been raised against these purified receptors.[106-108] It is envisaged that full-length amino acid sequences of CGRP receptors will be available in the near future. This should allow the development of specific receptor-based super agonists for CGRP. These agents can then be used on cardiovascular disorders in man, especially if they are organ or vascular specific.[109]

VII. CONCLUSION

Calcitonin gene-related peptide is a potent vasodilatory neuropeptide with positive chronotropic and inotropic effects. It is normally distributed throughout the central and peripheral nervous system. High-affinity CGRP receptors are similarly distributed. Peripherally, CGRP is located in neurons, forming a dense periadventitial plexus throughout the vasculature, including cerebral, coronary, and renal beds. Therefore, it is logical to speculate that CGRP plays a role in normal cardiac function, systemic blood pressure, and regional organ blood flow. Similarly, alterations in CGRP may be involved in the pathophysiology of a spectrum of cardiovascular diseases, including but not limited to cerebrovascular disease, coronary artery disease, congestive heart failure, and hypertension. In addition, the development of a simple, orally absorbable peptide agonist drug capable of activating CGRP receptors without down regulation of CGRP receptors may be an important therapeutic modality in cardiovascular disease.

ACKNOWLEDGMENTS

The authors wish to thank Ms. Vicki Isaacks for the excellent secretarial assistance. Donald J. DiPette is supported by NIH grant 1R01 HL44277-01A1 and a recipient of the Established Investigator Award of the American Heart Association. Sunil J. Wimalawansa was, in part, supported by the British Heart Foundation.

REFERENCES

1. Amara, S. G., Arriza, J. L., Leff, S. E., Swanson, L. W., Evans R. M., and Rosenfeld, M. G., Expression in brain of messenger RNA encoding a novel neuropeptide homologous to calcitonin gene-related peptide, *Science,* 229, 1094, 1982.
2. Rosenfeld, M. G., Mermod, J. J., Amara, S. G., Swanson, L. W., Sawchenko, P. E., Rivier, J., Vale, W. W., and Evans, R. M., Production of a novel neuropeptide encoded by the calcitonin gene via tissue-specific RNA processing, *Nature,* 304, 129, 1983.
3. Steenburgh, P. H., Hoppener, J. W. M., Zandberg, J., Van de Ven, W. J. M., Jansz, H. S., and Lips, C. J. M., Calcitonin gene-related peptide coding sequence is conserved in the human genome and is expressed in medullary thyroid carcinoma, *J. Clin. Endocrinol. Metab.,* 59, 358, 1984.
4. Wimalawansa, S. J., Morris, H. R., Etienne, A., Blench, I., Panico, M., and MacIntyre, I., Isolation, purification and characterization of β-hCGRP from human spinal cord, *Biochem. Biophys. Res. Commun.,* 167, 993, 1990.
5. Steenberg, P. H., Hoppener, J. W. M., Zandberg, J., Lips, C. J. M., and Jansz, H. S., A second human calcitonin/CGRP gene, *FEBS Lett.,* 183, 403, 1985.
6. Hoppener, J. W., Steenberg, P. H., Slebos, R. J., Visser, A., Lips, C. J. M., Janz, H. S., Bechet, J. M., Lenoirg, M., Born, W., and Haller-Berm, S., Expression of the second calcitonin/calcitonin gene-related peptide gene in Ewing sarcoma cell lines, *J. Clin. Endocrinol. Metab.,* 64, 809, 1987.
7. Ramana, C. V., DiPette, D. J., and Supowit, S. C., Localization and characterization of calcitonin gene-related mRNA in rat heart, *Am. J. Med. Sci.,* 304(6), 339, 1992.
8. Girgis, S. I., Macdonald, D. W. R., Stevenson, J. C., Bevis, P. J. R., Lynch, C., Wimalawansa, S. J., Self, C. H., Morris, H. R., and MacIntyre, I., Calcitonin gene-related peptide: potent vasodilator and major product of the calcitonin gene, *Lancet,* 2, 14, 1985.
9. Zaidi, M., Bevis, P. J. R., Abeyasekera, G., Girgis, S. I., Wimalawansa, S. J., Morris, H. R., and MacIntyre, I., The origin of calcitonin gene-related peptide in the rat, *J. Endocrinol.,* 110, 185, 1986.

10. Wimalawansa, S. J., Morris, H. R., and MacIntyre, I., Both α- and β-calcitonin gene-related peptides are present in plasma, cerebrospinal fluid and spinal cord in man, *J. Mol. Endocrinol.,* 3, 247-252, 1990.

11. Wimalawansa, S. J. and El-Kholy, A. A., A comparative study of distribution and biochemical characterization of brain CGRP receptors in five different species, *Neuroscience,* 54, 513, 1993.

12. Tschopp, F. A., Henke, H., Petermann, J. B., Tobler, H., Janzer, R., Hockfelt, T., Lundberg, J. M., Cuello, C., and Fischer, J. A., Calcitonin gene-related peptide and its binding sites in the human central nervous system and pituitary, *Proc. Natl. Acad. Sci. U.S.A.,* 82, 248, 1985.

13. Sigrist, S., Franco-Cereceda, A., Muff, R., Henke, H., Lundberg, J. M., and Fischer, J. A., Specific receptor and cardiovascular effects of calcitonin gene-related peptide, *Endocrinology,* 119, 381, 1986.

14. Wimalawansa, S. J., Emson, P. C., and MacIntyre, I., Regional distribution of calcitonin gene-related peptide and its specific binding sites in rats with particular reference to the nervous system, *Neuroendocrinology,* 46, 131, 1987.

15. Wharton, J., Gulbenkian, S., Mulderry, P. K., Ghatei, M. A., McGregor, M. P., Bloom, S. R., and Polak, J. M., Capsaicin induces a depletion of calcitonin gene-related peptide (CGRP)-immunoreactive nerves in the cardiovascular system of the guinea pig and rat, *J. Autonomic Nerv. Syst.,* 16, 289, 1986.

16. Skofitsch, G. and Jacobowitz, D. M., Calcitonin gene-related peptide: detailed immunohistochemical distribution in the central nervous system, *Peptides,* 6, 721, 1985.

17. Wanaka, A., Matsuyama, T., Yoneda, S., Kamada, T., MacIntyre, I., Emson, P. C., and Tohyama, M., Origin and distribution of calcitonin gene-related peptide-containing nerves in the wall of the cerebral arteries of the guinea pig with special reference to coexistence with substance P, *Cell. Mol. Biol.,* 33, 201, 1987.

18. Giuliani, S., Wimalawansa, S. J., and Maggie, C. A., Involvement of multiple receptors in the biological effects of calcitonin gene-related peptide and amylin in rat and guinea-pig preparations, *Br. J. Pharmacol.,* 107, 510, 1992.

19. Brain, S. D., Williams, T. J., Tippins, J. R., Morris, H. R., and MacIntyre, I., Calcitonin gene-related peptide is a potent vasodilator, *Nature,* 313, 54, 1985.

20. Brain, S. D., MacIntyre, I., and Williams, T. J., A second form of human calcitonin gene-related peptide which is a potent vasodilator, *Eur. J. Pharmacol.,* 124, 349, 1986.

21. DiPette, D. J., Schwarzenberger, K., Kerr, N., and Holland, O. B., Systemic and regional hemodynamic effect of calcitonin gene-related peptide in conscious rats, *Hypertension,* 9(Part 2), III142, 1987.

22. DiPette, D. J., Schwarzenberger, K., Kerr, N., and Holland, O. B., Dose dependent systemic and regional hemodynamic effects of calcitonin gene-related peptide, *Am. J. Med. Sci.,* 297, 65, 1989.

23. Lee, Y., Takami, K., Kawai, Y., Girgis, S., Hillyard, C. J., MacIntyre, I., Emson, P. C., and Tohyama, M., Distribution of calcitonin gene-related peptide in the rat peripheral nervous system with reference to its coexistence with substance P, *Neuroscience,* 15, 1227, 1985.

24. Asimakis, G., DiPette, D. J., Conti, V., Holland, O. B., and Zwischenberger, J. B., Hemodynamic action of calcitonin gene-related peptide in the isolated rat heart, *Life Sci.,* 41, 597, 1987.

25. Franco-Cereceda, A., Bengrsson, L., and Lundberg, J. M., Inotropic effects of calcitonin gene-related peptide, vasoactive intestinal polypeptide and somatostatin on the human right atrium *in vitro, Eur. J. Pharmacol.,* 134, 69, 1987.

26. Franco-Cereceda, A. and Lundberg, J., Calcitonin gene-related peptide (CGRP) and capsaicin-induced stimulation of heart contractile rate and force, *Arch. Pharmacol.,* 331, 146, 1985.

27. Ishikawa, T., Okamara, N., Saito, A., Masaki, T., and Goto, K., Positive inotropic effect of calcitonin gene-related peptide mediated by cyclic AMP in guinea pig heart, *Cir. Res.,* 63, 726, 1988.

28. McEwan, J., Chierchia, S., Davies, G., Stevenson, J. C., Brown, M., Maseri, A., and MacIntyre, I., Coronary vasodilation by calcitonin gene-related peptide, *Br. Heart J.,* 54, 643, 1985.

29. McEwan, J., Legon, S., Wimalawansa, S. J., Zaidi, M., Dollery, C. T., and MacIntyre, I., Calcitonin gene-related peptide: a review of its biology and relevance to the cardiovascular system, in *Endocrine Mechanisms in Hypertension,* Laragh, J. H., Brenner, B. M., and Kaplan, N. M., Eds., Raven Press, New York, 1989, 287.

30. Franco-Cereceda, A., Lundberg, J., Saria, A., Schreibmayer, W., and Tritthart, H., Calcitonin gene-related peptide: release by capsaicin and prolongation of the action potential in the guinea-pig heart, *Acta Physiol. Scand.,* 132, 181, 1987.

31. Miyauchi, T., Ishikawa, T., Sugishita, Y., Saito, A., and Goto, K., Effects of capsaicin on nonadrenergic noncholinergic nerves in the guinea pig atria: role of calcitonin gene-related peptide as cardiac neurotransmitter, *J. Cardiovasc. Pharmacol.,* 10, 675, 1987.

32. Miyauchi, T., Sano, Y., Hiroshima, O., Yuzuriha, T., Sugishita, Y., Ishikawa, T., Saito, A., and Goto, K., Positive inotropic effects and receptors of calcitonin gene-related peptide (CGRP) in porcine ventricular muscles, *Biochem. Biophys. Res. Commun.,* 155(1), 289, 1988.

33. Ohmura, T., Nishio, M., Kigoshi, S., and Muramatsu, I., Electrophysiological and mechanical effects of calcitonin gene-related peptide on guinea-pig atria, *Br. J. Pharmacol.,* 100, 27, 1990.

34. Wang, X. and Fiscus, R., Calcitonin gene-related peptide increases cAMP, tension, and rate in rat atria, *Am. J. Physiol.,* 256(25) R421, 1989.

35. Franco-Cereceda, A., Gennari, C., Nami, R., Agnusdei, D., Pernow, J., Lundberg, J., and Fischer, J., Cardiovascular effects of calcitonin gene-related peptides I and II in man, *Circ. Res.,* 60, 393, 1987.

36. Howden, C. W., Logue, C., Gavin, K., Collie, L., and Rubin, P. C., Hemodynamic effects of intravenous human calcitonin-gene-related peptide in man, *Clin. Sci.,* 74, 413, 1988.

37. Marshall, I., Al-Kazwini, S. J., Roberts, P. M., Shepperson, N. B., Adams, A., and Craig, R. A., Cardiovascular effects of human and rat CGRP compared in the rat and other species, *Eur. J. Pharmacol.,* 123, 207, 1986.

38. Tippins, J. R., Morris, H. R., Panico, M., Etienne, T., Bevis, P. J. R., Girgis, S., MacIntyre, I., Azria, M., and Attinger, M., The myotropic and plasma calcium modulating effects of calcitonin gene-related peptide (CGRP), *Neuropeptides,* 4, 425, 1984.

39. Kawasaki, H., Takasaki, K., Saito, A., and Goto, K., Calcitonin gene-related peptide acts as a novel vasodilator neurotransmitter in mesenteric resistance vessels of the rat, *Nature,* 335, 164, 1988.

40. Edvinsson, L., Fredhol, B. B., Hamel, E., Jansen, I., and Verrochia, C., Perivascular peptides relax cerebral arteries concomitant with stimulation or release of an endothelium-derived relaxing factor in the cat, *Neurosci. Lett.,* 58, 213, 1985.

41. Hanko, J., Hardebo, J. E., Kahlstrom, J. K., Owman, C., and Sundler, F., Calcitonin gene-related peptide is present in mammalian cerebrovascular nerve fibers and dilates pial and peripheral arteries, *Neurosci. Lett.,* 57, 91, 1985.

42. Hughes, A., Thron, S., Martin, G., and Sever, P., Endothelial-dependent relaxation of human arteries by peptide hormone, *Clin. Sci.,* 13(Suppl.), 88P, 1985.

43. Witherington, P. G., The differential actions of calcitonin gene-related peptide on the vascular and capsular smooth muscle of the dog spleen, *Br. J. Pharmacol.,* 88(Suppl.), 436P, 1986.

44. DiPette, D. J., Asimakis, G., and Holland, O. B., Comparison of calcitonin gene-related peptide, adenosine and calcitonin as coronary vasodilators in the isolated rat heart, *Fed. Proc.,* 2, 1817, 1988.

45. Gennari, C. and Fischer, J. A., Cardiovascular actions of calcitonin gene-related peptide in humans, *Calcif. Tissue Int.,* 37, 581, 1985.

46. Struthers, A. D., Brown, M. J., Macdonald, D. W. R., Beacham, J. L., Stevenson, J. C., Morris, H. R., and MacIntyre, I., Human CGRP: the most potent endogenous vasodilator in man, *Clin. Sci.,* 70, 389, 1986.

47. Fisher, L. A., Kikkawa, D. D., Rivier, J. E., Amara, S. G., Evans, R. M., Rosenfeld, M. G., Vale, W. W., and Brown, M. R., Stimulation of noradrenergic sympathetic outflow by calcitonin gene-related peptide, *Nature,* 305, 534, 1983.

48. Lappe, R. W., Todt, J. A., and Wendt, R. L., Cardiovascular effects of central calcitonin gene-related peptide in conscious rats, *Am. J. Hypertens.,* 1, 47, 1988.

49. Gardiner, S. M., Compton, A. M., and Bennett, T., Regional hemodynamic responses to intracerebroventricular administration of rat calcitonin gene-related peptide in conscious, Long-Evans and Brattleboro rats, *Neurosci. Lett.,* 88, 343, 1988.

50. Nguyen, K., Sills, M., and Jacobowitz, D., Cardiovascular effects produced by microinjection of calcitonin gene-related peptide into the rat central amygdaloid nucleus, *Peptides,* 7(2), 337, 1986.

51. Siren, A. and Feuerstein, G., Cardiovascular effects of rat calcitonin gene-related peptide in the conscious rat, *J. Pharmacol. Exp. Ther.*, 247(1), 69, 1988.

52. Gardiner, S. M., Compton, A. M., and Bennett, T., Regional hemodynamic effects of calcitonin gene-related peptide, *Am. J. Physiol.*, 256(25), R332, 1989.

53. Westermark, P., Wernstedt, C., Wilander, E., and Sletten, K., A novel peptide in the calcitonin gene-related peptide family as an amyloid fibril protein in the endocrine pancreas, *Biochem. Biophys. Res. Commun.*, 140, 827, 1987.

54. Westermark, P., Wernstedt, C., Wilander, E., Hayden, D. W., O'Brien, T. D., and Johnson, K. H., Amyloid fibrils in human insulinoma and islets of Langerhans of the diabetic cat are derived from a neuropeptide-like protein also present in normal islet cells, *Proc. Natl. Acad. Sci. U.S.A.*, 84, 3881, 1987.

55. Cooper, G. J. S., Willis, A. C., Clark, A., Turner, R. C., Sim, R. B., and Reid, K. B. M., Purification and characterization of a peptide from amyloid-rich pancreases of type 2 diabetic patients, *Proc. Natl. Acad. Sci. U.S.A.*, 84, 8628, 1987.

56. Morishita, T., Yamaguchi, A., Fugita, T., and Chiba, T., Activation of adenyl cyclase by islet amyloid polypeptide with COOH-terminal amide via calcitonin gene-related peptide receptors on rat liver plasma membranes, *Diabetes*, 39, 875, 1990.

57. McEwan, J., Wimalawansa, S. J., and MacIntyre, I., Amylin Amide is the Third CGRP and Activates Adenyl Cyclase, Abstr No. 845, presented at 71st Annu. Meet. American Endocrine Society, Seattle, 1989.

58. Brain, S. D., MacIntyre, I., Wimalawansa, S. J., and Williams, T. J., Amylin amide, which is structurally similar to calcitonin gene-related peptide (CGRP), stimulates increased blood flow in vivo, *Eur. J. Pharmacol.*, 183, 2221, 1990.

59. Brain, S. D., Wimalawansa, S. J., MacIntyre, I., and Williams, T. J., The demonstration of vasodilatory activity of pancreatic amylin in the rabbit, *Am. J. Pathol.*, 136, 487, 1990.

60. Datta, H. K., Zaidi, M., Wimalawansa, S. J., Ghatei, M. A., Beacham, J. L., Bloom, S. R., and MacIntyre, I., In vivo and in vitro effects of amylin amide on calcium metabolism in the rat and rabbit, *Biochem. Biophys. Res. Commun.*, 162, 876, 1989.

61. Zaidi, M., Datta, H. K. Bevis, P. J. R., Wimalawansa, S. J., and MacIntyre, I., Human amylin-amylin amide, a potent hypocalcemic peptide: possible physiological role in skeletal homeostasis, *J. Exp. Physiol.*, 75, 529, 1990.

62. Cooper, G. J. S., Leighton, B., Dimitriadis, G. D., Parry-Billings, M., Kowalchuk, J. M., Howland, K., Rothbard, J. B., Willis, A. C., and Reid, K. B. M., Amylin found in amyloid deposits in human type 2 diabetes mellitus may be a hormone that regulates glycogen metabolism in skeletal muscle, *Proc. Natl. Acad. Sci. U.S.A.*, 85, 7763, 1988.

63. Leighton, B. and Cooper, G. J. S., Pancreatic amylin and calcitonin gene-related peptide cause resistance to insulin in skeletal muscle in vitro, *Nature*, 335, 632, 1988.

64. Young, A. A., Deems, R. O., Deacon, R. W., McIntosh, R. H., and Foley, J. E., Effects of amylin on glucose metabolism and glycogenolysis in vivo and in vitro, *Am. J. Physiol.*, 177, 771, 1990.

65. Chance, W. T., Balasubramanium, A., Zhang, F. S., Wimalawansa, S. J., and Fischer, J. E., Anorexia following the introhypothalamic administration of amylin, *Brain Res.*, 539, 352, 1991.

66. Mulderry, P. K., Ghatei, M. A., Rodrigo, J., Allen, J., Rosenfeld, M. G., Polak, J., and Bloom, S. R., Calcitonin gene-related peptide in cardiovascular tissues in the rat, *Neurosciences*, 14, 947, 1985.

67. Wimalawansa, S. J. and MacIntyre, I., Calcitonin gene-related peptide and its specific binding sites in the cardiovascular system of rat, *Int. J. Cardiol.*, 20, 29, 1988.

68. Marshall, I., Al-Kazwini, S. J., Holman, J. J., and Craig, R. K., Human and rat alpha CGRP but not calcitonin cause mesenteric vasodilation in rats, *Eur. J. Pharmacol.*, 123, 217, 1986.

69. Wimalawansa, S. J., The relationship of immunoreactive CGRP in plasma and thyroid with the age of the rat, *Peptides*, 12, 1143, 1991.

70. Wimalawansa, S. J., Age-related changes of tissue content of immunoreactive calcitonin gene-related peptide, *Aging-Clin. Exp. Res.*, 4, 211, 1992.

71. Wimalawansa, S. J., Diurnal variation of plasma calcitonin gene-related peptide in man, *J. Neuroendocrinol.*, 3, 319, 1990.

72. Wimalawansa, S. J., Effects of in vivo stimulation on molecular forms of circulatory calcitonin and calcitonin gene-related peptide in man, *Mol. Cell. Endocrinol.,* 71, 13, 1990.

73. Datta, H. K., Wimalawansa, S. J., Rafter, P. W., Chen, Z. P., and MacIntyre, I., CGRP and amylin amide displays a proliferative effect on human umbilical-cord endothelial cells and osteoblast-like osteosarcoma cell-line, *Biochem. Soc. Trans.,* 18, 1276, 1990.

74. Haegerstrand, A., Dalsgaard, C. J. Jonzon, B., Larsson O., and Nilsson, J., Calcitonin gene-related peptide stimulates proliferation of human endothelial cells, *Proc. Natl. Acad. Sci. U.S.A.,* 87, 3299, 1990.

75. Girgis, S. I., Lunch, C., Hillyard, C. J., Stevenson, J. C., Hill, P. A., Macdonald, D. W. R., and MacIntyre, I., Calcitonin gene-related peptide: the diagnostic value of measurements in medullary thyroid carcinoma, *Henry Ford Hosp. Med. J.,* 35, 119, 1987.

76. Hillyard, C. J., Stevenson, J. C., and MacIntyre, I., Relative deficiency of plasma calcitonin in normal women, *Lancet,* 1, 961, 1978.

77. Goltzman, D. and Mitchell, J., Interaction of calcitonin and calcitonin gene-related peptide at receptor sites in target tissues, *Science,* 227, 1343, 1985.

78. Wimalawansa, S. J., Sensitive and specific radio-receptor assay for calcitonin gene-related peptide, *J. Neuroendocrinol.,* 1, 15, 1989.

79. Krahn, D. D., Gosnell, B. A., Levine, A. S., and Morley, J. E., Effects of calcitonin gene-related peptide on food intake, *Peptides,* 5, 861, 1984.

80. Tannenbaum, G. S. and Goltzman, D., Calcitonin gene-related peptide mimics calcitonin actions in brain on growth hormone release and feeding, *Endocrinology,* 116, 2685, 1985.

81. Newbold, P. and Brain, S. D., The modulation of inflammatory oedema by calcitonin gene-related peptide, *Brit. J. Pharmacol.,* 108, 705, 1993.

82. Brain, S. D., Tippins, J. R., Morris, H. R., MacIntyre, I., and Williams, T. J., Potent vasodilator activity of calcitonin gene-related peptide in human skin, *J. Invest. Dermatol.,* 87, 533, 1986.

83. Kjartansson, J. and Dalsgaard, C. J., Calcitonin gene-related peptide increases survival of a musculocutaneous critical flap in the rat, *Eur. J. Pharmacol.,* 142, 35, 1987.

84. Cambridge, H. and Brain, S. D., Calcitonin gene-related peptide increases blood flow and potentiates plasma protein extravasation in the rat knee joint, *Br. J. Pharmacol.,* 106, 746, 1992.

85. Hughes, S. R. and Brain, S. D., A calcitonin gene-related peptide (CGRP) antagonist ($CGRP_{8-37}$) inhibits microvascular responses induced by CGRP and capsaicin in skin, *Br. J. Pharmacol.,* 104, 738, 1991.

86. Shekhar, Y. C., Anand, I. S., Sarma, R., Ferrari, R., Wahi, P. L., and Poole-Wilson, P. A., Effects of prolonged infusion of human alpha calcitonin gene-related peptide on hemodynamics, renal blood flow, and hormone levels in congestive cardiac failure, *Am. J. Cardiol.,* 67, 732, 1991.

87. Resnick, L., Calciotropic hormones in human and experimental hypertension, *Am. J. Hypertens.,* 3, 171S, 1990.

88. DiPette, D. J., Westlund, K., and Holland, O. B., Dietary calcium modulates spinal cord content of calcitonin gene-related peptide in the rat, *Neurosci. Lett.,* 95, 335, 1988.

89. Westlund, K. N., DiPette, D. J., Carson, J., and Holland, O. B., Decreased neuronal content of calcitonin gene-related peptide in the spontaneously hypertensive rat, *Neurosci. Lett.,* 131, 183, 1991.

90. Supowit, S. C., Ramana, C. V., Westlund, K. N., and DiPette, D. J., Calcitonin gene-related peptide gene expression in the spontaneously hypertensive rat, *Hypertension,* 21, 1010, 1993.

91. Ando, K., Pegram, B., and Frohlich, E., Hemodynamic effects of calcitonin gene-related peptide in spontaneously hypertensive rats, *Am. J. Physiol.,* 258(27), R425, 1990.

92. Lappe, R., Todt, J., and Wendt, R., Regional vasodilator actions of calcitonin gene-related peptide in conscious SHR, *Peptides,* 8(4), 747, 1987.

93. DiPette, D. J., Westlund, K., and Supowit, S. C., Enhanced calcitonin gene-related peptide gene expression in mineralocorticoid-salt hypertensive rats, *Hypertension,* 18, 417, 1991.

94. Masuda, A., Shimamoto, K., Mori, Y., Nakagawa, M., Ura, N., and Limura, O., Plasma calcitonin gene-related peptide levels in patients with various hypertensive diseases, *J. Hypertens.,* 10, 1499, 1992.

95. Schifter, S., Krusell, L., and Sehested, J., Normal serum levels of calcitonin gene-related peptide (CGRP) in mild to moderate essential hypertension, *Am. J. Hypertens.*, 4, 565, 1991.

96. Edvinsson, L., Ekman, R., and Thulin, T., Reduced levels of calcitonin gene-related peptide (CGRP) but not substance P during and after treatment of severe hypertension in man, *J. Hum. Hypertens.*, 3, 267, 1989.

97. Schifter, S., Williams, E. D., Craig, R. K., and Hansen, H. H., Calcitonin gene-related peptide and calcitonin in medullary thyroid carcinoma, *Clin. Endocrinol.*, 25, 703, 1986.

98. Wimalawansa, S. J., Effects of neonatal capsaicin therapy on plasma contents and tissue levels of immunoreactive-CGRP, *Peptides*, 14, 247, 1993.

99. Wimalawansa, S. J., CGRP radioreceptor assay, a new diagnostic test for medullary thyroid carcinoma, *J. Bone Min. Res.*, 8, 467, 1993.

100. Bendtsen, F., Schifter, S., and Henriksen, J. H., Increased circulating calcitonin gene-related peptide (CGRP) in cirrhosis, *J. Hepatol.*, 12, 118, 1991.

101. Griffin, E. C., Aiyar, N., Siivak, M. J., and Smith, E. F., III., Effect of endotoxicosis on plasma and tissue levels of calcitonin gene-related peptide, *Circ. Shock*, 38, 50, 1992.

102. Brain, S. D., Petty, R. G., Lewis, J. D., and Williams, T. J., Cutaneous blood flow responses in the forearms of Raynaud's patients induced by local cooling and intradermal injections of CGRP and histamine, *Br. J. Clin. Pharmacol.*, 30, 853, 1990.

103. Arienta, C., Balbi, S., Caroli, M., and Fumagalli, G., Depletion of calcitonin gene-related peptide in perivascular nerves during acute phase of posthemorrhagic vasospasm in the rabbit, *Brain Res. Bull.*, 27(5), 605, 1991.

104. Edvinsson, L., Delgado-Zygmunt, T., Ekman, R., Jansen, I., Svendgaard, N,-A., and Uddman, R., Involvement of perivascular sensory fibers in the pathophysiology of cerebral vasospasm following subarachnoid hemorrhage, *J. Cereb. Blood Flow Metab.*, 10, 602, 1990.

105. Hongo, K., Tsukahara, T., Kassell, N., and Ogawa, H., Effect of subarachnoid hemorrhage on calcitonin gene-related peptide-induced relaxation in rabbit basilar artery, *Stroke*, 20, 100, 1989.

106. Wimalawansa, S. J., Isolation and characterization of calcitonin gene-related peptide receptors and raising monoclonal antibodies. Proceedings, First international symposium on calcitonin gene-related peptide, Graz, Austraia, *Regul. Peptides*, 34, 77, 1991.

107. Wimalawansa, S. J., Gunasekeri, R. D., and Zhang, F., Isolation, purification and characterization of calcitonin gene-related peptide receptor, *Peptides*, 14, 691, 1993.

108. Wimalawansa, S. J., Isolation, purification, and biochemical characterization of calcitonin gene-related peptide receptor (review), *Annals N.Y. Acad. Sci.*, 657, 70, 1992.

109. Wimalawansa, S. J., Calcitonin gene-related peptide, calcitonin and amylin: a peptide super family, *Crit. Rev. Neurobiol.*, (in press).

11

Cardiovascular Actions of Some Steroid Hormones

Jie Shan, Mario Barbagallo, and Peter K. T. Pang

CONTENTS

I. INTRODUCTION

Many hormones are important in the regulation of plasma calcium levels. Peptide hormones, such as parathyroid hormone (PTH) and calcitonin (CT) and their gene-related peptides — parathyroid hormone-related peptide (PTHrp) and calcitonin gene-related peptide (CGRP) — have been studied extensively. Steroid hormones, such as vitamin D_3 and its metabolites, and female sex steroids, including estrogen and progesterone, are also well recognized for their role in the regulation of plasma calcium homeostasis. These hormones are closely involved in calcium uptake from the gut, reabsorption and excretion from the kidney, and storage and release in bone. It is the equilibrium of the actions of these hormones at their target sites that provides the overall balance of calcium in the body. This balance is reflected in the plasma level of this important ion. Recently, these hormones also have been demonstrated to participate actively in another

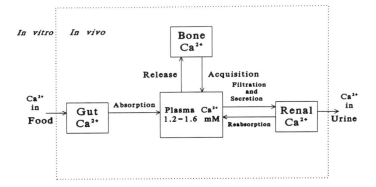

FIGURE 1   Schematic representation of the relationship among the four major components of calcium homeostasis in the body. Plasma Ca^{2+} level reflects the overall balance in the other three: bone, gut, and kidney. These three active contributors to Ca^{2+} homeostasis are closely regulated by calcium-regulating hormones such as PTH, CT, vitamin D, and female sex steroids.

physiological system, i.e., the cardiovascular system. Other chapters in this book deal with various cardiovascular aspects of CGRP and 1,25-dihydroxyvitamin D_3 [1,25$(OH)_2D_3$]. This chapter will concentrate on the female sex steroids, i.e., estrogen and progesterone, and another vitamin D_3 metabolite, 24,25-dihydroxyvitamin D_3 [24,25$(OH)_2D_3$].

In order to understand the overall role of steroids in cardiovascular functions, a general hypothesis will first be proposed to present an overall scheme of the regulation of calcium ions (Ca^{2+}). This hypothesis will explain how most, if not all, of the calcium-regulating hormones fit into the picture of calcium balance in the body.

In the classical description of calcium balance in the body, four compartments are usually considered: the storage site (bone), the absorption site (gut), the excretory site (kidney), and the transport site (blood). The plasma level of calcium is kept in a rather narrow range, reflecting the overall balance at the other three sites (Figure 1). Disturbances in this balance will result in either hypocalcemia or hypercalcemia. These sites are closely regulated by the calcium-regulating hormones such as PTH, CT, vitamin D, and sex steroids. In the present hypothesis, another aspect is introduced that involves the use of calcium by the remainder of the body tissues. The main rationale for this idea consists of a single question, i.e., what is the purpose of calcium in plasma? A constant plasma level of calcium provides a stable environment, which is the key issue for the overall homeostasis of calcium in our body. However, this has not been adequately considered in our understanding of calcium homeostasis. Calcium is no doubt important as a structural element in bone and cell components such as plasma membrane. However, calcium is also used by most, if not all, cells for proper functioning and survival. In order to better understand the implication of this hypothesis in relation to calcium-regulating hormones, the use of calcium by cells will first be delineated. How the cardiovascular tissues fit into the scheme will be explained. The roles of calcium-regulating hormones will then be described in general. Female sex steroids will be used as specific examples in both the normal and disease states.

Every cell in our body contains calcium, which serves several important, if not essential, functions such as those of being a cofactor in enzyme activity, a component of the plasma membrane, and an intracellular messenger. Cells respond to the needs of the body as a whole to provide proper functioning of the body in relation to internal and external environmental changes. The integration of bodily functions requires an efficient coordinating system that uses chemical messengers to direct the activity of individual cells and, eventually, the tissues. How do cells respond to the extracellular chemical messengers? It is essential that these messages outside the cells be translocated into cells so that proper responses can be elicited.

This is accomplished by intracellular second messengers. Calcium is one such messenger. The level of intracellular free calcium concentration ($[Ca^{2+}]_i$) serves as the message. The arrival of the extracellular message to the cell membrane produces changes in $[Ca^{2+}]_i$. Since many intracellular enzymes are sensitive to calcium, a change in $[Ca^{2+}]_i$ will initiate or decrease enzyme activity. Therefore, the regulation of $[Ca^{2+}]_i$ becomes the transmission of messages from the outside to the inside of cells.

To understand the intracellular calcium messenger system, the regulation of $[Ca^{2+}]_i$ must first be understood. The key point is the concentration gradient between extracellular and intracellular free calcium concentrations. Free calcium concentration outside a cell is around 1 to 2 mM, 10,000 or more times greater than that inside the cell, which is around 100 nM. The maintenance of such a great concentration gradient relies on the impermeability of the cell membrane to calcium. The prevention of free movement of calcium ions across the cell membrane is necessary to counteract the tremendous physical chemical force generated by the concentration gradient. However, $[Ca^{2+}]_i$ must be able to change in order to serve as the intracellular message. Several mechanisms have been described. One of the most important ways is through the activity of channels on the cell membrane. These channels are specific passages, some particularly for calcium, but some for divalent ions in general. These channels are tightly controlled. When opened, calcium ions will move from outside to inside the cell along the large concentration gradient. The closing of such channels will again render the membrane impermeable to calcium. Calcium channels are classified according to their physiochemical properties. In vascular smooth muscle cells (VSMC), there are two main types of calcium channels: voltage-operated (VOC) and receptor-operated (ROC). The VOCs are voltage sensitive. Depolarization of the cell membrane results in the opening of these channels. The two main types of VOC found on VSMC membrane depend on the range of voltage activating the channels, the duration of opening upon activation, and their response to pharmacological agents. The L or long-lasting type, once activated, remains open for a long time and shows peak activation around +20 mV. These channels are also sensitive to synthetic organic calcium antagonists such as dihydropyridines. The T or transient type will stay open only for a comparatively short period and can be maximally activated around –10 mV. These T channels are not sensitive to the organic calcium antagonists. The ROCs are rather ill-defined at this time. For VSMC, many vasoactive hormones interact with receptors, leading to changes in $[Ca^{2+}]_i$ and even VOC activity. However, in the truest sense, ROC activity should be affected by the agonists, independently of membrane voltage difference.

Another mechanism is through the activity of quickly mobilized pools of calcium in intracellular storage sites. In VSMC, the endoplasmic reticulum (ER) stores calcium to a concentration thousands of times higher than $[Ca^{2+}]_i$. The membrane around these organelles is, again, rather impermeable to calcium. However, there are channels on this membrane. The opening of these calcium channels will allow calcium to move from inside the organelle to the cytoplasm, thereby increasing $[Ca^{2+}]_i$. Some of these channels are sensitive to inositol-1,4,5-trisphosphate (IP_3). Extracellular messengers, after interacting with cell surface receptors, will activate phospholipase C (PLC), resulting in a cascade of enzyme stimulation and the eventual formation of IP_3. IP_3 will then interact with ER calcium channels and facilitate their opening and calcium movement from the ER store to the cytoplasm. Many vasoactive substances, such as norepinephrine (NE), angiotensin (ANG), and arginine vasopressin (AVP), act in this manner.

So far, the mechanisms of $[Ca^{2+}]_i$ increase have been described. It is also essential to lower $[Ca^{2+}]_i$. This is achieved by the active transport of calcium against a steep concentration gradient at two sites. On the plasma membrane, calcium pumps, such as the one with energy supplied by Ca^{2+}/Na^+ ATPase, move calcium from the inside to the outside of VSMC. On the membrane of the ER, active calcium pumps also transport calcium from the cytoplasm into the ER. These $[Ca^{2+}]_i$-lowering mechanisms are particularly important in terminating a

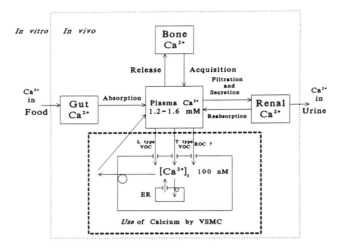

FIGURE 2   Schematic representation of the hypothesis that incorporates the use of calcium by cells as the major component in the overall consideration of calcium homeostasis in the body. In this hypothesis, the use of calcium is placed centrally and most prominently, not because of the size of the pool it represents but more for the importance of its role in the functioning of the body. The key point in this hypothesis is that plasma calcium is maintained quite constant by the activities of bone, gut, and kidney mainly for the purpose of supplying calcium to the use component of this scheme. Data from this chapter and other chapters in this volume suggest that calcium-regulating hormones, PTH, CT, vitamin D, and female sex steroids, regulate not only the bone, gut, and renal components but also the cell use component. The figure uses VSMC as an example, but the same can be applied to almost all other cells in the body. VOC = voltage-operated calcium channel; ROC = receptor-operated calcium channel; $[Ca^{2+}]_i$ = intracellular free calcium concentration; O = active calcium pump.

calcium signal. An increase in $[Ca^{2+}]_i$ provides the message, which must also terminated. The return of $[Ca^{2+}]_i$ to its normal level by these active transport mechanisms signifies the end of the message. These pumps are also important in the maintenance of basal $[Ca^{2+}]_i$ in a nonstimulated state. However impermeable the cell membrane may be, there is still a slow leak of calcium into cells because of the steep concentration gradient and, perhaps, because of some basal opening activity of calcium channels. The active efflux will remove the calcium that has gained entry by these means.

This brief description of cellular calcium regulation serves to indicate the dynamic use of calcium by target tissues. According to our hypothesis, this is probably a very important, if not the most important, aspect of calcium homeostasis in the body. It is proposed here that the use of calcium by most cells in their routine activities, though recognized and extensively studied, has not been fully incorporated into our thinking on overall calcium homeostasis. Plasma calcium concentration reflects the equilibrium among acquisition, storage, excretion and use. The use is the main issue in the whole picture. The acquisition, storage, and excretion are mainly there to ensure adequate supply for use. Figure 2 summarizes this hypothesis. There does not seem to be much discussion in the literature of this particular simple, logical, but rather significant aspect of calcium homeostasis. This concept is central to the theme of this monograph. The aspects of acquisition, storage, and excretion involve all of the calcium-regulating hormones: PTH, CT, vitamin D_3, and sex steroids. Should these same hormones also be involved in the use of calcium by target cells? It is logical that they should. In this book, the cardiovascular actions of calcium-regulating hormones are considered. Cardiovascular tissue is certainly a calcium-using tissue. Cardiac myocytes and VSMC determine the function of the cardiovascular system. It is known that $[Ca^{2+}]_i$ plays a key role in the activities of these cells. If our hypothesis is correct, the calcium-regulating hormones should be involved in the control of calcium use by these cells. In other words, these hormones should be regulating $[Ca^{2+}]_i$ through their actions on the various cellular sites. Indeed, the contents of the various chapters point to the extensive regulatory role of these calcium-regulating hormones in the cardiovascular system. In several chapters, the cellular effects, such as those on calcium channel activity and $[Ca^{2+}]_i$, are described. In this chapter, the vascular actions of some types of steroid hormones, i.e., female sex hormones and a vitamin D_3 metabolite — $24,25(OH)_2D_3$ — will be delineated. Some data on $[Ca^{2+}]_i$ regulation and cellular target sites, such as calcium channels and intracellular stores, will be discussed. The sex steroids, in addition to other calcium-regulating hormones, will be used as examples to support the hypothesis we have put forth here. These hormones are regulators of the use aspect of calcium homeostasis. It must be made clear that although calcium-regulating hormones including sex steroids may play a role in regulating the use of calcium by cells, they are by no means the only hormones performing that function. In fact, they may not be the most important regulator of the cardiovascular system. Various vasoactive substances, such as angiotensin II (ANG II), endothelin, arginine vasopressin (AVP), parathyroid hypertensive factor (PHF), atrial natriuretic factor (ANF), and others may have more prominent cardiovascular effects and may be equally effective in the regulation of calcium use. Nevertheless, the calcium-regulating hormones are particularly interesting because of their involvement in all the other components of calcium homeostasis, as shown in Figure 2.

II. FEMALE SEX STEROIDS AND CARDIOVASCULAR FUNCTION

Estrogen and progesterone are two major female sex hormones. Estrogens are secreted by the ovaries and the placenta. The progestins are involved in the maintenance of pregnancy and are produced by the ovaries and the placenta. Both of these hormones are steroids. In addition to their regulatory effect on the development of reproductive organs, estrogen and progesterone have widespread effects on many other physiological and metabolic processes. They are known to play roles in protecting against bone loss and in regulating the cardiovascular system through other vasoactive hormones, e.g., by increasing circulating levels of ANG II. In this chapter, evidence for their direct involvement in cardiovascular function will be described. The mechanism of action of this involvement will also be discussed.

A. Estrogen

1. Epidemiological Studies

Epidemiological studies show that blood pressure starts to increase progressively in post-menopausal women. There is little change in blood pressure with aging until approximately the time of menopause.[1-3] These changes may be related to the decrease in production of both estrogen and progesterone at the time of menopause (i.e., it is hormonally mediated).

The effect of estrogen replacement therapy on cardiovascular morbidity and mortality has not been completely clarified. Several epidemiological studies indicate that estrogen may have beneficial effects on cardiovascular morbidity and mortality,[4-8] while other studies have found an increase in cardiovascular morbidity among estrogen users. Wilson et al.[9] showed an increase in cardiovascular and cerebrovascular morbidity in estrogen use from the Framingham study. At the same time, Stampfer et al.[4] found a protective effect of estrogen for cardiovascular but not for cerebrovascular disease from a study conducted at Harvard. These two studies on the outcome of estrogen replacement therapy reached opposite conclusions probably due to the following — (1) Age factor: Wilson's study involved only women over 50, while Stampfer's study involved all ages (average, 51.47); nevertheless, Stampfer's study showed that the estrogen protection decreased with age. (2) Type of menopause: In Wilson's study, most women had a physiologic menopause (70 to 80% according to age group) while in Stampfer's study, the percentage is not specified, but the mean age may indicate that most of the women had surgical menopause.

In an update of the previous study from Stampfer's group,[8] the 10-year followup confirmed their findings. They found that the protective effect was limited to current users, while former users did not show protection. The beneficial effect in the older population decreased with age. Another important finding is that the protection is limited to the lower doses of estrogen, with an increased risk among women taking more than 1.25 mg/day of conjugated estrogen. Recently, in a prospective trial of 8881 postmenopausal females, Henderson et al.[7] reported a decrease in all-cause mortality in all categories of acute and chronic arteriosclerotic disease and cerebrovascular disease by estrogen replacement therapy.

Hyperestrogenemia may constitute a cardiovascular risk factor when it is pathologically present in males. It was suggested that hyperestrogenemia may be an important risk factor for myocardial infarction in males.[10] Other risk factors include high doses of estrogens in some pathological conditions[11] (prostatic cancer) and contraception.[12] In examining the potential effect of oral contraceptives on disease risk, it should be noted that this drug class has developed considerably during the last decade, particularly regarding progestin and estrogen type, dosage, and strength. Epidemiological research has contributed to these changes in oral contraceptives over time, since early reports have shown increased mortality and serious cardiovascular side effects[13-17] among oral contraceptive users. The increased risk seems to relate to thrombosis and to the action of estrogens on clotting factors.[18] Early epidemiologic evidence established that oral contraceptives caused a dose-dependent increase in the risk of both arterial and venous thromboembolic disease.[19] More recent data on the effect of newer pills on cardiovascular risk and mortality showed no increase among the users.[20,21]

Estrogen may be important in plasma lipid metabolism, thus indirectly affecting the development of cardiovascular disease.[22] Users of postmenopausal estrogen replacement therapy have consistently displayed higher levels of the protective high-density lipoprotein cholesterol (HDL-C) levels than did non-users.[5,9,23-26] These changes in plasma lipids induced by estrogens, although significant, have been shown in several studies to remain within normal physiologic limits.

2. Animal Studies

Animal studies also show contradicting results in the action of estrogen on the cardiovascular system. It was reported that administration of estrogen alone decreased,[27] increased,[28] or did not affect[29] blood pressure. The reported effects of estrogen on the pressor responses to some vasoconstrictors, such as ANG II, NE, and AVP, are also inconsistent.[30] Kando et al.[31] reported that estrogens were able to antagonize the hypertensive effect of NE in conscious rats. Yoshimura et al.[32] reported that prolonged estradiol treatment in ovariectomized rabbits decreased the pressor response to ANG II. Toba et al.[30] reported that chronic treatment of ovariectomized rats with estradiol reduced pressor responsiveness to AVP. It was also suggested that estrogen was unable to inhibit the pressor response to ANG II in conscious rats.[33,34] *In vitro* studies have suggested a direct effect of estrogen on the cardiovascular system. Raddino et al.[35] have shown that, in isolated rabbit heart, estrogen directly reduced myocardial contractility beginning at a concentration of 10^{-6} M and induced coronary vasodilation beginning at a concentration of 10^{-7} M. Specific estrogen receptors were located in the heart and various blood vessels,[36-41] and estrogen could affect the contractility of these blood vessels directly.[42-44] Estrogen also may have indirect effects on the cardiovascular system, e.g., through an interaction with the adrenergic nervous system.[45] The mechanism of the vascular

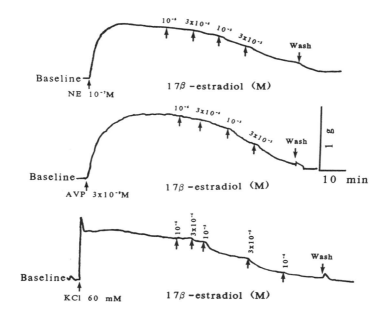

FIGURE 3 The effects of 17β-estradiol on SD rat tail artery helical strips precontracted by 10^{-9} M AVP, 10^{-7} M NE, or 60 mM KCl. Original recordings from three individual experiments are presented. The rat tail artery helical strip was stimulated by 10^{-7} M NE (upper), 3×10^{-9} M AVP (middle), or 60 mM KCl (bottom). In all cases, the tension was generated. Cumulative doses of 17β-estradiol were applied during the sustain phase of contractions. Dose-dependent relaxant effects of 17β-estradiol were observed in all three cases. (From Shan, J., Resnick, L., Liu, Q., Wu, X., Barbagallo, M., and Pang, P. K. T., unpublished data.)

action of estrogen remains unclear. Athough it was proposed that steroid sex hormones might interfere with calcium fluxes and/or calcium utilization,[38,46,47] there is little evidence to indicate that these steroid sex hormones directly affect membrane Ca^{2+} channels in VSMC.[48] The contradicting reports on estrogen action make it difficult to determine the action of this hormone on the cardiovascular system. The inconsistency of the reported results on the effect of estrogen could be due to species differences, experimental conditions, techniques, dosages of estrogen used, and the time after administration.

In a recent study conducted in our laboratory, we investigated the effects of estrogen on blood pressure *in vivo*, tail artery tension *in vitro*, and VSMC $[Ca^{2+}]_i$, and Ca^{2+} channel current in male SD rats.[49] The data showed that administration of estrogen (i.v., bolus injection) did not affect the basal blood pressure itself for up to 6 h in anesthetized SD rats. Estrogen started to inhibit the pressor response to NE 4 h after administration. In *in vitro* isolated denuded SD rat tail artery helical strips, pharmacological doses of (10^{-6} to 10^{-4} M) of estrogen relaxed the tonic contraction produced by the three vasoconstrictors (KCl, AVP, and norepinephrine, or NE) (Figure 3). It also decreased the phasic tension development induced by these three vasoconstrictors. The results of the *in vitro* tension study paralleled the overall depressor effect of estradiol *in vivo*.

As mentioned above, an interference by steroid sex hormones with Ca^{2+} influxes and/or Ca^{2+} utilization has been previously hypothesized but not clearly demonstrated. Recently, Rendt et al.[48] used the whole cell patch-clamp method to measure the Ca^{2+} currents (I_{Ca}) in myometrial cells from nonpregnant adult rats and immature rats injected with either estrogen or progesterone or estrogen plus progesterone. They found that I_{Ca} density was significantly different between the cells isolated from rats injected with progesterone and the cells isolated from control or estrogen-injected rats. This experiment suggested that the adminstration of sex steroids may change some properties of calcium channels in myometrial cells *in vivo* through a direct or indirect mechanism.

In order to obtain direct evidence, we carried out the experiment on cultured VSMC isolated from rat tail artery to determine the effect of estrogen on $[Ca^{2+}]_i$ using the Fura-II method, and calcium channel activity using the whole cell version of the patch-clamp technique. The tail artery was freshly isolated from SD rats (100 to 200 g body weight). The tail artery was enzymatically digested, and the VSMC obtained were cultured in Dulbecco's modified Eagle's medium (DMEM) for about 24 h. The cells were attached to the bottom of the culture dish in preparation for the patch-clamp study. To start the patch-clamp study, the DMEM medium was then replaced by an external solution containing 110 m*M* Tris, 5 m*M* CsCl, 20 m*M* HEPES, 30 m*M* glucose, 20 m*M* BaCl$_2$, and 0.5 µ*M* TTX. A polished pipette filled with the internal solution (75 m*M* Cs$_2$-aspartate, 10 m*M* EGTA, 2 m*M* ATP, 5 m*M* MgCl$_2$, 5 m*M* K-pyruvate, 5 m*M* K-succinate, 25 m*M* HEPES (N-[2-hydroxyethyl]piperazine-N′-[2-ethanesulfonic acid]), 5 m*M* creatine phosphate-Na$_2$, and 50 units/ml creatine kinase) was gently attached to the cell membrane using a Narishige hydraulic micromanipulator. Gentle suction was applied until a gigaseal was formed and the patch membrane was ruptured. When holding potential was set at –80 mV and testing potential was increased stepwise, an inward Ba^{2+} current (20 m*M* Ba^{2+} was used as the charge carrier) was recorded and showed the typical characteristic of a calcium channel current. The peak current appeared at around –10 mV. The control current was recorded for 15 min and estrogen was applied. One to 2 min later, the current started to decrease and reached the maximum at about 20 min (Figure 4).

For the Fura-II study, VSMC were cultured for about 24 h until they reached confluence. The cells were loaded with Fura-II AM for 45 min, and the DMEM culture medium was then replaced by 5 K buffer containing 145 m*M* NaCl, 5 m*M* KCl, 1 m*M* MgCl$_2$, 10 m*M* glucose, 1 m*M* CaCl$_2$, 0.5 m*M* NaH$_2$PO$_4$, and 10 m*M* HEPES at pH 7.4. The fluorescence measurements were made with a spectrofluorometer. $[Ca^{2+}]_i$ was then determined using the following equation:

$$[Ca^{2+}]_i \ (nM) = K_d \times (R - R_{min})/(R_{max} - R) \times b$$

where R was the ratio of the 510 nm fluorescence at the two excitation wavelengths, 340 nm and 380 nm. R_{max} was the fluorescence ratio determined by adding 2 µ*M* ionomycin. R_{min} was determined by subsequent addition of 5 m*M* EGTA. b was the ratio of fluorescence of Fura-II when excited at 380 n*M* in the zero and the saturating Ca^{2+}. K_d was the dissociation constant of Fura-II for Ca^{2+}, assumed to be 224 nM.[50] Estrogen itself did not affect the basal $[Ca^{2+}]_i$. To test the effect of estrogen on stimulated $[Ca^{2+}]_i$, the cells were stimulated by 15 m*M* KCl, and a transient increment of $[Ca^{2+}]_i$ was recorded as the control $[Ca^{2+}]_i$ increment. The cells were then washed with 5 K buffer, and estrogen was applied for 5 min. The cells were challenged again with 15 m*M* KCl, and the $[Ca^{2+}]_i$ increment, which was much less than the control increment, was recorded. After three washes, the cells were stimulated by 15 m*M* KCl, and this time the KCl response recovered (Figure 5).

The above studies clearly demonstrated that estrogen decreased calcium channel current, which correlated with its decreasing effect on the $[Ca^{2+}]_i$ increase induced by KCl depolarization. These vascular effects of estrogen were relatively delayed (1 to 2 min) compared with the effect of other vasoactive peptides (seconds). However, this is also different from the conventional genomic action of steroids, which takes longer than 1 to 2 min. It is possible that estrogen may affect protein synthesis in the time frame of our study since specific mRNA may already be present. Recently, the nongenomic action of some steroid hormones has received attention. The time-dependent effect of estrogen on the vascular system is consistent with that

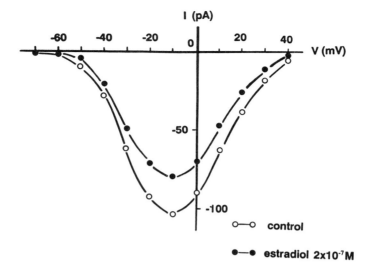

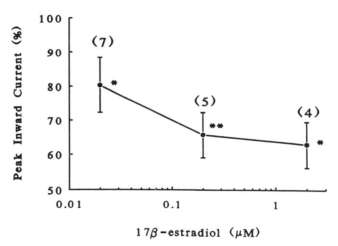

FIGURE 4   The effect of 17β-estradiol on calcium channel activity in VSMC isolated from rat tail artery. The upper panel shows the curves of the current/voltage (I/V) relationship. The peak current appears at the test pulse of –10 mV. The holding potential was –80 mV, the control I/V curve (empty circles) and the I/V curve after application of 17β-estradiol for 15 min (solid circles). The bottom panel shows the dose-dependent inhibitory effect of 17β-estradiol on calcium channel activity. The peak inward calcium current was determined at test pulses of –10 mv after application of 17β-estradiol for 15 min. The numbers in brackets are the numbers of experiments. Values are means ± SE percent of control current. *, **, significantly different from the control current change, $p < 0.05$ and $p < 0.01$, respectively. The mean control inward current is 46.89 ± 12.70 pA. (From Shan, J., Resnick, L., Liu, Q., Wu, X., Barbagallo, M., and Pang, P. K. T., unpublished data.)

of another steroid hormone, $1,25(OH)_2D_3$.[51] $1,25(OH)_2D_3$ increased the L-type Ca^{2+} current in cultured VSMC. The peak effect occurred at about 20 min. Accordingly, $1,25(OH)_2D_3$ also increased $[Ca^{2+}]_i$, and the peak effect occurred at about 30 min. *In vivo*, estrogen itself did not affect blood pressure for up to 6 h, and it started to affect the pressor response to NE 4 h after administration. *In vitro* (at the tissue or cellular level), estrogen exhibited acute effects (within 30 min). The difference in the timing of the effects between the *in vivo* and *in vitro* responses may be related to the difference in bioavailability between the *in vivo* and *in vitro* situations.

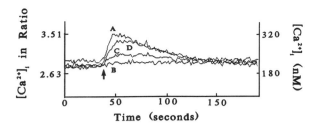

FIGURE 5   The effect of 17β-estradiol on the $[Ca^{2+}]_i$ increment induced by 15 mM KCl in VSMC isolated from rat tail artery. Original recordings were obtained from one typical experiment showing the effect of 15 mM KCl alone (A), 17β-estradiol (3×10^{-6} M) alone (B), 15 mM KCl after incubation with 17β-estradiol (3×10^{-6} M) for 15 min (C), and 15 mM KCl after washes (D). Note that the increment in $[Ca^{2+}]_i$ in trace C is much less than in trace A. After washes, the response to KCl recovered (D). These four tests were performed sequentially on the same group of cells. (From Shan, J., Resnick, L., Liu, Q., Wu, X., Barbagallo, M., and Pang, P. K. T., unpublished data.)

In the *in vivo* situation, the end result of the drug effect is more complicated. Several factors should be considered: (1) binding with carriers in blood transportation; (2) the blood pressure reflex mechanisms; (3) interaction with other vasoactive systems such as prostaglandins, histamine, and AVP; and (4) the genomic effect of estrogen.

Although the dosage of estrogen used in our studies is much higher than circulating levels, it is important to recognize the ability of estrogen to relax blood vessels. This action is consistent with epidemiological data. Overt or substantial changes were sought in our experimental situation. Much lower levels of steroid may be required *in vivo* to produce modulatory and more subtle effects. In summary, our studies suggest a correlation between the effect of estrogen in voltage-dependent Ca^{2+} channel activity and its effect in decreasing the $[Ca^{2+}]_i$ increment induced by membrane depolarization. In the *in vivo* situation, estrogen may affect $[Ca^{2+}]_i$ balance and, hence, tissue responsiveness to other vasoactive substances. This may suggest the protective effect of estrogen against cardiovascular diseases, which is in agreement with some previous epidemiological studies.

B. Progesterone

1. Epidemiological and Clinical Studies

Epidemiological studies showed that the decrease in production of both estrogen and progesterone may be responsible for the increasing incidence of cardiovascular diseases in postmenopausal women. A protective role of progesterone and of estrogen on blood pressure and on the cardiovascular system has been postulated, although the detailed mechanism(s) are not clear. Few studies have focused on the cardiovascular actions of progesterone. It has been reported that progesterone alone or in combination with estrogen may lower blood pressure in hypertensive and postmenopausal women.[52] In a placebo-controlled, double-blind crossover study in which natural progesterone was given by mouth in increasing doses (100, 200, 300 mg twice a day) to six men and four postmenopausal women with mild to moderate hypertension, progesterone caused a significant dose-dependent reduction of blood pressure when compared to blood pressure values recorded both before treatment and during administration of the placebo. It was then suggested that progesterone may be hypotensive. Another short term study[53] showed that neither estrogen nor progesterone alone was able to alter blood pressure, while a combination of the two decreased systolic, diastolic, and mean blood pressures. The investigators suggested that the combination of the two hormones may be more effective in lowering the blood pressure than each hormone alone.

2. Animal Studies

As with the investigation of estrogen, the effects of progesterone in animal studies are not conclusive. Nakamura et al.[54] reported that the pressor responses to graded doses of ANG II were significantly reduced in late pregnancy in conscious Wistar rats compared to those in nonpregnant rats. No effect of estradiol was found, but injection of progesterone alone or in association with estradiol significantly decreased the pressor response to ANG II. The authors suggested that the reduced pressor response to ANG II found in pregnancy may be mediated mainly by progesterone rather than by estrogen. In another report, Novak et al.[34] confirmed a reduction in the pressor response to ANG II in pregnancy, but in this study neither estrogen nor progesterone was able to reproduce this effect. They argued that the discrepancy in results between their experiments and those of Nakamura and co-workers was due to the difference in the species of rats (Long Evans vs.Wister) or the diet (sodium intake may alter pressor response to ANG II).

The precise mechanism(s) whereby progesterone modulates cardiovascular function is poorly understood. Progesterone receptors have been localized in the myocardium[55] and in vascular tissue.[41] It has been suggested that ions play an important role in this modulation.[44] Interference by steroid sex hormones with calcium fluxes and/or calcium utilization has been hypothesized.[38,56] However, as mentioned prviously, evidence for the direct effect of steroids on intracellular calcium mobilization is still lacking. A direct effect of progesterone on the adrenergic nervous system has been shown.[57] Also, a negative inotropic action of progesterone has already been suggested in the isolated rabbit heart.[56] It has also been suggested that progesterone, at least in some tissues, is able to stimulate cGMP production.[58]

As described above, we have investigated the vascular effects of estrogen in the *in vivo* whole animal, in *in vitro* isolated vascular tissue, and in *in vitro* cultured VSMC. Using the same experimental protocol and the same animal and experimental setup, we also studied the vascular effect of progesterone.[59] We found that increasing doses of progesterone (10 to 100 µg/kg) did not affect blood pressure. However, progesterone relaxed the vasoconstriction induced by other vasoconstrictors (KCl, AVP, or NE) in both isolated SD aorta and tail artery helical strips. The progesterone-induced relaxation was more intense in the tail artery than in aortic strips. The rat tail artery is a responsive blood vessel, and its contractility is similar to that of small resistance vessels.[60] This suggests that the resistance vessels might be more sensitive to progesterone than are capacitance vessels. We also found that progesterone at higher doses showed negative inotropic and chronotropic actions in the SD rat right atria preparation, which is in agreement with the results reported by Raddino et al.[56] These investigators suggested a negative inotropic action of progesterone in the isolated rabbit heart. Again, under our experimental conditions the observed cardiovascular effects could be nongenomic.

Using the same experimental protocol as described in the section on estrogen, we also found that progesterone blunted the $[Ca^{2+}]_i$ increment induced by 15 mM KCl in cultured VSMC isolated from SD rat tail artery. Accordingly, progesterone produced a dose-dependent decrease on the L-type calcium current in VSMC isolated from rat tail artery. Our results suggest that the effect of progesterone on the cardiovascular system may occur through an interference with intracellular calcium metabolism and calcium fluxes. Although we observed a reduction of calcium current by progesterone, it is not known whether the effect is a direct one or is mediated by an intracellular second messenger system. It is difficult to extrapolate its clinical significance. However, our study showed the pharmacological and/or physiological relevance. These results agree with the theory that progesterone is a protective female hormone.[52]

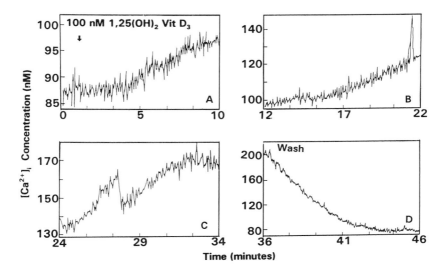

FIGURE 6   An actual recording of changes in intracellular free calcium concentration in a monolayer of vascular
smooth muscle cells. The cells were monitored at 2-min intervals for 34 min after application of
1,25(OH)$_2$D$_3$. A, B, and C each display 10 min of recording. 1,25(OH)$_2$D$_3$ was then removed by
changing the medium three successive times, and the cells were then recorded for another 10 min (D).
(From Shan, J., Resnick, L., Lewanczuk, R. Z., Karpinski, E., Li, B., and Pang, P. K. T., *American
Journal of Hypertension*, 6, 983, 1994. With permission.)

III. VITAMIN D$_3$ METABOLITES AND VASCULAR FUNCTION

Vitamin D is a prohormone for its more polar metabolites, such as 1,25(OH)$_2$D$_3$, 24,25(OH)$_2$D$_3$,
and others. It is well established that hydrophobic vitamin D$_3$ is the precursor of a steroid
hormone. The molecule vitamin D$_3$ is a sterol and displays the common chemical properties
characteristic of steroids, including steroid hormones. Vitamin D$_3$ is subject to a complex
series of metabolic conversions that generate some 37 separate metabolites. Most of these new
daughter compounds differ from the parent vitamin D by the presence of 1-3 hydroxyls, oxo,
or lactone functionalities.[61] Vitamin D$_3$ is first hydroxylized in the liver at the carbon-25
position and is further hydroxylized at the carbon-1 position in the kidney to become
1,25(OH)$_2$D$_3$, which is believed to be the active metabolite.[62] 1,25(OH)$_2$D$_3$ generates biological responses through both genomic and nongenomic pathways. The genomic pathway is
usually mediated through nuclear receptors. Over 60 systems and tissues possess a nuclear
receptor for 1,25(OH)$_2$D$_3$,[63] which may be responsible for the genomic response of 1,25(OH)$_2$D$_3$.
The nongenomic pathway may involve the regulation of [Ca^{2+}]$_i$ and calcium channels[51] and
protein kinase A and C signal transduction pathways.[64] In the kidney, through the renal P$_{450}$-
dependent 24-hydroxylase enzyme, 25(OH)$_2$D$_3$ is converted into another metabolite,
24,25(OH)$_2$D$_3$. The biological action of 24,25(OH)$_2$D$_3$ is not yet clear.

A. 1,25(OH)$_2$D$_3$

The cardiovascular effect of 1,25(OH)$_2$D$_3$ has been extensively reviewed in previous chapters
in this book. In this chapter, we will only describe some recent findings in our laboratory.[51]
Our study was designed to determine whether 1,25(OH)$_2$D$_3$ had any direct effect on VSMC.
We found that 1,25(OH)$_2$D$_3$ increased [Ca^{2+}]$_i$ in VSMC isolated from rat tail artery (Figure 6).
Such a change in [Ca^{2+}]$_i$ correlated well with the stimulatory effect of 1,25(OH)$_2$D$_3$ on L-type
calcium channel activity in the same type of VSMC (Figure 7). These data suggested that this
active vitamin D$_3$ metabolite might increase Ca^{2+} entry through calcium channels and produce

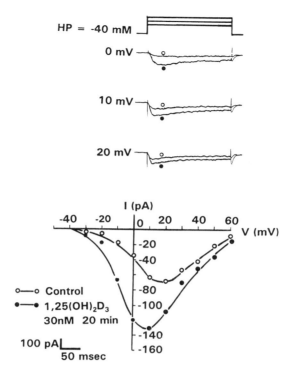

FIGURE 7   The effect of 1,25(OH)$_2$D$_3$ on the L-channel current in a smooth muscle cell. Top panel shows the original traces elicited from a holding potential of –40 mV to three different test potentials. Open circles represent the control traces, and the filled circles represent the traces 15 min after treatment of the cell with 30 nM 1,25(OH)$_2$D$_3$. The bottom panel shows the current/voltage (I/V) relations before and after the application of 1,25(OH)$_2$D$_3$. (From Shan, J., Resnick, L., Lewanczuk, R. Z., Karpinski, E., Li, B., and Pang, P. K. T., *American Journal of Hypertension*, 6, 983, 1994. With permission.)

an increase in [Ca^{2+}]$_i$. Although calcium has been implicated in the action of 1,25(OH)$_2$D$_3$,[66-70] our study provides evidence for such a direct effect. In both calcium channel activity and [Ca^{2+}]$_i$ studies, the effects were delayed, reaching their peak at approximately 30 min. In both studies, the effect occured in minutes and not in seconds, as is usually seen with peptides and catecholamines. It is difficult at this time to determine whether 1,25(OH)$_2$D$_3$ acts directly on calcium channels, since the effect takes more than 20 minutes to develop fully. It is believed that the effect may be mediated by a second messenger system. It was reported that 1,25(OH)$_2$D$_3$ stimulated lysophosphatidylinositol (LPI) formation, which might mediate the increase in [Ca^{2+}]$_i$ in hepatocytes.[68] Furthermore, our experiment showed that LPI also stimulated a delayed and long-lasting increase in [Ca^{2+}]$_i$ in rat tail artery.[71] However, LPI caused a delayed blood pressure increment in SD rats and an increment in tension in rat tail artery strips while 1,25(OH)$_2$D$_3$ did not. Such a difference argues against LPI being involved in the action of 1,25(OH)$_2$D$_3$.

Our study supports the involvement of 1,25(OH)$_2$D$_3$ in hypertension. The direct effect of the hormone on VSMC [Ca^{2+}]$_i$ regulation correlated well with its possible role in the development of hypertension as seen in the literature. However, 1,25(OH)$_2$D$_3$ may not behave like a classical vasoconstrictor (e.g., AVP or NE) that produces overt vasoconstriction and an increase in blood pressure. 1,25(OH)$_2$D$_3$ increased [Ca^{2+}]$_i$ by less than 100% of the basal level even at doses of 10^{-8} to 10^{-7} M. It is possible that this increase in [Ca^{2+}]$_i$ is too small to cause overt contraction of blood vessels and blood pressure changes. The mechanism involved in this dissociation between [Ca^{2+}]$_i$ increment and tension generation is not known at this time.

Our data also indicate that $1,25(OH)_2D_3$ increases $[Ca^{2+}]_i$ by promoting calcium influx through the opening of membrane calcium channels and does not involve intracellular stored calcium release, since IP_3 formation was not affected by $1,25(OH)_2D_3$ in rat tail artery. The dose used to produce the effect on $[Ca^{2+}]_i$ was much higher (about 1000-fold) than the circulating concentration of $1,25(OH)_2D_3$. It is possible that, in *in vitro* conditions, a much higher dose is required to produce observable responses. It is also possible that only low doses of $1,25(OH)_2D_3$ are required to affect basal $[Ca^{2+}]_i$ during chronic exposure to the hormone. Perhaps in an intact animal, the role of $1,25(OH)_2D_3$ is to elevate chronically basal $[Ca^{2+}]_i$ in VSMC by increasing calcium influx through voltage-dependent calcium channels. Such a chronic basal $[Ca^{2+}]_i$ effect may not by itself change the blood pressure, as was observed. It may, however, be capable in the long run of potentiating the actions of other vasoconstricting mechanisms. It may then increase vascular resistance and affect the blood pressure level. This would fit with a proposed long-term modulatory role of $1,25(OH)_2D_3$ in hypertension. Hypertension is a heterogeneous disease, and abnormal levels of vitamin D_3 may be only one of several factors involved and may be important in only some special forms of essential hypertension.

B. $24,25(OH)_2D_3$

$24,25(OH)_2D_3$ has been considered to be an inactive metabolite of vitamin D_3, although its concentration in normal individuals is much higher than that of $1,25(OH)_2D_3$. However, there is some evidence that $24,25(OH)_2D_3$ may play an important role in the development of endochondral bone.[72-74] Specific receptors for this metabolite are present in many tissues, such as parathyroid gland,[75] chondrocytes,[76] epiphyseal growth plates,[77] and limb bud mesenchymal cells.[78] It was reported[79] that both $1,25(OH)_2D_3$ and $24,25(OH)_2D_3$ might affect L-type calcium currents and the uptake of ^{45}Ca in rat osteosarcoma cells. It was demonstrated that $24,25(OH)_2D_3$ increased bone mineral concentrations in healthy rats[80] and decreased the number of osteoclasts and the area of bone resorption. The tendency for $24,25(OH)_2D_3$ to cause a positive Ca^{2+} balance and to favor bone mineralization, rather than breakdown, has been suggested. The vascular effects of $24,25(OH)_2D_3$ have not been reported so far. However, since $1,25(OH)_2D_3$ was shown to have a direct action on VSMC in our study, these findings led us to investigate the vascular effect of $24,25(OH)_2D_3$. Our study showed for the first time the direct effects of $24,25(OH)_2D_3$ on vascular tissue, although only at high pharmacological doses.[81] $24,25(OH)_2D_3$ directly relaxed tonic tension produced by vasoconstrictors (KCl or NE) in SD rat tail artery (Figure 8). Moreover, it also inhibited the phasic tension generated by NE, KCl, or AVP. The direct vasorelaxant effect of this vitamin D_3 metabolite, however, did not produce a hypotensive effect *in vivo*. The mechanism of its vascular action may be related to its effects on calcium influx and intracellular calcium release, as shown in the tension studies. The protocol was designed as follows: the rat tail artery helical strip was incubated in Kreb's buffer with normal calcium for 30 min. The buffer was then replaced by calcium-free Kreb's solution. Five minutes later, the tissue was challenged with a vasoconstrictor (KCl, AVP, or NE). In the case of NE, a brief transient tension was generated, which represented the vasoconstriction induced by calcium release from intracellular calcium store(s). Cumulative doses of $CaCl_2$ were applied, and in all three cases, a stepwise tension increment was recorded, which represented the vasoconstriction induced by extracellular calcium influx. Our experiments demonstrated that both KCl- and AVP-induced vasoconstrictions were exclusively dependent upon extracellular calcium influx.[82] $24,25(OH)_2D_3$ was applied 3 minutes before the vasoconstrictor; it inhibited the vasoconstriction dependent on extracellular Ca^{2+} influx and on the intracellular stored calcium release induced by various vasoconstrictors. The whole cell version of the patch-clamp technique was also used to demonstrate that $24,25(OH)_2D_3$ inhibited the L-type

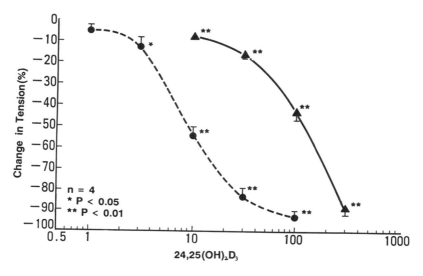

FIGURE 8   Dose-dependent relaxing effects of 24,25(OH)$_2$D$_3$ on SD rat tail artery helical strips precontracted by 10^{-7} M NE or 60 mM KCl. The tissue was precontracted by 10^{-7} M NE (circles) or 60 mM KCl (triangles). Values are means $\pm$ SE; n = number of tissues. (From Shan, J. and Pang, P. K. T., unpublished data.)

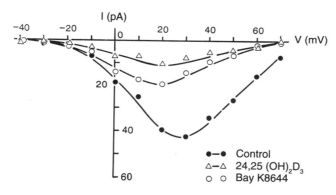

FIGURE 9   The effect of 24,25(OH)$_2$D$_3$ on the L-channel current in a VSMC isolated from SD rat tail artery. The curves of current/voltage (I/V) relations were presented. The control I/V curve (solid circles), the I/V curve after application of 5 $\times$ 10^{-6} M 24,25(OH)$_2$D$_3$ for 20 min (empty triangles), and the curve after application of a calcium channel agonist, Bay K-8644 (empty circles) are shown. (From Shan, J., Li, B., and Pang, P. K. T., unpublished data.)

voltage-dependent calcium current in cultured VSMC isolated from rat tail artery (Figure 9). 24,25(OH)$_2$D$_3$ also inhibited the [Ca^{2+}]$_i$ increment induced by 15 mM KCl in VSMC (Figure 10). Therefore, it may inhibit the increase in [Ca^{2+}]$_i$ stimulated by vasoconstrictors and the contraction of blood vessels. Eilam et al.[83] found that both 1,25(OH)$_2$D$_3$ and 24,25(OH)$_2$D$_3$ increased the initial rate of Ca^{2+} influx in primary cultures of rat bone cells through a mechanism insensitive to protein synthesis inhibition. It has been reported that in primary cultures of mouse osteoblasts, physiological concentrations of 1,25(OH)$_2$D$_3$ and 24,25(OH)$_2$D$_3$ rapidly induced significant increases in [Ca^{2+}]$_i$. The response to 1,25(OH)$_2$D$_3$ was dependent on Ca^{2+} influx, whereas 24,25(OH)$_2$D$_3$ mobilized Ca^{2+} from intracellular stores, as shown by the blockade experiments using Ca^{2+} channel antagonists and drugs affecting Ca^{2+} sequestration

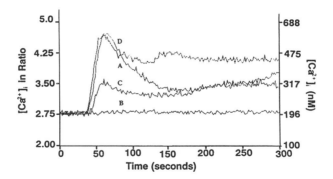

FIGURE 10 The effect of 24,25(OH)$_2$D$_3$ on the [Ca^{2+}]$_i$ increment induced by 15 mM KCl in VSMC isolated from rat tail artery. Original recordings were obtained from one typical experiment showing the effect of 15 mM KCl alone (A), 24,25(OH)$_2$D$_3$ (3 × 10^{-6} M) alone (B), 15 mM KCl after incubation with 24,25(OH)$_2$D$_3$ (3 × 10^{-6} M) for 15 min (C), and 15 mM KCl after washes (D). Note that the increment in [Ca^{2+}]$_i$ in trace C is much less than in trace A. After washes, the response to KCl recovered (D). These four tests were performed sequentially on the same group of cells. (From Shan, J., Wu, X., and Pang, P. K. T., unpublished data.)

by intracellular organelles.[64] These results contradict the present data, which show the inhibitory effect of 24,25(OH)$_2$D$_3$ on the increase in [Ca^{2+}]$_i$. The difference may be due to tissue specificity and/or experimental procedures.

24,25(OH)$_2$D$_3$ may be a nonspecific Ca^{2+} antagonist, since it blocked both Ca^{2+} influx and intracellular stored Ca^{2+} release. Patch-clamp data directly showed that it blocked the voltage-dependent Ca^{2+} channels. It is possible that 24,25(OH)$_2$D$_3$ inhibited Ca^{2+} channels on both the cell membrane and the intracellular organelle membrane. This would explain its effect on Ca^{2+} entry and intracellular stored Ca^{2+} release. As in the case of 1,25(OH)$_2$D$_3$, the effects of 24,25(OH)$_2$D$_3$ required minutes (10 to 20 min) to develop fully, suggesting the involvement of a second messenger system(s) that is independent of the genomic pathway.

Similar to estrogen, progesterone, and 1,25(OH)$_2$D$_3$, 24,25(OH)$_2$D$_3$ cannot produce an overt pressor response *in vivo*. The mechanisms may be similar to that of estrogen. It may affect the balance of [Ca^{2+}]$_i$ and its state of equilibrium. Therefore, it may modulate vasoconstriction induced by other endogenous vasoconstricting mechanisms and prevent the development of hypertension.

24,25(OH)$_2$D$_3$ may prevent some forms of hypertension, and 1,25(OH)$_2$D$_3$ may be related to the development of hypertension. However, apart from the supportive [Ca^{2+}]$_i$ data, results from blood pressure and vascular tension studies with 1,25(OH)$_2$D$_3$ are not consistent with its involvement in short-term blood pressure regulation. These data only suggest that the vitamin D$_3$ endocrine system may be important in the long-term regulation of blood pressure. Structurally, estrogen, progesterone, 1,25(OH)$_2$D$_3$, and 24,25(OH)$_2$D$_3$ have the same basic steroid nucleus. This may explain their common pharmacological actions at high doses, i.e., all of them are capable of modulating the actions of other vasoconstrictors. However, 1,25(OH)$_2$D$_3$ has the intrinsic property of increasing [Ca^{2+}]$_i$ at lower doses, thus indicating a possible modulatory role in hypertension.

IV. GENOMIC AND NONGENOMIC EFFECTS OF STEROID HORMONES

Thus far, we have emphasized the nongenomic effects of some steroid hormones. From a conventional point of view, the peptide hormones play a role through nongenomic pathways. They interact with membrane receptors on the cell surface. Hydrophilicity prevents the peptide from crossing the cell membrane. Therefore, it binds to specific receptors on the cell surface, and signal transduction systems are stimulated inside the cell to affect cellular processes. In contrast to the hydrophilic peptide hormones, steroid hormones can cross the cell membrane because of their hydrophobicity. In their respective target cells, steroid hormones bind with their own specific cytoplasmic receptors. The hormone-receptor binding is essential for hormonal activity. Some hormones (e.g., estradiol) possess more than one receptor protein in the target cell, and one cell may have receptors for several hormones (e.g., for estradiol and progesterone). One hormone may influence the number of receptors for other hormones. For example, estradiol can increase the number of progesterone receptors in progesterone target cells.

The short-term effects of steroid hormones are becoming more widely recognized. The mechanism of the short-term effects of steroids may not involve alteration of gene expression. The above evidence strongly suggests that all the steroid hormones thus far studied have a nongenomic short-term biological response. Norman et al.[65] have suggested that $1,25(OH)_2D_3$ may produce biological responses by utilizing a signal transduction pathway that is independent of the regulation of gene transcription. The hormone interacts with a putative membrane recognition element, which then, in some fashion, is coupled to the activity of calcium channels so that a rapid biological response can be initiated. The biological response appears within seconds to minutes after the application of $1,25(OH)_2D_3$. This is different from the 60 min or longer required for the genomic responses to be detectable. From our own studies, we suggest that the nongenomic pathway is probably common in steroid action, at least pharmacologically.

V. CONCLUSION

From the above discussion, it is obvious that steroids do have substantial effects on the cardiovascular system. While the study of most vasoactive substances, such as ANG II and AVP, starts with pharmacological and mechanistic investigations leading to clinical involvement and eventually epidemiological implications, in the case of steroids the first indications come from epidemiological studies, with little or no information on the mechanism of action of these hormones. Female sex steroids have been shown to be epidemiologically involved in preventing cardiovascular diseases. Vitamin D metabolite excess is correlated with the occurrence of hypertension. In both cases, there are few data on their actions on the target tissue, the cardiovascular tissue. This chapter describes some recent findings concerning the effect of these steroids on the vascular tissue (i.e., the vascular smooth muscle). The results further delineate the possible mechanisms of action. These findings show that, indeed, steroids do have cardiovascular effects. Their mechanism of action at least in part supports the previous epidemiological findings. In addition, some other interesting aspects have emerged and should be discussed.

First, the genomic and nongenomic possibilities should be reinvestigated. From the discussion above, the data point to a nongenomic mechanism simply by virtue of the rather fast onset of the effect. It is very unlikely that the actions described are due to changes in gene expression. However, it does not preclude the involvement of synthesis of new proteins from existing mRNA. The direct effect can also be produced by affecting the contractile mechanism through second messengers without additional protein synthesis. It is possible that a combination of these two rather rapid nongenomic responses plays an important role in the cardiovascular effect of steroids. Steroids are known to have profound effects on gene expression. The above studies do not address this issue. It is possible that steroids may affect the expression of genes, leading to gene production, which may affect the cardiovascular system. The estrogen effect on the angiotensinogen production has been reported. The profound disturbance in lipid metabolism produced by steroids can, no doubt, interfere with cardiovascular functions. Vitamin D metabolites can influence intestinal calcium absorption through many mechanisms, including carrier protein synthesis. Increases in the overall balance of calcium can perhaps directly and indirectly affect cardiovascular functions. It is conceivable that steroids may have both nongenomic and genomic mechanisms in their overall influence on the cardiovascular system.

Second, even with the nongenomic actions of steroids, there may be an acute and a chronic aspect. The effects of the steroids on VSMC calcium channels can potentially alter $[Ca^{2+}]_i$ enough to elicit acute or immediate responses, such as relaxation of blood vessels or a fall in blood pressure. As most of the data we obtained so far are with rather high pharmacological doses, these acute actions may have little real functional meaning. Nevertheless, these data do indicate the capability of steroids to influence $[Ca^{2+}]_i$. In reality, the actions of these steroids may be more involved in basal $[Ca^{2+}]_i$ regulation. In the body, steroids may not produce such drastic effects as seen in our assay systems. They may produce small but effective modulatory actions on the channels, thus shifting the basal equilibrium of $[Ca^{2+}]_i$. The change in $[Ca^{2+}]_i$ equilibrium will then alter the responsiveness of VSMC to other vasoconstrictors, which have more overt effects. Such long-term chronic actions of steroids seem to fit well with epidemiological observations. In the case of estrogen, its effect on the responsiveness to other vasoconstrictors 4 to 6 h after its application fits such a hypothesis.

Third, the present data clearly delineate the effects of steroids on $[Ca^{2+}]_i$ regulation. Their effects on calcium channels are exciting, because although peptides and other biologically active substances have been shown to affect calcium channels, such effects have seldom been reported for steroids. In fact, these results with VSMC may be the first for this type of cell. Another important aspect of the data is the confirmation of the channel results with $[Ca^{2+}]_i$ measurements. In order to measure calcium channel activities, sodium and potassium channels are blocked. The cells are dialyzed with EGTA to deplete intracellular calcium, and the cells are bathed with 20 mM Ba^{2+}, which acts as the charge carrier. Under such totally abnormal conditions, the effect of chemicals on the calcium channels is difficult to interpret. It is highly possible that the observations are artifactual. To confirm the channel data with $[Ca^{2+}]_i$ determinations in relatively undisturbed cells is therefore essential. In the case of estrogen and progesterone, the calcium channel blocking effect parallels that of $[Ca^{2+}]_i$ increased inhibition. In the case of $1,25(OH)_2D_3$, the calcium channel opening effect coincides with its ability to increase $[Ca^{2+}]_i$. Furthermore, the calcium channel effect temporally parallels that of the $[Ca^{2+}]_i$ effect. These cellular calcium effects of steroids are, therefore, biologically meaningful.

Fourth, in this book the main theme is the cardiovascular actions of calcium-regulating hormones. The other chapters on peptide hormones, such PTH, PTHrp, CGRP, etc., describe the evidence for their effect on the cardiovascular system. The active metabolite of vitamin D, $1,25(OH)_2D_3$, has been suggested to be involved in cardiovascular functions. In the present chapter, the other metabolite, $24,25(OH)_2D_3$, which is considered to be inactive, is shown to have effects opposite of those of $1,25(OH)_2D_3$. This is the first time the cardiovascular effect of such a metabolite has been observed. The other steroid hormones described are the female sex steroids, which play a regulating role in the cardiovascular system. A second conclusion is that all of these hormones affect $[Ca^{2+}]_i$ regulation. The effects of PTH and steroid hormones on calcium channels are also presented. These two conclusions are important, since they provide the necessary information to support the hypothesis put forth at the beginning of this chapter. In the overall homeostasis of calcium in the body, plasma calcium concentration represents the balance among uptake, storage, and excretion, as is generally understood. In the present hypothesis, it is suggested that the use of calcium by cells could be the most important aspect of calcium balance and should be included in the overall picture as shown in Figure 2.

It is further suggested that calcium-regulating hormones, which affect all the other aspects of calcium homeostasis in the body, should be effective in regulating the use of calcium by cells. Indeed, at least in the cardiovascular system studied here, calcium-regulating hormones are quite important in $[Ca^{2+}]_i$ regulation which, as described in the introduction, represents the use of calcium by cells to serve as an intracellular messenger. Thus far, the observations are consistent and supportive of the hypothesis. Initially, it may appear that this hypothesis is not that exciting, as calcium as a second messenger has been extensively studied in the mechanism of action of hormones, including the calcium-regulating hormones. However, this has never been considered as a use of calcium by cells and has therefore not been considered in the overall homeostasis of calcium. This hypothesis, although simple, is logical and provocative. It takes a well-known phenomenon, i.e., calcium as a second messenger for most hormones, and places it in its proper prospective in the overall calcium balance in the body. It would then become logical that the same hormones that affect all other aspects of calcium balance should affect the use of calcium by cells. Since cardiovascular functions are very much related to $[Ca^{2+}]_i$, it would therefore be logical that the calcium-regulating hormones should have a profound effect on the cardiovascular system.

REFERENCES

1. Weiss, N. S., Relationship of menopause to serum cholesterol and arterial blood pressure: the United States health examination survey of adults, *Am. J. Epidemiol.*, 96, 337, 1972.
2. Kannel, W. B., Hjortland, M. C., McNamara, P. M., and Gordon, T., Evaluation of cardiovascular risk in the elderly: the Framingham study, *Ann. Intern. Med.*, 85, 447, 1976.
3. Roberts, J. and Maurer, K., Blood pressure levels of persons 6 to 74 years, United States, 1971–74, *Vital Health Stat.*, 11, 203, 1977.
4. Stampfer, M. J., Willet, W. C., Colditz, G. A., Rosner, B., Speizer, F. E., and Hennekens, C. H., A prospective study of postmenopausal estrogen therapy and coronary heart disease, *N. Engl. J. Med.*, 313, 1044, 1985.
5. Bush, T. L., Barret-Connor, E., Cowan, L., Criqui, M. H., Wallace, R.B., Suchindran, C. M., Tyroler, H. A., and Rifkind, B. M., Cardiovascular mortality and noncontraceptive use of estrogen in women: results from the lipid research clinics program follow up study, *Circulation*, 75, 11029, 1987.
6. Petitti, D., Perlman, J. A., and Sidney, S., Non-contraceptive estrogen and mortality: long term follow up of women in the Walnut Creek Study, *Obstet. Gynecol.*, 70, 289, 1987.
7. Henderson, B. E., Paganini-Hill, A., and Ross, R. K., Decreased mortality in users of estrogen replacement therapy, *Arch. Intern. Med.*, 151, 75, 1991.
8. Stampfer, M. J., Colditz, G. A., Willet, W. C., Manson, J. E., Rosner, B., Speizer, F. E., and Hennekens, C. H., Postmenopausal estrogen therapy and cardiovascular disease. Ten-year follow-up from the nurses' health study, *N. Engl. J. Med.*, 325, 756, 1991.
9. Wilson, P. W. F., Garrison, R. J., and Castelli, W. P., Postmenopausal estrogen use, cigarette smoking and cardiovascular morbidity in women over 50, the Framingham study, *N. Engl. J. Med.*, 313, 1038, 1985.
10. Phyllips, G. B., Evidence for hyperestrogenemia as a risk factor for myocardial infarction in men, *Lancet*, 2, 14, 1976.
11. Veterans Administration Cooperative Urological Research Group, Treatment and survival of patients with cancer of the prostate, *Surg. Gynecol. Obstet.*, 124, 1011, 1967.
12. Mann, J. I. and Imman, W. H. W., Oral contraceptive and death from myocardial infarction, *Br. Med. J.*, II, 245, 1975.
13. Vessey, M. and Doll, R., Investigation of relation between use of oral contraceptives and thromboembolic disease, *Br. Med. J.*, 2, 199, 1968.
14. Royal College of General Practitioners' Oral Contraceptive Study: mortality among oral contraceptive users, *Lancet*, 2, 731, 1977.

15. Shapiro, S., Slone, D., Rosenberg, L., Kaufman, D. W., Stolley, D. D., and Miettinen, O. S., Oral contraceptive use in relation to myocardial infarction, *Lancet*, 1, 743, 1979.

16. Vessey, M., McPherson, K., and Hohson, B., Mortality among women participating in the Oxford Family Planning Association Contraceptive Study, *Lancet*, 2, 727, 1977.

17. Stadel, B. V., Oral contraceptives and cardiovascular disease, *N. Engl. J. Med.*, 305, 612, 1981.

18. Meade, T. W., Oral contraceptives, clotting factors and thrombosis, *Am. J. Obstet. Gynecol.*, 142, 758, 1982.

19. Inman, W., Vessey, M. P., Westerholh, M., and Engelund, A., Thromboembolic disease and the steroidal content of oral contraceptives: a report to the Committee on Safety of Drugs, *Br. Med. J.*, 2, 203, 1970.

20. Porter, J. B., Hunter, J. R., Jick, H., and Stergachis, A., Oral contraceptives and non-fatal vascular disease, *Obstet. Gynecol.*, 66, 1, 1985.

21. Porter, J. B., Hershel, J., and Walker, A. M., Mortality among oral contraceptive users, *Obstet. Gynecol.*, 70, 29, 1987.

22. Stokes, T. and Wynn, V., Serum lipids in women on oral contraceptives, *Lancet*, 2, 677, 1971.

23. Bradley, D. D, Wingerd, J., Petitti, D. B., Krauss, R. M., and Ramcharan, S., Serum HDL-cholesterol in women using oral contraceptives, estrogens and progestins, *N. Engl. J. Med.*, 299, 17, 1978.

24. Wallace, R., Walden, C., Barret-Connor, E., Rifkind B. M., Hunninghake, D. B., Mackenthun, A., and Heiss, G., Altered plasma lipid and lipoprotein levels associated with oral contraceptives and estrogen use, *Lancet*, 2, 112, 1979.

25. Knopp, R. H., Walden, C. E., Wahl, P. W., Hoover, J., Warnick, R. G., Albers, J. J., Ogilvie, J. T., and Hazzard, W. R., Oral contraceptives and postmenopausal hormone estrogen effect on lipoprotein triglyceride and cholesterol in an adult female population: relationship to estrogen and progestin potency, *J. Clin. Endocrinol. Metab.*, 53, 1123, 1981.

26. Wahl, P., Walden, C., Knopp, R., Hoover, J., Wallace, R., Heiss, G., and Rifdind, B., Effect of estrogen/progestin potency on lipid/lipoprotein cholesterol, *N. Engl. J. Med.*, 308, 862, 1983.

27. Hammond, C. B., Jelowsek, F. R., Lee, K. L., Creasman, W. T., and Parker, R. T., Effect of long term estrogen replacement therapy. I. Metabolic effects, *Am. J. Obstet. Gynecol.*, 133, 525, 1979.

28. Pfëffer, R. I. and Van der Noort, S., Estrogen use and stroke risk in postmenopausal women, *Am. J. Epidemiol.*, 103, 445, 1976.

29. Gow, S. and MacGillvray, I., Metabolic, hormonal, and vascular changes after synthetic oestrogen therapy in oophorectomized women, *Br. Med. J.*, 10, 73, 1977.

30. Toba, K., Crofton, J. T., Inoue, M., and Share, L., Effects of vasopressin on arterial blood pressure and cardiac output in male and female rats, *Am. J. Physiol.*, 261, R1118, 1991.

31. Kondo, K., Okuno, T., Eguchi, T., Suzuki, H., Nagahama, S., and Saruta, T., Vascular action of high dose estrogen in rats, *Endocrinol. Jpn.*, 27, 307, 1980.

32. Yoshimura, T., Ito, M., and Nakamura, T., Effect of pregnancy and estrogen on the angiotensin II pressor response of the rabbit using serial blood pressure measurement in the ear. *Clin. Exp. Hypertens*, B3, 97, 1984.

33. Nakamura, T., Kurokawa, T., and Orimo, H., Increased bone volume and reduced bone turnover in rabbits by high doses of 24R,25-dihydroxyvitamin D_3, *J. Bone Miner. Res.*, 4(Suppl.), S401, 1989.

34. Novak, K. and Kauffman, S., Effect of pregnancy, estradiol, and progesterone on pressor responsiveness to angiotensin II, *Am. J. Physiol.*, 261, R1164, 1991.

35. Raddino, R., Manca, C., Poli, E., Bolognesi, R., and Visioli, O., Effect of 17-beta-estradiol on the isolated rabbit heart, *Arch. Int. Pharmacodyn. Ther.*, 281, 57, 1986.

36. Stumpf, W. E., Sar, M., and Amuller, G., The heart: a target organ for estradiol, *Science*, 196, 319, 1977.

37. Collburn, P. and Buonassisi, V., Estrogen-binding sites in endothelial cell culture, *Science*, 201, 817, 1978.

38. Harder, D. R. and Coulson, P. B., Estrogen receptors and effect of estrogen on membrane electrical properties of coronary vascular smooth muscle, *J. Cell. Physiol.*, 100, 375, 1979.

39. Nakao, J., Chang, W. C., Murota, S.I., and Orimo, H., Estradiol-binding sites in rat aortic smooth muscle cells in culture, *Atherosclerosis*, 38, 75, 1981.

40. McGill, H. C. and Sheridan, P. J., Nuclear uptake of sex steroid hormones in the cardiovascular system of the baboon, *Circ. Res.*, 48, 234, 1982.

41. Horwitz, K. B. and Horwitz, L. D., Canine vascular tissues are targets for androgens, estrogens, progestins and glucocorticoids, *J. Clin. Invest.*, 69, 750, 1982.

42. McCalden, T. A., The inhibitory action of oestradiol-17-β and progesterone on venous smooth muscle, *Br. J. Pharmacol.*, 53, 183, 1975.

43. Silva, De Sa, M. F. and Meirelles, R. S., Vasodilating effect of estrogen on the human umbilical artery, *Gynecol. Invest.*, 8, 307, 1977.

44. Altura, B. M. and Altura, B. T., Influence of sex hormones, oral contraceptives and pregnancy on vascular muscle and its reactivity, in *Factors Influencing Vascular Reactivity*, Carrier, O. and Shibata, S. Eds., Igaku-Shoin, New York, 1977, 221.

45. Colucci, W. S., Gimbrone, M. A., Jr., McLaughlin, M. K., Halpern, W., and Alexander, R. W., Increased vascular catecholamine sensitivity and alpha adrenergic receptor affinity in female and estrogen treated male rats, *Circ. Res.*, 50, 805, 1982.

46. Batra, S. C., Effect of some estrogens and progesterone on calcium uptake and calcium release by myometrial mitochondria, *Biochem. Pharmacol.*, 23, 803, 1973.

47. Batra, S. C. and Bengtsson, B., Effect of diethylstilbestrol and ovarian steroids on the contractile responses and calcium movements in rat uterine smooth muscle, *J. Physiol.*, 276, 329, 1978.

48. Rendt, J. M., Toro, L., Stefani, E., and Erulkar, S. D., Progesterone increases calcium currents in myometrial cells from immature and non pregnant adult rats, *Am. J. Physiol.*, 262(31), C293, 1992.

49. Shan, J., Resnick, L. M., Liu, Q., Wu, X., Barbagallo, M., and Pang, P. K. T., Vascular effect of 17β-estradiol in male SD rats, *Am. J. Physiol.*, 266, H967, 1994.

50. Grynkiewicz, G., Poenie, M., and Tsien, R. W., A new generation of Ca^{2+} indicators with greatly improved fluorescence properties, *J. Biol. Chem.*, 260, 3440, 1985.

51. Shan, J., Resnick, L. M., Lewanczuk, R. Z., Karpinski, E., Li, B., and Pang, P. K. T., 1,25 Dihydroxyvitamin D as a cardiovascular hormone: effects on calcium current and cytosolic free calcium in vascular smooth muscle cells, *Am. J. Hypertens.*, 6, 983, 1994.

52. Rylance, P. B., Brincat, M., Lafferty, K., De Trafford, J. C., Brincat, S., Parson, V., and Studel, J. W. W., Natural progesterone and antihypertensive action. *Br. Med. J.*, 290, 13, 1985.

53. Regensteiner, J. G., Hiatt, W. R., Byyny, R. L., Pickett, C. K., Woodard, W. D., and Moore, L. G., Short-term effect of estrogen and progestin on blood pressure of normotensive postmenopausal women, *J. Clin. Pharmacol.*, 31, 543, 1991.

54. Nakamura, T., Matsui, K., Ito, M., Yoshimura, T., Kawasaky, N., Fujisaky, S., and Okamura, H., Effects of pregnancy and hormone treatments on pressor response to angiotensin II in conscious rats, *Am. J. Obstet. Gynecol.*, 159, 989, 1988.

55. Lin, A. L., McGill, H. C., and Shain, S. A., Hormone receptors of the baboon cardiovascular system. Biochemical characterization of aortic and myocardial cytoplasmic progesterone receptors, *Circ. Res.*, 50, 610, 1982.

56. Raddino, R., Poli, E., Pela, G., and Manca, C., Action of steroid sex hormones on the isolated rabbit heart, *Pharmacology*, 38, 185, 1989.

57. Williams, L. T. and Lefkowitz, R. J., Regulation of rabbit myometrial alpha-adrenergic receptors by estrogen and progesterone, *J. Clin. Invest.*, 60, 815, 1977.

58. Sancho, M. J., Gomez-Munoz, A., Sanchez-Bueno, A., Trueba, M., and Marlino, A., Glycogen phosphorylase activity is increased before protein synthesis activation by progesterone, *Exp. Clin. Endocrinol.*, 92, 154, 1988.

59. Barbagallo, M., Shan, J., and Pang, P. K. T., unpublished data, 1993.

60. Frost, B. R., Gerke, D. C., and Frewin, D. D., The effect of 2-phenylalanine-8-lysine vasopressin (octapressin) on blood vessels in the rat tail, *Aust. J. Exp. Biol. Med. Sci.*, 54, 403, 1976.

61. Henry, H. L. and Norman, A. W., Vitamin D: metabolism and mechanism of action, *Annu. Rev. Nutr.*, 4, 493, 1984.

62. Haussler, M. R., Vitamin D receptors: nature and function, *Annu. Rev. Nutr.*, 6, 527, 1986.

63. Walters, M. R., Newly identified action of the vitamin D endocrine system, *Endocr. Rev.*, 13(4), 719, 1992.

64. Lieberherr, M., Grosse, B., Duchambon, P., and Drueke, T., A functional cell surface type receptor is required for the early action of 1,25-dihydroxyvitamin D_3 on the phosphoinositide metabolism in rat enterocytes, *J. Biol. Chem.*, 264, 20403, 1989.

65. Norman, A. W., Nemere, I., Shou, L., Bishop, J. E., Lowe, K. E., Maiyar, A. C., Collins, E. D., Taoka, T., Sergeev, I., and Farach-Carson, M. C., 1,25$(OH)_2$-vitamin D_3, a steroid hormone that produces biologic effects via both genomic and nongenomic pathways, *J. Steroid Biochem. Mol. Biol.*, 41(3-8), 231, 1992.

66. Bukoskit, R. D., Nue, H., and McCarron, D. M., Effect of 1,25$(OH)_2$ vitamin D_3 and ionized Ca^{2+} on ^{45}Ca uptake by primary cultures of aortic myocytes of spontaneously hypertensive and Wistar-Kyoto normotensive rats, *Biochem. Biophys. Res. Commun.*, 146, 1330, 1987.

67. Walter, M. R., Llenchuk, T., and Claycomb, W. C., 1-25-Dihydroxyvitamin D_3 stimulates ^{45}Ca uptake by cultured adult rat ventricular cardiac muscle cells, *J. Biol. Chem.*, 262, 2536, 1987.

68. Baran, D. T. and Kelly, A. W., Lysophosphatidylinositol: a potential mediator of 1,24-dihydroxyvitamin D-induced increments in hepatocyte cytosolic calcium, *Endocrinology*, 122, 930, 1988.

69. Bukoski, R. D., Wang, D., and Weyman, D. W., Injection of 1,25$(OH)_2$ vitamin D_3 enhances resistance artery contractile properties, *Hypertension*, 16, 523, 1990.

70. Inoue, Y., Oike, M., Nakao, K., Kitamura, K., and Kuriyama, H., Endothelin augments unitary calcium channel currents on the smooth muscle cell membrane of guinea-pig portal vein, *J. Physiol.*, 4, 423, 171, 1990.

71. Resnick, L. M., Shan, J., and Pang, P. K. T., unpublished data, 1993.

72. Ornoy, A., Goodwin, D., Noft, D., and Edelstein, S., 24,25-Dihydroxyvitamin D is a metabolite of vitamin D essential for bone formation, *Nature*, 276, 517, 1978.

73. Endo, H., Kiyoki, M., Kawashima, K., and Marnohi, T., Vitamin D_3 metabolites and PTH synergistically stimulate bone formation of chick embryonic femur *in vitro*, *Nature*, 286, 262, 1980.

74. Malluche, H. H., Henry, H., Meyer-Saballek, W., Sherman, S., Massry, S. G., and Norman, A. W., Effects and interactions of 24,25$(OH)_2D_3$ and 1,25$(OH)_2D_3$ on bone, *Am. J. Physiol.*, 238, E494, 1980.

75. Merke, J. and Norman, A. W., Evidence for 24(R)25$(OH)_2D_3$ receptor in the parathyroid gland of the rachitic chicken, *Biochem. Biophys. Res. Commun.*, 100, 551, 1981.

76. Corvol, M. M., Ulmann, A., and Garabedian, M., Specific nuclear uptake of 24,25 dihydroxy-cholecalciferol, a vitamin D_3 metabolite biological active in cartilage, *FEBS Lett.*, 116, 273, 1980.

77. Sömjen, D., Sömjen, G. J., Harell, A., Mechanic, G. L., and Binderman, I., Partial characterization of a specific high affinity binding macromolecule for 24R,25dihydroxyvitamin D_3 in differentiating skeletal mesenchyme, *Biochem. Biophys. Res. Commun.*, 106, 644, 1982.

78. Sömjen, D., Sömjen, G. J., Weisman, Y., and Binderman, I., Evidence for 24,25-dihydroxycholecalciferol receptors in long bones of newborn rats, *Biochem. J.*, 204, 31, 1982.

79. Caffrey, J. M. and Farach-Carson, M. C., Vitamin D_3 metabolites modulate dihydropyridine-sensitive calcium currents in clonal rat osteosarcoma cells, *J. Biol. Chem.*, 264, 20265, 1989.

80. Nakamura, T., Kurokawa, T., and Orimo, H., Increase of bone volume in vitamin D-repleted rats by massive adminstration of 24R, 25$(OH)_2D_3$, *Calcif. Tissue Int.*, 43, 235, 1988.

81. Shan, J. and Pang, P. K. T., unpublished data, 1993.

82. Shan, J. and Pang, P. K. T., unpublished data, 1993.

83. Eilam, Y., Szydel, N., and Harell, A., Effects of vitamin D_3 metabolites on cellular Ca^{2+} and on Ca transport in primary cultures of bone cells, *Mol. Cell. Endocrinol.*, 19, 263, 1980.

12

The Vasculature as an Insulin-Sensitive Tissue: Implications of Insulin and Insulin-Like Growth Factors in Hypertension, Diabetes, Atherosclerosis, and Arterial Smooth Muscle Growth

Paul R. Standley, Jeffrey L. Ram, and James R. Sowers

CONTENTS

I. INTRODUCTION

Hypertension and accelerated atherosclerosis are associated with both non-insulin-dependent diabetes (type II) and obesity.[1-16] Both type II diabetes and obesity are characterized by resistance to insulin-stimulated glucose disposal, which has also been observed in patients with essential hypertension.[17-21] The mechanisms responsible for the link found in the resistance to insulin-induced glucose disposal, hypertension, and accelerated atherosclerosis, although currently being explored in a number of laboratories, remain poorly understood. This chapter reviews current knowledge obtained from both basic and clinical experimentation which impacts on this important relationship.

II. HYPERINSULINEMIA/INSULIN RESISTANCE AND HYPERTENSION

Increased peripheral vascular resistance and vascular hyperreactivity occurs in insulin-resistant states.[2-4,21] It has been suggested that hyperinsulinemia associated with type II diabetes, obesity, and essential hypertension may cause hypertension through effects which increase sympathetic nervous system activity[22-24] and renal tubular sodium reabsorption.[25,26] The latter two insulin effects may contribute to the salt sensitivity reported in hyperinsulinemic states;[63,64] however, Hall et al.[29] observed that hyperinsulinemia induced in dogs by chronic insulin infusion did not cause hypertension despite salt retention. Acute insulin infusion in normal human volunteers that produced physiologic hyperinsulinemia decreased peripheral vascular resistance even though sympathetic nerve activity was increased.[30] Indeed, insulin administration causes hypotension in the absence of a compensatory rise in sympathetic nerve activity,[31] and glucose ingestion associated with accompanying hyperinsulinemia does not acutely cause hypertension despite its relatively acute or subacute effects which increase sympathetic nervous system activity and renal sodium retention. Nevertheless, prolonged hyperinsulinemia may contribute to the development of hypertension in type II diabetes, overtreated type I diabetes, and essential hypertension by promoting atherosclerosis, vascular remodeling, and other mechanisms that have not been investigated.[3] Finally, the vasodilatory effects of insulin may not exist in the above-tested insulin-resistant states, as recently noted.[33,34] In fact, insulin resistance may be characterized by paradoxical vasoconstrictive responses to physiological hyperinsulinemia.[35]

III. BASIC STUDIES OF EFFECTS OF INSULIN ON VASCULAR TONE

Studies conducted in recent years have demonstrated that insulin can alter vascular smooth muscle responsiveness to various vasoactive substances, an action that is complex and still not well understood. Indeed, *in vitro* insulin is capable of both attenuating[35-40] and accentuating[35,37,40-43] adrenergically mediated contractile responses of arterial tissue and does so in vessels of various calibers (aorta, coronary, mesenteric, and tail arteries and renal arterioles). Knowledge is sparse concerning factors that mediate such opposite ("vasodilator" vs. "vasoconstrictor") effects of insulin on arterial vasculature. Except for the fact that both effects require sufficient elapsed time (30 min to 2 h *in vitro*) apparently due to dependence on protein synthesis,[38,39,42] both can be demonstrated with either low (physiological) or high (pharmacological) effects of insulin.[35-44]

Several studies have shown that physiological concentrations of insulin induce vasodilation in dogs and humans;[29-32] however, the precise mechanism and site of action of insulin has not been delineated. Endothelial cells, interstitial cells, and neuron terminals, as well as vascular smooth muscle cells (VSMC), could be involved in the attenuation of contraction of insulin. Several studies[45,46] have sought to determine whether insulin inhibits agonist-induced contraction at the level of the individual VSMC. Using a single-cell video-morphometric technique, incubation of short-term cultured VSMC with high physiological doses (100 μU/ml) of insulin for 60 min significantly inhibited the contractile responses to pressor doses of vasopressin.[45] Using similar methodology, other investigators[46] have shown that incubation of VSMC with physiological concentrations of insulin (40 μU/ml) for 20 min significantly attenuated the contractile responses to angiotensin II and serotonin. In that study, insulin's attenuation of

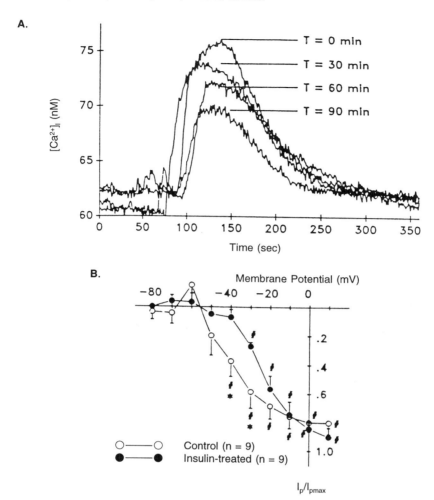

FIGURE 1 (A) Time course of the effect of insulin (100 μU/ml) on vasopressin (10 nM × 60 s) -induced rise in [Ca^{2+}]$_i$ in a7r5 VSMC. (B) Effects of insulin on voltage-dependent inward current. Graph illustrates summary of 18 cells (9 control, 9 treated 1.5 h with 100 μU/ml insulin) in which currents were normalized using individual cells' maximum elicited currents. * $p < 0.03$ ANOVA control vs. insulin treated. (From Standley, P. R. et al., *J. Clin. Invest.*, 88, 1230, 1991. With permission.)

agonist-induced contraction was not related to insulin-mediated glucose uptake because removal of glucose from the media did not alter the effect of insulin.[46] Insulin had no attenuating effect when contraction was induced by depolarization or when vasoactive hormone-induced contraction was studied in the presence of calcium channel antagonists and ouabain. These data are consistent with the notion that insulin decreases signal transduction by decreasing calcium (Ca^{2+}) influx across the VSMC membrane.[3]

IV. EFFECTS OF INSULIN ON CELLULAR CATION METABOLISM

A. Calcium

Insulin appears to exert important effects on VSMC intracellular Ca^{2+} levels ([Ca^{2+}]$_i$). Work conducted in our laboratory indicates that insulin attenuates VSMC Ca^{2+} influx by both receptor-mediated (e.g., vasopressin) and voltage-operated channels[47] (Figure 1). Hori et al.[48] have also demonstrated that insulin decreases VSMC [Ca^{2+}]$_i$ responses to vasoactive agonists by altering intracellular Ca^{2+} release and Ca^{2+} influx from the media. Insulin has been shown to stimulate Na^+,K^+-ATPase membrane pump activity,[49] and recent work from our laboratory demonstrated that insulin increases gene expression as well as activity of this membrane pump in cultured VSMC.[50] Insulin also has been demonstrated to be a regulator of the VSMC Ca^{2+}-ATPase pump;[3,4] regulation of this membrane pump is important in the sensitive (fine-tuning) process of modulating $[Ca^{2+}]_i$ levels. The cell membrane Na^+-H^+exchanger is also stimulated by physiological levels of insulin.[51] Thus, insulin can regulate cellular $[Ca^{2+}]_i$ and $[Na^+]_i$ concentrations by its multiple effects on cell membrane exchange systems (Figure 2).

In view of the role of insulin in modulating VSMC $[Ca^{2+}]_i$ metabolism and contractility, it is quite possible that the hypertension and increased vascular resistance seen in insulin-resistant and -deficient states may be related to decreased modulation by insulin of VSMC $[Ca^{2+}]_i$ metabolism[2-4] (Figure 2). In this regard, our investigative group has recently demonstrated that VSMC isolated from Zucker obese, insulin-resistant hypertensive rats have enhanced $[Ca^{2+}]_i$ responses to receptor-induced stimulation.[52] As the VSMC from Zucker obese rats did not differ from VSMC from lean littermates with respect to insulin or vasoactive agonist receptor properties, the conclusion was made that enhanced $[Ca^{2+}]_i$ responses represented a postreceptor abnormality. Furthermore, decreased activity of the Ca^{2+}-ATPase and Na^+,K^+-ATPase cell membrane pump has been associated with insulin-resistant obese states.[53-59] Decreased insulin action on VSMC may thus lead to reduced Na^+,K^+ and Ca^{2+}-ATPase activity and consequent elevations in $[Ca^{2+}]_i$, accounting for increased vascular resistance.

Insulin resistance may also indirectly cause altered cellular cation metabolism via associated hyperinsulinemia. The cell membrane Na^+-H^+ exchanger is stimulated by physiological levels of insulin.[51] Our investigative group has demonstrated increased sodium-lithium countertransport in insulin-resistant diabetic hypertensive blacks.[56] Canessa et al.[60] showed that young blacks with mild hypertension, hyperinsulinemia, and insulin resistance have elevated erythrocyte Na^+-H^+ exchange activity as compared to normotensive and hypertensive blacks without hyperinsulinemia and insulin resistance. The resultant increase in Na^+-H^+ exchange activity, along with decreased cellular Na^+,K^+-ATPase and Ca^{2+}-ATPase activity, could contribute to the increase in $[Ca^{2+}]_i$ and vascular resistance in insulin-resistant states of hypertension (Figure 2).

B. Role of Magnesium Deficiency

A number of studies suggest that individuals with hypertension and diabetes have extracellular[75] and intracellular[76-78] magnesium (Mg^{2+}) deficiency, as well as altered distributions of extracellular and intracellular Mg^{2+}.[77,78] These studies and other *in vitro* observations that Mg^{2+} deficiency can enhance vascular reactivity[79,80] suggest that Mg^{2+} deficiency may contribute to increased vascular tone associated with altered insulin action at the VSMC level. The mechanism by which reduced intracellular Mg^{2+} ($[Mg^{2+}]_i$) levels may account for this increased vascular reactivity is unclear, but likely involves an alteration in VSMC $[Ca^{2+}]_i$ metabolism. Mg^{2+} can decrease inward Ca^{2+} currents and reduce inositol phosphate generation,[81,82] both of which would result in decreased VSMC $[Ca^{2+}]_i$. Indeed, elevated $[Ca^{2+}]_i$ and suppressed $[Mg^{2+}]_i$ levels were observed together in patients having hypertension, diabetes, or both.

Insulin has been reported to increase the cellular uptake of Mg^{2+} in the erythrocyte.[83] In states of decreased cellular insulin action (types I and II diabetes mellitus), decreased insulin action might then account for reduced $[Mg^{2+}]_i$. Support for this notion is the observation of impaired erythrocyte magnesium uptake in type II diabetics.[87] Furthermore, both the impaired insulin-mediated Mg^{2+} uptake and the lower basal $[Mg^{2+}]_i$ values are closely related to the insulin resistance of essential hypertensives[76] and of type II diabetics.[84] Oral Mg^{2+} supplementation can improve insulin-mediated glucose metabolism as evidenced by significant reductions in glycosylated hemoglobin levels and improvement in enhanced platelet reactivity seen

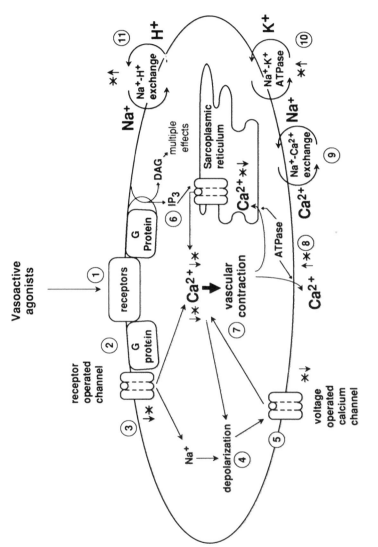

FIGURE 2   Schematic diagram depicting mechanisms regulating contraction in VSMC and proposed targets of insulin action. Pivotal steps in regulation of contraction are indicated by the circled numbers. (From Epstein, M. and Sowers, J. R., *Hypertension*, 19, 403, 1992. With permission.)

in type II diabetics.[77] Improved insulin secretion and improved insulin action following Mg^{2+} supplementation were also observed in another study.[85] Because enhanced platelet reactivity may contribute to thrombosis,[86] a primary Mg^{2+} deficiency could itself at least partially account for impaired insulin action and increased vascular disease associated with both diabetes and hypertension. According to this hypothesis, $[Mg^{2+}]_i$ deficiency could result in increased intracellular $[Ca^{2+}]_i$ levels,[78] which in turn would enhance vascular contractility, increase platelet reactivity, and impair cellular insulin action. All of these findings are characteristics of type II diabetes associated with hypertension and many individuals with essential hypertension.

V. GLUCOSE, INSULIN, AND VASCULAR TONE

Hyperglycemia, particularly postprandial, may exist in persons with obesity and essential hypertension, as well as in diabetic persons. Hyperglycemia in turn may contribute to the pathogenesis of hypertension. Glucose can be concentrated in the renal proximal tubule cells by an active process in which sodium and glucose cotransporters utilize the electrochemical potential of the sodium ion as an energy source.[71,72] Hyperglycemia results in hyperfiltration of glucose, which ultimately stimulates the proximal tubular sodium-glucose cotransporter.[72] This mechanism is insulin-independent and is rapidly operative, as evidenced by elevated proximal tubular cell sodium concentration and increased Na^+,K^+-ATPase activity within 4 d of inducing hyperglycemia in rats.[73] The resultant sodium retention caused by hypertension can explain the increased total exchangeable sodium seen in diabetic hypertensive patients.[2-4]

Chronic hyperglycemia may also contribute to hypertension via mechanisms related to hyperglycemia and atherosclerosis.[2-4] Toxic effects of elevated glucose may promote vascular endothelial dysfunction[2,4] which would then promote increased vascular tone. In addition, chronic hyperglycemia may contribute to vascular remodeling and rigidity and increased resistance by promoting vascular structural changes.[2-4] Recently it was shown that elevated glucose levels increase VSMC $[Ca^{2+}]_i$ and proliferation in cell culture.[74] This observation suggests that glucose has the potential to exert direct effects to increase vascular contraction and blood pressure.

Insulin resistance at the level of VSMC may play a role in the pathogenesis of hypertensive states such as type II diabetes, hypertension, obesity-related hypertension, and essential hypertension.[2-4] Insulin appears to have actions in VSMC similar to those in skeletal muscle tissue. Recent work in our laboratory has demonstrated that cultured VSMC display insulin-stimulated glucose transport (Figure 3).[61] We also demonstrated that VSMC cultured from an insulin-resistant hypertensive rat do not have altered insulin receptor functionality. Thus, if insulin-mediated action on the VSMC is decreased, it is likely that it represents a postreceptor phenomenon. In persons with essential hypertension, forearm skeletal muscle insulin resistance has been shown to be selective for nonoxidative glucose metabolism, likely related to impaired glucose conversion to glycogen.[62] Natali and co-workers suggested that this insulin resistance resulted from a postreceptor defect in insulin action.

Postbinding defects in insulin action may be associated with one or more important events mediating insulin stimulation of glucose transport. With insulin stimulation of fat and skeletal muscle cells, facilitative glucose transporters (specific integral membrane proteins) are translocated from an intracellular pool to the plasma membrane[62,63] where they help transfer glucose intracellularly via facilitated diffusion down a concentration gradient. Although the mechanisms involved in the translocation-activation of these transporters remain incompletely understood, insulin-receptor tyrosine kinase activation is necessary for insulin to stimulate glucose transport. Several insulin-resistant states are associated with a decrease in tyrosine kinase activity and an associated reduction in the number of glucose transporters translocated into the plasma membrane.[64-67]

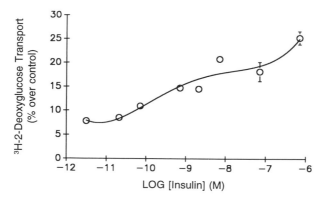

FIGURE 3 Effects of insulin on glucose transport in a7r5 VSMC. Insulin treatment (20 min) preceded addition of [³H]-2-deoxyglucose to confluent cultures of VSMC. Uptake was allowed to occur and cells were trypsinized, washed, and counted in a scintillation counter. All concentrations of insulin tested yielded statistically greater 2-deoxyglucose uptake vs. control. ($p < 0.05$, posthoc t-test.)

Preliminary data, using the insulin-resistant and hypertensive obese Zucker rat model, suggest a glucose transporter functional abnormality involving impaired translocation of transporters in skeletal muscle.[68] This abnormality may involve "docking" of vesicles at the plasma membrane so that they are physically juxtaposed but not fused, or partially fused, to the membrane. Partial fusion or altered configuration of transporters in the plasma membrane would render them cryptic, with inadequate exposure to the extracellular milieu, reduced activation of transporters, or increased inactivation of transporters.[64] Because guanosine triphosphate-binding proteins are involved in movement of the transporters to plasma membranes, altered function of these membrane-associated proteins, as occurs with aging, could help explain the glucose transport functional abnormalities that occur in skeletal muscle tissue. Although the insulin receptor B-subunit appears to be structurally unaltered in insulin-resistant states such as advanced age[67,69] and type II diabetes,[64,69] insulin-stimulated tyrosine kinase activity, as assessed by both autophosphorylation and phosphorylation of the synthetic substrate poly(Glu⁴-Tyr¹), is usually depressed.[63-71] It is quite possible that these glucose transport functional abnormalities may also be present in VSMC in insulin-resistant states such as obesity, type II diabetes mellitus, and essential hypertension. This is an extremely interesting investigative area for the next decade, particularly as it applies to mechanisms involved in the pathogenesis of hypertension associated with insulin-resistant states.

VI. INSULIN, INSULIN-LIKE GROWTH FACTORS, AND ATHEROSCLEROSIS

Growth of VSM may be stimulated by several circulating peptides, including insulin, insulin-like growth factors (IGF_1 and IGF_2), platelet-derived growth factors (PDGF), and epidermal growth factor (EGF).[2-4,87-93] Insulin may exert its atherogenic effects in part via its influence on both vascular endothelial and smooth muscle cells. Receptors for insulin are present on bovine endothelial cells cultured from pulmonary vessels (both arteries and veins), aorta, fat capillaries, and on human umbilical venous and arterial endothelium.[87,90,92] Some of these endothelial cells also bind IGF_1 and IGF_2 and multiplication-stimulating activity, a form of IGF_2.[95] It has been demonstrated that aortic endothelial cells take up and release insulin by transporting it across cells via an insulin receptor-mediated transport mechanism.[96] These studies have also demonstrated that aortic endothelium is capable of rapidly internalizing and releasing insulin with minimal degradation.[97] Similar experiments with IGF_2[98] have shown that there is greater channeling of IGF_2 than of insulin into a degradative (lysosomal) pathway within these cells. By employing the mechanism of differentially processing specific polypeptide hormones, endothelial cells modulate the delivery of circulating peptides to VSM tissue.

The hallmark of early atherosclerosis — smooth muscle hyperplasia in the arterial intima — is likely related to the responsiveness of smooth muscle cells to insulin and IGFs, because the mitogenic effects of the growth factors are additive at near-physiological concentrations.[99,100] High circulating levels of insulin, as exist with type II diabetes and essential hypertension and during aggressive insulin therapy for type I diabetes, may contribute directly or in conjunction with IGFs to the accelerated atherosclerosis associated with these conditions. Insulin in conjunction with IGFs also may be important to microvessel endothelial growth and repair mechanisms — processes very similar to those involved in the pathogenesis of atherosclerosis.[101]

A. Insulin as a Mitogenic Stimulus in Vascular Smooth Muscle Cells

Hyperplastic growth of VSMC is one mechanism by which the vasculature is remodeled in response to growth factors and injury. Insulin induces hyperplasia in several culture populations of VSMC. For example, bovine aortic VSMC grown in culture on an extracellular protein matrix (derived from bovine corneal endothelial cells) respond in a concentration-dependent manner to insulin treatment.[102] Maximal increase in cell number is achieved with 2500 ng/ml insulin, suggesting that at such supraphysiological insulin concentrations, the growth-promoting effects of insulin may be mediated in part by binding to IGF receptors (see below). King et al.[103] also demonstrated similar insulin-induced increases in calf aortic smooth muscle cell proliferation. In these studies, insulin at 10^{-7} and 10^{-6} M increased cellular hyperplasia by 30 to 50% over control media containing only 0.5% fetal calf serum after 3 to 6 d of hormone treatment. Additional work by Banskota et al.[87] showed that upon insulin receptor blockade [F(ab') fragments of the anti-insulin receptor antibody], insulin doubled the cell number of human renal artery VSMC. In contrast, upon IGF$_1$ receptor blockade (using antibody αIR$_3$) the effects of insulin on cellular hyperplasia were decreased by >90%, demonstrating that the growth-promoting effects of insulin are conferred via IGF membrane receptors.

A requisite step of the cell cycle prior to cytokinesis is passage of cells through the synthesis or S phase, during which DNA is synthesized. Many investigations focus on DNA synthesis when determining the temporal effects of various growth factors and differentiating between hyperplastic and hypertrophic growth responses. DNA synthesis is most commonly determined by measuring the rate of uptake of radiolabeled thymidine into cellular DNA during a 12 to 24 h "window" of time during growth factor additions to culture medium. Dose response studies conducted in our laboratory have demonstrated a peak stimulation of DNA synthesis in a7r5 VSMC at nonphysiological concentrations of insulin (Figure 4). Further, King et al.[103] reported that insulin ($1.7 \times 10^{-6} M$) increased by 240% ^{3}H-thymidine uptake in near-confluent calf aortic endothelial cells. Banskota et al.[87] demonstrated that maximal increase in thymidine incorporation in human arterial VSMC occurs at 1000 ng/ml insulin, a process which is effectively (90%) inhibited by IGF receptor blockade. Bornfeldt et al.[104] recently confirmed these insulin effects on thymidine incorporation in rat aortic VSMC, and further characterized the biologically active portion of insulin conferring those effects by demonstrating that an insulin analogue (made by replacing His 10 with Asp) was 100 times as potent as natant insulin in stimulating thymidine uptake in these cells. These authors suggest that the His $\rightarrow$ Asp alteration renders insulin more IGF$_1$-like, and the normal basic amino acid (His) of insulin is responsible for the decreased cellular actions of insulin as compared to IGF$_1$ and IGF$_2$.

The exact mechanism by which insulin stimulates cellular hyperplasia remains to be elucidated; however, a necessary first step in hyperplastic responses is induction of

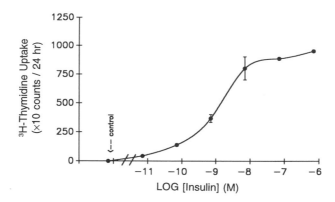

FIGURE 4   Effects of insulin on [^{3}H]-thymidine incorporation (a measure of DNA synthesis activity) in near-confluent cultures of a7r5 VSMC. Cells were treated with vehicle or indicated concentrations of insulin at the same time as [^{3}H]-thymidine addition. After 24 h, nuclear [^{3}H]-thymidine was assessed using scintillation counting.

protooncogenes such as c-*myc* and c-*fos*. Banskota et al.[105] demonstrated that insulin (1 × 10^{-7} *M*) and IGF$_1$ (1 × 10^{-9} *M*) both cause a five- to tenfold increase in c-*myc* RNA levels in human arterial smooth muscle cells. Surprisingly, these authors also demonstrated that, under conditions of selective IGF$_1$ receptor blockade (with antibody αIR$_3$), insulin stimulated c-*myc* RNA levels, but not DNA synthesis or cellular hyperplasia. These data suggest induction of c-*myc* does not entirely correlate with the growth effects of insulin or IGF$_1$.

In addition to proliferating, VSMC migrate from the media to the intima in the early stages of atherogenesis.[106] Although insulin itself does not induce VSMC migration, insulin does augment VSMC migration induced by 12-hydroxyeicosatetraenoic acid, a cellular chemotactic agent.[107] Thus, insulin may have yet another role in bringing about the rapid growth and migration of VSMC in diseased states such as hypertension and atherosclerosis.

A common finding of investigations dealing with insulin as a VSMC mitogen is that insulin interacts in a complex fashion with other growth factors to induce hyperplasia and DNA synthesis. For example, in some cells such as GH$_3$ pituitary cells and TM-4 Sertoli cells, the proliferative effects of insulin are seen only when IGF$_1$ is also present.[108,109] These data suggest that at least in some cells insulin and IGF$_1$ stimulate growth via different biochemical pathways. Similar data were obtained by Lonchampt et al.,[110] who showed that while endothelin-1 (ET-1) is capable of increasing VSMC thymidine incorporation, insulin (0.1 to 10 μg/ml) significantly enhances this effect. Similarly, arginine vasopressin-induced increases in thymidine incorporation in mesangial cells (smooth muscle-like cells) are greatly exaggerated by insulin treatment.[111] Further, in Swiss 3T3 cells, high insulin concentrations promote DNA synthesis, but in the presence of fibroblast growth factor (FGF), much lower concentrations of insulin (50 ng/ml) have similar mitogenic potency.[112,113] Similar data were reported for the synergistic effects of insulin with prostaglandin F$_{2α}$.[114] Thus, it is clear that insulin may be permissive for some growth factors in exerting their effects, while at the same time insulin can produce additive effects with other mitogens (Figure 5).

As detailed below, recent studies have demonstrated that VSMC produce and secrete IGF$_1$. An interesting set of studies points to insulin as a potent stimulator of VSMC IGF$_1$ production and secretion. Bornfeldt et al.[115] have shown that insulin (10 μ*M*) increases IGF$_1$ messenger RNA (mRNA) in rat aortic VSMC by some 46% after 3-h treatment. Interestingly, IGF$_1$ increased its own transcription by 65% in the same cells.[115] Whether insulin and IGF$_1$ promote these transcriptional events via binding to their own or each other's receptors remains to be elucidated.[116]

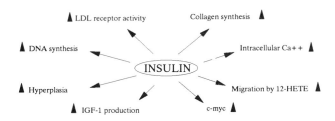

FIGURE 5   Growth-related effects of insulin in VSMC. Details regarding individual effects depicted are found in the text.

In addition to the aforementioned mitogenic properties, insulin regulates a number of other biochemical processes important in VSMC growth and formation of vascular lesions. Insulin is necessary for the production of experimental atherosclerosis in cholesterol-fed, alloxan diabetic rabbits. This finding may be a result of the ability of insulin to stimulate cholesterol synthesis and incorporation in cultured VSMC, and to enhance low-density lipoprotein (LDL) receptor activity in a number of cell types.[117] Further evidence suggesting a pivotal role for insulin in the development of atherosclerosis is that insulin (and IGF_1) directly exaggerate the production of collagen, a process that leads to decreased vessel distensibility and plaque formation[116] (see below). Finally, plaque formation and decreased plaque regression have correlated well with atherosclerosis.[116]

B.   Insulin-Like Growth Factor-1 as a Mitogenic Stimulus in Vascular Smooth Muscle Cells

For many years it was assumed that production of IGF_1 was limited to a few tissue types, most notably the liver.[118] In recent years, however, it has been shown that IGF_1 is produced and secreted by VSMC. Bornfeldt et al.[115] reported that IGF_1 stimulation of VSMC increases transcription of IGF_1 mRNA transcripts of 7.4, 1.7, and 0.8 to 1.1 kb in length by 50%. These data suggest that local production of IGF_1 in the vasculature is under autocrine/paracrine control and also may be involved in a positive feedback loop.

Insulin-like growth factor-1 is a potent mitogen for a variety of cell types,[119-123] including endothelial cells[102] and VSMC.[102,103,115,124,125] For example, IGF_1 stimulates VSMC hyperplasia by a pathway different than that shown for EGF and PDGF.[124] It is 10 to 100 times more potent in stimulating VSMC hyperplasia than insulin, causing *in vitro* cell doubling time to elapse in half the time demonstrated for insulin.[103] Human arterial smooth muscle cells also respond to IGF_1 in culture, a process almost completely dependent upon IGF_1 binding to its own receptor.[87]

As well as increasing hyperplasia, IGF_1 has been shown to increase thymidine incorporation in rat[115] and rabbit[125] aortic VSMC, a process that is greatly exaggerated in the presence of PDGF. Fibroblast growth factor-induced DNA synthesis is similarly amplified by treatment with IGF_1.[125] As with hyperplasia, the effects of IGF_1 on thymidine uptake is due to IGF_1 binding to its own receptor and not binding of the hormone to insulin receptors.[87] Thus, like insulin IGF_1 is an important modulator of vascular cell growth and remodeling,[126] but unlike insulin, the effects of IGF_1 are seen at physiological levels of the hormone and are mediated by its own receptor.

In addition to IGF_1, other factors modulate the local production, secretion, and binding of IGF_1 in VSMC. Injury (e.g., balloon angioplasty) increases IGF_1 production in porcine and rat aortic VSMC where an increase in IGF_1 receptors on VSMC precedes the induction of IGF_1

transcripts.[128,129] The finding that IGF_1 and its mRNA transcripts in VSMC derived from diabetic rats are altered suggest that local (smooth muscle cell) production of these factors is modulated by serum insulin, glucose levels, or both.[130] Angiopeptin and other analogues of somatostatin also decrease smooth muscle cell proliferation by decreasing smooth muscle cell-derived IGF_1.[131] The three growth factors, PDGF, EGF, and IGF_1, are additive in promoting DNA synthesis in porcine aortic cells, implying a complex interrelationship among the growth factors in α-granules of platelets on VSMC proliferation.

Other factors regulating smooth muscle cell-derived IGF_1 is smooth muscle cell-produced IGF binding proteins (IGFBPs).[132-134] Secretion of IGFBPs is increased by insulin,[135] demonstrating that insulin not only increases[130] but also decreases (via production of IGFBPs) IGF_1 effects at the level of VSMC. Giannella-Neto et al.[134] reported that PDGF decreases IGF_1 production in rat VSMC while concomitantly increasing production of IGFBP-4. It is suggested that these autocrine effects of IGF_1 are held in check by PDGF in order to limit the final magnitude of the PDGF response in smooth muscle cells.[134] Clearly, the effects of IGF_1 on VSMC growth are under multiple controls by a variety of locally produced growth factors and binding proteins.

Conflicting reports[136-139] were filed regarding the exact mechanism by which IGF_1 induces VSMC hyperplasia. Dempsey et al.[140] suggests that in neonatal pulmonary artery smooth muscle cells, IGF_1 stimulates hyperplasia via a protein kinase C (PKC) -independent pathway, although trace amounts of PKC activators are capable of synergistically augmenting this response. Additionally, it has been suggested that activation of c-*fos* (an early response gene as is c-*myc* described above) may be the initial trigger and final common pathway for both the PKC-dependent and -independent pathways leading to cellular hyperplasia.[136,141-142] It would not be surprising to find that the mechanisms underlying the insulin- and IGF_1-induced increases in VSMC growth were similar, because it is known that the actions of both hormones are mediated via a common receptor.[87,102,115]

C. Role of Calcium in Vascular Smooth Muscle Cell Mitogenesis

Buhler[143] depicts the current philosophy of using Ca^{2+} channel blockers in combating hypertension. It has been known for years that this class of drugs inhibits contraction of the vasculature by interrupting excitation-contraction coupling at the step of Ca^{2+} influx through plasma membrane calcium channels. Attenuation of vascular contraction is the primary mechanism by which Ca^{2+} channel blockers reduce vascular tone and thus blood pressure.[144] Many investigators have since shown that Ca^{2+} channel blockers such as nifedipine, diltiazem, and verapamil also decrease VSMC growth and proliferation. These culminated works suggest that Ca^{2+} is an important modulator of certain agonist-/growth factor-induced proliferation in these cells.

The Ca^{2+} antagonist, verapamil, inhibits proliferation of VSMC.[145,146] However, similar concentrations of this drug were shown to be without effect on basal thymidine incorporation, while they attenuate angiotensin II (AII) -induced increases in thymidine incorporation in smooth muscle cells.[34] Presumably, these antimitogenic effects of verapamil are a result of its ability to block voltage-mediated Ca^{2+} channels, but recent data from our laboratory suggests that this is not the case.[146] Using a7r5 aortic VSMC, we have shown that two enantiomers of verapamil, R+ and S−, equally inhibit VSMC hyperplasia (Figure 6). This is an interesting finding given that only the S−enantiomer is capable of blocking voltage-mediated Ca^{2+} currents.[146] These data suggest that, in the case of verapamil, there exists an antimitogenic property of this drug independent of its Ca^{2+} channel blocker properties. This notion is further supported by Kuriyama et al.,[145] who have demonstrated antimitogenic effects of verapamil, nifedipine, nicorandil, bunazocine, and labetalol. Because these drugs have presumably only

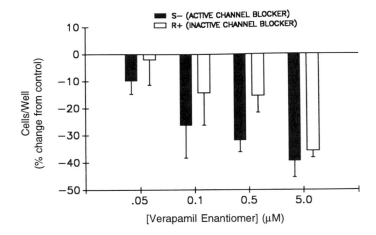

FIGURE 6   Effects of two verapamil enantiomers, S– and R+, on a7r5 VSMC proliferation. Data shown are cell numbers after 12 d of drug treatment, with refeeding of cells occurring every 48 h. Growth-inhibiting effects with both enantiomers were seen as early as 2 d into treatment.

an α-receptor antagonist property in common, the authors suggest that they act as proliferation inhibitors via this adrenergic receptor pathway, and that α-blockers may be useful in preventing hyperproliferation of VSMC commonly seen in the vascular walls of hypertensive patients. Further evidence that Ca^{2+} is involved in VSMC mitogenic responses comes from the similar work of Sato et al.[148] and Hirata et al.,[149] who demonstrated that other Ca^{2+} channel blockers such as nifedipine and diltiazem effectively inhibit DNA synthesis in these cells. Further, ET-1, a vasoconstrictor known to increase $[Ca^{2+}]_i$, induces DNA synthesis by a mechanism blockable by nifedipine.[149]

As stated previously, induction of the so-called mitogenic/early response protooncogenes such as c-*fos*, c-*myc*, and c-*jun* is a necessary first event in the proliferative responses in VSMC.[150] Vascular mitogens such as AII and ET-1 have been shown to increase transcription of these and other protooncogenes.[151,152] The fact that both of these vasoconstrictors/mitogens dramatically increases $[Ca^{2+}]_i$ suggests that a rise in $[Ca^{2+}]_i$ is a requisite step in inducing transcription of these genes. Further, induction of these genes can be achieved by treatment of VSMC with the Ca^{2+} ionophore A23187. These data suggest that any vasoconstrictor that increases $[Ca^{2+}]_i$ can increase oncogene transcription and consequent hyperplasia. This notion, however, is not supported by other works. For example, Hirosumi et al.[124] demonstrated that while an EGF-induced increase in VSMC proliferation depends upon a transient increase in $[Ca^{2+}]_i$, IGF_1-induced proliferation is not dependent on such calcium movement. Further, Parrott et al.[153] reported that while 5-hydroxytryptamine (5-HT) and AII increase phosphoinositol turnover and mobilize $[Ca^{2+}]_i$, only 5-HT increased DNA synthesis in porcine aortic VSMC grown in a serum-free medium. The latter two studies suggest that phosphoinositol turnover and increases in $[Ca^{2+}]_i$ are not sufficient to stimulate VSMC mitogenesis. Possible differences in VSMC mitogenic responses among growth factors/vasoconstrictors may be due to the stimulation of cytokines which may activate or potentiate transcriptional events necessary for mitogenesis.[154]

ACKNOWLEDGMENTS

We wish to thank Paddy Gavric for her excellent work in preparing this review chapter. Work supported by Grants HD24497 and VA Merit Review Grant 15E.

REFERENCES

1. Reaven, G. M. and Hoffman, B. B., Hypertension as a disease of carbohydrate and lipoprotein metabolism, *Am. J. Med.*, 87(Suppl. 6A), 2S, 1989.
2. Flack, J. M. and Sowers, J. R., Epidemiologic and clinical aspects of insulin resistance and hyperinsulinemia, *Am. J. Med.*, 91(Suppl. 1A), 11S, 1991.
3. Sowers, J. R., Standley, P. R., Ram, J. L., Zemel, M. B., and Resnick, L. M., Insulin resistance carbohydrate metabolism and hypertension, *Am. J. Hypertens.*, 4, 466S, 1991.
4. Epstein, M. and Sowers, J. R., Diabetes mellitus and hypertension, *Hypertension*, 19, 403, 1992.
5. Kaplan, N. M., The deadly quartet: upper body obesity, glucose intolerance, hypertriglyceridemia and hypertension, *Arch. Intern. Med.*, 149, 1514, 1989.
6. Julius, S., Jamerson, K., Mejia, A., Krause, L., Schork, N., and Jones, K., The association of borderline hypertension with target organ changes and higher coronary risk: Tecumseh Blood Pressure Study, *JAMA*, 264, 354, 1990.
7. Ruderman, N. B. and Haudenschild, C., Diabetes as an atherogenic factor, *Prog. Cardiovasc. Dis.*, 26(5), 373, 1984.
8. Butler, W. J., Ostrander, L. D., Jr., Carman, W. J., and Lamphiear, D. E., Mortality from coronary heart disease in the Tecumseh study. Long-term effect of diabetes mellitus, glucose tolerance and other risk factors, *Am. J. Epidemiol.*, 121, 541, 1985.
9. Pan, W. H., Cedes, L. B., Liu, K., Dyer, A., Schoenberger, J. A., Shekelle, R. B., Stamler, J. et al., Relationship of clinical diabetes and a symptomatic hyperglycemia to coronary heart disease mortality in men and women, *Am. J. Epidemiol.*, 123, 504, 1986.
10. Abbott, R. D., Donahue, R. P., MacMahon, S. W., Reed, D. M., and Yano, K., Diabetes and the risk of stroke. The Honolulu heart program, *JAMA*, 257, 949, 1987.
11. Pyoralu, K., Laakso, M., and Uusitupa, M., Diabetes and atherosclerosis: an epidemiologic view, *Diabetes/Metab. Rev.*, 3, 463, 1987.
12. Cambien, F., Warne, J. M., Eschwiege, E., Jecqueson, A., Richard, J. L., and Rosselin, G., Body mass, blood pressure, glucose, and lipids: does plasma insulin explain their relationship?, *Arteriosclerosis*, 7, 197, 1987.
13. Modan, M., Halkin, H., Almog, S., Lusky, A. L., Eshkol, A., Shefi, M., Shitrit, A., and Fuchs, Z., Hyperinsulinemia: a link between hypertension, obesity and glucose intolerance, *J. Clin. Invest.*, 75, 809, 1985.
14. Haffner, S. M., Stern, M. P., Hazuda, H. P., Mitchell, B. D., and Patterson, J. K., Cardiovascular risk factors in confirmed prediabetic individuals: does the clock for coronary heart disease start ticking before the onset of clinical diabetes?, *JAMA*, 263, 2893, 1990.
15. Stolar, M. W., Atherosclerosis in diabetes: the role of hyperinsulinemia, *Metabolism*, 37, 1, 1988.
16. Zavaroni, I., Bonora, E., Pagliara, M., Dall'Aglio, E., Luchetti, L., Buonanno, G., Bonati, P. A., Bergonzani, M., Gnudi, L., Passeri, M., and Reaven, G., Risk factors for coronary artery disease in healthy persons with hyperinsulinemia and normal glucose tolerance, *N. Engl. J. Med.*, 320, 702, 1989.
17. Ferrannini, E., Buzzigoli, G., Bonadonna, R., Giorico, M. A., Oleggini, M., Graziadei, L., Pedrinelli, R., Brandi, L., and Bevilacqua, S., Insulin resistance in essential hypertension, *N. Engl. J. Med.*, 317, 350, 1987.
18. Swislocki, A. L. M., Hoffman, B. B., and Reaven, G. M., Insulin resistance, glucose intolerance and hyperinsulinemia in patients with hypertension, *Am. J. Hypertens.*, 2, 419, 1989.
19. Manolio, T. A., Savage, P. J., Burke, G. L., Liu, K. A., Wagenknecht, L. E., Sidney, S., Jacobs, D. R., Roseman, J. M., Donahue, R. P., and Oberman, A., Association of fasting insulin with blood pressure and lipids in young adults: the Cardia study, *Arteriosclerosis*, 10, 430, 1990.
20. Pollare, T., Lithell, H., and Berne, C., Insulin resistance is a characteristic feature of primary hypertension independent of obesity, *Metabolism*, 39, 167, 1990.
21. Sowers, J. R., Relationship between hypertension and subtle and overt abnormalities of carbohydrate metabolism, *J. Am. Soc. Nephrol.*, 1, 539, 1990.
22. Landsberg, L. and Young, J. B., Insulin-mediated glucose metabolism in relationship between dietary intake and sympathetic nervous system activity, *Int. J. Obesity*, 9, 63, 1985.

23. Hwang, I. S., Ho, H., Hoffman, B. B., and Reaven, G. M., Fructose-induced insulin resistance and hypertension in rats, *Hypertension*, 10, 512, 1987.

24. Berne, C., Fagius, J., and Niklasson, F., Sympathetic response to oral carbohydrate administration. Evidence from microelectrode nerve recordings, *J. Clin. Invest.*, 84, 1403, 1989.

25. DeFronzo, R. A., Cooke, C. R., Andres, R., Faloona, G. R., and Davis, P. J., The effect of insulin on renal handling of sodium, potassium, calcium and phosphate in man, *J. Clin. Invest.*, 55, 845, 1975.

26. Baum, M., Insulin stimulates volume absorption in the rabbit proximal convoluted tubule, *J. Clin. Invest.*, 79, 1104, 1987.

27. Rocchini, A. P., Katch, V., Kveselis, D., Moorehead, C., Martin, M., Lampman, R., and Gregory, M., Insulin and renal sodium retention in obese adolescents, *Hypertension*, 14, 367, 1989.

28. Rocchini, A. P., Key, J., Bondie, D., Chico, C., Moorehead, C., Katch, V., and Martin, M., The effect of weight loss on the sensitivity of blood pressure to sodium in obese adolescents, *N. Engl. J. Med.*, 321(Suppl. 9), 580, 1989.

29. Hall, J. E., Coleman, T. G., and Mizelle, H. L., Does chronic hyperinsulinemia cause hypertension?, *Am. J. Hypertens.*, 2, 171, 1989.

30. Anderson, E. A., Hoffman, R. P., Balon, T. W., Sinkey, C. A., and Mark, A. L., Hyperinsulinemia produces both sympathetic neural activation and vasodilation in normal humans, *J. Clin. Invest.*, 87, 2246, 1991.

31. Mathias, C. J., da Costa, D. F., Fosbraey, P., Christensen, N. J., and Bannister, R., Hypotensive and sedative effects of insulin in autonomic failure, *Br. Med. J.*, 295, 161, 1987.

32. Jansen, R., Penterman, B., Van Lier, H. J., and Hoenagels, W. H., Blood pressure reduction after oral glucose loading and its relation to age, blood pressure and insulin, *Am. J. Cardiol.*, 60, 1087, 1987.

33. Laakso, M., Edelman, S. V., Brechtel, G., and Baron, A. D., Decreased effect of insulin to stimulate skeletal muscle blood flow in obese man, *J. Clin. Invest.*, 85, 1844, 1990.

34. Doria, A., Fioretti, P., Avogaro, A., Carraro, A. et al., Insulin resistance is associated with high sodium-lithium countertransport in essential hypertension, *Am. J. Physiol.*, 261, E684, 1991.

35. Peuler, J. D., Johnson, B. A., Phare, S. M., and Sowers, J. R., Sex-specific effects of an insulin secretogogue in stroke-prone hypertensive rats, *Hypertension*, 22, 214, 1993.

36. Sowers, J. R., Khoury, S., Standley, P., and Zemel, P., Zemel, M. B., Mechanisms of hypertension in diabetes, *Am. J. Hypertens.*, 4, 177, 1991.

37. Alexander, W. D. and Oake, R. J., The effect of insulin on vascular reactivity to norepinephrine, *Diabetes*, 26, 611, 1977.

38. Zemel, M. B., Reddy, S., Shehin, S. E., Lockette, W., and Sowers, J. R., Vascular reactivity in Zucker obese rats: role of insulin resistance, *J. Vasc. Med. Biol.*, 2, 82, 1990.

39. Zemel, M. B., Reddy, S., and Sowers, J. R., Insulin attenuation of vasoconstrictor responses to phenylephrine in Zucker lean and obese rats, *Am. J. Hypertens.*, 4, 537, 1991.

40. Juncos, L. A., Ito, S., and Carretero, O. A., Disparate effects of insulin on isolated rabbit afferent (Af-Art) and efferent arterioles (Ef-Art), *Hypertension*, 20(Abstr.), 403, 1992.

41. Yanagisawa-Miwa, A., Ito, H., and Sugimoto, T., Effects of insulin on vasoconstriction induced by thromboxane A_2 in porcine coronary artery, *Circulation*, 81, 1654, 1990.

42. Barber, D. A. and Tackett, R. L., Insulin enhances vasoreactivity by a mechanism dependent on protein synthesis in vasoconstrictor but not vasorelaxant responses, *FASEB J.*, 6(Abstr.), A970, 1992.

43. Townsend, R. R., Yamamoto, R., Nickols, M., DiPette, D. J., and Nickols, G. A., Insulin enhances pressor responses to norepinephrine in rat mesenteric vasculature, *Hypertension*, 19(Suppl. II), 105, 1992.

44. Chan, T. M., Hsueh, W. A., and Wu, H. Y., Insulin and insulin-like growth factor-1 enhance agonist-induced vasocontraction, *Hypertension*, 20(Abstr.), 421, 1992.

45. Ram, J. L., Fares, M. A., Standley, P. R., Therrell, L. L., Thyagaranjan, R. V., and Sowers, J. R., Insulin inhibits vasopressin-elicited contraction of vascular smooth muscle cells, *J. Vasc. Med. Biol.*, 4, 250, 1993.

46. Kahn, A. M., Seidel, C. L., Allen, J. C., O'Neil, R. G., Shelat, H., and Song, T., Physiological insulin concentration inhibits the agonist-induced intracellular Ca^{2+} transient and contraction of individual VSM cells, *Hypertension*, 22, 735, 1993.

47. Standley, P. R., Zhang, F., Ram, J. L., Zemel, M. B., and Sowers, J. R., Insulin attenuates vasopressin-induced calcium transients and a voltage dependent calcium response in rat vascular smooth muscle cells, *J. Clin. Invest.*, 88, 1230, 1991.
48. Hori, M. T., Fittinghof, M., and Tuck, M. L., Insulin attenuates angiotensin II-mediated calcium mobilization in cultured rat vascular smooth muscle by depletion of intracellular calcium stores, *Clin. Res.*, 39, 270A, 1991.
49. Lytton, J., Lin, J. C., and Guidotti, G., Identification of two molecular forms of (Na$^+$ + K$^+$)-ATPase in rat adipocytes: relation to insulin stimulation of the enzyme, *J. Biol. Chem.*, 260, 1177, 1985.
50. Tirupattur, P. R., Ram, J. L., Standley, P. R., and Sowers, J. R., Modulation of alpha-2 isoform of the Na$^+$, K$^+$ - ATPase gene expression by insulin in vascular smooth cells, *Am. J. Hypertens.*, 6, 626, 1993.
51. Moore, R. D., Stimulation of Na:H exchange by insulin, *Biophys. J.*, 33, 203, 1981.
52. Standley, P. R., Ram, J. L., and Sowers, J. R., Insulin attenuation of vasopressin-induced calcium responses in arterial smooth muscle from Zucker rats, *Endocrinology,* 133, 1693, 1993.
53. Levy, J., Zemel, M. B., and Sowers, J. R., Role of cellular calcium metabolism in abnormal glucose metabolism and diabetic hypertension, *Am. J. Med.*, 87(Suppl. 6A), 7, 1989.
54. Wong, E. C., Sacks, D. B., Laurino, J. P., and McDonald, J. M., Characteristics of calmodulin phosphorylation by the insulin receptor kinase, *Endocrinology*, 123, 1830, 1988.
55. Levy, J., Sowers, J. R., and Zemel, M. B., Abnormal Ca^{2+}-ATPase activity in erythrocytes of non-insulin dependent diabetic rats, *Horm. Metab. Res.*, 22, 136, 1990.
56. Johnson, B. A., Sowers, J. R., Zemel, P., Luft, F. C., and Zemel, M. B., Increased sodium-lithium countertransport in black non-insulin dependent diabetic hypertensives, *Am. J. Hypertens.*, 3, 563, 1990.
57. Levy, J., Avioli, L. V., Roberts, M. L., and Gavin, J. R., III, (Na$^+$ + K$^+$)-ATPase activity in kidney basolateral membranes of non-insulin-dependent diabetic rats, *Biochem. Biophys. Res. Commun.*, 139, 1313, 1986.
58. De Luise, M., Blackburn, G. L., and Flier, J. S., Reduced activity of red-cell sodium-potassium pump in human obesity, *N. Engl. J. Med.*, 303, 1017, 1980.
59. Sowers, J. R., Whitfield, L. A., Beck, F. et al., Role of enhanced sympathetic nervous system activity and reduced Na$^+$ + K$^+$-dependent adenosine triphosphatase activity in the maintenance of elevated blood pressure in obesity; effects of weight loss, *Clin. Sci.,* 63, 1215, 1982.
60. Canessa, M., Falkner, B., and Hulman S., Red blood cell NaH exchanger (EXC) activity is elevated in young hypertensive blacks, *Hypertension*, 18(Abstr.), 378, 1991.
61. Standley, P. R., Rose, K., Tirupattur, P. R., and Sowers, J. R., Insulin stimulated glucose transport in vascular smooth muscle cells: possible implications of GLUT-4 in the vasculature, *Physiologist*, 35, A13, 1992.
62. Natali, A., Santoro, D., and Palombo, C., Impaired insulin action on skeletal muscle metabolism in essential hypertension, *Hypertension*, 17, 170, 1991.
63. Caro, J., Sinha, M. K., Raju, S. M. et al., Insulin receptor kinase in human skeletal muscle from obese subjects with and without noninsulin dependent diabetes, *J. Clin. Invest.*, 79, 1330, 1987.
64. Kahn, B. B., Facilitative glucose transporters: regulatory mechanisms and dysregulation in diabetes, *J. Clin. Invest.*, 89, 1367, 1992.
65. Klip, A. and Douen, A. G., Role of kinases in insulin stimulation of glucose transport, *J. Membr. Biol.*, 111, 1, 1989.
66. Obermaier-Kusser, B., White, M. F., Pongratz, D. E., Su, Z., Ermel, B., Muhlbacher, C., and Haring, H. U., A defective intramolecular autoactivation cascade may cause the reduced kinase activity of the skeletal muscle insulin receptor from patients with non-insulin dependent diabetes mellitus, *J. Biol. Chem.*, 264, 9497, 1989.
67. Barnard, R. J., Lawani, L. O., Martin, D. A., Youngren, J. F., Singh, R., and Scheck, S. H., Effects of maturation and aging on the skeletal muscle glucose transport system, *Am. J. Physiol.*, 262, 619, 1992.
68. Horton, E. D., King, P. A., Hirshman, M. F., and Horton, E. S., Failure of insulin to stimulate glucose transporter translocation in skeletal muscle from obese (fa/fa) Zucker rat, *Diabetes*, 39, 83A, 1990.

69. Kono, S., Kuzuya, H., Okamoto, M., Nishimura, H., Kosaki, A., Kakehi, T., Okamoto, M., Inoue, G., Maeda, I., and Imura, H., Changes in insulin receptor kinase with aging in rat skeletal muscle and liver, *Am. J. Physiol.*, 259, 27, 1990.

70. Scheck, S. H., Barnard, R. J., Lawani, L. O., Youngren, J. F., Martin, D. A., and Singh, R., Effects of NIDDM on the glucose transport system in human skeletal muscle, *Diabetes Res.*, 16, 111, 1991.

71. Wright, E. M., Turk, E., Zabel, B., Mundlos, S., and Dyer, J., Molecular genetics of intestinal glucose transport, *J. Clin. Invest.*, 88, 1435, 1991.

72. Harris, R. C., Brenner, B. M., and Seifter, J. L., Sodium-hydrogen exchange and glucose transport in renal microvillus membrane vesicles from rats with diabetes mellitus, *J. Clin. Invest.*, 77, 724, 1986.

73. Kumar, A. M., Gupta, R. K., and Spitzer, A., Intracellular sodium in proximal tubules of diabetic rats. Role of glucose, *Kidney Int.*, 33, 792, 1988.

74. Koibuchi, Y., Lee, W. S., and Pratt, R. E., Glucose directly stimulates the growth of vascular smooth muscle cells in culture, *Hypertension*, 6(Suppl. 4) (Abstr.), 10, 1992.

75. Gunn, I. and Burns, E., Plasma ultrafiltrable magnesium in insulin dependent diabetes, *J. Clin. Pathol.*, 40, 294, 1987.

76. Resnick, L. M., Gupta, R. K., Gruenspan, H., Alderman, M. H., and Laragh, J. H., Hypertension and peripheral insulin resistance: possible mediating role of intracellular free magnesium, *Am. J. Hypertens.*, 3, 373, 1990.

77. Nadler, J., Malayan, S., Luong, H., Shaw, S., Natarajan, R., and Rude, R., Intracellular free magnesium deficiency plays a role in increased platelet reactivity in type II diabetes mellitus, *Diabetes Care*, 15, 835, 1992.

78. Resnick, L. M., Laragh, J. H., Sealey, J. E., and Alderman, M. H., Divalent cations in essential hypertension. Relations between serum ionized calcium, magnesium, and plasma renin activity, *N. Engl. J. Med.*, 309, 888, 1983.

79. Altura, B. M. and Altura, B. T., New perspectives on the role of magnesium in the pathophysiology of the cardiovascular system. II. Experimental aspects, *Magnesium*, 4, 245, 1985.

80. Rude, R., Manoogian, C., Ehrlich, L., DeRusso, P., Ryzen, E., and Nadler, J., Mechanisms of blood pressure regulation by magnesium in man, *Magnesium*, 8, 266, 1989.

81. White, R. E. and Hartzell, H. C., Effects of intracellular free magnesium on calcium current in isolated cardiac myocytes, *Science*, 239, 778, 1988.

82. Roth, B. L., Modulation of phosphatidylinositol-4-5-biphosphate hydrolysis in rat aorta by guanidine nucleotide, calcium and magnesium, *Life Sci.*, 41, 629, 1987.

83. Paolisso, G., Sgambato, S., Passarriello, B., Giugliano, D., Scheen, A., D'Onofrio, F., and Lefebvre, P. J., Insulin induces opposite changes in plasma and erythrocyte magnesium concentrations in normal man, *Diabetologia*, 29, 644, 1986.

84. Paolisso, G., Sgambato, S., Giugliano D., Torella, R., Varricchio, M., Scheen, A. J., D'Onofrio, F., and Lefebvre, P. J., Impaired insulin-induced erythrocyte magnesium accumulation is correlated to impaired insulin, insulin mediated glucose disposal in type 2 (non-insulin-dependent) diabetic patients, *Diabetologia*, 31, 910, 1988.

85. Paolisso, G., Sgambato, S., Pizza, G., Passariello, N., Varricchio, M., and D'Onofrio, F., Improved insulin response and action by chronic magnesium administration in aged NIDDM subjects, *Diabetes Care*, 12, 265, 1989.

86. Colwell, J., Winocur, P., and Halushka, P., Do platelets have anything to do with diabetic microvascular disease?, *Diabetes*, 32, 14, 1983.

87. Banskota, N. K., Taub, R., Zellner, K., Olsen, P., and King, G. L., Characterization of induction of protooncogene c-*myc* and cellular growth in human cellular smooth muscle cells by insulin and IGF-1, *Diabetes*, 38, 123, 1989.

88. Berk, B. C., Brock, T. A., Webb, R. C., Taubman, M. B., Atkinson, W. J., Gimbrone, M. A., and Alexander, R. W., Epidermal growth factor, a vascular smooth muscle mitogen, induces rat aortic contraction, *J. Clin. Invest.*, 75, 1083, 1985.

89. Pfeifle, B. and Ditschuneit, H., Effect of insulin on growth of cultured human arterial smooth muscle cells, *Diabetologia*, 20, 155, 1981.

90. Pfeifle, B. and Ditschuneit, H., Two separate receptors for insulin and insulin-like growth factors on arterial smooth muscle cells, *Exp. Clin. Endocrinol.*, 81, 280, 1983.

91. Reilly, C. F., Fritze, L. M. S., and Rosenberg, R. D., Antiproliferative effects of heparin on vascular smooth muscle cells are reversed by epidermal growth factor, *J. Cell Physiol.*, 131, 149, 1987.

92. Scott-Burden, T., Resink, T. J., Baur, I., Burgin, M., and Buhler, F. R., Epidermal growth factor responsiveness in smooth muscle cells from hypertensive and normotensive rats, *Hypertension*, 13, 295, 1989.

93. Weinstein, R., Stemerman, M. B., and Maciag, T., Hormonal requirements for growth of arterial smooth muscle cells in vitro: an endocrine approach to atherosclerosis, *Science*, 212, 818, 1981.

94. Bark, R. S. and Boes M., Distinct receptors for IGF-I, IGF-II, and insulin are present on bovine capillary endothelial cells and large vessel endothelial cells, *Biochem. Biophys. Res. Commun.*, 124, 203, 1984.

95. King, G. L., Kahn, C. R., Rechler, M. M., and Nissley, S. P., Direct demonstration of separate receptors for growth and metabolic activities, of insulin and multiplication stimulating activity (an insulin-like growth factor) using antibodies to the insulin receptor, *J. Clin. Invest.*, 66, 130, 1980.

96. King, G. L. and Johnson, S. M., Receptor-mediated transport of insulin across endothelial cells, *Science*, 227, 1583, 1985.

97. Jialal, I., King, G. L., Buckwald, S. et al., Processing of insulin by bovine endothelial cells in culture. Internalization without degradation, *Diabetes*, 33, 794, 1984.

98. Hachiya, H. L., Carpentier, J. L., and King, G. L., Comparative studies on insulin-like growth factor II and insulin processing by vascular endothelial cells, *Diabetes*, 35, 1065, 1986.

99. Rechler, M. M., Podskalny, J. M., Goldfine, I. D., and Wells, C. A., DNA synthesis in human fibroblasts: stimulation by insulin and by nonsuppressible insulin-like activity (NSILA-S), *J. Clin. Endocrinol. Metab.*, 39, 512, 1974.

100. King, G. L., Buzney, S. M., Kahn, C. R., Hetu, N., Buchwald, S., Macdonald, S. G., and Rand, L. I., Differential responsiveness to insulin of endothelial and support cells from micro- and macrovessels, *J. Clin. Invest.*, 71, 974, 1983.

101. Vinters, H. V. and Berliner, J. A., The blood vessel as an insulin target issue, *Diabetic Metab.*, 13, 294, 1987.

102. Gospodarowicz, D., Herabayashi, K., Giguere, L., and Tauber, J. P., Factors controlling the proliferative rate, final cell density, and life span of bovine vascular smooth muscle cells in culture, *J. Cell Biol.*, 89, 568, 1981.

103. King, G. L., Goodman, A. D., Buzney, S., Moses, A., and Kahn, C. R., Receptors and growth promoting effects of insulin and insulin-like growth factors on cells from bovine retinal capillaries and aorta, *J. Clin. Invest.*, 75, 1028, 1985.

104. Bornfeldt, E., Gidlof, R. A., Wasterson, A., Skottner, A., and Arnqvist, A. J., Binding and biological effects of insulin, insulin analogues and insulin-like growth factors in rat aortic smooth muscle cells. Comparison of maximal growth promoting activities, *Diabetologia*, 34, 307, 1991.

105. Banskota, N. K., Taub, R., Zellner, K., and King, G. L., Insulin, insulin-like growth factor 1 and platelet-derived growth factor interact additively in the induction of the protooncogene c-*myc* and cellular proliferation in cultured bovine aortic smooth muscle cells, *Mol. Endocrinol.*, 3, 1183, 1989.

106. Stout, R. W., Insulin as a mitogenic factor: role in the pathogenesis of cardiovascular disease, *Am. J. Med.*, 90(Suppl. 2A), 62S, 1991.

107. Nakao, J., Ito, H., Kanayasu, T., and Murota S. I., Stimulatory effect of insulin on aortic smooth muscle migration induced by 12-L-hydroxy-5,8,10,14-eicosatetraenoic acid and its modulation by elevated extracellular glucose levels, *Diabetes*, 34, 185, 1985.

108. Barnes, D. and Sato, G., Methods for growth of cultured cells in serum-free medium, *Anal. Biochem.*, 102, 255, 1980.

109. Hayashi, I., Larner, J., and Sato, G., Hormonal growth control of cells in culture, *In Vitro*, 14, 23, 1978.

110. Lonchampt, M. O., Pinelis, S., Goulin, J., Chabrier, P. E., and Braquet, P., Proliferation and Na$^+$/H$^+$ exchange activation by endothelin in vascular smooth muscle cells, *Am. J. Hypertens.*, 4, 776, 1991.

111. Ganz, M. B., Pekar, S. K., Perfetto, M. C., and Sterazal, R. B., Arginine vasopressin promotes growth of rat glomerular mesangial cells in culture, *Am. J. Physiol.*, 255, F898, 1988.

112. Holley, R. W. and Kiernan, J. A., Control of the initiation of DNA synthesis in 3T3 cells: low molecular weight nutrients, *Proc. Natl. Acad. Sci. U.S.A.*, 71, 2908, 1974.

113. Jimenez de Asua, L., Clingan, D., and Rudland, P. S., Initiation of cell proliferation in cultured mouse fibroblasts by prostaglandin F2 alpha, *Proc. Natl. Acad. Sci. U.S.A.*, 72, 2724, 1975.

114. Smith, J. A. and Martin, L., Do cells cycle?, *Proc. Natl. Acad. Sci. U.S.A.*, 70, 1263, 1973.

115. Bornfeldt, K. E., Arnqvist, H. J., and Norstedt, G., Regulation of insulin-like growth factor-I gene expression by growth factors in cultured vascular smooth muscle cells, *J. Endocrinol.*, 125, 381, 1990.

116. DeFronzo, R. A. and Ferraninni, E., Insulin resistance; a multifaceted syndrome responsible for NIDDM, obesity, hypertension, dyslipidemia, and atherosclerotic cardiovascular disease, *Diabetes Care*, 14, 173, 1991.

117. Standl, E., Clinical sequelae of hyperinsulinemia in diabetes mellitus, *Klin. Wochenschr.*, 69(Suppl. 29), 63, 1992.

118. Froesch, E. R., Schmid, S., Schwander, J., and Zapf, J., Actions of insulin-like growth factors, *Annu. Rev. Physiol.*, 47, 443, 1985.

119. Barnes, D. and Sato, G., Serum-free cell culture: a unifying approach, *Cell*, 22, 649, 1980.

120. Bottenstein, J., Hayashi, I., Hutchings, S., Masui, H., Mather, J., McClure, D. B., Sugayuki, O., Rizzino, A., Sato, G., Serrero, G., Wolfe, R., and Wu, R., The growth of cells in serum-free hormone-supplemented media, *Methods Enzymol.*, 58, 94, 1979.

121. Gospodarowicz, D., Mescher, A., and Birdwell, C. R., Control of cellular proliferation by fibroblast and epidermal growth factors in gene expression and regulation in cultured cells, *NCI Monogr.*, 48, 109, 1978.

122. Gospodarowicz, D., Moran, J., and Braun, D., Control of proliferation of bovine vascular endothelial cells, *J. Cell. Physiol.*, 91, 377, 1977.

123. Sato, G. and Reid, L., Replacement of serum in cell cultures by hormones, *Int. Rev. Biochem.*, 20, 219, 1978.

124. Hirosumi, J., Ouchi, Y., Wantabe, M., Kusunoki, J., Nakamura, T., and Orimo, H., Effects of growth factors on cytosolic free calcium concentration and DNA synthesis in cultured rat aortic smooth muscle cells, *Tohuku J. Exp. Med.*, 157, 289, 1989.

125. Morisaki, N., Koyama, N., Mori, S., Kanzaki, I., Koshikawa, I., Saito, Y., and Yoshida, S., Effects of smooth muscle derived growth factor (SDGF) in combination with other growth factors on smooth muscle cells, *Atherosclerosis*, 78, 61, 1989.

126. Badesch, D. B., Lee, P. D., Parks, W. C., and Stenmark, K. R., Insulin-like growth factor I stimulates elastin synthesis by bovine pulmonary arterial smooth muscle cells, *Biochem. Biophys. Res. Commun.*, 160, 382, 1989.

127. Delafontaine, P., Lou, H., and Alexander, W., Regulation of insulin-like growth factor I messenger RNA levels in vascular smooth muscle cells, *Hypertension*, 18, 742, 1991.

128. Cercek, B., Fishbein, M. C., Forrester, J. S., Helfant, R. H., and Fagin, J. A., Induction of insulin-like growth factor I mRNA in rat aorta after balloon denudation, *Circ. Res.*, 66, 1755, 1990.

129. Bornfeldt, K. E., Arnqvist, H. J., and Capron, L., In vivo proliferation of rat vascular smooth muscle in relation to diabetes mellitus, insulin-like growth factor I and insulin, *Diabetologia*, 35, 104, 1992.

130. Murphy, L. J., Ghahary, A., and Chakrabarti, S., Insulin regulation of IGF-I expression in rat aorta, *Diabetes*, 39, 657, 1990.

131. Lundergan, C. F., Foegh, M. L., and Ramwell, P. W., Peptide inhibition of myometrial proliferation by angiopeptin, a somatostatin analogue, *J. Am. Coll. Cardiol.*, 17(Suppl. 6B), 132B, 1991.

132. McCusker, R. R. and Clemmons, D. R., Insulin-like growth factor binding protein secretion by muscle cells: effect of cellular differentiation and proliferation, *J. Cell. Physiol.*, 137, 505, 1988.

133. McCusker, R. H., Camacho-Hubner, C., and Clemmons, D. R., Identification of the types of insulin-like growth factor binding proteins that are secreted by muscle cells in vitro, *J. Biol. Chem.*, 264, 7795, 1989.

134. Giannella-Neto, D., Kamyar, A., Sharafi, B., Pirola, C. J., Kupfer, J., Rosenfeld, R. G., Forrester, J. S., and Fagin, J. A., PDGF isoforms decrease IGF$_1$ gene expression in rat vascular smooth muscle cells and selectively stimulate the biosynthesis of IGF binding protein-4, *Circ. Res.*, 71, 646, 1992.

135. Clemmons, D. R., Interaction of circulating cell-derived and plasma growth factors in stimulating cultured smooth muscle cell replication, *J. Cell. Physiol.*, 121, 425, 1984.

136. Blackshear, P. J., Insulin-stimulated protein biosynthesis as a paradigm of protein kinase C-independent growth factor, *Clin. Res.*, 37, 15, 1989.

137. Buchou, T., Charollais, R. H., Fagot, D., and Mester, J., Mitogenic activity of phorbol esters and insulin-like growth factor in a chemically transformed mouse fibroblast BP-A31; independent effects and differential sensitivity to inhibition by 3-isobutyl-1-methyl xanthine, *Exp. Cell Res.*, 182, 129, 1989.

138. Froesch, E. R., Schmid, C., Schwander, J., and Zapf, J., Action of insulin-like growth factors, *Annu. Rev. Physiol.*, 47, 443, 1985.

139. Taylor, A. M., Dandona, P., Morrell, D. J., and Preece, M. A., Insulin-like growth factor-I, protein kinase-C, calcium and cyclic AMP: partners in the regulation of chondrocyte mitogenesis and metabolism, *FEBS Lett.*, 236, 33, 1988.

140. Dempsey, E. C., Stenmark, K. R., McMurty, I. F., O'Brien, R., Voelkel, N. F., and Badesch, D. B., Insulin-like growth factor I and protein kinase C activation stimulate pulmonary artery smooth muscle cell proliferation through separate but synergistic pathways, *J. Cell. Physiol.*, 144, 159, 1990.

141. Marx, J. L., The *fos* gene as "master switch" — *fos* gene activity may be central to the cell's ability to convert short-term stimulation to long-term responses such as growth and memory formation, *Science*, 237, 854, 1987.

142. Bolander, F. F., *Molecular Endocrinology,* Academic Press, San Diego, 1989, 290.

143. Buhler, F. R., The case for calcium antagonists as first-line treatment of hypertension, *J. Hypertens.*, 10, S17, 1992.

144. Morgan, K. G., Papageorgiou, P., and Jiang, M. J., Pathophysiologic role of calcium in the development of vascular smooth muscle tone, *Am. J. Cardiol.*, 64, 35F, 1989.

145. Kuriyama, S., Nakamura, K., Kaguchi, Y., Kimura, M., Tamura, H., Tamai, K., Hashimoto, J., and Miyahara, I., The effects of vasoactive agents on the proliferation of vascular smooth muscle cells grown in vitro, *J. Hypertens.*, 6, S154, 1988.

146. Simpson, L. L., Standley, P. R., Zhang, F., Ram, J. L., Weir, M. R., and Sowers, J. R., Role of calcium in vascular smooth muscle proliferation: antiproliferative effects of verapamil enantiomers' independence from calcium channel blockade, submitted.

147. Sachinidis, A., Ko, Y., Graak, G. K., Wieczorek, A. J., and Vetter, H., Action of mesoprolol, enalapril, diltiazem, verapamil, and nifedipine on cell growth of vascular smooth muscle cells, *J. Cardiovasc. Pharmacol.*, 19(Suppl. 2), S60, 1992.

148. Sato, M., Abe, K., Yasujima, M., Omata, K., Fang, S., Tsunoda, K., Kudo, K., Takeuchi, K., Hagino, T., Kanazawa, M. et al., Inhibitory effect of cicletanine on vascular smooth muscle cell proliferation, *Arch. Mal. Coeur Vaiss.*, 82, 63, 1989.

149. Hirata, Y., Takagi, Y., Fukuda, Y., and Marmo, F., Endothelin is a potent mitogen for rat vascular smooth muscle cells, *Atherosclerosis*, 78, 225, 1989.

150. Mark, A. R., Calcium channels expressed in vascular smooth muscle, *Circulation*, 86(Suppl. 6), III61, 1992.

151. Naftilan, A. J., The role of angiotensin II in vascular smooth muscle cell growth, *J. Cardiovasc. Pharmacol.*, 20(Suppl. 1), 537, 1992.

152. Bobik, A., Grooms, A., Millar, J. A., Mitchell, A., and Grinpukel, S., Growth factor activity of endothelin on vascular smooth muscle, *Am. J. Physiol.*, 258, C408, 1990.

153. Parrott, D. P., Lockey, P. M., and Bright, C. P., Comparison of the mitogenic activity of angiotensin II and serotonin on porcine arterial smooth muscle cells, *Atherosclerosis*, 88, 213, 1991.

154. Campbell, J. H., Tachas, G., Black, M. J., Cockerill, G., and Campbell, G. R., Molecular biology of vascular hypertrophy, *Basic Res. Cardiol.*, 86(Suppl. 1), 3, 1991.

13

Calcium-Regulating Hormones and Human Hypertension

Lawrence M. Resnick

CONTENTS

I. INTRODUCTION

The critical role of mineral ions in muscle contraction has been appreciated for over 100 years, since Ringer[1] first described the heart's requirement for extracellular calcium. It is now understood that calcium acts as a final common factor in mediating cellular responses to a wide variety of physiological stimuli, including both stimulus-contraction coupling in cardiac, skeletal, and smooth muscle and stimulus-secretion coupling in endocrine hormone and neural transmitter release.[2] As such, calcium participates in the regulation of all aspects of blood pressure homeostasis, including the role of central and peripheral sympathetic nervous system

0-8493-8661-6/95/$0.00+$.50

activity, cardiac output and peripheral vascular resistance, and the numerous "classic" blood pressure hormone systems such as the renin-aldosterone system. Thus, gross pathologic deviations of circulating calcium may have cardiovascular consequences, as hypocalcemia is associated with hypotension and heart failure, and hypercalcemia with peripheral vasoconstriction, increased myocardial contractility, and an increased incidence of hypertensive disease.[3,4]

Hence, the clinical problem of hypertension — in which well-documented alterations of sympathetic neural, cardiac and peripheral smooth muscle, and endocrine mechanisms have all been demonstrated — suggests the simultaneous dysfunction of cellular calcium-dependent processes diffusely in many tissues. Indeed, our group has formulated an ionic hypothesis of cardiovascular and metabolic disease, in which alterations in cellular calcium and magnesium metabolism represent the common, underlying biological link between different disease states, alternatively expressed clinically as hypertension, accelerated atherosclerotic disease, obesity, cardiac hypertrophy, insulin resistance, and/or diabetes mellitus — disease components of the syndrome complex often referred to as "Syndrome X".[5]

Research into the mechanisms for this diffuse alteration in calcium-related processes in hypertension has usually been focused at the cellular level, where primary genetic differences as well as structural and functional differences in transduction system components such as protein kinase species, G-proteins, phospholipases, membrane fluidity and composition, etc., have been elucidated over the past decade. At the environmental level, much accumulated epidemiological evidence points to consistent relations between dietary mineral intake and hypertension. Insufficient dietary calcium, magnesium, and potassium intake are thus closely related to the incidence of clinical hypertension in a variety of Western population groups. Interestingly, despite the emphasis on dietary NaCl as a factor in hypertension, it appears that salt may play a role only in the presence of insufficient dietary calcium or other ion intake; i.e., in subjects with adequate calcium intake, there is no relation between dietary salt and blood pressure.[6]

In all of these research activities, however, little attention has been paid to the potential role in hypertension of calcium-regulating hormones, whose normal physiological function is to monitor and alter the state of circulating and cellular calcium in response to environmental dietary mineral and other signals (Figure 1). Thus, parathyroid hormone (PTH), calcitonin, and 1,25-dihydroxyvitamin D [1,25(OH)$_2$D], as well as more recently described calcium-related hormones such as parathyroid hypertensive factor (PHF) and calcitonin gene-related peptide (CGRP), may all affect the intra- and extracellular distribution of calcium and its companion ions, magnesium, potassium, and sodium. These hormones also seem to have direct cardiovascular actions. It is reasonable, therefore, to investigate the extent to which the function of these calcium hormone species may be altered in hypertensive disease states. Accordingly, the purpose here is to review what is known about calcium-regulating hormones in hypertension, how their actions may alter blood pressure homeostasis, and to what extent alterations of circulating calcium-regulating hormones may be involved in the pathophysiology of the hypertensive process.

Resnick[7] developed the working hypothesis that calcium-regulating hormones, rather than dietary access to or circulating levels of calcium per se, serve to mediate the contribution of calcium to blood pressure homeostasis. Furthermore, these hormone systems are linked to other blood pressure hormone systems such as the renin-angiotensin-aldosterone system. Together they coordinately regulate cellular monovalent (sodium and potassium) and divalent (calcium and magnesium) cation metabolism. By regulating cytosolic free calcium, intracellular free magnesium, and other ion content, the hormone systems determine the metabolic set point for cellular responsiveness of the wide variety of tissues involved in the control of blood pressure. Additionally, it appears that deviations in the renin-aldosterone system and in

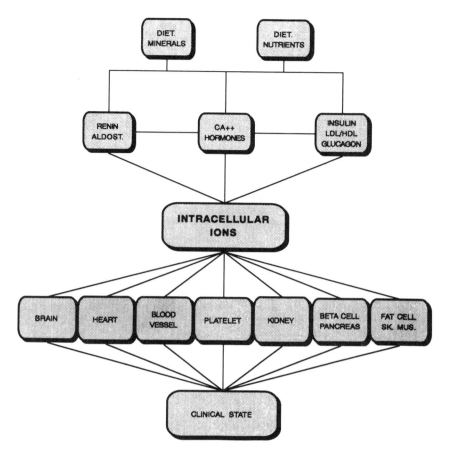

FIGURE 1   Schematic representation of homeostatic mechanisms, in which hormonal signals transduce environmental stimuli at the cellular level. The resultant alterations in steady-state ion activities are expressed
as altered organ system function, producing the clinical state characterizing that individual's response
to the initial stimulus. Differing metabolic-hormonal set points in different individuals determine which
of the possible clinical states results.

calcium-regulating hormones identify specific forms of hypertensive disease such as low-
renin and salt-sensitive hypertension. Measurement of these calcium-regulating hormones
may thus be used diagnostically to indicate the selective benefit of particular dietary and drug
regimens in the treatment of hypertension.

II. PARATHYROID HORMONE

Both primary and secondary hyperparathyroidism are associated with a variety of hypertensive
states.[8-10] While this clinical association suggests a role for PTH in the pathophysiology of the
hypertensive process, the precise nature of its participation and whether PTH directly contributes to or rather serves to retard elevated blood pressure remain controversial. Thus, almost
70 years ago, Canadians Collip and Clark[11] observed the vasodilatory effects of parathyroid
extracts injected into dogs[11]. All but forgotten until it was rediscovered by Charbon and
associates[12] four decades later, this vascular effect has since been confirmed by many other
workers,[13,14] leading to the suggestion that PTH functions physiologically as a vasodilator to
regulate peripheral vascular tone. Conversely, clinical hypertensive disease is often a feature

of primary hyperparathyroidism and is present in this form of hypercalcemia more than in other hypercalcemic syndromes.[8] These data suggest the opposite — that PTH somehow causes or at least predisposes to the excess peripheral vasoconstriction characteristic of hypertension.[15] A similar paradox appears at the cellular level. Despite evidence that PTH can increase cellular calcium accumulation in many tissues such as heart, kidneys, and even red blood cells,[16,17] electrophysiologic patch clamp studies and direct cellular measurement of cytosolic free calcium levels reveal PTH to possess calcium channel blocking properties.[18] These observations highlight the still unresolved role of PTH in vascular homeostasis.

A. Cellular Actions of Parathyroid Hormone

The chief cells of the parathyroid glands, in response to circulating calcium-related signals, produce an 84-amino acid long peptide, PTH. This peptide is derived from successive hydrolytic cleavage of longer, inactive precursor molecules, preproPTH and proPTH, reflecting a common mechanism for intracellular processing of proteins for storage and subsequent cellular export. Although native, intact PTH-(1-84) is the most commonly secreted species, other peptides comprising N-terminal and/or C-terminal portions of the molecule also circulate, resulting from parathyroid gland secretion and from peripheral metabolism. Although it is generally believed that the amino terminal, 1-34 amino acid sequence is necessary for most biological functions of PTH,[19] recent evidence suggests that C-terminal amino acid sequences of PTH may also possess biological activity.[20] Each of these PTH fragment species, intact (1-84), N-terminal (1-34), or mid-molecule/C-terminal, is utilized for currently available PTH assays. In most clinical situations the immunoradiometric assay for intact PTH provides the most physiologic information, although the longer half-life of circulating mid-portion and C-terminal fragments may in some cases better reflect the average secretory activity of the parathyroid gland.

   The physiologic actions of PTH at various target organ sites depend on and are in turn mediated by its binding to one or more receptor subtypes associated with activation of cytosolic free calcium-dependent-, adenyl cyclase-dependent-, or both, transduction systems. Hesch has termed the classic, adenyl cyclase-dependent PTH receptor the type I receptor. Some actions of PTH, especially in the renal tubule, may not be mediated as much by adenosine 3':5'-cyclic phosphate (cAMP) as by cellular calcium activation, attributed to PTH binding to a second, type II receptor.[21] Further evidence in favor of the functional (if not structural) separation of PTH receptor subtypes comes from amino-terminal modified (3-34) and selective methionine-oxidized PTH fragments, which may activate calcium-dependent (type II receptor) PTH events, but may at the same time inhibit PTH binding and/or activation of cAMP-dependent (type I receptor) events.[22]

   The cAMP-dependent actions of PTH are presumably mediated by the activation of protein kinase A and subsequently protein phosphorylation. As direct and indirect stimulation of cAMP generation in vascular tissue is associated with vasodilation, the acute vasodilatory effects of PTH are presumably consequent to and depend on cAMP stimulation.[23] This has been supported by direct electrophysiologic patch clamp-derived data, in which the action of PTH to block L-channel-type calcium current in vascular smooth muscle could be replicated by cAMP analogues.[14,18,24]

   Other documented postreceptor effects of PTH may result in altered vascular responses, either vasoconstrictive or vasodilatory in nature. Thus, PTH has been observed to either stimulate or inhibit Na,K-ATPase.[25,26] Parathyroid hormone also may inhibit sodium hydrogen exchange,[27] perhaps explaining its action to inhibit proximal renal tubular bicarbonate reabsorption. This hormone also may impair potassium tolerance, either decreasing cellular potassium uptake and/or efflux from cells,[28] or it may lower serum potassium levels.[29] The ability of PTH to stimulate calcium uptake into brain, heart, and red blood cells underlies the hypothesis that PTH plays a critical role in the toxicity of chronic renal failure, in which PTH levels are extraordinarily elevated.[30]

As a result of these various adenyl cyclase-dependent and cellular ionic actions of PTH, a variety of tissue and organ responses occur. In vascular studies *in vitro* and *in vivo*, PTH possesses acute vasodilatory properties that are apparent within the first 1 to 3 min and resolve over 5 to 20 min.[24] These effects correspond to the time course of PTH stimulation of cAMP, which is independent of changes in circulating calcium itself. In contrast, longer term vascular effects of PTH may relate more to its cellular ionic actions and its peripheral hypercalcemic effects. Hypercalcemia itself causes peripheral and renal vasoconstriction,[31] and calcium infusions in hypocalcemic animals increase cardiac output and blood pressure. Conversely, chronic hypocalcemia has negative inotropic effects and can result in frank congestive heart failure.[3] Lastly, although circulating calcium raises pressure by increasing cardiac output when ambient calcium concentrations are low, when calcium levels are elevated above normal limits, circulating calcium continues to raise pressure by increasing peripheral resistance without further changing cardiac output.[32]

A more indirect connection between PTH and blood pressure involves the effects of PTH on the renin-aldosterone system and the sympathetic nervous system. Thus, in the absence of any significant change in circulating calcium levels, PTH appears to directly increase renin secretion from the juxtaglomerular apparatus.[33] Interestingly, unlike most other hormone systems (except for PTH itself), renin secretion is stimulated by decreased rather than increased cytosolic free calcium levels. This mechanism functions as a final common pathway by which baroreceptor, macula densa, neural, and other direct hormonal and ionic inputs are integrated into a net signal stimulating or inhibiting renin secretion.[34] The mechanism of PTH stimulation of renin is thus presumably cAMP-mediated, analogous to its calcium channel blocking properties in other smooth muscle tissues, resulting in a fall in cytosolic free calcium. Furthermore, and independently of its effect on renin secretion, PTH also may potentiate aldosterone secretion, either alone or in conjunction with other aldosterone secretagogues such as angiotensin II.[35] Unlike its cAMP-mediated stimulatory action on renin secretion, this action of PTH may depend more on stimulation of cellular calcium uptake because aldosterone secretion, like most other hormones, is stimulated by increases in cytosolic free calcium. Work by Campese[36] also suggested that PTH enhances norepinephrine release and more generally, sympathetic tone. Thus, acting as a calcium ionophore, PTH stimulates cardiac inotropy and chronotropy and alters sympathetic neural tone as well as neurotransmitter release in synaptosomal preparations. Taken together, these effects of PTH on other hormone secretory systems would tend to raise blood pressure or contribute to elevations of blood pressure (or both) observed in the setting of increased PTH levels, such as primary hyperparathyroidism (see below).

Indirect effects of PTH on calcium metabolism and direct effects of PTH on ion metabolism of minerals other than calcium may contribute to its impact on vascular tone. At the renal level PTH decreases tubular reabsorption of phosphate, increasing phosphate clearance and decreasing serum phosphate levels;[37] it also decreases proximal tubular bicarbonate reabsorption, producing metabolic acidosis.[38] There is now also evidence of direct effects of PTH on potassium metabolism, although it is not clear whether its net effect is to increase or decrease cellular potassium stores. Parathyroid hormone activates the renal proximal tubular enzyme, 25-hydroxyvitamin D hydroxylase (25-OHD-1α-hydroxylase), increasing the conversion of circulating 25-OHD to the active circulating hormonal form of vitamin D, 1,25-dihydroxyvitamin D [$1,25(OH)_2D$].[39] This effect is regulated by circulating phosphate and calcium levels themselves, lower phosphate levels enhancing and higher calcium inhibiting this effect of PTH.[40] 1,25-Dihydroxyvitamin D, as well as altered acid-base balance, hypophosphatemia, and potassium balance, may each have direct effects on mechanisms of peripheral vasoconstriction.

Vascular effects of PTH may also result indirectly from its action on insulin and glucose metabolism which have been linked increasingly to cardiovascular disease. Recent evidence suggests that PTH suppresses pancreatic insulin release. This has been studied both *in vivo* and *in vitro* by Massey and colleagues,[40a] who have postulated that the glucose intolerance of chronic renal failure may result from chronic suppression of insulin secretion by high circulating PTH levels. Thus, the ability of $1,25(OH)_2D$ and of parathyroidectomy to improve glucose tolerance in subjects with end stage renal disease may result from the net effect of these maneuvers to lower circulating PTH levels.

B. Parathyroid Hormone in Experimental and Human Hypertension

1. Spontaneously Hypertensive Rat and Other Experimental Models

Evidence has accumulated that consistently and extensively documents a spectrum of abnormalities in calcium metabolism in the spontaneously hypertensive rat (SHR) model as well as other rat models of hypertension.[41] Increased parathyroid gland weight, decreased serum ionized calcium, and decreased circulating phosphate levels have all been demonstrated, implying the presence of secondary hyperparathyroidism in the SHR. Consistent with this, hypercalcuria, either on an absolute basis or relative to urinary sodium and/or creatinine excretion, has been noted in SHR, DOCA-NaCl, and two-kidney, one-clip Goldblatt hypertensive rat models. Controversy continues, however, as to what extent this hypercalciuria represents a primary renal defect or an appropriate renal response to elevated blood pressure per se.[42] Nevertheless, hyperparathyroidism in these hypertensive models is secondary to and appropriate for a presumed primary calcium deficit, based perhaps on renal loss or, more generally, due to the cytosolic free calcium excess, cellular magnesium depletion, and thus the redistribution of calcium between extra- and intracellular spaces characteristic of hypertension.

Regardless of its physiological appropriateness, the critical and as yet unanswered question remains: Does PTH contribute to or does it tend to offset the development of hypertension in these animal models? Because PTH possesses direct vasodilating action, some suggest that PTH both compensates for the lower circulating calcium levels seen in SHR and other models and acts as a vasodilator in hypertension, tending to ameliorate the hypertension.[43] Other groups suggest that PTH has at least a permissive role in the development of hypertension.[44] Thus, in the DOCA-saline hypertensive model, Bertollot and Garrard[45] reported that parathyroidectomized animals develop hypertension to a lesser degree and over a more prolonged period of time as compared to control animals with intact parathyroid glands. This occurred even though circulating calcium levels were kept in the normal range. Similarly, in normotensive animals salt loading stimulated N-terminal but not mid-portion or C-terminal PTH levels when salt increased blood pressure.[46]

Supporting its ameliorative role, evidence also suggests decreased PTH action is involved in hypertension. Parathyroid hormone infusions in the SHR produce less of a rise in urinary cAMP excretion as compared to the same dose in normotensive control animals.[47] This relative PTH resistance of hypertension has been supported further by studies demonstrating a blunted PTH stimulation of 25-OHD-1α-hydroxylase in hypertensive vs. normotensive animals, despite no differences in the renal phosphaturic response to PTH being noted.[48] Furthermore, an altered adenyl cyclase-related stimulatory G-protein, G_s, has been reported in SHR vs. WKY animals, in association with a blunted cAMP response to PTH. Hence, it is reasonable to wonder if in hypertension an imbalance exists among vasodilatory, cAMP-related PTH actions, and cellular calcium-related vasoconstrictive actions of PTH, due to a partial "pseudohypoparathyroidism". This would further contribute to the secondary hyperparathyroidism of hypertension, vasoconstriction being the price to pay for adequate or marginal calcium homeostasis.

2. Human Hypertension

Higher circulating PTH levels, lower serum ionized calcium and serum phosphorus levels, and hypercalciuria were also reported in human essential hypertension.[9,49,50] A primary defect in renal calcium handling as well as a primary cellular redistribution of calcium between extracellular and intracellular pools in many tissues, including the kidney, were hypothesized, resulting in appropriate secondary hyperparathyroidism and elevated 1,25(OH)$_2$D, and parathyroid hypertensive factor (PHF) levels which have been reported in essential hypertension.[50a] Unlike SHR, however, urinary cAMP concentrations may be increased in human hypertension, and no evidence of pseudohypoparathyroidism has been reported.[51] Nevertheless, hypertension is a prominent clinical feature of patients with pseudohypoparathyroidism type IA, where the stimulatory G$_s$ protein is deficient, and in which PTH cellular binding is uncoupled from cAMP stimulation.[52]

These data may be explained on the basis of an appropriate PTH response to decreased circulating calcium levels, in which PTH offsets and compensates not only for the lower calcium levels but for the elevated blood pressure as well. However, in hypertensive subjects with chronic renal failure, in whom PTH levels are clearly elevated, the hypotensive response to beta blockade correlated best with the ability of beta blockers to lower PTH levels. This is more consistent with the opposite hypothesis — that PTH is somehow contributing to the increased pressure as it is appropriately attempting to compensate for the observed decreased circulating ionized calcium levels.

Our group has suggested that the role of calcium-regulating hormones in hypertension is different in different pathophysiological types of hypertensive disease. Thus, essential hypertensive subjects with low plasma renin activity values have higher levels of circulating PTH, while high PTH levels were not observed in normal to high renin patients.[53] These higher PTH levels in low renin patients are appropriate for the lower ionized calcium observed predominantly in this hypertensive subgroup.[54] Similarly, the highest levels of PTH and the lowest ionized calcium levels were observed in subjects with primary hyperaldosteronism, the lowest renin, most salt-sensitive form of human hypertension.[10] In support of the linkage between increased parathyroid gland activity and low renin, salt-sensitive hypertension studies have shown that salt loading in black human subjects stimulates PTH.[55,56] Thus, whether PTH itself directly contributes to salt-sensitive hypertension or whether it serves as a marker for other, more active agents such as PHF or 1,25(OH)$_2$D remains unresolved.

3. Hypertension of Primary Hyperparathyroidism

Although not initially suspected,[57] hypertension is now appreciated as a frequent clinical finding in primary hyperparathyroidism, occurring in 40 to 75% of patients.[8] This "hyperparathyroid hypertension" was one of the first observations to suggest a link between calcium-regulating hormones and the regulation of blood pressure. Although it was initially thought that renal damage secondary to chronic nephrocalcinosis was the underlying mechanism in milder forms of primary hyperparathyroidism without overt renal damage, hypertension is still recognized as a primary feature of the syndrome.

Alterations of the renin-angiotensin system may also contribute to the mechanism of hypertension in primary hyperparathyroidism;[58] this condition is associated with a greater prevalence (up to 40%) of increased plasma renin activity as compared to essential hypertension (10 to 15%). In our experience, few primary hyperparathyroid subjects have normal plasma renin activities; patients either have inappropriately low or high renin forms of hypertension. This again contrasts with the distribution of renin activity in essential hypertension, in which approximately half of the patients have values similar to normotensive subjects. This skewing of renin activity values in hyperparathyroidism in both directions away from

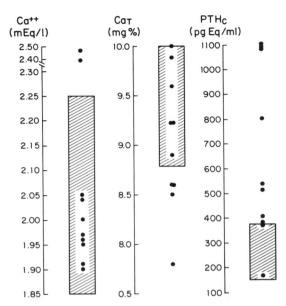

FIGURE 2   Secondary hyperparathyroidism and possible tertiary hyperparathyroidism in patients with primary hyperaldosteronism. (From Resnick, L. M. and Laragh, J. H., *Am. J. Med.*, 78, 385, 1985. With permission.)

average normotensive values supports a primary and/or secondary role for the renin-angiotensin system in this form of hypertension.[59] Thus, the secondary hyperparathyroidism observed most often in low renin states, such as low renin essential hypertension and primary aldosteronism (Figure 2), may over many years result in parathyroid gland autonomy in some subjects. Primary hyperparathyroidism with concurrent hypertension in low renin individuals may therefore represent low renin essential hypertension with subsequent tertiary hyperparathyroidism. Conversely, because PTH itself may directly stimulate renin secretion, primary hyperparathyroidism of high renin hypertension patients implies the effects of excess circulating PTH values on renin activity. This working hypothesis helps to explain the heterogeneous blood pressure responses to surgical correction of "primary" hyperparathyroidism; some published series report lowered blood pressure, others report an elevation in 20 to 30% of patients. These data are also consistent with the notion that PTH may have been serving a compensatory role, consistent with its vasodilatory effects, either offsetting prior long-standing hypertensive disease or the hypertensive effects of PTH-induced renin and angiotensin II levels. If this notion is correct, surgical correction of primary hyperparathyroidism would benefit mainly higher renin individuals in whom PTH would cause hypertension. On the other hand, no effect or even higher pressures would result in low renin hyperparathyroid subjects, where PTH elevations are compensatory.

Finally, the existence of the recently described PHF in the peripheral blood of hypertensive primary hyperparathyroid subjects,[60] and the direct link between the disappearance of PHF from the circulation post-parathyroidectomy and the resolution of hypertension strongly suggests its contribution to the pathogenesis of hypertension in this disease.

4. Summary

Parathyroid hormone affects a wider range of target organs than have been previously suspected, including heart and blood vessels. It possesses potent vasoactive properties, which are dependent on multiple postreceptor effects, and changes sodium, hydrogen, potassium, and calcium ion movements across cell membranes. Circulating PTH levels may be elevated in experimental and human hypertension, including SHR, Dahl-S, and DOCA-saline rats, and in primary hyperaldosteronism and low renin-essential hypertension. When present, this secondary hyperparathyroidism appears to appropriately respond to a perceived calcium deficit. Available evidence suggests that PTH may have a compensatory, offsetting effect on the elevated blood pressure, that it may have a primary pathogenetic role in causing elevated blood pressure, or that it is a marker for increased parathyroid gland activity. Thus, blood pressure changes may be more directly mediated by other parathyroid substances such as PHF, or by parathyroid-dependent substances such as 1,25(OH)$_2$D. This issue remains unresolved, and perhaps should best be considered in the particular types of hypertensive disease in which it may serve any of these roles.

Whatever its particular role in the pathogenesis of hypertensive disease, it is clear that PTH coordinately is linked to the function of the renin-aldosterone system, to sympathetic nerve activity, and thus to the control not only of blood pressure but of monovalent and divalent ion metabolism.

III. CALCITONIN

Calcitonin is secreted as an intact 32-amino acid peptide from the parafollicular or C cells of the thyroid, and circulates in monomeric and various polymeric forms. Calcitonin receptors are diffusely distributed among many tissues of the body, including brain, liver, and kidney. Although the overall function of calcitonin in human metabolism remains unclear, most attention has focused on its action on bone and calcium metabolism. Because calcitonin, both acutely and longer term, decreases bone reabsorption and thus may decrease serum calcium levels, it has been used therapeutically in emergency hypercalcemic syndromes, and in the treatment of metabolic bone disorders such as Paget's disease of the bone and osteoporosis.[61] Its action on bone, however, seems to represent a more general effect of calcitonin at other tissue sites to alter calcium uptake, distribution, and release. In the brain, calcitonin increases calcium uptake into some nuclei, while actually decreasing calcium uptake into other nuclei.[62] In the liver, calcitonin facilitates calcium uptake in a specific, apparently L-channel-dependent manner, because this effect is blocked by calcium channel blockade with verapamil.[63]

We have investigated the cellular mechanism of calcitonin action in a kidney slice model, studying juxtaglomerular cell release of renin. In this system, calcitonin seems to interact with the voltage-operated calcium channels. Thus, in the basal state calcitonin was observed to suppress renal renin secretion, an effect also blocked by the calcium channel blocker verapamil[64] (Figure 3). However, when the JG cells were incubated in a 50-mm KCl-containing medium, the resulting, expected suppression of renin secretion due to depolarization and calcium influx through voltage-operated calcium channels was blunted by calcitonin.[65] Furthermore, this occurred with concentrations of calcitonin that in the nondepolarized JG cell preparation appeared to facilitate calcium entry. These findings seem to indicate that in the basal state, in the absence of membrane depolarization, calcitonin increases cellular calcium accumulation through specific, voltage-dependent L-channels. However, in a state of cell depolarization, calcitonin has the opposite effect, appearing to act as a calcium channel blocker. This ability of calcitonin to alter calcium entry in either direction according to the membrane potential of the tissue suggests that calcitonin may function as an endogenous calcium-buffering hormone, modulating otherwise more dramatic changes in cytosolic calcium resulting from acute cell stimulation.

In parallel experiments in intact humans, salmon calcitonin infused in graded doses (10^{-4} to 10^1 U) to normotensive and hypertensive subjects had either vasodilatory or vasoconstrictive effects, as measured by forearm plethysmography.[66] This alternative, opposite vascular responsiveness to calcitonin seemed to be a function of pretreatment initial serum ionized calcium concentrations and of dietary salt intake. Calcitonin was most vasodilatatory when

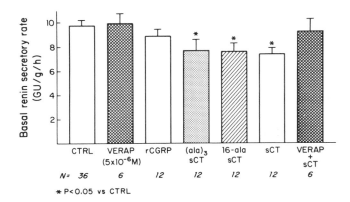

FIGURE 3   Effects of calcitonin and calcitonin analogues to suppress basal renin secretion in rat kidney slices; these effects are prevented by verapamil pretreatment. (From Resnick, L. M. et al., *Am. J. Hypert.*, 2, 453, 1989. With permission.)

serum ionized calcium levels were lower and was vasoconstrictive the higher the average level of ionized calcium. In addition, higher dietary salt intakes (200 vs. 100 vs.10 mEq NaCl per day) were associated with decreased forearm blood flow, while less of a decrease or even an increase in forearm flow, often in the same individual subject, was observed on lower dietary salt intakes.[67] These heterogeneous clinical peripheral vascular effects of calcitonin in humans may thus parallel its similar apparently opposite, calcium-dependent effects at the cellular level in altering renal renin secretion.

The vascular effects of calcitonin must also be distinguished from possible overlap effects mediated by cross-binding of calcitonin to CGRP receptors. Both species appear to have independent vascular actions; however, calcitonin directly increases smooth muscle tone and blood pressure in humans,[68] but CGRP decreases smooth muscle tone and blood pressure in the rat.[69,70] Furthermore, CGRP did not suppress renin secretion under the same conditions as calcitonin. Although capable of acting as a vasodilator under some conditions, perhaps at doses that may activate CGRP receptors, calcitonin at more physiologic levels and in the absence of other stimuli to cellular depolarization may contribute to the vasoconstriction of the hypertensive state.

The calcium-dependent vascular effects of calcitonin also may be clinically relevant. In hypertension in the SHR, elevated levels of calcitonin have been observed prior to the onset of significant hypertension.[71] Because circulating calcium levels at this early stage of development in the SHR were reported to be higher, normal, or lower than in normotensive control rats of the same age, it is not clear whether these elevated levels of calcitonin are secondary and appropriate for the calcium level. Interestingly, stimulation of renal sodium excretion, a well-known effect of exogenous calcitonin, is blunted in the SHR.[72] This effect is consistent with chronically higher circulating levels and secondary down-regulation of calcitonin receptors, with a primary lesion of altered target-organ responsiveness to calcitonin, or both. Levels of calcitonin in human essential hypertensive subjects, similar to those of other calcium-regulating hormones we have studied, are heterogeneously deviated among different renin subgroups of hypertensives. Thus, low renin essential hypertensives had lower average serum ionized calcium values and appropriately lower levels of calcitonin as compared to high renin essential hypertensives who had higher average ionized calcium levels and appropriately higher circulating levels of calcitonin[53] (Figure 4). In human essential hypertension, therefore, the distribution of calcitonin values is altered, but seems to be appropriate for the parallel deviations in serum ionized calcium that we previously observed in these different renin subgroups.

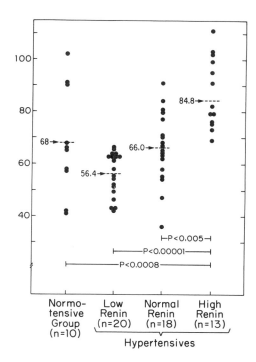

FIGURE 4 Calcitonin levels in normotensive and different renin subgroups of essential hypertensive subjects. (From Resnick, L. M., Maller, F. B., and Laragh, J. H., *Ann. Intern. Med.*, 105, 649, 1986. With permission.)

It seems reasonable to conclude that calcitonin is a vasoactive hormone, although the role of calcitonin in human physiology generally remains unclear. The basis for at least some of its effects seems to depend on altering the distribution of calcium between the intracellular and extracellular spaces, and even within the same tissue it may specifically stimulate or inhibit calcium influx according to the ambient tissue membrane potential. Clinically, this cellular action may be expressed in the effect of calcitonin on the peripheral vasculature, either increasing or decreasing vascular resistance depending on the underlying state of calcium metabolism and salt balance, which also differ among different renin subgroups of hypertension. However, whether the altered distribution of calcitonin values found in human essential hypertensives and in experimental rat models of hypertension reflect any direct contribution of calcitonin to the hypertensive process is unknown and warrants further study.

IV. CALCITONIN GENE-RELATED PEPTIDE

Two messenger RNA (mRNA) species may be transcribed from the calcitonin gene, based on alternate gene splicing, which result in RNAs encoding for both calcitonin and the 37-amino acid protein, CGRP.[73] In tissues expressing this gene, a predominance of one or the other species may be found. Thus, in thyroid C-cells, calcitonin is synthesized in excess of CGRP (95:1), whereas CGRP is produced almost exclusively relative to calcitonin in brain, peripheral sympathetic and parasympathetic ganglia, cardiac atria, mesenteric vasculature, the kidney, and endocrine tissues.[74] Two forms of CGRP, α- and β-CGRP, have been described, differing in humans by only three amino acid residues[75,76] and possessing functionally similar properties. This peptide is an exceptionally powerful vasodilator, being 17 times more potent than prostacyclin and also more potent than atrial natriuretic factor (ANF).[77-79] Its active vasodilatory properties reside at the N-terminal portion of the molecule,[80-82] and its cellular

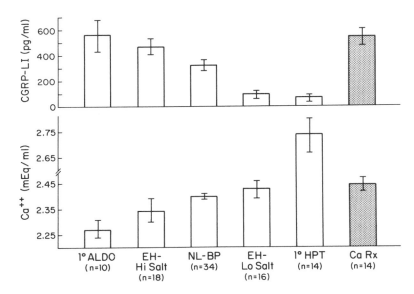

FIGURE 5 Levels of CGRP and of serum ionized calcium in different clinical subgroups of hypertensive men. (From Resnick, L. M., Preibisz, J. J., and Laragh, J. H., in *Salt and Hypertension,* Ganten and Reitch, Eds., Springer-Verlag, New York, 1989, 190. With permission.)

mechanism of action has been linked to cAMP via the CGRP type I receptor,[83] nitric oxide formation,[84-86] adensoine triphosphate-dependent potassium channels,[87] calcium channel blocking effects,[65] and its stimulatory action on ANF release.[88] Recent observations also implicated CGRP in adrenal cortical function. Calcitonin gene-related peptide can increase cortisol production independently of adrenocorticotropic hormone.[89] It also can suppress aldosterone production, despite increased adrenocorticotropic hormone and plasma renin activity,[90] even in the presence of hypotension.[91]

Whether by its direct vasodilatory effects or by indirect inhibition of aldosterone secretion, accumulating circumstantial evidence supports a role for CGRP in blood pressure regulation in general, and in the pathophysiology of hypertension in particular. Thus, even at doses that do not alter blood pressure, CGRP can increase forearm blood flow[92] and inhibits the pressor response to angiotensin II.[93] Circulating levels of CGRP exhibit a circadian rhythm, peaking between 11 p.m. and 12 midnight. Higher levels correspond to the lower pressures at night,[94] and precede the rise in ANF, cortisol, renin, etc.[95] Decreased circulating CGRP and increased hypothalamic and aortic tissue CGRP levels are found in the SHR rat model.[96] A decreased number of CGRP-containing neurons in the mesenteric vasculature and spinal cord of the SHR have been reported.[97-99] A decreased responsiveness to exogenous CGRP has also been demonstrated in diabetes, a condition predisposing to the development of hypertension.[100] In human essential hypertension, CGRP levels were reported to be normal, decreased,[101] and increased.[102] High levels of circulating CGRP were reported in pheochromocytoma and primary aldosteronism, returning to normal postadrenalectomy.[103]

We studied the relation of CGRP to human hypertensive disease by measuring circulating concentrations of CGRP in male and female normotensive and hypertensive subjects under different dietary and pathophysiologic conditions[104,105] (Figure 5). We found no significant differences among free-living male and female normotensive and essential hypertensive individuals; all had immunoreactive CGRP values averaging 250 to 350 pg/ml. These serum values are somewhat higher than the plasma values of normotensive volunteers, averaging 25 pmol/l (approximately 100 pg/ml). This difference between serum and plasma values has been consistently observed utilizing five different antibodies raised to human CGRPα (and not cross-reacting with calcitonin),[106] and it now appears that the circulating CGRP species detected by immunoreactive measurements with CGRP antibodies is not identical to native monomeric α-CGRP, but probably also represents polymeric forms of CGRP. Thus, the measurements reported here should be properly termed CGRP-like immunoreactivity (CGRP-LI).

With this limitation in mind, different distributions of CGRP-LI were found in hypertensive subjects according to the state of calcium and sodium metabolism. First, CGRP-LI levels were suppressed on a low dietary sodium intake and were stimulated by dietary salt loading in the same patients. Second, a continuous, positive relationship was observed in free-living essential hypertensives, but not in normotensives, between CGRP-LI and urinary sodium excretion. Third, average CGRP-LI levels were elevated in the hypertension of primary aldosteronism. Hence, stimulation of circulating CGRP-LI levels seems characteristic of the sodium-volume expanded state. Altered calcium metabolism also seemed to affect circulating CGRP-LI levels. Thus, low levels were observed in hypertensive primary hyperparathyroid subjects. Furthermore, for all unmedicated hypertensive subjects as a group, the lower the serum ionized calcium, the greater the CGRP-LI levels measured. This was true also of hypertensive patients who were normotensive on therapy with calcium channel blockers, which produced increased serum ionized calcium values and reduced CGRP-LI levels. Because CGRP-LI levels in hypertensives were positively related to the level of blood pressure itself, we cannot determine whether the fall in CGRP-LI with nitrendipine therapy is specific for the drug, reflects the inverse relation of CGRP-LI with circulating ionized calcium, or is related directly to lowered blood pressures.

These sodium- and calcium-linked alterations in CGRP-LI emphasize the more general linkage between sodium and calcium metabolism and hypertension and suggest a role for endogenous CGRP in the reciprocal ("see-saw") variations in sodium and calcium metabolism that appear to operate in essential hypertension, especially the salt-sensitive type. Thus, salt-induced changes in calcium metabolism may mediate the pressor response to salt loading in essential hypertension,[107] while the blood pressure-lowering effects of oral calcium loading are best observed in salt-loaded states.[108-110] We have long postulated that the mechanism of this relation between calcium and sodium metabolism is mediated by calcium-regulating hormones such as $1,25(OH)_2D$.[111,112] As an extension of this overall hypothesis, we consider it likely that CGRP functions as a sodium-calcium responsive vasodilating hormone in hypertension. Indeed, the calcium channel blocking properties exhibited by CGRP *in vitro*[65] and its anatomic localization in sympathetic neurovasculature suggest that it serves a similar role endogenously, either responding directly to sodium- and calcium-related signals, or indirectly to the impact of these mineral systems on higher sympathetic nerve centers.

V. 1,25-DIHYDROXYVITAMIN D

1,25-Dihydroxyvitamin D is the hormonally active form of vitamin D and is derived endogenously from the sequential steroid metabolism of cholesterol in the skin upon exposure to sunlight radiation, producing vitamin D, in the liver where it is hydroxylated at the C-25 position and in the proximal tubular epithelium of the kidney, where a specific mitochondrial 1α-hydroxylase further hydroxylates 25-OHD to $1,25(OH)_2D$. Alternative hydroxylation of the precursor 25-OHD results in the formation of other, less active compounds, including $24,25(OH)_2D$, and $1,24,25(OH)_3D$ by this enzyme. Although other tissues of the body, especially cells of the lymphoreticular system, are capable of a similar 1α-hydroxylation reaction, the majority of the hormone $1,25(OH)_2D$ is made in the kidney. Under normal dietary circumstances and with access to adequate sunlight and/or with supplemental oral intake of vitamin D, the availability of the circulating 25-OHD substrate is not rate limiting. The conversion of 25-OHD to $1,25(OH)_2D$ via 1α-hydroxylase, rather than to $24,25(OH)_2D$, etc., is a closely regulated step, with lower circulating phosphate, lower calcium, and higher PTH

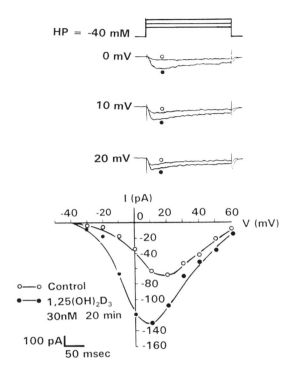

FIGURE 6   Effects of 1,25(OH)$_2$D on L-channel calcium current in vascular smooth muscle cells. (From Shan, J. et al., *Am. J. Hypert.*, 6, 983, 1993. With permission.)

levels, the main factors stimulating 1,25(OH)$_2$D production. In addition, a variety of other hormones, including growth hormone, prolactin, insulin, and calcitonin, have also been shown to influence 1α-hydroxylase activity and thus the renal production of 1,25(OH)$_2$D.[113]

Although not historically emphasized as classic target tissues, the presence of specific intracellular 1,25(OH)$_2$D receptors in cardiovascular tissues and the contribution of altered vitamin D metabolism to the pathophysiology of hypertensive disease have become increasingly apparent. Thus, both cardiac[114] and smooth muscle[115] have been identified as potential vitamin D steroid target organs, where 1,25(OH)$_2$D increases calcium uptake into skeletal muscle, cardiac muscle,[116] and vascular smooth muscle[117] associated with specific 1,25(OH)$_2$D hormone binding to cytosolic receptors. Furthermore, increased cardiac and vascular smooth muscle contractile function in the presence of vitamin D steroids suggests specific physiologic effects of vitamin D in these tissues.[118] Thus, 1,25(OH)$_2$D potentiates vascular smooth muscle contractile responses to norepinephrine, vasopressin, and angiotensin II.[119,120] Furthermore, chronic nonhypercalcemic doses of 1,25(OH)$_2$D that maintain circulating levels within the physiologic range can also elevate blood pressure in intact animals, indicating a direct effect of the steroid itself rather than of perturbed circulating calcium levels.[119] This direct action of 1,25(OH)$_2$D is supported by observations that the noncalcemic analogue of 1,25(OH)$_2$D, 22-oxacalcitriol, possessed similar vascular effects.[120]

The cellular basis of these 1,25(OH)$_2$D-dependent vascular effects remains incompletely understood. Electrophysiologically, utilizing whole cell patch clamp techniques, our group showed that 1,25(OH)$_2$D activates L-type calcium channel current and increases cytosolic free calcium in vascular smooth muscle cells[121] (Figure 6). 1,25-Dihydroxyvitamin D action classically requires binding to its specific cytosolic receptor followed by gene activation and subsequent protein synthesis-dependent events. Thus, one report[122] demonstrates that cells from patients lacking cytosolic vitamin D receptors did not exhibit a $1,25(OH)_2D$-induced rise in cytosolic free calcium.[122] Alternatively, a liponomic hypothesis has been put forward in which direct, nonreceptor-mediated alterations of membrane lipids are responsible for rapid early vitamin D hormone-related effects.[123] Baran and Kelly[124] isolated phospholipid components which are produced by $1,25(OH)_2D$ action and which, even in the absence of $1,25(OH)_2D$ itself, mimic its effects and cause rapid calcium influx in hepatic cells in tissue culture. Via *in vitro* membrane lipid fragment incubation we have confirmed the role of these phospholipase-dependent components in vascular smooth muscle cells, observing a rise in cytosolic free calcium indistinguishable from the action of $1,25(OH)_2D$. Furthermore, administration of these agents to the intact animal elevated blood pressure. Regardless of the mechanism by which these effects occur, smooth muscle function as well as cardiac function must now routinely be considered vitamin D-dependent events.

VI. VITAMIN D METABOLISM IN HYPERTENSION

Alterations of circulating vitamin D levels and of vitamin D-mediated actions have been reported in both experimental and clinical hypertension.[125-128] In the SHR rat model, no change or even increased levels of $1,25(OH)_2D$ have been reported early in life,[129,130] although after 12 weeks of age, despite lower average serum ionized calcium, lower average phosphorus, and higher average PTH activity, suppressed levels of $1,25(OH)_2D$ were observed. Similarly, recent studies demonstrated lower $1,25(OH)_2D$-induced intracellular calcium-binding protein mRNA and protein synthesis in the SHR model. Accordingly, these data have led to the suggestion of a primary defect in $1,25(OH)_2D$ formation, metabolic clearance, and/or action in this experimental hypertensive rat model. However, in the Dahl-S hypertensive rat model, on standard, low, and high salt diets, the lower average serum ionized calcium observed is associated with an appropriately higher level of $1,25(OH)_2D$ as compared to its normotensive control animal, the Dahl-R rat.[131]

Abnormalities of vitamin D metabolism have also been reported in human hypertensive disease, which more directly suggests a role for $1,25(OH)_2D$ in the pathophysiology of the hypertensive process. When we measured $1,25(OH)_2D$ levels in different renin subgroups of essential hypertensive disease, we found that $1,25(OH)_2D$ levels were altered, but were appropriate for parallel changes in serum ionized calcium[53] (Figure 7). This finding was similar to the results obtained with PTH and calcitonin. Thus, low renin essential hypertensives with lower average serum ionized calcium and higher average PTH values had significantly higher $1,25(OH)_2D$ levels as compared to high renin hypertensive patients, who had higher average calcium levels and relatively suppressed levels of $1,25(OH)_2D$ (Figure 8). The same calcium metabolic profile that is characteristic of the low renin patient, similar to the Dahl-S rat — lower ionized calcium and higher $1,25(OH)_2D$ levels — could be produced dynamically by dietary salt loading.[107] Salt induced a significant fall in circulating serum ionized calcium, especially in salt-sensitive subjects, in whom blood pressure rose proportionately to the concomitant elevations in circulating $1,25(OH)_2D$ levels. This has now also been shown to result in a transfer of extracellular calcium intracellularly; cytosolic levels of free calcium rose and free magnesium levels fell reciprocally.[132,133] Consistent with its actions to stimulate inward L-channel calcium current and cytosolic free calcium levels in vascular smooth muscle, a role was postulated for $1,25(OH)_2D$ in mediating the salt-induced cellular accumulation of calcium, and thus the pressor effects of dietary salt.[112]

The hypothesis that $1,25(OH)_2D$ directly contributes to at least some forms of human hypertension has been supported further by recent data utilizing dietary calcium supplementation in hypertension. We observed that dietary calcium loading can offset dietary salt-induced hypertension, and that this effect is closely linked to its ability to suppress salt-

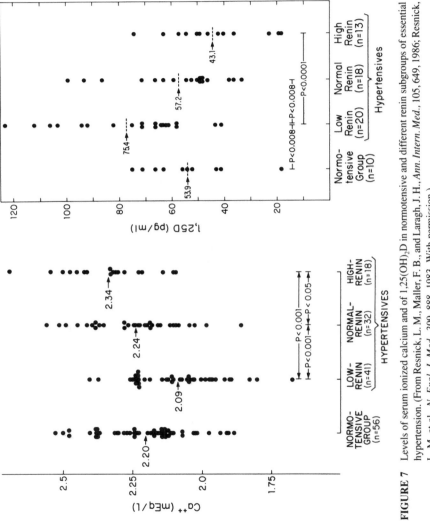

FIGURE 7 Levels of serum ionized calcium and of 1,25(OH)$_2$D in normotensive and different renin subgroups of essential hypertension. (From Resnick, L. M., Maller, F. B., and Laragh, J. H., *Ann. Intern. Med.*, 105, 649, 1986; Resnick, L. M. et al., *N. Engl. J. Med.*, 309, 888, 1983. With permission.)

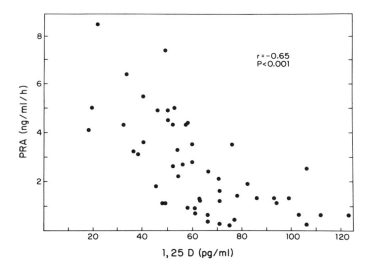

FIGURE 8 Inverse relation of circulating 1,25(OH)₂D (1,25 D) levels and plasma renin activity (PRA) values in normal and essential hypertensive subjects. (From Resnick, L. M., Maller, F. B., and Laragh, J. H., *Ann. Intern. Med.,* 105, 649, 1986. With permission.)

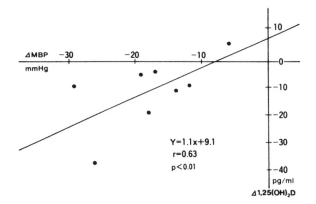

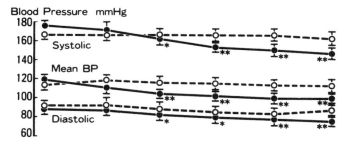

FIGURE 9 Parallel related effects of calcium supplementation to lower blood pressure and to suppress circulating levels of 1,25(OH)₂D [Δ1,25(OH)₂D]. (From Tabuchi, Y. et al., *J. Clin. Hypert.,* 3, 254, 1986.)

induced elevations in 1,25D levels.[109] Similarly, the ability of oral calcium loading to lower blood pressure in essential hypertensive patients was more pronounced in low renin subjects, who possess lower serum ionized calcium levels and higher basal levels of 1,25(OH)₂D.[134] This has also been supported by other studies, in which the ability of oral calcium

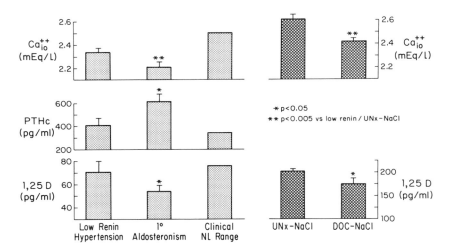

FIGURE 10   Abnormal lack of 1,25(OH)$_2$D (1,25 D) stimulation in syndromes of mineralocorticoid excess. (From Resnick, L. M., Germer, J. M., and Laragh, J. H., *J. Hypertens.*, 5(Suppl. 5), 599, 1987. With permission.)

supplementation to lower pressure in elderly hypertensives was best predicted by initial 1,25(OH)$_2$D levels, i.e., the greater the basal 1,25(OH)$_2$D level and the greater the calcium-induced fall in 1,25(OH)$_2$D, the greater the hypotensive response to calcium supplementation[135] (Figure 9). Additional evidence in favor of a critical role for 1,25(OH)$_2$D in mediating salt-sensitive, low renin, lower ionized calcium, higher basal 1,25(OH)$_2$D forms of hypertension comes from experiments in which feeding calcium alone, as compared to the combination of calcium with oral administration of 1,25(OH)$_2$D, produced opposing results. The blood pressure effects of calcium alone were reversed by the addition of 1,25(OH)$_2$D to the calcium, despite a further fall in circulating PTH levels with the combination.[136] Hence, 1,25(OH)$_2$D seems important in explaining the blood pressure effects of dietary calcium. Lastly, the hypotensive effect of calcium channel blockade is proportional to its effects on circulatory 1,25(OH)$_2$D levels, but not to the levels of calcium.[137] Therefore, vitamin D hormones themselves, rather than circulating calcium, PTH levels, or both, may determine the effects of calcium metabolism on blood pressure.

The mechanism of these 1,25(OH)$_2$D-mediated effects may not only derive from its direct effects on cellular calcium uptake in vascular smooth muscle and heart, causing vasoconstriction and elevated blood pressure, but may also derive from its linkage with the renin-aldosterone system. In syndromes of mineralocorticoid excess — both primary aldosteronism and the DOCA-saline hypertensive rat model — we observed that despite lower circulating calcium levels and appropriately higher circulating PTH levels, 1,25(OH)$_2$D levels were in each case inappropriately suppressed[138] (Figure 10). Indeed, levels of 1,25(OH)$_2$D in patients with primary aldosteronism were lower than those with low renin essential hypertension, and levels in the DOCA-saline hypertensive rat model were lower than in uninephrectomized saline controls not given deoxycorticosterone, even though renin was further suppressed and ionized calcium and PTH levels were further stimulated by mineralocorticoid excess.[10] Moreover, instead of the normal negative feedback relationship between PTH and 1,25(OH)$_2$D levels, in which PTH stimulates 1,25(OH)$_2$D production, an inverse relationship was observed in patients with primary aldosteronism: the higher the 1,25(OH)$_2$D, the lower the PTH. It thus appears that in these syndromes excess mineralocorticoid per se, whether as a direct effect or by virtue of its effects on sodium metabolism in the kidney, results in a primary suppression of 1,25(OH)$_2$D formation. This suppression is independent of otherwise physiologically compelling circulating calcium and PTH-related signals. This primary action on 1,25(OH)$_2$D

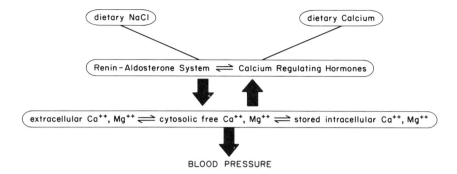

FIGURE 11   Overall scheme in which the coordinated, interacting effects of calcium-regulating hormones and the renin-aldosterone system on steady-state cellular ion content determine smooth muscle vascular tone and thus blood pressure. Each hormone system influences the blood pressure by altering either the extracellular availability of calcium to the cell (calcium hormones) or the recruitment of calcium from intracellular stores (angiotensin II). (From Resnick, L. M., *Am. J. Med.*, 82(Suppl. IB), 16, 1987. With permission.)

would then result in feedback suppressive effects of $1,25(OH)_2D$ on PTH[139] rather than the usually primary direct stimulatory effect of PTH on $1,25(OH)_2D$ levels.

In summary, both peripheral vascular and cardiac tissues appear to be target organs for the vitamin D steroid hormone, $1,25(OH)_2D$. In these tissues, $1,25(OH)_2D$ mediates calcium influx, stimulates contraction, and may potentiate contractile responses to other circulating agonists. A role for $1,25(OH)_2D$ in low renin, salt-sensitive forms of hypertensive disease seems likely, mediating the pressor response to dietary salt loading and, conversely, the antihypertensive effects of dietary calcium loading.

VII. ROLE OF THE CALCIOTROPIC HORMONES AND RENIN-ALDOSTERONE SYSTEM IN BLOOD PRESSURE HOMEOSTASIS: THE IONIC HYPOTHESIS OF HYPERTENSION

We have developed an overall hypothesis, consistent with experimental and clinical observations, in which all forms of hypertension are associated with and dependent on cytosolic free calcium excess, intracellular magnesium depletion, or both (Figure 11). What underlies the different pathophysiologies present in different forms of hypertensive disease — and clinically what determines the broad heterogeneity of hypertensive responses to similar dietary and drug therapies — is the extent to which this distortion of cellular cations is due to extracellular vs. intracellular ionic events.[140] In "pure" extracellular calcium-dependent hypertension (identified clinically with low renin, salt-sensitive forms of hypertension), the operative mechanism is excess net cellular calcium accumulation from the extracellular space, mediated by the actions of calcium-regulating hormones such as $1,25(OH)_2D$, and PHF. In this situation, elevations of PTH and CGRP, and/or lower calcitonin and suppressed renin values are secondary, appropriate, and compensatory mechanisms that either directly promote vasodilation or withdraw additional vasoconstrictive mechanisms.

The opposite, pure intracellular calcium-dependent hypertension, is mediated and clinically characterized by excess circulating renin activity and increased angiotensin II levels. Here, the excess cytosolic free calcium is not a result of accumulation from extracellular sources but is from angiotensin II-mediated release of calcium into the cytosol from storage sites in the endoplasmic reticulum or calciosomes. This mechanism involves the well-studied angiotensin II-induced activation of protein kinase C and the production of inositol triphosphate, with subsequent calcium release into the cytoplasm and reciprocal sequestration of free magnesium ions into the same storage areas, and thus out of the cytosolic pool. Adequate extracellular calcium levels are maintained in this condition by this intracellular mobilization and subsequent equilibration across the cellular plasma membrane. The result is that PTH, $1,25(OH)_2D$, and PHF levels are either suppressed or indistinguishable from those in normotensive subjects. This is exactly the calcium hormonal profile observed in high renin hypertension.

Because in most hypertensive subjects neither pure mechanism entirely determines the blood pressure, it is important to consider calcium-regulating hormones coordinately with the renin-aldosterone system as regulators of blood pressure and ion homeostasis, linking the humoral control of monovalent and divalent cation metabolism. Thus, the blood pressure effects of dietary mineral signals, whether of salt, calcium, potassium, etc., are transduced at the cellular level by their effect on these hormone systems. The resultant hormone-mediated steady-state alterations in the distribution of calcium, for example, between intracellular and extracellular compartments and within different intracellular sites alters cardiac hemodynamic function, central nervous and peripheral vasoactive hormone release, peripheral smooth muscle vasoconstrictor tone, and the resultant blood pressure.

Clinically, how does this work? Different genetic or acquired alterations in cellular ion transport systems result in the metabolic set points of the renin-aldosterone system and of calcium-regulating hormones among different individuals. Hypertension results only when the availability of dietary salt, potassium, calcium, or magnesium are so altered as to either enhance or suppress these hormonal set points. Therefore, high dietary salt intake in the setting of high endogenous $1,25(OH)_2D$, PHF, or both would result in accelerated cellular calcium uptake, and thus the vasoconstriction, enhanced cardiac output, and increased central sympathetic outflow often observed in salt-sensitive hypertension. In the absence of this skewed metabolic profile, dietary salt loading would result in no blood pressure elevation.

The above scheme describes the cardiovascular consequences of an environmental manuever, mediated by the metabolic set point of monovalent and divalent cation regulating hormones, which in turn function to alter the steady-state cellular distribution of mineral ions. The scheme provides a unified perspective for understanding the biochemical and clinical heterogeneity of human hypertension as well as the linkage of hypertension with other components of Syndrome X, more descriptively termed "generalized cardiovascular and metabolic disease".[5] The detailed mechanisms of calcium-regulating hormone involvement in these related metabolic and vascular syndromes await many future studies.

REFERENCES

1. Ringer, S., A third contribution regarding the infusion of the inorganic constituents of the blood on the ventricular contraction, *J. Physiol.*, 4, 222, 1983.
2. Rubin, R. P., The role of calcium in the release of neurotransmitter substances and hormones, *Pharmacol. Rev.*, 22, 389, 1970.
3. Connor, T. B., Rosen, B. L., Blaustein, M. P., Applefield, M. M., and Doyl, L, A., Hypocalcemic precipitating congestive heart failure, *N. Engl. J. Med.*, 307, 869, 1982.
4. Marone, C. et al., Acute hypercalcemic hypertension in man: role of hemodynamics, catecholamines, and renin, *Kidney Int.*, 20, 92, 1980.
5. Resnick, L.M., Ionic basis of hypertension, insulin resistance, vascular disease, and related disorders: the mechanism of "Syndrome X", *Am. J Hypertens.*, 6, 123s, 1993.
6. Hamet, P., Daignault-Gelinas, M., Lambert, J., Ledoux, M., Whissell-Cambiotti, L., Bellevance, F., and Mongeau, E., Epidemiological evidence of an interaction between calcium and sodium intake impacting on blood pressure: a Montreal study, *Am. J. Hypertens.*, 5, 378, 1992.
7. Resnick, L. M., Uniformity and diversity of calcium metabolism in hypertension: a conceptual framework, *Am. J. Med.*, 82(Suppl. IB), 16, 1987.

8. Rosenthal, F. D. and Roy, S., Hypertension and hyperparathyroidism, *Br. Med. J.*, 4, 396, 1972.
9. McCarron, D. A., Pingree, P. A., Rubin, R. J., Gaucher, S. M., Molitch, M., and Krutzik, S., Enhanced parathyroid function in essential hypertension: a homeostatic response to a urinary calcium leak, *Hypertension,* 2, 162, 1980.
10. Resnick, L. M. and Laragh, J. H., Calcium metabolism and parathyroid function in primary aldosteronism, *Am. J. Med.,* 78, 385, 1985.
11. Collip, J. B. and Clark, E. P., Further studies on the physiological action for parathyroid hormone, *J. Biol. Chem.,* 64, 485, 1925.
12. Charbon, G. A., Brummer, F., and Reneman, R.S., Diuretic and vascular action of parathyroid extracts in animals and man, *Arch. Int. Pharmacodyn. Ther.,* 171, 1, 1968.
13. Nakamura, R., Watanabe, T. X., and Sokabe, H., Acute hypotensive action of parathyroid hormone (1-34) fragments in hypertensive rats, *Proc. Soc. Exp. Biol. Med.,* 168, 168, 1981.
14. Pang, P. K. T., Tenner, T. E., Jr., Yee, J. A., Yang, M., and Janssen, H. F., Hypotensive action of parathyroid hormone preparations on rats and dogs, *Proc. Natl. Acad. Sci. U.S.A.,* 77, 675, 1980.
15. Langford, H. G., Nainby-Luxemoore, J. C., Nelson, M. C. et al., Hyperparathyroidism is associated with hypertension and may be causal, *Clin. Res.,* 28, 333a, 1980.
16. Bogin, E., Massey, S. G., and Harary, L., Effect of parathyroid hormone on rat heart cells, *J. Clin. Invest.,* 67, 1215, 1981.
17. Bogin, E., Massey, S. G., Levi, J., Djaideti, M., Bristol, G., and Smith, J., Effect of parathyroid hormone on osmotic fragility of human erythrocytes, *J. Clin. Invest.,* 69, 1017, 1982.
18. Pang, P. K. T., Yang, M. C. M., and Shan, J. S. K., Parathyroid hormone and calcium entry blockade in a vascular tissue, *Life Sci.,* 42, 1395, 1988.
19. Parsons, J. A., Physiology of parathyroid hormone, in *Endocrinology,* Vol. 2, DeGroot, J., Ed., Grune & Stratton, New York, 1979, 621.
20. Murray, T. M., Rao, L. G., Muzzafer, S. A., and Ly, H., Human parathyroid hormone carboxyterminal peptide (53-84) stimulates alkaline phosphatese activity in dexamethane-treated rat osteosarcoma cells in vitro, *Endocrinology,* 124, 1097, 1989.
21. Herrmann-Erlee, M. P. M., Nijweide, P. J., Meer, J. M., and Van der Ooms, M. A. C., Action of BPTH and bPTH-fragments on embryonic bone in vitro: dissociation of the cyclic AMP and bone resorbing response, *Calcif. Tissue Int.,* 35, 70, 1983.
22. Hesch, R. D., Herrmann, G., Ferris, A. D., and Atkinson, M. J., Type II PTH receptor operated calcium channel and its importance for PTH peptide elevations in coronary artery disease, *Am. J. Nephrol.,* 6(Suppl. 1), 155, 1986.
23. Nickols, G. A., Increased CAMP in cultured vascular smooth muscle cells and relaxation of aortic strips by parathyroid hormone, *Eur. J. Pharmacol.,* 116, 137, 1985.
24. Pang, P. K. T., Yang, M. C. M., Shew, R., and Tenner, T. E., Jr., The vasorelaxant action of parathyroid hormone fragments on isolated rat tail artery, *Blood Vessels,* 22, 57, 1985.
25. Acceto, R. and Weder, A. B., Parathyroid hormone and verapamil inhibit the Na^+, K^+ pump in human erythrocytes, *Clin. Res.,* 35, 437a, 1987.
26. De Luise, M. and Harker, M., Parathyroid 33. Hormone stimulation of the Na^+/K^+ pump in rat clonal osteosarcoma cells, *J. Endocrinol.,* 111, 61, 1986.
27. Kahn, A. M., Zimmer, R. A., and Navran, S. S., Parathyroid hormone inhibits Na^+/H^+ exchange in cultured vascular smooth muscle cells, *Kidney Int.,* 33(Abstr.), 298, 1988.
28. Sugannan, A. and Kahn, T., Parathyroid hormone impairs extrarenal potassium tolerance in the rat, *Am. J. Physiol.,* 254, F385, 1988.
29. Neuser, D., Schulte-Brinkmann, R., Knorr, A., and Kazda, S., Long-term hypotensive effect of parathyroid hormone in stroke prone spontaneously hypertensive rats, *Eur. J. Pharmacol.,* 182(3), 569, 1990.
30. Collins, J., Massey, S. G., and Campese, V. M., Parathyroid hormone and the altered vascular response to norepinephrine in uremia, *Am. J. Nephrol.,* 5, I10, 1985.
31. Benabe, J. E. and Martinez-Maldonado, M., Hypercalcemic nephropathy, *Arch. Intern. Med.,* 138, 777, 1978.
32. Drop, L. J. and Scheidegger, D., Plasma ionized calcium concentration: important determinant of the hemodynamic response to calcium infusion, *J. Thorac. Cardiovasc. Surg.,* 79, 425, 1980.

33. Smith, J. M., Mouse, D. R., and Vander, A. J., Effect of parathyroid hormone on plasma renin activity and sodium excretion, *Am. J. Physiol.,* 236, F311, 1979.

34. Davis, J. O. and Freeman, R. H., Mechanisms regulating renin release, *Physiol. Rev.,* 56, 1, 1976.

35. Olgaard, K., Dangaard, H., and Egfjord, M., Parathyroid hormone enhances the stimulatory effect of Ca^{2+} on aldosterone secretion, *Kidney Int.,* 29(Abstr.), 168, 1986.

36. Campese, V. M., Calcium, parathyroid hormone, and sympathoadrenal system, *Am. J. Nephrol.,* 6(Suppl. 1), 29, 1986.

37. Mizzola, C. L. and Quamme, G. A., Renal handling of phosphate, *Physiol. Rev.,* 54, 431, 1985.

38. Karlinskv. M. L. et al., Effect of parathormone and cyclic adenosine monophosphate on renal bicarbonate reabsorption, *Am. J. Physiol.,* 277, 1226, 1974.

39. Norman, A. W., Roth, J., and Orei, L., The vitamin D endocrine system: steroid metabolism, hormone receptors, and biological response, *Endocr. Rev.,* 3, 331, 1982.

40. Hulter, H. N., Halloran, B. P., Toto, R. D., and Peterson, J. C., Long-term control of plasma calcitriol concentration in dogs and humans, *J. Clin. Invest.,* 76, 695, 1985.

40a. Sahai, A., Fadda, G. Z., Massry, S. G., Parathyroid hormone activates protein kinase C of pancreatic islets, *Endocrinology,* 131, 1888, 1992.

41. Young, E. W., Bukowski, R. D., and McCarron, D. A., Calcium metabolism in experimental hypertension, *Proc. Soc. Exp. Biol. Med.,* 187, 123, 1988.

42. Barbagallo, M., Resnick, L. M., Sosa, R. E., Corbett, M. L., and Laragh, J. H., Renal divalent cation excretion in secondary hypertension, *Clin. Sci.,* 83, 561, 1992.

43. Kawashima, H., Altered vitamin D metabolism in the kidney of the spontaneously hypertensive rat, *Biochem. J.,* 237, 893, 1986.

44. Hulter, H. N., Melby, J. C., Peterson, J. C., and Cooke, C. R., Chronic continuous PTH infusion results in hypertension in normal subjects, *J. Clin. Hypertens.,* 2, 360, 1986.

45. Bertollot, A. and Garrard, A., Parathyroid hormone and deoxycorticosterone acetate-induced hypertension in the rat, *Clin. Sci.,* 58, 365, 1980.

46. Doris, P. A., Harvey, S., and Pang, P. K. T., Parathyroid hormone in sodium-dependent hypertension, *Life Sci.,* 41, 1383, 1987.

47. Pettinger, W. A., Umemura, S., and Smyth, D. D., The role of renal catecholamines in hypertension, *Am. J. Kidney Dis.,* 5, A23, 1985.

48. Kurtz, T. W., Portele, A. A., and Morris, R. C., Jr., Evidence for a difference in vitamin D metabolism between spontaneously hypertensive rats and Wistar Kyoto rats, *Hypertension,* 8, 1015, 1986.

49. Strazullo, P., Nunziata, V., Cirillo, M. et al., Abnormalities of calcium metabolism in essential hypertension, *Clin. Sci.,* 65, 137, 1985.

50. Ljunghall, S. and Hedstrand, H., Serum phosphate inversely related to blood pressure, *Br. Med. J.,* 1, 553, 1977.

50a. Resnick, L. M., Lewanczuk, R. Z., Laragh, J. H., and Pang, P. K. T., Parathyroid hypertensive-like activity in human essential hypertension: relationship to plasma renin activity and dietary salt sensitivity, *J. Hypert.,* 11, 1235, 1993.

51. Ellison, D. H., Shneidman, R., Morris, C., and McCarron, D. A., Effect of calcium infusion on blood pressure in hypertensive and normotensive humans, *Hypertension,* 8, 487, 1986.

52. Sowers, J. R., Brickman, A. S., Asp, N., Tuck, M. L., Jasberg, K., and Magnone, S., Altered dopaminergic modulation of prolactin and aldosterone secretion in pseudohypoparathyroidism, *J. Clin. Endocrinol. Metab.,* 52, 914, 1981.

53. Resnick, L, M., Maller, F. B., and Laragh, J. H., Calcium regulating hormones in essential hypertension: relation to plasma renin activity and sodium metabolism, *Ann. Intern. Med.,* 105, 649, 1986.

54. Resnick, L. M., Laragh, J. H., Sealey, J. E., and Alderman, M. H., Divalent cations in essential hypertension. Relations between serum ionized calcium, magnesium, and plasma renin activity, *N. Engl. J. Med.,* 309, 888, 1983.

55. Zemel, M. B., Geraldoni, S. M., Walsh, M. F., Konnenicky, P., Standley, P., Johnson, D., Fitter, W., and Sowers, J. R., Effects of sodium and calcium on calcium metabolism and blood pressure regulation in hypertensive black adults, *J. Hypertens.,* 4(Suppl. 5), S364, 1986.

56. Zemel, M. B. and Sowers, J. R., Salt sensitivity and systemic hypertension in the elderly, *Am. J. Cardiol.*, 61, 7H, 1988.

57. Cope, O., Hyperparathyroidism: diagnosis and treatment, *Am. J. Surg.*, 99, 394, 1960.

58. Brinton, G. S., Jubig, W. M., and Lagerquist, L. D., Hypertension in primary hyperthyroidism: the role of the renin-angiotensin system, *J. Clin. Endocrinol. Metab.*, 41, 1025, 1975.

59. Zawada, E. T., Jr., Brickman, A. S., Maxwell, M. H., and Tuck, M., Hypertension associated with hyperparathyroidism is not responsive to angiotensin blockade, *J. Clin. Endocrinol. Metab.*, 50, 912, 1980.

60. Lewanczuk, R. Z. and Pang, P. K. T., Expression of parathyroid hypertensive factor in hypertensive primary hyperparathroid patients, *Blood Pressure*, 2, 22, 1993.

61. Stewart, A. F. and Broadus, A. E., Mineral metabolism, in *Endocrinology and Metabolism*, 2nd ed., Felig, P., Baxter, J. P., Broadus, A. E., and Frohman, L. A., Eds., McGraw-Hill, New York, 1987, 1337.

62. Koida, M., Yamamoto, Y., Nakamuta, H., Matsuo, J., Okamoto, M., Morimoto, T., Seyler, J. K., and Orlowski, R. C., A novel effect of salmon calcitonin on in vitro calcium uptake by rat brain hypothalamus: the regional and hormonal specificities, *Jpn. J. Pharmacol.*, 32, 981, 1982.

63. Yamaguchi, M. and Yoshida, H., Participation of calcium channel in liver calcium regulation by calcitonin in rats, *Acta Endocrinol.*, 110, 239, 1985.

64. Resnick, L. M., Churchill, M. C., Churchill, P. C., Laragh, J. H., and Orlowski, R., The effects of calcitonin, calcitonin analogs and calcitonin-gene-related peptide on basal, in vitro renin secretion: *Am. J. Hypert.*, 2, 453, 1989.

65. Resnick, L. M., Churchill, P. C., Churchill, M., Laragh, J. H., Orlowski, R., The direct effect of calcitonin (CT), calcitonin analogs, and calcitonin gene-related peptide (CGRP) on renin secretion: evidence for calcium channel antagonism, *Clin. Res.*, 34, 552A, 1986.

66. Resnick, L. M., Maller, F. B., Nicholson, J. P., and Laragh, J. H., Hormonal and Hemodynamic Effects of Graded Calcitonin Infusion in Hypertensive Man, presented at the 7th Int. Congr. Endocrinology, Québec City, June 1984.

67. Resnick, L. M., Millier, F. B., Nicholson, J. P., and Laragh, J. H., Calcitonin is a vasoactive hormone in hypertensive man, *Clin. Res.*, 32, 523A, 1984.

68. Gnaedinger, M. P., Uehlinger, D. E., Weidmann, P., Sha, S. G., Muff, R., Born, W., Rascher, W., and Fischer, J. A., Distinct hemodynamic and renal effects of calcitonin gene-related peptide and calcitonin in men, *Am. J. Physiol.*, 257(6, Part 1), 848, 1989.

69. Peguero-Rivera, A. M. and Corder, C. N., Hemodynamic effects of calcitonin in the normal rat, *Peptides*, 13(3), 571, 1992.

70. Chakder, S. and Rattan, S., (Tyr0)-calcitonim gene-related peptide 28-37 (rat) as a putative antagonist of calcitonin gene-related peptide responses on opossum internal anal sphincter smooth muscle, *J. Pharmacol. Exp. Ther.*, 253(1), 200, 1990.

71. Binders, R. J. M., van den Broeck, A. M., Janger, M. J. M., Hacking, W. H. L., Lewik, C. W. G., and van Os, C. H., Increased plasma calcitonin levels in young spontaneously hypertensive rats: role in disturbed phosphate homeostasis, *Pfluegers Arch.*, 40B, 395, 1987.

72. Brin, V. B. and Tsabolova, Z. T., The effect of calcitonin on the mechanisms of urine formation and sodium excretion in normotensive and spontaneously hypertensive rats, *Byull. Eksp. Biol. Med.*, 111(2), 118, 1991.

73. Amara, S. G., Jones, V., Rosenfeld, M. G., Ing, E. S., and Evans, R. M., Alternative RNA processing in calcitonin gene expression generates mRNAs encoding different polypeptide products, *Nature*, 198, 240, 1982.

74. Goodman, E. C. and Iverson, L. L., Calcitonin gene-related peptide: novel neuropeptide, *Life Sci.*, 38, 2169, 1986.

75. Krootila, K., Uusitalo, H., and Palkama, A., Intraocular and cardiovascular effects of calcitonin gene-related peptide (OGRP)-I and II in the rabbit, *Invest. Ophthalmol. Vis. Sci.*, 32(12), 3084, 1991.

76. Tippins, J. R., DiMarzo, V. D., Panico, M., Morris, H. R., and MacIntyre, I., Investigation of the structure/activity relationship of human calcitonin gene-related peptide (CGRP), *Biochem. Biophys. Res. Commun.*, 134, 1306, 1986.

77. Fisher, L. A., Kikkawa, D. O., Rivier, J. E., Amara, S. G., Evans, R. M., Rosenfeld, M. D., Vale, W. W., and Brown, M. R., Stimulation of noradrenergic sympathetic outflow by calcitonin gene-related peptide, *Nature,* 305, 534, 1983.

78. Stones, R. W., Thomas, D. C., and Beard, R. W., Suprasensitivity to calcitonin gene-related peptide but not vasoactive intestinal peptide in women with chronic pelvic pain, *Clin. Autom. Res.,* 2(5), 343, 1992.

79. Ando, K., Ito, Y., Ogata, E., and Fujita, T., Vasodilating actions of calcitonin gene-related peptide in normal man: comparison with atrial natriuretic peptide, *Am. Heart J.,* 123(1), 111, 1992.

80. Gardiner, S. M., Compton, A. M., Kemp, P. A., Bennett, T., Bose, C., Foulkes, R., and Hughes, B., Human alpha-calcitonin gene-related peptide (CGRP)-(8-37), but not -(28-37), inhibits carotid vasodilator effects of human alpha-CGRP in vivo, *Eur. J. Pharmacol.,* 199(3), 375, 1991.

81. Gardiner, S. M., Compton, A. M., Kemp, P. A., Bennett, T., Bose, C., Foulkes, R., and Hughes, G., Antagonistic effect of human, alpha-CGRP [8-37] on the in vivo regional haemodynamic actions of human alpha-CGRP, *Biochem. Biophys. Res. Commun.,* 171(3), 938, 1990.

82. Maggi, C. A., Rovero, P., Giuliani, S., Evangelista, S., Regoli, O., and Meli, A., Biological activity of N-terminal fragments of calcitonin gene-related peptide, *Eur. J. Pharmacol.,* 179(1-2), 217, 1990.

83. Krootila, K., Uusitalo, H., and Palkama, A., Intraocular and cardiovascular effects of calcitonin gene-related peptide (OGRP)-I and II in the rabbit, *Invest. Ophthalmol. Vis. Sci.,* 32(12), 3084, 1991.

84. Lambrecht, N., Burchert, M., Respondek, M., Muller, K. M., and Peskar, B. M., Role of calcitonin gene-related peptide and nitric oxide in the gastroprotective effect of capsaicin in the rat, *Gastroenterology,* 104(5), 1371, 1993.

85. Anderson, S. E., Gilibenclamide and L-NG-nitro-arginine methyl ester modulate the ocular and hypotensive effects of calcitonin gene-related peptide, *Eur. J. Pharm.,* 224(1), 89, 1992.

86. Abdelrahman, A., Wang, Y. X., Chang, S. D., and Pang, C. C., Mechanism of the vasodilator action of calcitonin gene-related peptide in conscious rats, *Br. J. Pharmacol.,* 106(1), 45, 1992.

87. Hood, J. S., McMahon, T. J., and Kadowitz, P. J., Influence of lemakalim on the pulmonary vascular bed of the cat, *Eur. J. Pharmacol.,* 202(1), 101, 1991.

88. Gennari, C., Nami, R., Agnusdai, D., Maioli, E., and Gonnelli, S., Calcitonin gene-related peptide stimulates secretion of atrial natriuretic factor in men, *J. Hypertens. Suppl.,* 9(6), S252, 1991.

89. Bloom, S. R., Edwards, A. V., and Jones, C. T., Adrenal responses to calcitonin gene-related peptide in conscious hypophysectomized calves, *J. Physiol.,* 409, 29, 1989.

90. Murakami, M., Suzuki, H., Nakamoto, H., Kageyama, Y., Naitoh, M., Sakamaki, Y., and Saruta, T., Calcitonin gene-related peptide modulates adrenal hormones in conscious dogs, *Acta Endocrinol.,* 124(3), 346, 1991.

91. Pralong, P., Corder, R., and Gaillard, R. C., Responses of the rat pituitary-adrenal axis to hypotensive infusions of corticotropin-releasing factor, vasoactive intestinal peptide and other depressor agents, *Regul. Peptides,* 32(2), 217, 1991.

92. Jernbeck, J., Edner, M., Dalsgaard, C. J., and Pernow, B., The effect of calcitonin gene-related peptide (CGRP) on human forearm blood flow, *Clin. Physiol.,* 10(4), 335, 1990.

93. Fujioka, S., Sasakawa, O., Kishimoto, H., Tsumura, K., and Morii, H., The antihypertensive effect of calcitonin gene-related peptide in rats with norepinephrine- and angiotensin II-induced hypertension, *J. Hypertens.,* 9(2), 175, 1991.

94. Portaluppi, F., Trasforini, G., Margutti, A., Vergnani, L., Ambrosio, M. R., Rossi, R., Bagni, B., Pansini, R., and Degli Uberti, E. C., Circadian rhythm of calcitonin gene-related peptide in uncomplicated essential hypertension, *J. Hypertens.,* 10(10), 1227, 1992.

95. Trasforini, G., Margutti, M., Ambrosis, M. R., Bagni, B., Pansini, R., and Degli Uberti, E. C., Circadian profile of plasma calcitonin gene-related peptide in healthy man, *J. Clin. Endocrinol. Metab.,* 73(5), 945, 1991.

96. Xu, D., Wang, X. A., Wang, J. P., Yuan, Q. X., Fiscus, R. R., Chang, J. K., and Tang, J. A., Calcitonin gene-related peptide (CGRP) in normotensive and spontaneously hypertensive rats, *Peptides,* 10(2), 309, 1989.

97. Kawasaki, H., Saito, A., Soto, K., and Takasaki, K., Age-related changes in calcitonin gene-related peptide (OGRP)-mediated neurogenic vasodilation of the mesenteric resistance vessel in SHR, *Clin. Exp. Hypertens. A, Theory Pract.* 13(5), 745, 1991.

98. Westlund, K. N., DiPette, D. J., Carson, J., and Holland, O. B., Decreased spinal cord content of calcitonin gene-related peptide in the spontaneously hypertensive rat, *Neurosci. Lett.,* 131(2), 183, 1991.

99. Kawasaki, H., Saito, A., and Takasaki, K., Age-related decrease of calcitonin gene-related peptide-containing vasodilator innervation in the mesenteric resistance vessel of the spontaneously hypertensive rat, *Circ. Res.,* 67(3), 733, 1990.

100. Mathison, R. and Davison, J. S., Attenuated plasma extravasation to sensory neuropeptides in diabetic rats, *Agents Actions,* 38(1–2), 55, 1993

101. Portaluppi, F., Trasforini, G., Margutti, A., Vergnani, L., Ambrosio, M. R., Rossi, R., Bagni, B., Pansini, R., and Degli Uberti, E. C., Circadian rhythm of calcitonin gene-related peptide in uncomplicated essential hypertension, *J. Hypertens.,* 10(10), 1227, 1992.

102. Masuda, A., Shimamoto, K., Mori, Y., Nakagawa, M., Ura, N., and Iimura, O., Plasma calcitonin gene-related peptide levels in patients with various hypertensive diseases, *J. Hypertens.,* 10(12), 1499, 1992.

103. Herrera, M. F., Stone, E., Deitel, M., and Asa, S. L., Pheochromocytoma producing multiple vasoactive peptides, *Arch. Surg.,* 127(1), 105, 1992.

104. Resnick, L. M., Preibisz, J. J., and Laragh, J. H., Calcitonin gene-related peptide-like immunoreactivity in hypertension: relation to blood pressure, sodium, and calcium metabolism, in *Salt and Hypertension,* Ganten, D. S., and Reitch, R., Eds., Springer-Verlag, New York, 1989, 190.

105. Preibisz, J. J., Calcitonin gene-related peptide and regulation of human cardiovascular homeostasis, *Am. J. Hypertens.,* 6, 434, 1993.

106. Girgis, S. I., Stevenson, J. C., Lynch, C., Self, C. H., MacDonald, D. W. R., Bevis, P. J. R., Wimalewansa, S. J., Morns, H. R., and MacIntyre, I., Calcitonin gene-related peptide: potent vasodilator and major product of calcitonin gene, *Lancet,* 2, 14, 1985.

107. Resnick, L. M., Nicholson, J. P., and Laragh, J. H., Alterations in calcium metabolism mediate dietary salt sensitivity in essential hypertension, *Trans. Assoc. Am. Phys.,* 98, 313, 1985.

108. McCarron, D. A., Lucas, P. A., Schneideman, R. J., LeCour, B., and Druecke, T., Blood pressure development of the spontaneously hypertensive rat after concurrent manipulation of dietary Ce+ and Na+, *J. Clin. Invest.,* 76, 1147, 1985.

109. Resnick, L. M., DiFabio, B., Marion, R. M., James, G. D., and Laragh, J. H., Dietary calcium modifies the pressor effects of dietary salt intake in essential hypertension, *J. Hypertens.,* 4(Suppl. 6), S679, 1986.

110. Resnick, L. M., Sosa, R. E., Corbett, M. L., Germer, J. M., Sealey, J. E., and Laragh, J. H., Effects of dietary calcium on sodium volume vs. renin-dependent forms of experimental hypertension, *Trans. Assoc. Am. Phys.,* 99, 172, 1986.

111. Resnick, L. M., Dietary calcium and hypertension, *J. Nutr.,* 117, 1806, 1987.

112. Resnick, L. M., Calcium and vitamin D metabolism in the pathophysiology of human hypertension, in *Nutrition '87,* Levander, O. A., Ed., American Institute of Nutrition, Washington, D.C., 1987, 110.

113. Fraser, D. R., Regulation of the metabolism of vitamin D, *Physiol. Rev.,* 60, 551, 1980.

114. Walters, M. R., Wicki, D. C., and Riggle, P. C., 1,25 Dihydroxy-vitamin D_3 receptors identified in the rat heart, *J. Mol. Cell. Cardiol.,* 18, 67, 1986.

115. Marks, J., Hofmann, W., Goldenschmidt, D., and Ritz, E., Demonstration of 1,25 $(OH)_2$ vitamin D_3 receptors and actions in vascular smooth muscle cells in vitro, *Calcif. Tissue Int.,* 41, 112, 1987.

116. Wrzolkowa, T., Rudzinska-Kisiel, T., and Klosowska, B., Calcium content of serum and myocardium in vitamin D-induced cardionecrosis, *Bone Min.,* 13(2), 111, 1991.

117. Bukoski, R. D. and Kremer, O., Calcium regulating hormones in hypertension: vascular actions, *Am. J. Clin. Nutr.,* S4(Suppl. 1), 2209, 1991.

118. Bukoski, R. D., Li, J., Bo, J., Effect of long-term administration of 1,25 $(OH)_2$ vitamin D_3 on blood pressure and resistance artery contractility in the spontaneously hypertensive rat, *Am. J. Hypertens.,* 6, 944, 1993.

119. Bukoski, R. D. and Xue, H., On the vascular inotropic action of 1,25-(OH)$_2$ vitamin D$_3$, *Am. J. Hypertens.*, 6(5, Part 1), 388, 1993.

120. Shimosawa, T., Ando, K., and Fujita, T., Enhancement of vasoconstrictor response by a noncalcemic analogue of vitamin D$_3$, *Hypertension*, 21(2), 253, 1993.

121. Shan, J., Resnick, L. M., Lewanczuk, R. Z., Karpinski, E., Pang, P. K. T., 1,25 Dihydroxyvitamin D as a cardiovascular hormone: effects on calcium current and cytosolic free calcium in vascular smooth muscle cells, *Am. J. Hypert.*, 6, 983, 1993.

122. Barsony, J. and Marx, S. J., Receptor mediated rapid action of I alpha 25-dihydroxycholecataprol-increase of intracellular CGMP in human skin fibroblasts, *Proc. Natl. Acad. Sci. U.S.A.*, 85, 1223, 1988.

123. Matsumoto, T., Fontaine, O., and Rasmussen, H., Effect of 1,25 dihydroxyvitamin D$_3$ on phospholipid metabolism in chick duodenal mucosal cell. Relationship to its mechanism of action, *J. Biol. Chem.*, 256, 3354, 1981.

124. Baran, D. T. and Kelly, M., Lysophosphatide-inositol: a potential mediator of 1,25 dihydroxy-vitamin D-induced increments in hepatocyte cytosolic calcium, *Endocrinology*, 122, 930, 1988.

125. Hsu, C. H., Yang, C.-S., Patel, S. R., and Stevens, M. G., Calcium and vitamin D metabolism in spontaneously hypertensive rats, *Am. J. Physiol.*, 253, F712, 1987.

126. Lucas, P. A., Brown, R. C., Druecke, T., LaCour, B., Metz, J. A., and McCarron, D. A., Abnormal vitamin D metabolism, intestinal calcium transport, and bone calcium status in the spontaneously hypertensive rat compared with its genetic control, *J. Clin. Invest.*, 78, 221, 1986.

127. McCarron, D. A., Is calcium more important than sodium in the pathogenesis of essential hypertension?, *Hypertension*, 7, 607, 1985.

128. Kawashima, H., Altered vitamin D metabolism in the kidney of the spontaneously hypertensive rat, *Biochem. J.*, 237, 893, 1986

129. Druecke, T., Lucas, P.A., Bourgouin, P., Pointillart, A., Merke, J., Garabedian, M., Thomasset, M., LaCour, B., Ritz, E., and McCarron, D. A., Changes in calcitriol status and related parameters in the young hypertensive rats, *Kidney Int.*, 33(Abstr.), 294, 1988.

130. Lau, K. and Eby, B., The role of calcium in genetic hypertension, *Hypertension*, 7, 657, 1985.

131. Kotchen, T. A., Ott, C. E., Resnick, L. M., and Blebschmidt, N. G., Calcium and Salt-Sensitive Hypertension, paper presented at the 70th Annu. Meet. Endocrine Society, New Orleans, June, Abstr No. 128, 1988.

132. Oshima, T., Matsuura, H., Matsumoto, K., Kido, K., Kajiyama, G., Role of cellular calcium in salt sensitivity of patients with essential hypertension, *Hypertension*, 11, 703, 1991.

133. Shingu, T., Matsuura, H., Kusaka, M., and Shingu, M., Significance of intracellular free calcium and magnesium and calcium-regulating hormones with sodium chloride loading in patients with essential hypertension, *J. Hypertens.*, 9, 1021, 1991.

134. Resnick, L. M., Nicholson, J. P., and Laragh, J. H., Calcium metabolism and essential hypertension — relationship to altered renin system activity, *Fed. Proc.*, 45, 2739, 1986.

135. Tabuchi, Y., Ogihara, T., Hashigawa, D., Saito, H., and Kumahara, Y., Hypotensive effect of long-term oral calcium supplementation in elderly patients with essential hypertension, *J. Clin. Hypertens.*, 3, 254, 1986.

136. Resnick, L. M. and Laragh, J. H., Does dihydroxyvitamin D (1,25 D) cause low renin hypertension?, *Hypertension*, 6, 792, 1984.

137. Resnick, L. M., Nicholson, J. P., and Laragh, J. H., The antihypertensive effects of calcium channel blockade: role of sodium and calcium metabolism, *J. Cardiovasc. Pharmacol.*, 12(Suppl. 6), s114, 1988.

138. Resnick, L. M., Germer, J. M., and Laragh, J. H., Abnormal vitamin D metabolism in primary aldosteronism and experimental mineralocorticoid excess, *J. Hypertens.*, 5(Suppl. 5), S99, 1987.

139. Russell, J., Lettieri, D., and Sherwood, L. M., Suppression by 1,25 (OH)$_2$ D$_3$ of transcription of the preproparathyroid hormone gene, *Endocrinology*, 119, 2864, 1986.

140. Resnick, L. M. and Laragh, J. H., Calcium metabolism in hypertension: clinical evidence and cellular hypothesis, in *Essential Hypertension 2*, Aoki, K., Ed., Springer-Verlag, New York, 1989, 355.

Epilogue

As editors, we have attempted to offer our readers a most comprehensive updated review of "Calcium-Regulating Hormones and Cardiovascular Function", with full recognition that time limitations and constraints imposed by redaction obligations necessarily compromise our efforts in this regard. Although the nature and control of the PTHrP receptor in vascular smooth muscle are still uncertain, it had previously been observed that PTHrP-(141) stimulated cAMP in vascular smooth muscle cells (VSMC)[1] and that N-terminal PTHrP fragments induced vasorelaxation.[2] More recently, Okano et al., in studies designed to use the PTH/PTHrP receptor DNA to characterize the regulation of its messenger RNA in both VSMC and UMR osteoblastic-like cells, elegantly demonstrated that the expression and activity of the PTH/PTHrP receptor are regulated in a cell-specific manner.[3] The authors interpret these differences in PTH/PTHrP receptor regulation in the two tissue types as essential to coordination of distinct temporal biological responses in vascular and skeletal tissues.[3] Deftos et al., who had previously demonstrated that PTHrP is a secretory product of atrial myocytes,[4] recently quantitated the concentration of PTHrP in the rat cardiovascular system and relative levels of PTHrP messenger RNA utilizing region-specific radioimmunoassay and competitive polymerase chain reaction procedures and demonstrated that the atria, aorta, and vena cava contained the greatest amount of PTHrP in the cardiovascular system.[5] Their additional finding of a discrepancy between PTHrP concentrations and the presence of PTHrP mRNA in the aorta and vena cava also were consistent with the hypothesis that both PTHrP and its mRNA may be subjected to separate regulatory control mechanisms.[5] Intriguing observations of Watson et al.[6] demonstrating that 25-hydroxycholesterol, though apparently not 1,25-dihydroxyvitamin D_3, stimulates certain vascular cells (exclusive of VSMC and endothelial cells) to calcify have also been recorded after this volume was submitted for publication. Since these findings are consistent with the hypothesis that vascular intimal cells possess "osteoblastic" potential, further exploration of the comparative roles of calciotropic hormones on cardiovascular and skeletal function is certainly an essential priority for investigators analyzing those pathogenetic mechanism(s) that initiate and/or condition disorders of cardiovascular and skeletal function.

Louis V. Avioli, M.D.
M. F. Crass, III, Ph.D.

REFERENCES

1. Wu, S., Pirola, C. J., Green, J., Yamaguchi, D. T., Okano, K., Jueppner, H., Forrester, J. S., Fagin, J. A., and Clemens, T. L., Effects of N-terminal, midregion, and C-terminal parathyroid hormone-related peptides on adenosine 3',5'-monophosphate and cytoplasmic free calcium in rat aortic smooth muscle cells and UMR-106 osteoblast-like cells, *Endocrinology*, 133, 2437, 1993.
2. Mok, L. L. S., Nickols, G. A., Thompson, J. C., and Cooper, C. W., Parathyroid hormone as a smooth muscle relaxant, *Endocr. Rev.*, 10, 420, 1989.
3. Okano, K., Wu, S., Huang, X., Pirola, C. J., Jueppner, H., Abou-Samra, A-B., Segre, G. V., Iwasaki, K., Fagin, J. A., and Clemens, T. L., Parathyroid hormone (PTH)/PTH-related protection (PTHrP) receptor and its messenger ribonucleic acid in rat aortic vascular smooth muscle cells and UMR osteoblast-like cells: cell-specific regulation by angiotensin-II and PTHrP, *Endocrinology*, 135, 1093, 1994.
4. Deftos, L. J., Burton, D. W., and Brandt, D. W., Parathyroid hormone-like protein is a secretory product of atrial myocytes, *J. Clin. Invest.*, 92, 727, 1993.

5. Burton, D. W., Brandt, D. W., and Deftos, L. J., Parathyroid hormone-related protein in the cardiovascular system, *Endocrinology*, 135, 253, 1994.

6. Watson, K. E., Boström, K., Ravindranath, R., Lam, T., Norton, B., and Demer, L. L., TGF-β1 and 25-hydroxycholesterol stimulate osteoblast-like vascular cells to calcify, *J. Clin. Invest.*, 93, 2106, 1994.

Index

A

acetylcholine, 58

actin, 176

adenosine, 54

adenosine 3':5'-cyclic phosphate. *See* cAMP

adenylate cyclase activation, 59–60,112, 120, 146–147, 241

adenylyl cyclase, 15

adrenal blood flow, 48

α-adrenergic agonists, 241

β-adrenergic agonists, 144, 148, 241

age

    changes in calcitonin gene-related peptide, 244

    and vitamin D, 228–229

alkaline phosphatase, 19, 20

1α-hydroxylase, 10, 21, 120, 122

altitude, and cardiovascular disease, 220–222

amygdaloid, 242

amylin, 8, 243

angiotensin II, 154

antagonist compounds of calcium, 54, 66–67, 147

atherogenesis, 283

atherosclerosis, 245, 281–286

atrial natriuretic factor (ANF), 305

atrial natriuretic peptide (ANP), 158

AU (adenine and uracil)-rich motifs, 135–136

autocrine/paracrine function of PTHrP, 135, 136

B

B-channel, 83

biomechanical stretch, 136

blocking agents, effects on PTH vasodilator activity, 49. *See also* calcium, channel blocking

blood flow, 48, 132–133, 137, 139–141. *See also* coronary blood flow

    responses to parathyroid hormone, 48–55

blood lactate, 68

blood lipids, and vitamin D, 227

blood pressure, 103–104, 105f, 106f, 119f. *See also* parathyroid hormone (PTH), cardiodynamic effects of

    effects of estrogen on, 259

    and vitamin D, 227

blood vessels, expression and action of PTHrP in, 139. *See also* vasodilatory effects

blood volume, expression of parathyroid hormone-related protein (PTHrP) on, 155–156

bone formation, 19, 20

bone remodeling, 3, 20, 120

bone resorption, 3–4, 15, 18–19, 120, 135

induced by vitamin D, 18–19, 20

    suppression by calcitonin, 8, 13, 150, 150f

bone target cells, 18–21

bPTH-(1–34), 85–99, 86f, 87f, 89f, 90f, 138–139, 147

bPTH-(3–34), 88, 95, 99

bradykinin, 53–55, 54f

C

calbindin D, 22

calcification, role of noncollagenic proteins in, 20

calciotropic hormones, 1–44. *See also* calcitonin; calcitonin gene-related peptide (CGRP); parathyroid hormone (PTH); parathyroid hormone-related protein (PTHrP); vitamin D

    cellular actions of, 18–24, 134–135

calcitonin, 6–8, 10, 136, 137

    and bone resorption, 8, 150, 150f

    cardiovascular actions of, 67–68

    cellular actions of

        in bone, 19–20

        in kidney, 21–22

        in nonclassic target cells, 23

    gene, 6, 7f

    mechanism of target cell activation, 12–13

    metabolism of, 6–8

    radioimmunoassay procedures, 6–8

    receptors, 11, 12–13

    secretion, 6

    signal transduction, 17

    structure, 6, 7f

    synthesis of, 6

calcitonin gene-related peptide (CGRP), 6, 23, 59, 239–252. *See also* CGRP-(1–37); CGRP-(8–37)

    agonists, 246

    amino acid sequence homology, 243f, 243–244

    and cAMP, 8, 95, 99

    cardiac output, 245

    and cardiovascular pathophysiology, 244–247

    and cerebrospinal fluid, 8

    chronotropic and inotropic effects of, 241–242

    circadian rhythm, 244

    modulation of endothelial function, 245

    distribution in gastrointestinal tract, 244

    and hypertension, 244–247, 305–307

    immunoreactivity, 240

    radioimmunoassay procedures, 242

    receptors, 240–241, 243–244

    structure, 305–306

    and total peripheral resistance, 245

    and vasodilatory effects, 242–243

323